D1442803

MENTAL HEALTH SERVICES

A Public Health Perspective

SECOND EDITION

Edited by

BRUCE LUBOTSKY LEVIN
DR.P.H., M.P.H., FABHM

JOHN PETRILA
J.D., LL.M.

KEVIN D. HENNESSY
Ph.D

OXFORD
UNIVERSITY PRESS
2004

OXFORD

UNIVERSITY PRESS

Oxford   New York
Auckland   Bangkok   Buenos Aires   Cape Town   Chennai
Dar es Salaam   Delhi   Hong Kong   Istanbul   Karachi   Kolkata
Kuala Lumpur   Madrid   Melbourne   Mexico City   Mumbai
Nairobi   São Paulo   Shanghai   Singapore   Taipei   Tokyo   Toronto

Published by Oxford University Press, Inc.
198 Madison Avenue, New York, New York, 10016
http://www.oup.com

Oxford is a registered trademark of Oxford University Press

Library of Congress Cataloging-in-Publication Data
Mental health services : a public health perspective /
edited by Bruce Lubotsky Levin, John Petrila, Kevin D. Hennessy.—2nd ed.
p. cm.   Includes bibliographical references and index.
ISBN-13 978-0-19-515395-8
ISBN 0-19-515395-2
1. Mental health services—United States.
2. Mental health policy—United States.
I. Levin, Bruce Lubotsky.
II. Petrila, John. III. Hennessy, Kevin D., 1957-
RA790.6.M445 2004   362.2′0973—dc22   2003056532

The contents of this volume represent the opinions and views of the editors and the chapter
contributors, and not necessarily those of the institutions with which they are affiliated.

9 8 7 6 5 4 3 2

Printed in the United States of America
on acid-free paper

Foreword

The pace of change in the field of mental health has quickened dramatically during the past decade. We have moved rapidly from national health care reform, through managed behavioral health care, to quality and accountability, and now into large-scale state budget deficits. In this swirl of activities, it is important to keep our eyes on the key issues so that we can weather the storm. This can be accomplished by adhering to key principles that can serve as guides to informed action.

Below, I outline these key principles. They can apply to each of us individually, as well as to our field as a whole.

Principle 1: *Planning.* One must have a clear plan of action, and this plan must be shared broadly across the field. Fortunately, such a plan is available from the Institute of Medicine. However, many of us in the mental health field are not familiar with the Institute of Medicine's *Crossing the Quality Chasm*, a landmark work published in 2001 that provides a blueprint for the future of health care in the United States, including mental health care. Services are to be guided by key principles, including consumer-centric care. Systems of care are to be organized so that key issues are addressed, including equity, efficiency, and effectiveness. Finally, evidence-based practices are to be implemented by a well-trained workforce, and quality measures are to be collected through the use of appropriate information technology. As a first step, we need to understand and embrace this planning framework and make it our own.

Principle 2: *Goal Attainment.* Value must be a driving goal every day. Clearly, value from the consumer and family viewpoint—the perception that care has achieved desired effects—is essential. For some, these effects may be recovery or resiliency; for others, they may be improved job performance, better interpersonal relationships, or greater life stability. In all instances, however, we must adopt the consumer and family viewpoint in defining value, and we must seek to add value every day.

Principle 3: *Adaptation.* It is important to remain flexible as the context continues to change. Current changes are profound. Long-standing boundaries are breaking down. Mental health services are increasingly provided in primary health care settings; mental health and substance abuse services are frequently linked; and mental health is part of public health in a post September 11 world. In this changing context, we require new knowledge, and our services need retooling for the new demands that will be placed on them. Until these needed developments have taken place, it is important to remain flexible, open to new organizational and service arrangements as they arise.

Principle 4: *Training.* Improved training and retooling are essential for success in the future. *Mental Health, United States, 2000* shows that our field consists of nearly 1 million active providers and several thousand providers-in-training. Adaptation to the new demands of continuous quality improvement, initiation of new evidence-based practices, and better quality measurement all dictate the need for a new model of training. This new model can perhaps be described best as continuous quality training. It is very likely that it will be implemented through Internet technology. Because new demands are already on us, the time for new training is at hand.

Principle 5: *Collegiality.* The mental health field must undertake joint action, guided by a common vision and mission. All too often in the past, the collegiality essential for joint action failed us at critical junctures. This led to very negative consequences for consumers, family members, communities, and our field. We can initiate and sustain common action only if we communicate with our colleagues. Such dialogues need to be started now.

By this time, you may think that I am overly pessimistic about our future. Nothing could be further from the truth. I think that the mental health field has a great deal to offer: real value for children, adults, and their families. In the article "Mental Health in a Social Context," published in *Cosmos* (2003), I wrote that the catastrophic events of September 11 have accentuated both the need for and the effectiveness of mental health care.

Let me now turn to some potent forces in our environment that can have very salutary effects upon the future of our joint endeavor to add value by promoting positive mental health.

First, President George W. Bush has proposed a New Freedom Initiative to encourage persons with disabilities to participate in community life. In this initiative, the president has articulated very clearly what consumers and family members have been telling us for years: consumers want jobs, housing, social supports, and community services in order to become full community members. The mental health field has pioneered services in each of these areas for the past quarter century. Hence, we are poised to participate fully in the president's initiative.

Second, the president has created a New Freedom Commission on Mental Health, the first such commission since President Jimmy Carter initiated one in 1977. President Bush has asked the Commission to identify problems in the mental health system and to propose workable solutions. Once available, the Commission recommendations will provide a basis for undertaking needed reforms in our field.

Third, the field has embraced *resiliency* and *recovery* as overarching themes. Although these goals have been a very long time in coming, their importance cannot be overemphasized. They offer hope to a generation of consumers and family members where none existed before. The quality improvements we make and the value we add can be guided effectively by these key themes.

Fourth, we now have treatments that work, and we know how to configure services into systems that also work. The Surgeon General has documented both of these assertions in the landmark 1999 *Report on Mental Health*. We must help to ensure that these services and systems are available in every community in the United States.

Let me stop and ask how we are going to move from the turmoil that we are currently experiencing to effective services in every community in this country. Before we can implement the principles, before we can work effectively with the new initiatives and approaches, we ourselves need to have a fundamental knowledge of the current state of our field. Bruce Lubotsky Levin, John Petrila, and Kevin Hennessy provide that fundamental knowledge in this book. Written by nationally known researchers, academicians, and practitioners in both the mental health and substance abuse fields, this book reflects both the breadth and the depth necessary to become well grounded in the current realities of the field. Congratulations to the editors for providing this most important service. It is a "must read" for all who consider themselves part of the mental health field.

Ronald W. Manderscheid, Ph.D.
Center for Mental Health Services
Substance Abuse and Mental Health Services Administration

Preface

When the first edition of *Mental Health Services: A Public Health Perspective* was published 8 years ago, the difficulties involved in the organization, financing, and delivery of mental health services were great, and the proposed solutions for these public health problems were remarkably diverse. Many of these problems, particularly those related to the cost and insurance coverage of mental health services, remain very controversial, are debated in political arenas, and are largely unresolved. And yet the pace of change in both mental health systems and mental health services research has increased steadily since 1996.

This second edition builds on the original volume by examining the critical issues in the organization, financing, delivery, and evaluation of mental health services in the United States. While it covers what we consider to be the core issues in mental health services delivery, providing a detailed examination of epidemiological, treatment, and policy issues in selected populations at risk, this edition also includes new chapters on special areas (criminal justice, co-occurring disorders, psychopharmacology, and mental health informatics) that have emerged as key concerns.

The development of this second edition text has been influenced by our (B.L.L.) experiences in teaching graduate-level courses in the Graduate Studies in Behavioral Health (GSBH) Program here at the University of South Florida (USF) as well as consulting with mental health professionals and services researchers throughout the United States (J.P. and K.H.). The new GSBH Program is a collaborative teaching initiative that was established between the USF Louis de la Parte Florida Mental Health Institute and the Department of Community and Family Health at the USF College of Public Health to provide students an opportunity to pursue a variety of advanced degrees in public health (including the master of public health, the master of science in public health, and the doctor of philosophy in public health) with a concentration in behavioral health.

As stated in the preface for the first edition, we have found that many academies in the various disciplines that comprise the mental health sciences are reluctant to take a multidisciplinary approach to the education of their graduate students in mental health services delivery. We strongly believe that issues in mental health services may be more comprehensively presented and integrated within a public health framework.

Like the first edition, the second draws its strength from a group of nationally prominent experts in mental health services research and delivery. It represents a continuing effort to provide an integrated textbook that can be used by graduate students in public health, social work, psychiatric nursing, psychology, applied anthropology, public administration, and others in the behavioral health fields. It has also been designed to serve as a handy reference for applied academicians, researchers, practitioners, policy makers, and administrators involved with mental health and substance abuse services delivery at the local, state, and national levels.

Organization of the Second Edition

The book is divided into four parts: I—Service Delivery Issues, II—Selected Populations at Risk, III—Special Issues, and IV—Managing Mental Health Systems. The first five chapters describe the basic characteristics of mental health services delivery systems in the United States. Levin, Hennessy, and Hanson discuss prevention, primary care integration, and parity issues in mental health. In Chapter 2, Conti, Frank, and McGuire examine the direct and indirect costs of mental illness to individuals and society and review the public and private financing of mental health care, as well as describe the organization of the treatment of mental illness under managed care. Petrila and Levin, in Chapter 3, discuss the various ways in which the law has influenced and defined mental health services and policy since the mid-1960s. In Chapter 4, Urff explores the heterogeneity of the organization and delivery of state mental health services. Hennessy and Green-Hennessy describe the recovery movement in the United States in Chapter 5.

Part II deals with the unique epidemiological, services delivery, and policy issues in selected populations at risk. Its eight chapters are divided into four sections: A—Children and Adolescents, B—Adults, C—Older Adults, and D—Substance Abuse. Section A provides a discussion of the epidemiology of mental disorders in children by Costello and colleagues (Chapter 6) and an examination of children's mental health systems and policy issues by Friedman and colleagues (Chapter 7). In Section B, Kessler and colleagues (Chapter 8) offer a selective overview of the epidemiology of mental disorders in the United States based on data from the Epidemiologic Catchment Area (ECA) and the National Collaborative Study (NCS) studies, plus some preliminary results from the NCS-Revised survey. Young and Magnabosco (Chapter 9) then discuss the major adult psychiatric disorders and their treatment, emphasizing severe mental illness and homelessness. In Section C, Hybels and Blazer (Chapter 10) introduce some of the challenges in studying the epidemiology of mental disorders in older adults, and in Chapter 11 Bartels and colleagues provide an overview of the major policy issues related to the mental health of older adults. In Section D, Gfroerer (Chapter 12) discusses the epidemiology of substance abuse in the United States, while McCarty and Edmundson (Chapter 13) review the organization and financing of services for the treatment of alcohol and drug abuse.

Part III consists of four chapters on special issues in mental health. In Chapter 14, Borum reviews the prevalence of severe mental illness in U.S. jails and prisons and discusses key issues related to the availability of mental health services in the criminal justice system. Ihara and Takeuchi (Chapter 15) review the preva-

lence of mental disorders and the use of mental health services by racial and ethnic minorities and the implications for services delivery. In Chapter 16, Osher
highlights the outcomes associated with co-occurring disorders, the need for assessment, and the heterogeneity of the population with comorbid conditions, as
well as the barriers to the delivery of services to patients. Chapter 17, by Miller
and colleagues, addresses psychopharmacology and its impact on the design and
delivery of mental health services to individuals with serious and persistent mental disorders.

The last part of the book examines financial management, informatics, and the
evaluation of alcohol, drug abuse, and mental disorders. Chapter 18 (Sorensen)
will give readers a fundamental understanding of the financial management of a
public mental health system. Hanson and Levin (Chapter 19) examine the history
and evolution of information systems used in mental health services, as well as selected applications of information and communication technologies to mental
health services delivery. In Chapter 20, Orwin and Goldman review the basic elements in the evaluation of alcohol, drug abuse, and mental health services.

We readily acknowledge that it is impossible to examine all the relevant issues
in mental health services delivery in a single volume. Nevertheless, this second
edition underscores the importance of continuing to use a multidisciplinary framework for the study of mental health services within a public health context.

Throughout the preparation of this second edition, a number of individuals have
provided encouragement and continued support, including Drs. Robert Friedman
and David Shern. We would also like to acknowledge Ms. Ardis Hanson, who contributed numerous valuable suggestions during the preparation of this edition, including the creation of the comprehensive index. Special thanks should also be
given to Ms. Tamara Lee for her invaluable support in the final preparation of
this volume. We also would like to express our gratitude to Mr. Jeffrey House and
Ms. Edith Barry of Oxford University Press, who made numerous valuable suggestions during the editing of the second edition. Finally, we would like to thank
our families for their never-ending love, their deep understanding, and their
tremendous support during the book's preparation.

Tampa, Florida   B.L.L.
                                                                                    J.P.
                                                                                    K.H.

Contents

Contributors

ADRIAN ANGOLD, M.R.C.PSYCH
Associate Professor and Director, Center for Developmental Epidemiology
Department of Psychiatry and Behavioral Sciences
Duke University Medical School
Durham, NC

MARY I. ARMSTRONG, M.S.W., M.B.A.
Associate Director of Research and Programs
Department of Child and Family Studies
Louis de la Parte Florida Mental Health Institute
University of South Florida
Tampa, FL

C. BRUCE BAKER, M.D., J.D.
Assistant Professor and Deputy Director
Treatment Research Program
Department of Psychiatry
Yale University School of Medicine
New Haven, CT

STEPHEN J. BARTELS, M.D., M.S.
Associate Professor of Psychiatry, Dartmouth Medical School
Director, Aging Services Research
New Hampshire-Dartmouth Psychiatric Research Center
Lebanon, NH

KATHERINE A. BEST, M.S.W., M.P.H.
Graduate Assistant
Department of Child and Family Studies

Louis de la Parte Florida Mental Health Institute
University of South Florida
Tampa, FL

DAN G. BLAZER, M.D.
J.P. Gibbons Professor of Psychiatry
Department of Psychiatry and Behavioral Sciences
Center for the Study of Aging and Human Development
Duke University Medical Center
Durham, NC

RANDY BORUM, PSY.D.
Associate Professor
Department of Mental Health Law and Policy
Louis de la Parte Florida Mental Health Institute
University of South Florida
Tampa, FL

RENA CONTI
Ph.D. Student in the Department of Health Policy
Harvard Medical School
Boston, MA

E. JANE COSTELLO, PH.D.
Professor of Medical Psychology
Developmental Epidemiology Program
Department of Psychiatry and Behavioral Sciences
Duke University Medical School
Durham, NC

M. LYNN CRISMON, PHARM.D.
Professor
College of Pharmacy
The University of Texas
Austin, TX

ALBERT J. DUCHNOWSKI, PH.D.
Professor
Department of Child and Family Studies
Louis de la Parte Institute
University of South Florida
Tampa, FL

ARICCA R. DUMS, B.A.
Research Assistant
New Hampshire-Dartmouth Psychiatric
   Research Center
Department of Community and Family
   Medicine
Dartmouth Medical School
Lebanon, NH

ELDON EDMUNDSON, PH.D.
Associate Professor
Department of Public Health and Preventive
   Medicine
Oregon Health Sciences University
Portland, OR

MARY E. EVANS, R.N., M.S.N.,
PH.D., FAAN
Associate Dean for Research and Doctoral
   Studies
College of Nursing
University of South Florida
Tampa, FL

RICHARD G. FRANK, PH.D.
Margaret T. Morris Professor of Health
   Economics
Department of Health Care Policy
Harvard Medical School
Boston, MA

ROBERT M. FRIEDMAN, PH.D.
Professor and Chairperson
Department of Child and Family Studies
Louis de la Parte Florida Mental Health
   Institute

University of South Florida
Tampa, FL

JOSEPH GFROERER, M.A.
Director, Division of Population Surveys
Office of Applied Studies
Rockville, MD

HOWARD H. GOLDMAN, M.D.,
PH.D.
Professor of Psychiatry
University of Maryland School of Medicine
Potomac, MD

SHARON GREEN-HENNESSY, PH.D.
Assistant Professor
Department of Psychology
Loyola College in Maryland
Baltimore, MD

CATHERINE S. HALL, PHARM.D.
Instructor/Research
Division of Schizophrenia and Related
   Disorders, Department of Psychiatry
University of Texas Health Science Center at
   San Antonio
San Antonio, TX

ARDIS HANSON, M.L.S.
Library Director
Louis de la Parte Florida Mental Health
   Institute
University of South Florida
Tampa, FL

KEVIN D. HENNESSY, PH.D.
Senior Health Policy Analyst
Office of the Assistant Secretary for Planning
   and Evaluation
U.S. Department of Health and Human
   Services
Washington, DC

MARIO HERNANDEZ, PH.D.
Associate Professor
Department of Child and Family Studies
Louis de la Parte Florida Mental Health
   Institute
University of South Florida
Tampa, FL

SHARON HODGES, PH.D., M.B.A.
Assistant in Research
Department of Chlid and Family Studies
Louis de la Parte Florida Mental Health
   Institute
University of South Florida
Tampa, FL

CELIA F. HYBELS, PH.D.
Assistant Research Professor
Department of Psychiatry and Behavioral
   Sciences
Center for the Study of Aging and Human
   Development
Duke University Medical Center
Durham, NC

EMILY S. IHARA, M.S.W., M.A.
W.K. Kellogg Fellow in Health Policy Research
Doctoral Candidate
The Heller School for Social Policy and
   Management
Brandeis University
Waltham, MA

GORDON KEELER, M.S.
Statistician
Center for Developmental Epidemiology
Department of Psychiatry and Behavioral
   Sciences
Duke University Medical School
Durham, NC

RONALD C. KESSLER, PH.D.
Professor of Health Care Policy
Department of Health Care Policy
Harvard Medical School
Boston, MA

DOREEN KORETZ, PH.D.
Associate Director for Prevention
Chief, Developmental Psychopathology and
   Prevention Research Branch
National Institute of Mental Health
Bethesda, MD

KRISTA B. KUTASH, PH.D., M.B.A.
Research Associate Professor
Louis de la Parte Florida Mental Health
   Institute

University of South Florida
Tampa, FL

BRUCE LUBOTSKY LEVIN, DR.P.H.,
   M.P.H., FABHM
Associate Professor and Head
Graduate Studies in Behavioral Health
Louis de la Parte Institute and College of
   Public Health
University of South Florida
Tampa, FL

JENNIFER L. MAGNABOSCO, PH.D.
Associate Policy Researcher
RAND Corporation
Santa Monica, CA

RONALD MANDERSCHEID, PH.D.
Chief, Survey and Analysis Branch
Substance Abuse and Mental Health Services
   Administration
Rockville, MD

DENNIS MCCARTY, PH.D.
Professor
Department of Public Health and Preventive
   Medicine
Oregon Health Sciences University
Portland, OR

THOMAS G. MCGUIRE, PH.D.
Professor
Department of Health Care Policy
Harvard Medical School
Boston, MA

KATHLEEN R. MERIKANGAS, PH.D.
Senior Investigator
Section on Developmental Genetic
   Epidemiology
National Institute of Mental Health
Bethesda, MD

ALEXANDER L. MILLER, M.D.
Professor of Psychiatry and Pharmacology
University of Texas Health Science Center
Director of Clinical Research, San Antonio
   State Hospital
San Antonio, TX

SARAH MUSTILLO, PH.D.
Research Associate
Center for Developmental Epidemiology
Department of Psychiatry and Behavioral
  Sciences
Duke University Medical School
Durham, NC

ROBERT G. ORWIN, PH.D.
Senior Study Director
Substance Abuse Research Group
Westat
Rockville, MD

FRED C. OSHER, M.D.
Associate Professor and Director
Center for Behavioral Health, Justice, and
  Public Policy
Department of Psychiatry
University of Maryland School of Medicine
Jessup, MD

JOHN PETRILA, J.D., LL.M.
Professor and Chairperson
Department of Mental Health Law and Policy
Louis de la Parte Florida Mental Health
  Institute
University of South Florida
Tampa, FL

DENNIS G. SHEA, PH.D.
Associate Professor
Department of Health Policy and
  Administration
Penn State University
University Park, PA

JAMES E. SORENSEN, PH.D., C.P.A.
John J. Gilbert Endowed Professor of
  Accountancy
Daniels College of Business
University of Denver
Denver, CO

DAVID TAKEO TAKEUCHI, PH.D.
Professor
School of Social Work
Department of Sociology
University of Washington
Seattle, WA

JENIFER URFF, J.D.
Senior Policy Counsel
National Association of State Mental Health
  Program Director, and Consultant
Donahue Institute
University of Massachusetts
Hadley, MA

PHILIP S. WANG, M.D. DR.P.H.
Instructor in Medicine
Harvard Medical School
Division of Pharmacoepidemiology and
  Pharmacoeconomics
Brigham and Women's Hospital
Boston, MA

ALEXANDER S. YOUNG, M.D.,
  M.S.H.S.
Assistant Professor in Residence, UCLA
  Department of Psychiatry
Associate Director, Department of Veterans
  Affairs
West LA VA Healthcare Center
Los Angeles, CA

Part I

SERVICE DELIVERY ISSUES

1

Overview of Prevention, Integration, and Parity

BRUCE LUBOTSKY LEVIN
ARDIS HANSON
KEVIN D. HENNESSY

At the beginning of the twenty-first century, alcohol, drug abuse, and mental disorders remain significant public health problems. Mental disorders (Chapter 8), substance abuse (Chapter 12), and co-occurring addictive and mental disorders (Chapter 16) are highly prevalent in the general population. During a 12-month period, approximately 23% of the U.S. population appears to have a diagnosable mental disorder, and about 5% of adults have a serious mental illness (Kessler et al., 1996; U.S. Department of Health and Human Services, 1999). The World Health Organization has estimated that approximately 450 million people world-wide have mental and behavioral disorders (World Health Organization, 2001).

The impact of mental illness on health and productivity in the United States and throughout the world has long been seriously underestimated. According to the Global Burden of Disease Study (Murray and Lopez, 1996), mental disorders accounted for more than 15% of the total burden of disease in industrialized countries and represented 4 of the 10 leading causes of disability for individuals 5 years of age and older. Using the disability-adjusted life years (DALY)s measure, major depression was the leading cause of disability, while suicide was one of the leading preventable causes of death in the United States. Mental disorders rank second only to cardiovascular diseases in the magnitude of disease burden. Furthermore, the World Health Organization (2001) concluded that mental disorders account for 25% of all disability in major industrialized countries.

Meanwhile, the organization, financing, and provision of mental health and substance abuse services in the United States remain a complex and confusing assortment of uncoordinated public and private delivery systems (Norquist and Regier, 1996). Today, these de facto mental health service delivery systems are fragmented, largely consisting of (1) the primary medical care sector (including primary medical care practitioners and health care facilities), (2) the specialty behavioral health sector (including mental health, alcohol, and drug abuse practitioners and public and private facilities), (3) the human services sector (including social services, school-based counseling services, rehabilitation services, criminal justice services, and the clergy), and (4) the voluntary support network sector including self-help groups (U.S. Department of Health and Human Services, 1999).

In addition, the provision and financing of mental health services are generally separate from rather than integrated with somatic health services. This lack of integration between somatic health and mental health services has contributed to the development of a number of dubious public health policies, including insurance providers' unequal coverage of mental health services vis-à-vis somatic health services (Levin et al., 2000).

Moreover, the historical reliance on the public sector for long-term mental health care and on the private sector for acute mental health care has limited the overall continuity of care for mental health services (Elpers and Levin, 1996). Increasingly, mental health services have been financed through multiple (public and private) payers and public and private providers of mental health care (Frank and McGuire, 1996).

The chapters in this book attempt to present the latest knowledge in a variety of areas related to the organization, delivery, and financing of mental health services. This first chapter highlights three key issues that are at the forefront of mental health policy discussions: the prevention of mental disorders, the integration of mental health services with primary care, and the impact of mental health parity legislation on benefits plans.

Prevention

Primary, secondary, and tertiary prevention are well-known underlying principles for avoiding or controlling public health problems. Nevertheless, these concepts are more difficult to apply in mental health because the causes of most mental disorders continue to be unknown, incompletely known, or of multiple etiology. True primary prevention, the avoidance of the occurrence of an illness, is elusive in the field of mental health. Recent genetic discoveries may allow the prevention of such diseases as Huntington's chorea and early-onset Alzheimer's disease through genetic counseling or gene therapy, but the genetic predispositions of most mental disorders are complex and far from being completely understood. A great deal of *social engineering* has been attempted to prevent the occurrence of mental disorders, but there is little evidence that these efforts have been successful.

Secondary prevention, the avoidance of disease recurrences or exacerbations after disease diagnosis, is somewhat more possible in mental health. It is well known that with early identification and intervention, many mood disorders can be stabilized, allowing patients to lead productive, relatively unimpaired lives. Early intervention in other diagnostic groups has varying chances of success, but considering the magnitude of the disabilities, such intervention is certainly justifiable. Many areas of children's mental health operate largely on this premise, and the need in this area for high-quality program evaluation (as discussed in Chapter 20) is very great.

Finally, there is tertiary prevention—the reduction of disability or rehabilitation. Here is where one must classify a substantial portion of mental health care for individuals with serious mental disorders. The mental health field can document considerable success through community support programs, positive assertive community treatment, psychosocial rehabilitation, agencies that use an integrated services approach, and the many variations and permutations of such programs, all of which are combinations of clinical treatment and rehabilitation with proven effectiveness (Anthony and Liberman, 1986; Meisel et al., 1993; Stein and Test, 1978). However, while mental health professionals may readily justify costs in terms of preventing human misery in individuals and their families, the cost-benefit ratios of mental health treatment have been more difficult to prove both to the general public and to state and federal lawmakers. The funding of public mental health programs is a political process, and public mental health leaders can best fulfill their responsibilities to their clientele by articulately defining and defending these programs with convincing data.

During the past decade, there have been a number of important reports that may alter both the interest in and the complexity of the prevention field in the years ahead. One report was an interesting compendium prepared by the Committee on Prevention of Mental Disorders of the Institute of Medicine's Division of Biobehavioral Sciences and Mental Disorders (Institute of Medicine, 1994). Titled *Reducing Risks for Mental Disorders*, this report made recommendations about terminology, reviewed the available research on prevention, and set an ambitious agenda for prevention research in the future. This agenda included building an infrastructure to coordinate prevention research across all relevant governmental agencies, training and supporting new investigators, and conducting well-evaluated preventive interventions.

One intriguing aspect of the report is a recommendation that the traditional public health model of primary, secondary, and tertiary prevention terminology be discarded. Instead, the term *prevention* would be used for those interventions that occur before the initial onset of disorders. The report also recommended the use of Gordon's classification of preventive interventions (Gordon, 1987) with slight modifications. Briefly, *universal* interventions are those targeted to the general public, not related to individual risk factors. *Selective* preventive interventions are targeted to individuals or subgroups of the population whose risk of developing mental disorders is significantly higher than average. Finally, *indicated* preventive interventions are targeted to high-risk individuals who have early signs or symptoms or biological markers but do not meet diagnostic criteria. All other interventions would fall under either *treatment* (case identification and standard treatments) or *maintenance* (long-term care to prevent relapses and rehabilitation).

The two models of prevention (public health and mental health) have very similar overall goals: to reduce morbidity and mortality. However, while the public health prevention model examines problems, issues, and diseases from a population-based perspective, the Institute of Medicine's (1994) newer definitions for prevention within a mental health model focuses more on specific target populations. This may be more effective than targeting the whole population, as identifying risk factors plays an integral part in disease development. However, the Institute of Medicine's re-conceptualization of the terminology for prevention has not been widely accepted, recognized, or used in public health, mental health, and managed health care delivery systems. This may create added challenges regarding efforts to integrate preventive mental health efforts with primary prevention (somatic) health care delivery initiatives.

A second report, titled *Report to Congress on the Treatment and Prevention of Co-Occurring Substance Abuse and Mental Disorders* (Substance Abuse and Mental Health Services Administration, 2002), examined the prevention and treatment of co-occurring disorders in the estimated 7 to 10 million individuals in the United States who have at least one mental disorder and an alcohol or drug use disorder (U.S. Department of Health and Human Services, 1999). The report emphasized the characteristics and unique service needs of this population; prevention opportunities for children and adolescents, adults, and older adults; and evidence-based practices for co-occurring disorders (for additional information on co-occurring disorders, see Chapter 16).

The combined impact of these reports may well be stronger support for more research to increase the understanding of mental disorders and to develop more effective preventive interventions in the decade ahead. Undoubtedly, a major impetus of these efforts is the belief that enough new information about genetics, brain function, and mental disorders is becoming available so that prevention is now an attainable goal, at least for some mental disorders.

Integration with Primary Care

Efforts to integrate mental health care with primary (somatic) health care coincide with the concept of *managing* health care in the early-twentieth-century United States. This initiative was pioneered with the evolution of the prepaid group practice plan prototype of the Kaiser Foundation in California (Levin, 1992). Since then, efforts by Congress to enact legislation affecting mental health policy have included (*1*) creation of commissions and advisory groups at a federal level to influence mental health policy and research, (*2*) efforts to create and expand service capacity, (*3*) establishment of financing mechanisms for mental health services, and (*4*) creation of a set of principles to govern state planning of mental health services. However, these legislative and policy initiatives have, for the most part, fostered the creation of separate service delivery systems for the treatment of substance abuse and mental disorders quite apart from somatic services delivery (for additional readings in mental health law and policy, see Chapter 3).

In 1988, an Institute of Medicine report acknowledged that an underdeveloped relationship existed between public health and mental health. The report, titled *The Future of Public Health*, stated the need to strengthen the linkages between public health and mental health service delivery systems. One strategy for accomplishing this would be to encourage the integration of mental health services and primary health care, since the majority of individuals with emotional and behavioral disorders either (*1*) do not seek treatment or (*2*) if they do seek treatment are seen by primary health care providers rather than mental health care specialists (U.S. Department of Health and Human Services, 1999).

Primary health care providers and settings are important for the identification and treatment of mental disorders in children, adolescents, adults, and the elderly (U.S. Department of Health and Human Services, 1999). Primary health care providers and settings offer a variety of advantages vis-à-vis specialty mental health care, including increased geographic proximity and convenience, affordability, and coordination of health and mental health care. Nevertheless, the vast majority of these advantages have yet to be realized in American health care systems. Historically, primary care providers have not been interested or well trained in assessment, diagnosis, treatment (including knowledge of psychopharmacology), and the application of new models of mental health services delivery for individuals with serious mental disorders (U.S. Department of Health and Human Services, 1999).

Within the workplace setting, Melek (2000) has suggested that employers, through their purchasing decisions, are the driving force in the health care system. The literature shows that employers are focusing on maintaining the health of their employees rather than on simply treating injury and disease. From an employer's perspective, the integration of mental health and substance abuse services into primary care settings under managed care arrangements would assist in recovering lost productivity days as well as creating a healthier workforce. This major structural change within the health care system was supported by the Surgeon General's *Report on Mental Health* (U.S. Department of Health and Human Services, 1999), the first Surgeon General's report ever to address mental health issues.

As a result of this report, a meeting on the integration of mental health services and primary health care was held in Atlanta in 2000 (U.S. Department of Health and Human Services, 2001). At the meeting, Surgeon General David Satcher emphasized the use of a *balanced partnership* that provides an opportunity for the coordination and integration of patient care. He envisioned the health team, led by the primary care physician, as working with the family to ensure continuity of care that, in turn, ensures comprehensive, high-quality care. "Not only is family involvement therapeutic for the patient, but it is the key to sustaining continuity of care and providing high-quality care" (p. 2).

There are several major design challenges to the integration of mental health services with primary health care. With an average visit of 13 to 16 minutes and with patients averaging six problems a visit, primary care providers have limited time to attend to each patient's needs (Williams et al., 1999). Somatic and mental health care providers also have different cultures, including different styles of communication, duration of office visits, and level of interaction with patients (Herman et al., 2002). Providers see integrated programs as too expensive, with too little demand, and with limited evidence for cost neutrality or cost offsets (e.g., lower overall health care costs, lower disability costs, or improved worker productivity) (Melek, 1999).

The clinical research and the economic research appear to be at odds when discussing the effectiveness of integrating somatic and mental health services (Melek,

1999, 2000). For example, the separation of somatic and mental health funding focuses on different outcomes, different ways of looking at cost–effectiveness (acute
and chronic care and support services), and different ways of providing treatment
(carve-in vs. carve-out). The different methods of treatment do have implications
for access to services. In addition, many of the cost–effectiveness studies on managed behavioral health examine carve-out benefits. Of particular note in these studies is the pattern of increased use, increased care within the managed behavioral
health organization network, and long-term cost reductions. Goldman et al. (1999)
state that the mechanisms of managed care[1] appear to be sufficient to contain costs
over the long term, and over this long period of time the management of care may
be the critical factor, not benefit design.

Olfson et al.'s (1999) cross-sectional study of the cost impact of global service
expansions in behavioral health found little support for the cost-offset effect. They
identified in the literature three patient groups who yielded cost offsets: (1) distressed elderly medical inpatients, (2) primary care outpatients with multiple un-
explained somatic complaints, and (3) nonelderly adults with alcoholism. They also
found that cost offsets were unlikely in mental health treatment of persons with
schizophrenia, bipolar disorder, or other severe mental illnesses; persons with severe mental illnesses who received insufficient or inadequate medical care; and so-
cioeconomically disadvantaged or underserved groups who have limited access to
medical care. However, they emphasized that (1) cost offsets were important because they represent cost–effective practices to improve health, (2) information
about reducing costs from inappropriate general medical care by providing timely
mental health treatments will improve the quality of health care, and (3) managed
behavioral health care can use data from cost-offset studies to target use management of high users and in specific conditions for which specific mental health interventions would be most cost–effective, thereby allowing the most effective continuum of care for the patient.

Parity

The promotion and enactment of mental health parity has been one of the top legislative and policy priorities among individuals with mental disorders and those
who advocate for their interests (Mental Health Liaison Group, 2002a). *Parity*,
which in its most basic form is a call for equal benefit coverage for mental and
general medical disorders, has been described as a "step in the right direction"
(Frank et al., 2001) or a "sequential step" (Hennessy and Goldman, 2001) toward
the larger goal of achieving fairness in access to quality treatment for mental disorders. Given that insurance parity is consistent with the broader objective of reducing discrimination against individuals with mental illness, it is not surprising
that mental health advocacy organizations almost universally support parity (Mental Health Liaison Group, 2002b).

Over the past decade, the efforts of individuals and advocacy groups have contributed to the enactment of 33 state parity laws as well as a federal law mandating partial parity (NAMHC, 2000). However, as of 2003, the goal of a national law

ensuring full parity for mental health benefits relative to coverage for general medical care remains elusive. Despite substantial support in both houses of the U.S. Congress for a bill that would provide full parity and the endorsement by President George W. Bush of some extension of the parity law, sufficient opposition from several key interest groups and legislators has prevented its passage.

Opponents of a federal parity law have expressed concerns about mandating additional insurance benefits as well as the potential costs associated with such a mandate. In 2001, however, the Congressional Budget Office projected that the cost of a full parity bill would result in premium increases of less than 1% (CBO, 2001). This estimate factored in the likelihood that potential increases in mental health service use might be balanced by a more widespread application of managed care to contain the costs associated with such changes in use. This balancing appears to have occurred in several states that implemented parity laws in the past decade. In these states, the application of managed care strategies resulted in minimal cost increases related to parity and, in some cases, even net reductions in costs (NAMHC, 1998, 2000).

There is a great deal of variation in existing state parity laws, including the populations covered, the extent of covered services, and the nature of exclusions from coverage based on factors such as individual diagnosis and company size (Levin et al., 2001). While the differences among states may reflect a lack of consensus in defining the parity concept, it is equally (if not more) likely that these variations are a product of political realities, namely, that certain provisions of parity laws either were or were not acceptable to political decision makers or influential stakeholders within a given state. Thus, in some states only individuals with severe or biologically based mental disorders are afforded parity benefits, while those with less severe but equally disabling mental illnesses are denied such coverage. Further, the ability of companies that self-insure their employees' health benefits to avoid state mandates under the Employee Retirement Income Security Act (ERISA) of 1974 results in a lack of parity coverage for the approximately 130 million individuals covered by such plans in this country. In sum, the current patchwork of state laws leaves most individuals without parity coverage by virtue of their diagnosis or the self-insurance status of their employer.

Several years ago, the federal government, through the U.S. Office of Personnel Management (OPM), addressed this problem for federal employees and their dependents by implementing full parity for both mental health and substance abuse benefits within all plans participating in the Federal Employees Health Benefits (FEHB) Program (OPM, 1999). With approximately 200 distinct health plans and roughly 8.5 million beneficiaries, the FEHB Program has been characterized as the largest employer-sponsored health benefit system in the United States. Given the number of individuals affected, it is not surprising that OPM's decision to implement full parity for mental health and substance abuse benefits was seen by some as a "historic undertaking that breaks new ground for employer-sponsored health care programs" (WBGH, 2000).

Parity, as defined by OPM, is fairly inclusive in that a plan's coverage for mental health and substance abuse must be identical to that of traditional medical care with regard to deductibles, coinsurance, copayments, and day and visit limitations

(OPM, 2000). While plans retain a good deal of discretion in the design of their benefits, OPM's guidance to participating health plans strongly recommended that parity benefit proposals include "an appropriate care-management structure" (OPM, 2000). Such a structure could take various forms, including the use of managed behavioral health care organizations, gatekeeper referrals to network providers, authorized treatment plans, precertification of inpatient services, concurrent review, discharge planning, case management, retrospective review, and disease management programs. In providing guidance to the FEHB plans, OPM conveyed its belief, based on research evidence, that parity delivered under management could expand access to care with a minimal impact on cost. At present, OPM has partnered with the U.S. Department of Health and Human Services to conduct a comprehensive evaluation of the impact of this important policy change (Hennessy and Barry, in press).

The Surgeon General's *Report on Mental Health* (1999) has confirmed that the majority of persons suffering from a mental disorder do not seek or receive treatment for their condition, despite the presence of various effective treatments that promote remission and, in many cases, recovery from mental illness (U.S. Department of Health and Human Services, 1999). From a clinical perspective, the reasons for failing to seek needed treatment can be complex. Some of these reasons are internal and include shame, fear, ignorance, denial, resistance, or profound hopelessness. In many respects, these internal obstacles can be far more powerful and prohibitive than any external obstacles, such as lack of parity between mental health and medical benefits. Unfortunately, some of the external obstacles can be easily embraced by these individuals as further evidence of society's belief that mental illnesses are somehow less real, less debilitating, and less worthy of treatment than physical health conditions. With regard to passage of a national parity law, policy makers in the United States are faced with a choice that can either ultimately reinforce or refute the feelings of inferiority and discrimination felt by millions of individuals in this country who struggle daily with untreated mental illnesses (for an additional discussion of parity, see Chapters 2, 3, 11, and 13).

Implications for Mental Health Services

Prevention

A recent report, *Priority Areas for National Action: Transforming Health Care Quality* (Institute of Medicine, 2003), reiterates that chronic conditions account for the majority of the nation's health care. In addition, the report proposes a consumer-oriented framework that encompasses four domains of care: preventive care, acute care, chronic care, and palliative care. These domains cover the range of staying healthy, getting better, managing disease (living with illness or disability), and coping with the end of life. However, a fifth category, cross-cutting system interventions, was added to address critical issues in coordination of care, an issue that spans all aspects of disease treatment and management. The report also recommended that the U.S. Department of Health and Human Services focus on care coordination, self-management and health literacy, screening and treatment of major depression, and treatment of severe and persistent mental illness in the public sector.

Expanded definitions of prevention and promotion now appear in the literature and in research. These include the prevention of relapse, especially in the area of substance abuse, and the promotion of positive developmental strengths and resilience to stress. By using prevention and promotion together, prevention and promotion research slowly enters a new, and promising, stage of development and application to services delivery.

Another emerging area is the combination of specific interventions for greater impact and how culture, social class, and gender affect the success of these programs. With increased use of evidence-based practice in policy and practice, one of the major questions is how small, successful, scientifically researched programs can be adapted for large-scale use in public health and mental health. This becomes more complex as one considers adapting a successful intervention developed in one country for use in another country.

If the recommendations from *Priority Areas for National Action* (Institute of Medicine, 2003) are adopted by health professionals, the fifth category, crosscutting system interventions, would foster the further development of an integrated approach for somatic and behavioral health care.

Integration

There are many opportunities for integrating somatic and mental health care (Melek, 1999). Mental health professionals could be considered on-site members of the primary medical care team within the health care plan or on-site consultants to the primary care physician. Increased coordination and transition between the somatic and mental health portions of care would create the awareness among users of care that the different providers are part of the same treatment program or team and would improve interdepartmental and interclinic care planning, case management, and program development. Of interest is that the research indicates that prevention and promotion may be one avenue to further integration, with the use of patient self-management and awareness programs and case-finding programs for early intervention. Integration of somatic and mental health services would be enhanced by ensuring that mental health providers have a professional degree, state licensure, and active membership on key provider panels.

Another challenge in the integration of mental health and somatic health is the delegation of roles and responsibilities of primary care physicians and other behavioral and prevention professionals (Katon et al., 2001; Wise, 2001). Finally, the need for common integrated information technologies for medical records, scheduling, billing, and reporting must be met as we move toward an electronic health record and standards for outcomes assessment (Melek, 2000).

Historically, somatic health services are based on acute care service delivery models, and long-term care treatment environments generally do not include psychosocial rehabilitation or supportive services such as housing, education, or employment. The largest unmet needs of persons with severe mental illness involve community rehabilitation and long-term services that are typically not covered by private health insurance policies (Mechanic, 1998). One of the largest challenges for integration of somatic and mental health services may actually come at the level of insurance benefits design.

Parity

In *Can't Make the Grade* (National Mental Health Association, 2003), the National Mental Health Association State Mental Health Assessment Project evaluated state policy makers' work in mental health parity. Not only did Vermont receive an A, it also received the highest marks for its comprehensive parity law, which includes all mental health and substance abuse diagnoses and prohibits all forms of insurance discrimination in the provision of mental health treatment. Other states that received an A included Connecticut, Maryland, and Minnesota. Despite the fact that most states have passed some form of mental health parity law, efforts to do so at the national level appear to have stalled, and it is unclear at present what it may take to further advance the parity agenda on the national stage. However, it can be argued that the absence of a federal law continues to send a message to those with mental disorders regarding the degree to which their conditions are perceived as worthy of equitable coverage and treatment relative to those with other chronic health conditions.

In sum, prevention, integration with primary care, and parity are issues of continuing discussion and debate in both mental health and health policy circles more broadly. Further progress in each of these areas is essential to advancing our efforts both to effectively treat mental disorders in those with a current illness and prevent the emergence of such disorders in the larger population.

NOTES

1. Specifically, prospective and concurrent clinical reviews, substitution of benefits, individualized treatment planning, provider networks, fixed rates of reimbursement, and use of intermediary levels of care.

REFERENCES

Anthony WA, Liberman RP. The practice of psychiatric rehabilitation: historical, conceptual, and research base. *Schizophrenia Bulletin*, 12:542, 1986.

Congressional Budget Office. *Cost Estimate for S.543—Mental Health Equitable Treatment Act of 2001*. Washington, DC: Congressional Budget Office, 2001.

Elpers JR, Levin BL. Mental health services: epidemiology, prevention, and service delivery systems. In: Levin BL, Petrila J (eds). *Mental Health Services: A Public Health Perspective*. New York: Oxford University Press, pp. 5–22, 1996.

Frank RG, Goldman HH, McGuire TG. Will parity in coverage result in better mental health care? *New England Journal of Medicine*, 345(23):1701–1704, 2001.

Frank RG, McGuire TG. Introduction to the economics of mental health payment systems. In: Levin BL, Petrila J (eds). *Mental Health Services: A Public Health Perspective*. New York: Oxford University Press, pp. 23–37, 1996.

Frank RG, McGuire TG. Economics and mental health. In: Culyer A, Newhouse JP (eds.). *Handbook of Health Economics*. Amsterdam: Elsevier, pp. 894–954, 2000.

Goldman W, McCulloch J, Cuffel B, et al. More evidence for the insurability of managed behavioral health care. *Health Affairs*, 18(5):172–185, 1999.

Gordon R. An operational classification of disease prevention. In: Steinberg JA, Silverman MM (eds). *Preventing Mental Disorders*. Rockville, MD: U.S. Department of Health and Human Services, pp. 20–26, 1987.

Hennessy KD, Barry CL. Parity in the Federal Employees Health Benefits (FEHB) program: an overview. In: Manderscheid RM, Henderson MJ (eds). *Mental Health, United States, 2002*. Rockville, MD: Substance Abuse and Mental Health Services Administration, in press.

Hennessy KD, Goldman HH. Full parity: steps toward treatment equity for mental and addictive disorders. *Health Affairs*, 20(4):58–67, 2001.

Herman H, Trauer T, Warnock J. The roles and relationships of psychiatrists and other service providers in mental health services. *Australian and New Zealand Journal of Psychiatry*, 36(1):75–80, 2002.

Institute of Medicine. *The Future of Public Health*. Washington, DC: National Academy Press, 1988.

Institute of Medicine. *Reducing Risks for Mental Disorders: Frontiers for Preventive Intervention Research*. Washington, DC: National Academy Press, 1994.

Institute of Medicine. *Priority Areas for National Action: Transforming Health Care Quality*. Washington, DC: National Academy Press, 2003.

Katon W, Von Korff M, Lin E, et al. Rethinking practitioner roles in chronic illness: the specialist, primary care physician, and the practice nurse. *General Hospital Psychiatry*, 23(3):138–144, 2001.

Kessler RC, Berglund PA, Zhao S, et al. The 12-month prevalence and correlates of serious mental illness. In: Manderscheid RW, Sonnenschein MA (eds). *Mental Health, United States, 1996*. DHHS Pub. No. (SMA) 96-3098. Washington, DC: U.S. Government Printing Office, pp. 59–70, 1996.

Levin BL. Managed mental health care: a national perspective. In: Manderscheid RW, Sonnenschein MA (eds). *Mental Health, United States, 1992*. DHHS Pub. No. (SMA) 92-1942. Rockville, MD: Center for Mental Health Services, pp. 208–216, 1992.

Levin BL, Hanson A, Coe R: *Mental Health Parity: National and State Perspectives 2001*. Tampa, FL: University of South Florida: The Louis de la Parte Mental Health Institute, 2001.

Levin BL, Hanson A, Coe R, Kuppin SA: *Mental Health Parity: National and State Perspectives 2000*. Tampa, FL: University of South Florida, The Louis de la Parte Florida Mental Health Institute, 2000.

Mechanic D. Emerging trends in mental health policy and practice. *Health Affairs*, 17(6):82–98, 1998.

Meisel J, McGowen M, Patotzka D, et al. *Evaluation of AB3777 Client and Cost Outcomes/July 1990 through March 1992*. Available from the California State Department of Mental Health, Falls Church, VA: Lewin-VHI, 1993.

Melek SP. *Financial, Risk and Structural Issues Related to the Integration of Behavioral Healthcare in Primary Care Settings under Managed Care*. Washington, DC: Milliman & Robertson, 1999. Available at: http://www.milliman.com/health/publications/research_reports/hrr41.pdf Accessed 3 May 2003.

Melek SP. Integrating behavioral healthcare into managed care settings. *Broker World*, 20(6):32–38, 2000.

Mental Health Liaison Group (MHLG). *Parity Fact Sheet: Pass Mental Health Parity*. Washington, DC: MHLG, 2002a.

Mental Health Liaison Group (MHLG). *Mental Health Equitable Treatment Act (S.543): List of Supporting Organizations.* Washington, DC: MHLG, 2002b.

Murray CJ, Lopez AD (eds). *The Global Burden of Disease: A ComprehensiveAssessment of Mortality and Disability from Diseases, Injuries, and Risk Factors in 1990 and Projected to 2020.* Cambridge, MA: Harvard University Press, 1996.

National Advisory Mental Health Council (NAMHC). *Parity in Financing Mental Health Services: Managed Care Effects on Cost, Access, and Quality.* Report to Congress by the National Advisory Mental Health Council: Bethesda, MD: National Institutes of Health, 1998.

National Advisory Mental Health Council (NAMHC). *Insurance Parity for Mental Health: Cost, Access, and Quality.* Final report to Congress by the National Advisory Mental Health Council. Bethesda, MD: National Institutes of Health, 2000.

National Mental Health Association. *Can't Make the Grade: NMHA State Mental Health Assessment Project: Executive Summary.* Alexandria, VA: National Mental health Association, 2003. Available at: http://www.nmha.org/cantmakethegrade/execSummary. pdf   Accessed May 6, 2003.

Norquist GS, Regier DA. The epidemiology of psychiatric disorders and the de facto mental health care system. *Annual Review of Medicine,* 47:473–479, 1996.

Office of Personnel Management (OPM). *Mental Health and Substance Abuse.* FEHB Program Carrier Letter No. 1999-027. Washington, DC: OPM, 1999.

Office of Personnel Management (OPM). *Call Letter for Contract Year 2001—Policy Guidance.* FEHB Program Carrier Letter No. 2000-17. Washington, DC: OPM, 2000.

Olfson M, Sing M, Schlesinger HJ. Mental health/medical care cost offsets: opportunities for managed care. *Health Affairs,* 18(2):79–90, 1999.

Regier DA, Goldberg ID, Taube CA. The de facto U. S. mental health services system: a public health perspective. *Archives of General Psychiatry,* 35:685–693, 1978.

Stein LI, Test MA (eds). *Alternatives to Mental Hospital Treatment.* New York: Plenum, 1978.

Substance Abuse and Mental Health Services Administration. *Report to Congress on the Treatment and Prevention of Co-Occurring Substance Abuse and Mental Disorders.* Washington, DC: U.S. Department of Health and Human Services, 2002. Available at: www.samhsa.gov/reports/congress2002/index.html   Accessed May 1, 2003.

U.S. Department of Health and Human Services. *Mental Health: A Report of the Surgeon General.* Rockville, MD: Substance Abuse and Mental Health Services Administration, National Institute of Mental Health, 1999.

U.S. Department of Health and Human Services. *Report of a Surgeon General's Working Meeting on the Integration of Mental Health Services and Primary Health Care.* Rockville, MD: Office of the Surgeon General, 2001.

Washington Business Group on Health (WBGH). *Large Employer Experiences and Best Practices in Design, Administration, and Evaluation of Mental Health and Substance Abuse Benefits: A Look at Parity in Employer-Sponsored Health Benefit Programs.* Washington DC: WBGH, 2000.

Williams JW, Ross K, Dietrich AJ, et al. Primary care physicians' approach to depressive disorders: effects of physician specialty and practice structure. *Archives of Family Medicine,* 8(1):58–67, 1999.

Wise EA. Primary care physician survey on accessing mental health services: roles for psychologists in health care systems. *Journal of Psychotherapy in Independent Practice* 2(4):57–72, 2001.

World Health Organization. *The World Health Report, 2001. Mental Health: New Understanding, New Hope.* Geneva: World Health Organization, 2001.

2

Insuring Mental Health Care in the Age of Managed Care

RENA CONTI
RICHARD G. FRANK
THOMAS G. McGUIRE

Private health insurance has long served different functions in the financing of mental health care than it has in general health services. It is typically more limited in its level and extent of coverage (Buck, et al, 1997), it covers care used by the less severely ill among people suffering from mental illnesses, and its costs have received disproportionate attention. Public commitment to directly finance and provide mental health care to the most seriously impaired citizens also sets mental health apart (Goldman and Skinner, 1989; Grob, 1994). A fundamental reason why financing and organization are different for mental health care is that the basic economic forces causing market failures in health insurance, moral hazard, and adverse selection have special force in the mental health sector (Frank and McGuire, 2000; Newhouse et al., 1993).

This chapter examines the impact that evolving institutions associated with managed care in the United States have on the economics of mental health care delivery. We stress the following: in comparison to physical health, the organization and financing of the treatment of mental illness in the age of managed care have led to the use of specialty *carve-out* arrangements, dramatic reductions in costs, and state governments' delegation of management responsibilities to private management firms.

The chapter begins with a discussion of mental illnesses' direct and indirect costs to individuals and society and then reviews the public and private financing of care. Using recent empirical evidence, we describe the organization of the treatment of mental illness under managed care and its effects on use, costs, and state delegation. We rely on fundamental principles of economic theory to aid our understanding of the evolution of these unique features and the effects of managed behavioral health care. Finally, we discuss the policy implications of this framework and the challenges ahead.

Costs and Who Pays

Mental and addictive disorders are costly to society both in terms of direct spending on treatment and in terms of indirect costs resulting from the disorders. Spending on mental health and substance abuse care (MH/SA) in 1995 was estimated to be about $75 billion, amounting to about 8.3% of personal health expenditures (Triplett, 1998). Overall spending on MH/SA in the United States (including specialty and general care) grew at a rate of 13% per year during 1963–72, at 14% per year during 1972–80, and at 9.3% per year during 1980–95. Total health care spending grew at yearly rates of 11.5%, 13.7%, and 9.9% for the three time intervals, respectively. This suggests that MH spending tracked overall spending quite closely over the 1963–95 period (Triplett, 1998). Other evidence suggests that spending for MH treatment grew more slowly than health care spending in general, increasing by approximately 7% annually compared with health care's overall annual rate of more than 9% (Mark et al., 1998).

Among the fastest-rising expenses for MH services are those for outpatient prescription drugs, accounting for approximately 10% of direct costs (DHHS, 1999). Although the health care market in general has experienced dramatic increases in the use of prescription drugs over the past decade, 6 of the 20 best-selling drugs on the market are for mental illness (IMS Health, 2001). This growth reflects the tremendous expansion in scientific understanding and increasing availability and application of medications in treating mental disorders. Estimates from the National Ambulatory Medical Care Survey suggest that the annual number of visits during which psychotropic medication was prescribed increased from approximately 33 million to 46 million from 1986 to 1994. Psychiatrists prescribe only one-third of psychotropic medications, with two-thirds prescribed by primary care physicians and other medical specialists. This pattern reflects dramatic change in the treatment of mental illness over the past 40 years in terms of site of care (from inpatient to outpatient) and the provider's responsible for care. Outcomes evaluations suggest that several professions trained in psychotherapy produce comparable clinical gains to patients (Knesper, 1989). There is also evidence that for certain illnesses, pharmaceutical treatments can substitute effectively for psychotherapy (Elkin et al., 1989; Kupfer et al., 1992).

Spending for treatment is concentrated on people with the most disabling conditions. In 1990, nearly 30% of spending on MH/SA care was accounted for by 5% of the users of care (Frank et al., 1994). In 1993, for example, the mean level of spending on treatment of MH/SA conditions in a large insured population was $100 per enrollee per year, while the mean cost of treating someone with a diagnosis of manic depression was about $6700 annually (Frank et al., 1994). People with a history of MH care use also tend to incur higher levels of general health expenditures than do others (Cuffel et al., 1998; Frank et al., 2000). Further, a large segment of individuals who receive the most intense care do so because, in part, they are compelled by the legal system.

Spending on MH/SA care displays a different pattern than that of the health sector overall. Table 2.1 shows the composition of spending on health and MH/SA

Table 2.1 Mental Health (MH) and Substance Abuse (SA) Spending by Source of Payment, United States, 1996

Payer	MH/SA (%)	All Health (%)
Private insurance	25.8	31.0
Private out-of-pocket	15.1	18.1
Medicare	14.0	21.0
Medicaid	18.8	14.8
Other federal	3.9	4.3
Other state/local	19.4	7.2
Other private	2.7	3.3
Total	100	100

Note: Percentages may not sum due to rounding.
Source: McKusick et al. (1998).

care in the United States (all numbers in this paragraph cite McKusick et al., 1998). Among the most important differences is the role of government as a direct funder of care. The other federal (block grants) and other state and local categories comprise 23.3% of all MH/SA spending compared to 11.5% of overall health care spending. In addition, Medicaid plays a somewhat larger role in MH/SA spending, 18.8% versus 14.8%. Finally, Medicare plays a considerably smaller role in funding MH/SA than it does for all other health services. Thus, state and local governments generally allocated more resources for MH/SA, 42.1% (summing block grant, state/local and Medicaid funding), than for health services generally, 26.3%. This highlights the differing division of labor between federal and state governments. Whereas the federal government funds over 25% of health spending, it accounts for less than 20% of MH/SA expenditures. Table 2.1 indicates that private health insurance accounts for a smaller share of MH/SA spending than for all other health care (25.8% vs. 31%). The table also suggests that private out-of-pocket spending makes up a smaller share of nonpublic funding for MH/SA care than for overall health care. Similar patterns of mental health compared to general health spending are reported in the *Surgeon General's Report* (1999).

This brief profile leads to three conclusions. First, it is likely that underuse and overuse of care are present simultaneously in the private and public systems. These patterns provide room for more rationalized organization and use of resources devoted to MH/SA. Second, there has been tremendous growth in knowledge regarding the effective treatment of mental disorders using therapy and pharmacological modalities. There is also great variation and uncertainty in treatment. Thus, there may be wide latitude for managed care to substitute lower-cost providers and treatments for higher-costs ones. Third, the social costs of mental and addictive disorders are concentrated in the 4% of the population that experience the more severe forms of the disorders. The costs associated with the treatment and care of this population are enormous and put great financial pressure on state budgets in an era of cost containment policy. New treatment modalities and ways of organizing care present opportunities to rationalize the public provision of mental health care, enhancing value and quality.

Managed Behavioral Health Care

Managed care is transforming the health care sector generally and may be having a larger impact on MH care than on health care in general. Employers, government and other purchasers are bargaining for lower prices and monitoring treatment patterns. The response to the new policy of prudent purchasing of health care services has been acceleration in the growth of managed care organizations. Preferred provider organizations (PPOs), point-of-service (POS) plans, and health maintenance organizations (HMOs) accounted for 73% of the insured population in 1995. State governments have moved to strengthen the bargaining power of health care buyers by encouraging the creation of purchasing alliances that enable smaller purchasers of group health insurance to command more choice at more advantageous prices. While enrollment in managed care for Medicare beneficiaries (the Medicare + Choice program) has slowed in recent years, state Medicaid plans continue to expand enrollment of beneficiaries in managed care organizations bearing significant financial risk.

A striking development in MH/SA has been the development of so-called managed behavioral health care (MBHC) carve-outs. Traditionally, the purchaser, usually an employer, contracted with a single insurance plan to cover a full range of health risks. Increasingly, however, purchasers of health insurance are offering beneficiaries a range of plans. Purchasers may also carve out certain benefits, which means that they separate the health insurance function by disease or service category and contract separately for the management of those risks. This carve-out in insurance need not be associated with managed care, but it virtually always is.

There are three forms of carve-outs found in the MH/SA health subsector, with potentially distinct economic impacts: (*1*) payer specialty carve-outs from all health plans; (*2*) payer specialty carve-outs from only indemnity and PPO-type arrangements; and (*3*) individual health plan carve-outs to specialty vendors. The two forms of payer carve-outs are illustrated in Figures 2.1 and 2.2. In Figure 2.1, enrollees can choose between a traditional indemnity insurance plan and managed care plans (e.g., an HMO and a PPO). The payer in this case writes a separate contract with a specialty vendor for the carved-out service (e.g., behavioral health) to manage a segment of the risk in the traditional plan. Some well-known carve-out programs are of this type, such as the Massachusetts Medicaid plan (Beinecke

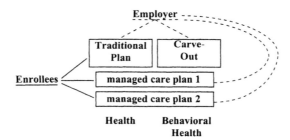

Figure 2.1   Partial payer carve-out.

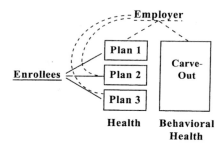

Figure 2.2   Full payer carve-out.

et al., 1997; Callahan, et al., 1995; Frank and McGuire, 1997) and the Massachusetts Group Insurance Commission (GIC) (Huskamp, 1997; Ma and McGuire, 1998; Merrick, 1997). In this case, a carve-out eliminates a traditional indemnity plan for behavioral health care, ensuring that all behavioral health care will be managed. The payer also intervenes in the competitive process by preventing the traditional plan from competing on the basis of the behavioral health benefit (or other service carve-outs).

The payer may entirely remove the carved-out service from the market for otherwise competing integrated health plans. Figure 2.2 shows the situation in which enrollees choose from among competing health plans for their entire health care except for the carved-out service. Behavioral health care for the State of Ohio employees and for employees and dependents of Pacific Bell are organized in such a fashion (Goldman et al., 1998). Enrollees are not given a choice of plan for the carved-out service, although a payer would typically use a competitive process to choose the carve-out vendor.

Figure 2.3 illustrates the third major carve-out arrangement. In this case, enrollees can choose a health plan for all services. Health plans manage certain services such as MH or cancer care by subcontracting with a specialized managed care organization. In this case, the carve-out is an element of the competitive strategy adopted by a health plan. The payer may set general requirements for plans to

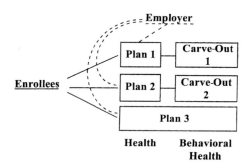

Figure 2.3   Plan carve-out.

meet but does not specify the organizational form. For example, an employer might contract with the Prudential HMO in St. Louis, which in turn carves out MH/SA to Merit Behavioral Health, Inc.

In 1999, almost 177 million Americans with health insurance (72%) were enrolled in managed behavioral health organizations. This represents an increase in enrollment of 9% over 1998 (OSS, 2002). It is difficult to know exactly how many people are enrolled in various forms of carve-out plans. According to Oss (1997), approximately 53 million people are enrolled in carve-out programs of all types. Between 20 and 25 million people are enrolled in so-called risk-based carve-out contracts (whereby the carve-out vendor assumes some or all of the financial risk for claims), which account for about 60% of the total revenue of firms that manage MH/SA benefits. Carve-outs are more common among larger firms than smaller firms. One recent report estimated that 35% of employers with more than 5000 employees have created payer carve-outs, while only 5% of firms with fewer than 500 employees have adopted them (Mark et al., 1998). A survey of 50 large HMOs revealed that roughly half of their enrollees chose carve-out plans (OSS, 2002). Umland (1995) reports that 35% of employers with 5000 or more employees contracted with a specialty MH/SA carve-out vendor compared with about 3% of firms with fewer than 500 employees.

Theoretically, carve-outs could be used for many different medical services. The preponderance of carve-outs in MH care, however, is a unique organizational feature. To understand why carve-outs are specifically part of the MH/SA landscape and what their effects are, we now consider insurance market failures and their implications for the traditional indemnity insurance market and the age of managed care.

Market Failure in Mental Health Care—Theory and Evidence Under Indemnity Insurance

Theory

It has long been appreciated that the primary difference between markets for health care and markets for other goods is the presence of significant asymmetry of information between patients, providers, and insurance companies (Arrow, 1963). Asymmetry in the presence of therapeutic uncertainty leads to two market failures in health insurance: moral hazard and adverse selection.

Moral hazard results from the insurance-caused reduction in the price of care for patients. In response to this reduction, patients demand (and providers may supply) more care. The extra costs to insurers associated with this care is referred to as a *moral*, or behavioral, hazard. In the conventional economic interpretation, this extra consumption produces a welfare loss, since services are consumed with benefits valued at less than their costs. A full evaluation of insurance recognizes the risk protection conferred. At actuarially fair prices, insurance effectively allows individuals to transfer purchasing from healthy states to sick ones, ensuring their ability to maintain consumption levels even in the presence of unexpected health care costs.

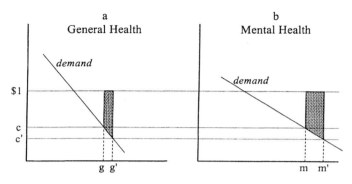

Figure 2.4   Welfare cost of insurance.

The degree of patients' demand response to free or low-cost care may vary among services. Empirical evidence discussed below suggests that MH services are particularly prone to moral hazard. We illustrate the differential effect of demand response for general and MH care to insurance provision in Figure 2.4. This figure shows demand curves for general health (a) and MH (b). On the vertical axis is the cost of each service, normalized at $1, and on the horizontal axis is the level of spending for each service. At an initial cost of c, set equal for each service, spending for general health care would equal g, while for MH care it would equal m. If the cost is reduced to c' due to health insurance, the quantity demanded for MH care would increase more than the quantity demanded for general health services. This is measured graphically as the distance between m' and m and g' and g, respectively. The key issue is that the demand for MH care is more responsive to price reductions than the demand for general health care. In this schema, we can visualize explicitly the implicit trade-off between gains from protection and losses from moral hazard in insurance mentioned above. To see this, note that the social cost is the area under the $1 line (since $1 of spending costs society $1). The efficiency loss is the excess of social cost over consumer benefits and is illustrated as the shaded region in parts a and b. Comparing the losses associated with MH and general care, there is more inefficiency associated with the former since the demand for MH is greater, and thus lower-value services are added to consumption when the price decreases.

Adverse selection refers to the enrollment of beneficiaries in different insurance plans based on their private knowledge of their propensity to use services (Rothschild and Stiglitz, 1976). Attempts to avoid costly enrollees by plans can undermine the efficiency of health insurance. In the extreme case, adverse selection may cause premiums to spiral and ultimately destroy the market for insurance (Cutler and Zeckhauser, 1998). Insurance plans may also distort the type or quality of their services to attract the well and shun the sick (Glazer and McGuire, 2000). This behavior produces welfare loss for consumers since individuals may be unable to enroll in plans that are best for them, given their preferences and illness, or may enroll but receive an inefficient level of treatment. Further, to the extent that the choice of provider is valued, particularly for sicker patients, patients may pay more money or use other resources (like their time or their caretaker's effort) to see physicians who will not actively avoid them, even though their illness is not under their control.

Evidence Under Indemnity Insurance

Virtually all areas of health care are subject to moral hazard to some degree. However, extensive empirical investigation has established that under indemnity insurance, demand for outpatient MH care is more responsive to insurance than demand for general health care. From the 1960s to the 1980s, numerous studies investigated the price response for MH services (Horgan, 1986; McGuire, 1981; Scheffler and Watts, 1986; Taube et al., 1986; Watts et al., 1986). Generally, these studies produced the same finding: ambulatory MH services are highly responsive to cost sharing. Typically, early studies could not make a direct comparison to responsiveness in health care, but they concluded that demand for ambulatory MH care was more responsive to cost sharing than ambulatory medical services based on nonexperimental designs. The major problem with these studies was that they were subject to selection problems, biasing the results. The RAND Health Insurance Experiment (HIE) improved on earlier studies of demand response by randomly assigning families to insurance conditions, thereby reducing selection biases. The HIE also made dramatic improvements in the measurement of key variables. Rather than relying on patient or provider reports about use, the HIE directly observed what was used and when, as well as using measures of health and MH status. Keeler et al. (1988) examined the demand of a subset of users in the RAND HIE who began MH (or general health) treatment while far away (in dollar terms) from the limit on out-of-pocket expenses. They assumed that individuals would foresee, at the initiation of care, all the care that would eventually be used in a given episode of care, but that individuals would not foresee that they might exceed the out-of-pocket limit from other episodes. They showed that individuals in families with full insurance (free care) coverage used about four times more ambulatory MH care than those with virtually no coverage (95% cost sharing). This is roughly double the response reported using a similar methodology for ambulatory medical care. In sum, nearly all the available empirical evidence points to a greater price response for ambulatory MH care than for other health care services. The magnitudes of the price responses vary considerably by study; however, the relative response compared to ambulatory medical care is quite consistent when comparison is possible.

As in the case of moral hazard, evidence suggests that the forces of adverse selection may work more powerfully in MH than in health care. The experience of the Federal Employees Health Benefit Program (FEHBP) during the 1960s and 1970s provides an early example. Plans offering more generous MH/SA benefits quickly attracted individuals who wanted to avail themselves of these services. Individuals not expecting to use these services enrolled in plans with more limited coverage. Ultimately, one of the plans experiencing spiraling health costs associated with adverse selection, AETNA, dropped out of the insurance options for FEHBP beneficiaries (Reed, 1975). Further evidence of adverse selection in the FEHBP comes from comparing responses to the price of MH/SA care under the

FEHBP and the RAND HIE (Newhouse et al., 1993). Individuals who were randomly assigned to health insurance plans in the Rand HIE had an observed price response to differential coverage substantially lower than that observed in the FEHBP (Newhouse et al., 1993). The differences in price response suggest that where plan choice was possible (under FEHBP), the high-option (lower-priced) plan differentially attracted higher-risk individuals, making it appear that the plan with slightly more generous coverage induced much higher use of MH/SA care. More recent evidence has confirmed selection's powerful effect. Deb et al. (1996) found that individuals with a family member with a mental illness were more likely than otherwise similar members of the U.S. population to choose coverage with more generous MH care provisions.

There is also evidence suggesting that MH care users consume more general health services as well, making them bad risks from a health plan's overall perspective. For example, data from Michigan Medicaid indicate that the average person had health care expenditures of $1873 per year over a 3-year period (1991–93) compared to $3722 (including MH care) for individuals with any treatment for mental illness during that time period (Frank et al., 2000). Cuffel et al. (1998) report that MH care users spend nearly 90% more on general medical care than do nonusers. Ellis (1988) examined the persistence of spending over time and its implications for choice of health plan. He found that individuals with a history of MH care use had persistently higher levels of spending than did otherwise similar enrollees. He also found that a history of MH use had a significant impact on individuals' choice of plan. A higher level of prior-year MH spending increases the likelihood that an enrollee will choose a low-deductible plan. This suggests choice based on anticipated spending such that the expected deductible payments exceed the differences in plan premium differentials. Frank et al. (2000) found highly correlated prior and future demands for MH services in the Michigan Medicaid program compared to other services. Cao and McGuire (2002) found evidence for service level selection in MH care in the federal Medicare program.

Together these results suggest that users of MH care are more predictably higher-cost users overall than otherwise similar people, putting plans attracting MH care users at a financial disadvantage. Further, evidence suggests that persons with MH/SA disorders select health plans that offer more generous coverage for behavioral health treatment. These ingredients imply that adverse selection due to variation in MH care coverage and provision generosity is a serious concern in a managed care setting.

The presence of these market failures impacted the structure of MH benefit design in the traditional indemnity insurance market. Generally, traditional private health insurance responded to moral hazard through demand-side cost sharing—copayments, limits, and deductibles that required consumers to bear a share of the cost of their health care consumption. The principle behind these practices was to make consumers more sensitive to the initiation of care and the volume of care provided. Typically, private insurance limited the number of reimbursable days of inpatient MH care to 30 and the number of outpatient visits to between 20 and 30 (all data in this paragraph are from the Employee Benefit Survey, BLS, 2000). Outpatient care generally involved 50% cost sharing in the majority of policies.

Lifetime spending limits were present in 40% of health plans for both inpatient and outpatient MH care. During the 1970s and 1980s, competition to avoid adverse selection took the form of limiting coverage for treatment of mental and addictive disorders. Generally, most Americans who obtained health insurance through their employers had some coverage for MH/SA treatment, but rarely on the same terms as for other medical care. Large companies tend to offer insurance plans with more restrictive coverage for MH care than for other services 86% of the time for inpatient benefits and 97% of the time for outpatient benefits. The corresponding figures for small companies were 85% and 99%. Approximately 22 states counteracted measures aimed at avoiding high risks by mandated benefit statutes, specifying a minimum level of coverage for MH/SA care (Frank, 1989; McGuire and Montgomery, 1982). These statutes generally specified coverage minimums in terms of coinsurance, limits on outpatient visits and hospital days, and deductibles. Since benefit design features were the key provisions of an insurance contract determining coverage, regulation of these components of coverage was potentially effective in limiting market failure associated with adverse selection. However, the impact of mandated benefit statutes was limited to non-self-insured companies offering insurance coverage to their workers under the Employee Retiree Income Security Act (ERISA) of 1974, a federal law that exempts self-insured companies from state insurance mandates.

Rationing in Managed Care

In the face of rapidly escalating medical costs—double-digit rates for almost a decade—the U.S. health care system has undergone a dramatic shift to managed care. This trend is particularly acute for the management of MH services. Managed care in general and MBHC in particular address cost containment by rationing care without relying on prices paid by consumers (Glied, 2000; Mechanic et al., 1995). Although there is wide variation, managed care arrangements generally rely on payment of a prospectively set budget for serving a defined number of individuals. The contracted plan is thus responsible for controlling costs under the budget while providing needed services to enrolled beneficiaries. Features of rationing within MBHC organizations include establishment of a network of providers selected to provide services to enrollees with potentially less costly practice styles and who are willing to provide services at discounted rates; directing individuals to levels of care based on clinical criteria about appropriate matches of clinical circumstances and provider capabilities; writing contracts to providers including financial incentives to limit care or costs; application of a medical necessity criterion to determine the need for and benefits from continuing treatment at different levels of care; and information feedback to providers on their own treatment patterns in relation to their peers and clinical norms. The organization makes these choices in the context of markets where potential enrollees may choose from among plans based on quality indicators, prices and reputation, and/or regulatory standards set by payers that require health plans to achieve particular levels of performance in terms of process or outcome measures.

From the very beginning of research on health economics, it was assumed that rationing occurred in an economically rational fashion (Pauly, 1968). Under standard economic models, consumers were assumed to be utility maximizers and price takers of insurance premiums, implying that consumers bought as much care or coverage as desired given their budget constraint. At a given price, then, the services that were rationed out had the least value to consumers. The validity of these assumptions has generated thousands of academic journal articles, particularly in the MH/SA context. Whatever the reader's opinion of this standard paradigm, under managed care the assumption of a price-taking, utility-maximizing consumer is not easily maintained. In fact, the essence of managed care is its ability to offer enrollees risk protection while effectively rationing care through alternative methods, not relying on money prices faced by consumers.

At present, there is no generally shared paradigm governing our thinking about rationing in managed care. To date, economists have taken two approaches. One approach is to view managed care as setting the quantity of services provided—that is, specifying what a person with a given demand curve would get under managed care (Baumgardner, 1991; Ramsey and Pauly, 1997). A strict rationing system would set a low quantity; a looser one would set a higher quantity. Note that if different types of patients get the same quantity of services, managed care rations inefficiently. Thus, in this case, shifting resources from consumers with low valuation to those with high valuation could improve welfare. The other approach is to view managed care as setting a shadow price for each service (Frank et al., 2000; Glazer and McGuire, 2002; Keeler et al., 1998). The shadow price describes the results of rationing and functions as a convenient composite measure of the many mechanisms managed care uses to allocate services to enrollees with varying demands for care. It is as if consumers were charged this price, and the managed care plan gave them all the services that had a value to them above the shadow price and denied care for all uses for which the value was below the shadow price. In this view, clinicians and patients have considerable latitude in choosing quantities of services that will be beneficial, but they must do so subject to a number of financial and administrative pressures to manage their care economically. Conceptually, we can describe the intensity of rationing by the level at which shadow prices are set. Once computed, the intensity of rationing between services may be compared.

How should the shadow price paradigm be applied to the demand curves we discussed earlier for general and MH care? Assume that consumers have the same willingness to pay for care under managed care than they did under indemnity insurance arrangements but now face rationing of a different kind, represented by a shadow price. Figures 2.5a and 2.5b represent the demand curves from Figures 2.4a and 2.4b and impose a shadow price equal to p to ration both general and MH care. Initially, the managed care plan would provide $\$g$ of general health care and $\$m$ of MH care given these demand curves. Now a slightly higher shadow price p' for each area is shown, representing stricter rationing and leading to offered quantities of g' and m', respectively. Note that because demand for MH/SA is more responsive to price, more rationing leads to a larger cutback in the spending on MH/SA for other services.

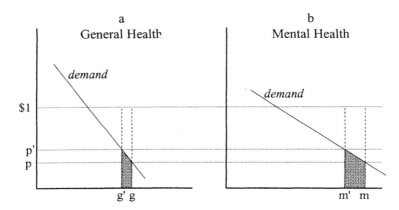

Figure 2.5   Managed care rationing by shadow prices.

When the shadow price is raised, what are the efficiency implications for consumers? Here is the key difference between managed care and indemnity coverage: the shadow price is a virtual price. The consumer is not actually paying the price, and thus there is no increase in the financial risk imposed on the consumer by this "as if" increase from p to p'. In fact, this is the appeal of managed care: nonprice rationing imposes no financial risk on the consumer, while the efficiency benefit accrues to the health plan if the initial price was below \$1 (the social cost of spending). Thus, the trade-off between insurance protection and moral hazard discussed above is altered by managed care to impose a risk on suppliers to produce care efficiently rather than on patients' demand for appropriate care. This may reduce spending from \$$g$ to \$$g'$ and consequently may reduce health plan premiums. Since consumers do not value spending between g and g' at the cost of providing it, this reduction in premiums makes the plan more attractive from the consumers' point of view. This argument may apply to other health services in addition to MH care. However, the shadow price rise for both general health and MH may be efficiency enhancing if both lead to cutbacks in low-value spending.

What about adverse selection? Health plans have the same incentives to discourage membership of persons with high health care costs that they did under indemnity insurance. Indeed, with the renaissance of risk-bearing contracts for health plans under managed care, if anything the incentives may be enhanced. In a market in which plans bear financial risk, adverse selection will lead plans to distort rationing devices away from efficient levels. This may take the form of the underprovision of certain services to avoid bad risks, a practice Ellis (1998) labels *skimping* and Newhouse et al. (1997) call *stinting*. The plan might also provide too many of the services used to treat the less seriously ill in order to attract low-risk consumers. Hence, in the presence of selection-related incentives, financial risk bearing and managed care market forces may generate too little care in some areas and too much in others (Frank et al., 2000). Thus, selection incentives will tend to raise shadow prices for areas of care, like MH/SA care, that "loser" enrollees value.

There are two general points to make about this problem. First, we know very little about the process of rationing in managed care. In general, decision making in managed care is poorly understood. The services that would be affected by selection-related incentives have not been identified. One candidate is MH/SA, but surely there are others. In general, all areas of care cannot be discriminated against in the relative sense. Can we expect MH/SA to fare less well than average? What evidence is there to bear on this point in terms of costs and use? We review the empirical evidence in the next section. Second, even if MH/SA care were distorted by selection-driven competition among managed care plans, what could be done about it? When insurers used benefit design features such as copayments and deductibles to ration care, for all their disadvantages at least regulators knew what to regulate and how. The problem of setting policy has become much more difficult under managed care.

There are two market-based approaches that may be used to counter selection-related incentives to distort the delivery of care: managed behavioral carve-outs and risk adjustment. Although managed behavioral carve-outs are usually regarded as cost-control devices, they may also have a role in diminishing selection-related incentives. The economic role of carve-out programs can differ significantly, depending on its specific form. For example, the carve-outs shown in Figure 2.3 are chosen by the health plan and can be viewed as an organizational structure that helps the health plan implement its desired rationing scheme. Viewed in this manner, carve-outs that are simple subcontractors of health plans may have little impact on selection because consumers continue to choose from among integrated health plans where the implementation of rationing rules across services can affect enrollment patterns. The incentives to ration MH/SA care to the organization are present with and without a carve-out contract. In contrast, the type of carve-out program depicted in Figure 2.2 separates MH/SA services from overall health care and as such removes it as a dimension of competition among health plans for enrollees. This can have potentially large impacts on the incentive to provide services. Carving out a service, MH/SA in this case, isolates that aspect of medical care from selection-related incentives. Rationing will be determined by the contract between the payer and the specialty managed behavioral health care organization (MBHO). It is also important to note that the rationing for any one service depends on all the other service demands. Thus, carving out any one service will affect the degree of rationing for all others. Of course, carve-out programs have other problems that must be considered along with the potential gains related to selection, including high administrative costs (estimated to be between 8% and 15%), difficulties in coordination with care between, for instance, general and MH providers, and an incentive to shift responsibility of care across insurance segments.

The other methodology for stemming selection-related incentives in managed care is risk adjustment. The basic idea behind risk adjustment is that if plans are paid more to care for enrollees likely to be costly, the plans will not actively avoid these enrollees. Most risk adjustment systems rely on demographic factors and clinical information on individuals from past time periods. The clinical information usually consists of diagnoses and procedures arranged in clusters based on clinical judgments regarding the complexity and intensity of past treatment (Weiner et al., 1996). If individuals choose from among plans based in part on predictable medical expenses, then a risk adjustment scheme able to predict this spending may be able to address some potential distortion. Although research is ongoing, risk adjustment methodologies currently in place explain only 7% of general health care spending, and little attention has been paid to MH/SA (Newhouse et al., 1997). To date, two initial evaluations of risk adjusters for MH/SA have been completed. Ettner and Notman (1997) evaluated the predictive power of the ambulatory care group (ACG) classification system, a set of diagnostic clusters and age and sex groupings using data on approximately 30,000 Medicaid enrollees in New Hampshire for fiscal years 1993 and 1994. Evaluating the explanatory power of the classification systems for predicting total individual health care spending and individual MH/SA spending, the results revealed the following: First, none of the classification systems studied explained more than 4% of variance in total health spending. Second, in the MH/SA area, the maximum explanatory power was 13% of the variance. Third, in the analysis of MH/SA spending, the results suggest that including age and sex along with a set of variables indicating whether an individual had 1, 2, or 3+ separate MH/SA disorders from claims data during the previous year provided greater explanatory power than any other method. In a second analysis, Ettner et al. (1998) examined several commonly used risk adjusters within a larger data set of privately insured employees and their dependents (totaling approximately 450,000 enrollees) for 1992 and 1993. To study the predictive ability of each system for total MH/SA spending, the authors made use of actual health plan choices of employees to assess how well each classification system would account for naturally occurring selection into plans in the absence of risk adjustment. The 1992 patterns of illness were used to classify enrollees and to predict 1993 spending. As in the case of New Hampshire, no classification system displayed strong predictive ability, and the results from the analysis of naturally occurring selection across plans for two large employer groups contained in the data illuminated the weaknesses of all the classification systems. Thus, to date, the potential for the existing risk adjustment methodologies to minimize selection is unlikely to be met.

Some recent theoretical work has suggested that quality and access distortions associated with rationing in the shadow price framework may be alleviated with better risk adjustment schemes (Glazer and McGuire, 2002). Glazer and McGuire (2002) propose a method, called *minimum variance optimal risk adjustment* (MVORA), that may be used to calculate weights minimizing variance in plan-predictable health care costs not accounted for in current risk adjustment schemes. Conditions for optimal risk adjustment are derived from the means and covariences among risk adjuster variables and elements of health care spending. Then a statistical fit criterion is applied to select from among the weights satisfying conditions for efficient quality. Application of the methodology requires that the distribution of health care spending in a population be available at the level of service and in aggregate, including diagnosis, location of services, and type of provider (general or specialty), information typically available in most claims data. Some work needs to be done to classify health care encounters into services, but once this is completed, the scheme may be readily applied by regulators, public providers, or private insurers. Essentially, MVORA is a tool that may be used to align the private incentives of managed care providers to maximize profit with the social objectives of minimizing quality and use distortions due to selection pressure. Further research is needed to test MVORA empirically and assess its practical ability to mitigate selection incentives in actual datasets.

In order to reduce further the adverse consequences of market failures, direct regulation of managed care contracts and efforts to measure and pay on quality have been proposed. Direct regulation of contracts has been suggested in state legislatures and elsewhere. However, rationing within managed care is a complex, and poorly understood business. We believe that rationing involves hundreds of decision points within managed care organizations. This is likely to make direct regulation of these practices costly, complex, difficult to monitor, and probably subject to endless litigation. More important, given our meager understanding of rationing in managed care, it is not clear that the distortions created by incomplete regulation would improve or hinder the fair and efficient provision of MH/SA care. Second, quality measurement is in its infancy. Direct measurement of health plan performance is currently a subject of active research. Measuring the quality of specific services such as MH care lags behind the overall effort (IOM, 1997). Using these measures to consider relative rationing offers a still greater challenge. Development of quality indicators to regulate rationing remains a distant goal. Given the state of these measures, we are left to assess the impact of carve-outs and risk adjustment schemes in stemming the effects of moral hazard and adverse selection.

Empirical Evidence on Managed Behavioral Health Organizations

Literature about the effect of managed care practices on MH costs and use is relatively recent. The initial experiences reported by employers include some instances of large reductions in the costs of MH/SA care. Hodgkin (1992) reviewed the early literature on the effects of utilization management, finding very few studies offering evaluation methods that could produce convincing results. The lone study that we judge to be methodologically sound showed savings in the neighborhood of 10% to 15% on total claims costs. The CHAMPUS program experimented with an *at-risk* PPO for behavioral health services during the late 1980s in the Tidewater, Virginia, area, which is known to be a high-cost MH/SA region. The demonstration achieved significant savings, totaling approximately 31% below expected costs, stemming largely from reduced use of inpatient care. In spite of the reported savings, there were clearly areas of considerable waste in expenditures and difficulties in running the program effectively (Coulam and Smith, 1990). A number of private corporations also adopted specialty MBHC carve-out programs in the late 1980s. In studies assessing these corporations' experience, it is fairly common to see reports of reductions in claims costs of 40% to 50%.

The interpretation of these changes is quite difficult. Often more than one change is made; thus, attributing cause and effect is challenging. Within a plan, there can be considerable year-to-year variation for unknown reasons (Dickey and Azeni, 1992; McGuire, 1994). Finally, a version of the *file-drawer* problem in research may be at work; only "good" (i.e., publishable) experiences may see the light.

With these limitations in mind, we review the reports of the performance of managed behavioral carve-out arrangements in the private sector. Key aspects of these studies are summarized in Table 2.2. As the table indicates, each of these natural experiments has taken place in the context of different risk-sharing arrangements. The GIC contract shifted only a small amount of risk to the MBHC vendor, while the Pacific Bell contract involved no financial risk at all to the vendor. Table 2.2 reports impressive reductions in mental health spending relative to fee-for-service arrangements (the comparison condition for all the studies). The estimated reductions in spending range from -17% to -43%, smaller than those observed in prepaid groups but consistent with theory. The reductions, for the most part, took place in the context of programs that had historically experienced high levels of spending on MH services. While the observed savings across studies were

Table 2.2   Private Insurance Carve-Out Impacts

Study	Population	MBHO	Spending Type	Cost Impact
Goldman et al. (1998)	Nonelderly employees of Pacific Bell enrolled in HMO and FFS plans	UBH	Specialty inpatient, outpatient, IOP, residential MH/SA claims	-43%
Huskamp (1997)	Nonelderly FFS and PPO enrollees from among Massachusetts state government employees	OPTIONS	Outpatient check	-25% (year 1) -16% (year 2) (outpatient vs. prior spending
Ma and McGuire (1998)	Nonelderly FFS and PPO enrollees from among Massachusetts state government employees	OPTIONS	Inpatient, outpatient, IOP, residential MH/SA claims	-30% to -40%
Grazier et al. (1993)	Employees enrolled in PPO/POS	PNA	Outpatient claims for visits with an ICD-9 MH/SA diagnosis	-30% to -42%
Sturm et al. (1998)	Enrollees covered by State of Ohio health plans	UBH	Specialty inpatient, outpatient, IOP, residential MH/SA claims	Non-HMO -38% HMO 0%
Brisson et al. (1998)	Nonelderly enrollees in an HMO carve-out	PNA	All MH/SA claims defined by ICD-9 and procedures	-48%

FFS: fee-for-service plan; HMO: health maintenance organization; ICD-9: International Classification of Diseases, Version 9; IOP: intensive outpatient; MBHO: managed benefits health organization; MH/SA: mental health/substance abuse; PNA: ; POS: point-of-service organization; PPO: preferred provider organization; UBH: United behavioral health.

in many respects achieved by similar shifts in services utilization patterns, there are some important differences. Savings were realized primarily by (*1*) reductions in the use of inpatient hospital care (all studies), (*2*) reductions in nominal prices paid to providers (Goldman et al., 1998; Ma and McGuire, 1998), and (*3*) reduced duration of outpatient treatment (Goldman et al., 1998, Huskamp, 1997).

The studies in Table 2.2 reflect changes in rates of utilization of any MH and SA care for the insured populations. Important differences in the utilization patterns were observed across studies. In the Pacific Bell study, a significant increase (17%) in the percentage of enrollees using any behavioral health care was estimated. In contrast, the Massachusetts GIC experienced very large reductions (20% to 30%) in the percentage of the population using behavioral health care. It is interesting to note that some companies, such as Sterling-Winthrop, reported dramatic increases in access to care (50%) due to expanded use of outpatient care at the same time that claims cost were falling. Reductions in rates of use create concern because they may be indicative of reductions in access to care for individuals who may benefit substantially from treatment. The studies discussed also reflect heterogeneous populations and differences in other institutional features. For this reason, there are no clear explanations for why the percentage of the population using managed health care may vary so strongly.

Some have questioned whether carve-outs truly result in cost savings or if the dramatic reductions are actually attributable to new avenues for cost shifting. In particular, anecdotal evidence suggests that carve-out plans are especially prone to adopt pharmacotherapeutic strategies because the drug benefit represents an off-budget set of treatments. Brisson et al. (1998) found a higher propensity for individuals with a history of SA treatment to be hospitalized in a general medical setting following introduction of a carve-out plan (Dickey and Azeni, 1992). Greater therapeutic variation, discussed above, may feed organizational opportunities for cost shifting from more intensive (and expensive) therapy-based regimes to treatments based on drugs.

Selective behavior by MH users is currently an active area of research. In one study, Sturm et al. (1994) analyzed the treatment of depression across health plans as part of the RAND's Medical Outcomes Study. They observed more frequent health plan switching among depressed individuals. Those receiving care from MH providers were more likely to migrate from managed care to fee-for-service (FFS) plans. They also found that those switching were at risk for poorer outcomes.

Analysis of adverse selection is incomplete without the recognition that health plans are not innocent bystanders, but rather may design their product in order to produce favorable selection (Frank et al., 2000; Glazer and McGuire, 2000; Miller and Luft, 1997; Newhouse, 1996). That plans may tightly ration or distort the quality of services attracting high-cost enrollees, while loosely rationing services associated with favorable selection, is a primary implication of the shadow price framework discussed above. Empirical tests of this hypothesis have been applied to data from the Michigan Medicaid program and, more recently, to Medicare claims (Cao and McGuire, 2002; Frank et al., 2000). Analysis of Michigan Medicaid claims data suggests that services attracting primarily high-cost enrollees, *particularly MH/SA* enrollees, may be subject to tighter rationing than other services attracting relatively healthy enrollees such as those seeking maternity care (Frank et al., 2000). In the Medicare study, the authors find further support for the idea that HMOs ration the quality of different services in different directions (Cao and McGuire, 2002). Hospital services, especially treatment for mental illness, and some Part B services including psychiatry, appear to be more rationed than average within HMOs. Primary care, in contrast, appears to be less rationed. This is consistent with a HMO gatekeeper model in which freer access to primary care is used to manage patients and control access to more costly specialized services.

Evidence on the quality of MH care in managed care is limited. Generally, studies comparing FFS to capitated managed care plans have not revealed a uniform quality impact one way or the other (Miller and Luft, 1997). There is some consistent evidence that quality of care for the sickest and poorest patients suffers under managed care (Miller and Luft, 1997; Newhouse et al., 1993). Specifically for MH, two studies have found that quality may be adversely affected in HMO-style managed care (Lurie et al., 1992; Wells, 1996).

As we argued above, managed behavioral carve-outs may ameliorate quality distortions due to adverse selection. However, one controversial question is whether MH/SA care is delivered more effectively when integrated with medical care via a primary care physician. In theory, integrated care is better than fragmented care. In practice, a separate MH system has some advantages. Primary care physicians tend to overlook mental illness in their patients (Jencks, 1985; Morlock, 1989). When mental illnesses are recognized, primary care physicians often fail to provide appropriate treatment (Shapiro et al., 1987; Wells et al., 1996). Merrick (1997) studied the pattern of claims for persons hospitalized for major depression prior to and after the carve-out plan in the GIC plan noted above. Her findings pointed to more appropriate patterns of care under the carve-out plan. Readmission rates did not rise, and contact with outpatient providers following discharge improved.

In sum, although much work remains to be done on the magnitude of savings that can be expected in particular circumstances and on the connections between savings, contract features, and cost shifting, it seems clear that managed care can substantially reduce moral hazard in MH/SA care. Evidence suggests that managed care plans do ration MH services more tightly to select lower-risk enrollees. Based on limited evidence to date, managed behavioral carve-outs may ameliorate the resulting quality distortions.

States' Experience in Managing Mental Health Care

Throughout the 1990s, states increasingly delegated responsibility for the supply of MH services to low income individuals in need of treatment to private organizations in combination with general services or alone (for additional information on state mental health systems, see Chapter 4). As of 1999, all but one state Medicaid agency relied on some managed care arrangement for the care of beneficiaries (Donohue et al., 1999). Further, 36 states were operating or had received approval to implement Medicaid waiver programs for MBHC programs as of 1998 (The Lewin Group, 2000).

Dorwart and Epstein (1993) defined *privatization* as expanded reliance on markets and competition for the provision of MH services. Perhaps a broader definition of privatization is "the delegation of public duties to private organizations" (Donahue, 1998). Government or public responsibilities may include the production and financing of services and/or the management of a system. In the MH system, privatization has usually referred to changes in the production of services, meaning government purchasing of services for delivery by private organizations. The 1990s, however, saw privatization of a number of other duties traditionally performed by the public MH system, including privatization of financing and management. Privatization of financing occurs when private mechanisms, such as insurance, substitute for public funding of MH care. Finally, privatization of management occurs when public agencies delegate responsibility for the monitoring, oversight, and administration of the MH system to private organizations. Managed care organizations, including behavioral health care carve-out programs servicing state Medicaid programs, are examples of the privatization of the production, insurance protection, and management of mental health services (Callahan et al., 1995).

One basic motive behind privatization of the delivery of MH care is to reduce the budgetary claims of these services. When the delivery of services is privatized, the cost is often less than it would be if government continued to deliver the service in accordance with civil service and other regulations. These changes have also allowed states to slow the growth of MH-related state expenditures. Generally, Medicaid MH carve-outs studied in the literature have realized cost savings consistent with those in the private sector. Among the most prominent examples of studies of private managed care in public MH systems are studies from Colorado, Massachusetts, Utah, and Tennessee (Table 2.3). These studies have documented a range of experiences with respect to use and cost savings (Alegria et al., 2002;

Table 2.3   Public Insurance Carve-Out Impacts

Study	Population	MBHO	Spending Type	Cost Impact
Callahan et al. (1995)	Mass Medicaid	MHMA	Specialty inpatient, outpatient, residential MH/SA claims	−22%
Frank and McGuire (1997)	Mass Medicaid	MHMA	Specialty inpatient, outpatient, residential MH/SA claims	−26%
Norton et al. (1997)	Mass Medicaid	MHMA	Specialty inpatient, outpatient, residential MH/SA claims	−24%
Christianson et al. (1995)	Utah Medicaid	CMHCs	Specialty inpatient and outpatient claims	−17%
Stoner et al. (1997)	Utah Medicaid	CMHCs	Specialty inpatient and outpatient claims	−17%
Bloom et al. (1998)	Colorado Medicaid	CMHC/MBHO partnerships	Specialty inpatient and outpatient care, including state hospitals	−27%

CMHC: community mental health center; MBHO: managed benefits health organization; MHMA: mental health of Massachusetts.

Bloom et al., 1998; Chang et al., 1998; Donohue et al., 1999; Frank and McGuire, 1997; Manning et al., 1999; Stoner et al., 1997). In general, cost savings seem to be particularly concentrated in shifting the location of care from inpatient to outpatient treatment, consistent with the general trend in deinstitutionalization. Evidence on overall use suggests little change, although one study found that MBHC increased the use of specialty services for the nonpoor while maintaining the same level of use for the poor in the public sector (Alegria et al., 2001a). In terms of rationalizing use, there has been little empirical work investigating managed care's impact. One study (Alegria et al., 2001b) tested whether managed MH care had a differential impact by level of need. The authors found that managed care did not succeed in reallocating resources from the unlikely to the definite needers.

Privatization has also been motivated by the desire to improve the quality and coordination of care and to increase flexibility in the production and administration of the treatment system. New technology in the treatment of the severely mentally ill has both helped this transition and fed the desire for privatization. One often stated criticism of public mental health systems is their apparent resistance to innovation (Mechanic, 1987). Successful innovations in the treatment of mental illness may require novel ways of organizing and coordinating the various elements of care for individuals with severe mental disorders (Dill and Rochefort, 1989; Schwartz et al., 1982; Stein and Test, 1980; Taube et al., 1990). There is also some evidence that the shift may be motivated in part by the desire to answer widespread criticisms of access and quality in traditional state Medicaid programs. Further, there may be economy-of-scale gains in increased volume of services provided by a group of providers with expertise in providing services to low-income MH care users. To date, there has been little empirical work testing these effects, due in part to inherent difficulties in measurement.

Reliance on managed behavioral carve-outs in the public sector may also provide political advantages, such as the potential to increase the number of enrollees covered for MH/SA services; ensure that equivalent resources are used for MH/SA services as for general health; and enable a vendor to do something the state government may not want to do due to political pressures, such as excluding certain providers from the network (Frank et al., 1995, 1996b). Finally, as we saw above in discussing the private sector, carve-outs at the state level may counter selection incentives for general health provider contracting.

The effectiveness of state delegation to managed care providers in attaining these goals depends on how the arrangement is structured and to what extent potential detriments are managed. To date, there is wide variation in how managed care is organized to serve MH clients. Some potential disadvantages to delegation of MH provision in the public sector include increases in administrative costs that may be over and above those incurred in the private sector. Reduced coordination with other social services may be particularly severe in the care of low-income beneficiaries and those with severe mental illness in the public sector. Most worrisome, moral hazard on the provider side may be aggravated by the widespread adoption of managed care techniques. Theoretically, services for which the optimal quantity and quality of care are largely unobservable to patients and/or subject to large professional uncertainty in diagnosis and treatment, the possibility of stinting maybe greatest. Mental health and substance abuse care fits these conditions well. Further, persons for whom asymmetric information is more severe, such as the severely mentally ill, may be more vulnerable to egregious practices with little respite. Concerns regarding information asymmetries and their implications for quality of care, access, provider–patient relationships, and patient choice lie at the heart of the criticisms levied against Medicaid managed care for people with severe mental disorders. Given the potentially serious implications, there is remarkably little empirical evidence that this has been a problem in public arrangements. As in the private sector, better risk adjustment methods and quality measures may help reduce these concerns.

Implications for Mental Health Services

The 1990s experienced fundamental changes in the way MH care is rationed in the United States and in the institutions charged with rationing care. Managed competition became the dominant model for organizing and financing health care. Thus the reliance on competitive insurance markets in both the private and public sectors grew during the 1990s. The MBHC carve-out emerged as a key institution for managing MH/SA services. As we have shown, these new institutions were successful in dramatically altering patterns of MH care and, in some cases, reducing MH spending.

The rapid diffusion of new institutions into both private insurance and public mental health arenas has altered the policy landscape for MH care financing. The cost control successes of MBHC have provided policy makers and managers with a new and powerful tool. The enormous complexity and diversity of managed care arrangements have made rationing of MH care far less amenable to either public or private regulation. In private insurance, the ability to control the cost and utilization of MH/SA care using mechanisms other than benefit design features has offered policy makers new options for trading off cost control and the generosity of insurance coverage. The implication is that the additional costs of expanding insurance coverage for MH/SA that have long served as an impediment to enacting mandated benefit statutes or parity laws no longer create as difficult a dilemma for policy makers seeking to address the desire to expand insurance coverage for MH/SA care.

The main economic rationale for public policy makers to seek expanded MH/SA coverage is to attend to failures in competitive insurance markets. In the world of indemnity insurance, adverse selection created strong incentives for health insurance plans to design benefits that would protect them from a disproportionate number of high-cost people, such as MH/SA care users. Avoiding adverse selection of enrollees led insurers to compete in offering MH benefits that would not be attractive to people with MH care needs. This form of inefficiency caused a number of state governments to regulate insurance coverage for MH/SA care. These efforts took the form of mandated benefit statutes in the 1970s and 1980s (Frank, 1989; McGuire and Montgomery, 1982). More recently, state parity laws and federal parity initiatives have been the focus of regulation of MH/SA insurance coverage.

The new institutions of the MH sector weaken the cost argument against expansion of insurance coverage for MH/SA care. In addition, MBHC weakens the effectiveness of regulations aimed at promoting comparable rationing for MH/SA and other medical services within private health insurance. The arguments we have made above have a number of implications for the continuing debate over parity for MH/SA care in private insurance. First and most important, managed care, by changing the terms of rationing in health care, offers the potential to efficiently provide enrollees better financial protection against the risk of mental and addictive disorders. By shifting control of moral hazard from the demand to the supply side, MH/SA services do not require special cost sharing, limits, and deductible provisions, unlike traditional indemnity coverage. The case for parity under managed care is far stronger than it was in the indemnity insurance context. The ability of parity to accomplish its goals has also changed. As discussed above, health plans have the same, if not greater, incentives to discourage membership of persons with high health care costs that they had under indemnity insurance. Excessive rationing thus could be driven by a desire to avoid unattractive enrollees even in the presence of parity in benefit design. It is in this sense that parity laws are necessary but not sufficient to ensure that efficient levels of access and quality of MH care will result in competitive insurance markets (Frank et al., 1997).

The implication for efforts to improve access to quality MH care in private insurance is that policies in addition to parity or mandated benefits are required. Risk adjustment of health care premiums and quality-of-care regulation offer some promise. However, none of these mechanisms is sufficiently well developed to offer much improvement in the near term. Risk-sharing contracts and carve-out arrangements may be the best short-term approaches to address selection-related incentives. Both of these mechanisms may be unattractive to payers and health plans for other reasons (for additional discussion of parity, see Chapters 1, 3, 11, and 13).

In the public MH sector, the rise of Medicaid as the dominant payer for MH/SA care coupled with the adoption of managed care and MBHC carve-outs has privatized a great deal of the management of MH/SA services and moved the oversight of the new institutions away from the state mental health authority. In the case where competitive HMOs are the dominant model of Medicaid managed care, all the incentive problems associated with adverse selection arise. In those Medicaid programs, one might well expect MH/SA services to be especially tightly rationed as a means of competing to avoid enrollment of people with the costliest MH problems.

Many state Medicaid programs have adopted carve-out arrangements that tend to limit selection incentives. Privatizing management of the public MH system under Medicaid means that contract oversight and regulation lie with Medicaid agencies that frequently have only limited expertise in the MH/SA area. Thus, ensuring that there is sufficient accountability in MH service delivery and that contracts are written that align the public interest and carve-out financial interests may rely on segments of state government that are not well prepared for the task. There have been some recent failures in Medicaid MBHC arrangements that were due in part to such oversight failures (Chang et al., 1998). The implication is that delegation of care for low-income and disabled populations with relatively high levels of mental disorders requires care and attention to incentives and accountability mechanisms. Managed behavioral health care organizations have developed tools to improve the efficiency of the MH system, but they will not necessarily pursue the public interest without clear guidance. Understanding health plan rationing and what tools of policy affect that rationing is today's work in the cause of a fair and efficient MH care system.

REFERENCES

Alegria M, McGuire T, Vera M, et al. Changes in access to mental health care for the poor and the non-poor with managed care: results from the health care reform in Puerto Rico. *American Journal of Public Health*, 91(9):1431–1434, 2001a.

Alegria M, McGuire T, Vera M, et al. Does managed mental health care reallocate resources to those with greater need for services? *Journal of Behavioral Health Services and Research*, 28(4):439–455, 2001b.

Alegria M, McGuire T, Vera M, et al. The impact of managed care on the use of outpatient mental health and substance abuse services in Puerto Rico. *Inquiry*, 38(4):381–395, 2002.

Arrow KJ. Uncertainty and the welfare economics of medical care. *American Economic Review*, 53:941–969, 1963.

Baumgardner J. The interaction between forms of insurance contract and types of technical change in medical care. *RAND Journal of Health Economics*, 22(1):36–53, 1991.

Beinecke RH, Shepard DS, Goodman M, et al. Assessment of the Massachusetts managed behavioral health program: year three. *Administration and Policy in Mental Health*, 24(3):191–204, 1997.

Bloom JR, Hu T, Wallace N. Mental health costs and outcomes under alternative capitation systems in Colorado: early results. *Journal of Mental Health Policy and Economics*, 1:3–114, 1998.

Brisson AS, Frank RG, Norman ES, Gazmararian JA, et al. *A Case Study in the Impact of Managed Care on Utilization and Costs of Behavioral Health Care in an HMO.* NBER Working Paper #6242, 1997.

Buck JA, Umland B. Trends: covering mental health and substance abuse services. *Health Affairs*, 16(4):120–126, 1997.

Bureau of Labor Statistics. *Tabulations from Employee Benefits in Medium and Large Private Establishments*, Washington, DC: U.S. Government Printing Office, 2000.

Callahan JJ, Shepard DS, Beinecke RH, et al. Mental health/substance abuse treatment in managed care: the Massachusetts medicaid experience. *Health Affairs*, 14(3):173–184, 1995.

Cao Z, McGuire TG. *Service-Level Selection by Medicare HMOs.* Unpublished paper, 2002.

Chang CF, Kiser LJ., Bailey JE, et al. Tennessee's failed managed care program for mental health and substance abuse services. *Journal of American Medical Association*, 279(11):864–869, 1998.

Christianson JB, Manning W, Lurie N, Stoner TJ, Gray DZ, Popkin M, Marriott S. Utah's prepaid mental health plan: the first year. *Health Affairs*, 14(3):160–172, 1995.

Coulam G, Smith J. *Evaluation of the CPA-Norfolk Demonstration: Final Report, Department of Defense, Contract MDA 907-87-C-0003.* Cambridge, MA: Abt Associates, 1990.

Cuffel B, Goldman W, Schlesinger H. *The Effects of Increased Mental Health Benefits and a MBHC Carve-Out on General Medical Costs.* Unpublished paper, 1998.

Cutler D, Zeckhauser R. The anatomy of health insurance. In: Cuyler A, Newhouse J (eds). *Handbook of Health Economics*. Amsterdam: North Holland, pp. 563–644, 1998.

Deb P, Rubin J, Wilcox-Gok V, et al. Choice of health insurance by families of the mentally ill. *Health Economics*, 5(1):61–76, 1996.

Dickey B, Azeni H. Impact of managed care on mental health services. *Health Affairs*, 11(3):97–226, 1992.

Dill AP, Rochefort D. The challenge of coordination. In: Rochefort D (ed). *From Poor Houses to Homelessness*. Westport, Ct: Auburn House, pp. 133–148, 1993.

Donahue J. *The Privatization Decision: Public Ends, Private Means*. New York: Basic Books, 1998.

Donohue JM, Hanson KW, Huskamp HA. *Medicaid Managed Care and the Disabled*. A report prepared for the Robert Wood Johnson Foundation. 1999. Unpublished manuscript.

Dorwart RA, Epstein SS. *Privatization and Mental Health Care: A Fragile Balance*. Westport, CT: Auburn House, 1993.

Elkin I, Shea T, Watkins JT, et al. National Institute of Mental Health Treatment of Depression Collaborative Research Program: General effectiveness of treatments. *Archives of General Psychiatry*, 46:971–982, 1989.

Ellis RP. The effect of prior-year health expenditures on health coverage plan choice. In: Scheffler RM, Rossiter LF (eds). *Advances in Health Economics and Health Services Research*. Greenwich, CT: JAI Press, pp. 149–170, 1988.

Ellis RP. Creaming, skimping and dumping: provider competition on the intensive and extensive margins. *Journal of Health Economics*, 17(5):537–556, 1998.

Ettner SL, Frank RG, McGuire TG, et al. Risk adjustment of mental health and substance abuse payments. *Inquiry*, 35(2):223–239, 1998.

Ettner SL, Notman EH. How well do ambulatory care groups predict expenditures of mental health and substance abuse patients? *Journal of Administration and Policy in Mental Health*, 24(4):339–358, 1997.

Frank RG. Regulatory policy and information deficiencies in the market for mental health services. *Journal of Health Politics, Policy and Law*, 14(3):477–503, 1998.

Frank RG, Glazer J, McGuire TG. Measuring adverse selection in managed health care. *Journal of Health Economics*, 19:829–854, 2000.

Frank RG, Huskamp HA, McGuire TG, et al. Some economics of a mental health carve out. *Archives of General Psychiatry*, 53:933–957, 1996a.

Frank RG, Koyanagi C, McGuire TG. Political economy of "parity" for mental health in insurance. *Health Affairs*, 16(4):108–119, 1997.

Frank RG, McGuire TG. Savings from a Medicaid carve-out for mental health and substance abuse services in Massachusetts. *Psychiatric Services*, 48(9):1147–1152, 1997.

Frank RG, McGuire TG. The economic functions of carve-out in managed care. *The American Journal of Managed Care*, 4(SP):SP31–SP39, 1998a.

Frank RG, McGuire TG. Economics and mental health. In: Cuyler A, Newhouse J (eds). *Handbook of Health Economics*. Amsterdam: North Holland, pp. 893–954, 2000.

Frank RG, McGuire TG, Newhouse JP. Risk contracts in managed mental health care. *Health Affairs*, 14(3):50–64, 1995.

Frank RG, McGuire TG, Notman EH, et al. Developments in Medicaid behavioral health care. In: Manderscheid R, Sonnenschein MA (eds): *Mental Health U.S., 1996*. Washington, DC: U.S. Government Printing Office, pp. 138–153, 1996b.

Frank RG, McGuire TG, Regier DA, et al. Paying for mental health and substance abuse care. *Health Affairs*, 13(1):337–342, 1994.

Frank, RG. Regulatory responses to information deficiencies in the market for mental health services. In: Taube C, Mechanic D, Hohmann A (eds). *The Future of Mental Health Services Research*. Rockville, MD: USDHHS, NIMH, USGPO, 1989.

Glazer J, McGuire TG. Optimal risk adjustment of health insurance premiums: an application to managed care. *American Economics Review*, 90(4):1055–1071, 2000.

Glazer J, McGuire TG. Setting health plan premiums to ensure efficient quality in health care: minimum variance optimal risk adjustment. *Journal of Public Economics*, 84:153–173, 2002.

Glied S. Managed care. In: Cuyler A, Newhouse J (eds). *Handbook of Health Economics*. Amsterdam: North Holland, pp. 707–754, 2000.

Goldman HH, Skinner A. Specialty mental health services: research on specialization and differentiation. In: Taube C, Mechanic D, Hohmann A (eds). *The Future of Mental Health Services Research*. Washington, DC: U.S. Government Printing Office, pp. 23–38, 1989.

Goldman W, McCulloch J, Sturm R. Costs and use of mental health services before and after managed care. *Health Affairs*, 17(2):40–52, 1998.

Grazier KL, Scheffler RM, Bender-Kitz S, Chase P. The effect of managed mental health care on use of outpatient mental health services in an employed population. *Advances in Health Economics and Health Services Research*, 14:71–86, 1993.

Grob GN. Government and mental health policy: a structural analysis. *The Milbank Memorial Fund Quarterly*, 72(3):471–499, 1994.

Hodgkin D. The impact of private utilization management of psychiatric care: a review of the literature. *Journal of Mental Health Administration*, 19(2):143–157, 1992.

Horgan CM. The demand for ambulatory mental health services from specialty providers. *Health Services Research*, 21(2):291–320, 1986.

Huskamp HA. The Impact of a Managed Behavioral Health Care Carve-Out and Benefit Expansion on Outpatient Spending for Mental Health and Substance Abuse Services. Doctoral dissertation, Harvard University, 1997.

IMS Health. *Data Indices, 2001*. Available at: http://www.imshealth.com. Accessed July 2002.

Institute of Medicine. *Managing Managed Care: Quality Improvement in Behavioral Health*. Washington, DC: National Academy of Sciences Press, 1997.

Jencks SF. Recognition of mental distress and diagnosis of mental disorder in primary care. *Journal of American Medical Association*, 253(13):1903–1907, 1985.

Keeler EB, Carter GM, Newhouse JP. A model of the impact of reimbursement schemes on health plan choice. *Journal of Health Economics*, 17(3):297–320, 1998.

Keeler EB, Manning WG, Wells KB. The demand for episodes of mental health services. *Journal of Health Economics*, 7(2):369–392, 1988.

Knesper DJ. Substitution in production as the basis for research and policy relevant to mental health specialists. In: Taube C, Mechanic D, Hohmann A (eds). *The Future of Mental Health Services Research*. Washington, DC: U.S. Government Printing Office, pp. 63–80, 1989.

Kupfer DJ, Frank E, Perel JM, et al. Five year outcomes for maintenance therapies in recurrent depression. *Archives of General Psychiatry*, 49(10):769–773, 1992.

Lewin Group *Review of the Medicaid 1915(c) Home and Community Based Services Waiver Program Literature and Program Data*, 2000. Available at: http:www.quintiles.com Accessed July 2002.

Lurie N, Moscovice IS, Finch M, et al. Does capitation affect the health of the chronically mentally ill? Results from a randomized trial. *Journal of the American Medical Association*, 267(24):3300–3304, 1992.

Ma CA, McGuire TG. Costs and incentives in a behavioral health carve out. *Health Affairs*, 17(2):53–69, 1998.

Manning WG, Liu CF, Stoner TJ, et al. Outcomes for Medicaid beneficiaries with schizophrenia under a prepaid mental health carve-out. *Journal of Behavioral Health Services and Research*, 26(4):442–450, 1999.

Mark T, McKusick D, King E, Harwood H, Genuardi J. *National Expenditures for Mental Health, Alcohol and other Drug Abuse Treatment, 1996*. Rockville, MD: U.S. Department of Health and Human Services, Substance Abuse and Mental Health Services Administration, 1998.

McGuire TG. *Financing Psychotherapy: Costs Effects and Public Policy*. Cambridge, MA: Ballinger Publishing Company, 1981.

McGuire TG, Montgomery J. Mandated mental health benefits in private health insurance policies. *Journal of Health Politics, Policy and Law*, 7(2):380–406, 1982.

McGuire TG. Predicting the costs of mental health benefits. *Milbank Memorial Fund Quarterly: Health and Society*, 72(1):3–23, 1994.

McKusick D, Mark T, King E, et al. Spending for mental health and substance abuse treatment 1996. *Health Affairs*, 17(5):147–157, 1998.

Mechanic D. Correcting misperceptions in mental health policy: strategies for improved care of the seriously mentally ill. *Milbank Memorial Fund Quarterly*, 73:19–55, 1987.

Mechanic D, Schlesinger M, McAlpine D. Management of mental health and substance abuse services: state of the art and early results. *Milbank Memorial Fund Quarterly*, 73:19–55, 1995.

Merrick EL. Impact of a Behavioral Health Carve Out on Treatment of Major Depression. Doctoral dissertation, Barndeis University, 1997.

Miller RH, Luft HS. Does managed care lead to better or worse quality of care? *Health Affairs*, 16(5):7–25, 1997.

Morlock LL. Recognition and treatment of mental health problems in the general sector. In: Taube C, Mechanic D, Hohmann H (eds). *The Future of Mental Health Services Research*. Washington, DC: U.S. Government Printing Office, pp. 39–62, 1989.

Newhouse JP. Reimbursing health plans and health providers: selection versus efficiency in production. *Journal of Economic Literature*, 34(3):1236–1263, 1996.

Newhouse JP, Beeuwkes Buntin M, Chapman JD. Risk adjustment and Medicare: taking a closer look. *Health Affairs*, 16:26–43, 1997.

Newhouse JP, the Insurance Experiment Group (Archibald RW, Bailit HL, Brook RH, et al.). *Free for All? Lessons from the RAND Health Insurance Experiment*. Cambridge, MA: Harvard University Press, 1993.

Norton EC, RC Lindrooth, Dickey B. Cost shifting in a mental health carve out for the AFDC population. *Health Care Financing Review*, 18(3):95–108, 1997.

Oss M. *Managed Behavioral Health Market Share in the United States*. Gettysburg, PA: Open Minds, 1997.

Oss M. *Yearbook of Managed Behavioral Health and Employee Assistance Program Market Share in the United States 2000–2003*. Gettysburg, PA: Open Minds, 2002.

Pauly MV. The economics of moral hazard: comment. *American Economic Review*, 58:531–537, 1968.

Ramsey S, Pauly MV. Structure incentives and adoption of medical technologies in HMO and fee-for-service Health Insurance Plans. *Inquiry*, 34:228–236, 1997.

Reed K. *Coverage and Utilization of Care for Mental Health Conditions Under Health Insurance , Various Studies 1973–74*. Washington, DC: American Psychiatric Association, 1975.

Rothschild M, Stiglitz J. Equilibrium in competitive insurance markets: an essay in the economics of imperfect information. *Quarterly Journal of Economics*, 90:629–649, 1976.

Scheffler RM, Watts CA. Inpatient mental health use among the heavily insured. *Journal of Human Resources*, 21(3):338–358, 1986.

Shapiro S, German P, Skinner A, et al. An experiment to change detection and management of mental health morbidity in primary care. *Medical Care*, 25(4):327–339, 1987.

Stein LI, Test MA. Alternative to mental hospital treatment. *Archives of General Psychiatry*, 37:392–397, 1980.

Stoner TJ, Manning WG, Christianson J, et al. Expenditures for mental health services in the Utah prepaid mental health plan. *Health Care Financing Review*, 18(3):73–93, 1997.

Sturm R, McCulloch J, Goldman W. Mental health and substance abuse parity: a case study of Ohio's state employee program. *Journal of Mental Health Policy and Economics*, 1:129–134, 1998.

Sturm R, Meridith LS, Wells KB, et al. Provider Choice and Continuity for the Treatment of Depression. Santa Monica, CA: Rand Paper DRU-692-AHCPR, 1994.

Taube CA, Kessler LG, Burns BJ. Estimating the probability and level of ambulatory mental health services use. *Health Services Research*, 21(2):321–340, 1986.

Taube CA, Murlock L, Burns BJ, Santos AB. New directions in research on assertive community treatment." *Hospital and Community Psychiatry*, 41(6):642–647.

Triplett JE. What's different about health? Human repair and care repair in national accounts. In: Cutler DM, Berndt ER (eds). *Medical Care Output and Productivity*. Chicago: University of Chicago Press, 1998.

Umland B. Behavioral healthcare benefit strategies of self-insured employers. *Behavioral Healthcare Tomorrow*, 4(6):65–70, 1995.

U.S. Department of Health and Human Services. *Mental Health: A Report of the Surgeon General*. Rockville, MD: National Institute of Mental Health, 1999.

Watts CA, Scheffler RM, Jewell NP. Demand for outpatient mental health services in a heavily insured population: the case of the Blue Cross and Blue Shield Association's Federal Employees Health Benefits Program. *Health Services Research*, 21(2):267–290, 1986.

Weiner JP, Dobson A, Maxwell SL, et al. Risk-adjusted capitation rates using ambulatory and inpatient diagnoses. *Health Care Financing Review*, 17(3):77–99, 1996.

Wells KB, Sturm R, Sherbourne CD, et al. *Caring for Depression*. Cambridge, MA: Harvard University Press, 1996.

3

Mental Disability Law, Policy, and Service Delivery

JOHN PETRILA
BRUCE LUBOTSKY LEVIN

As a discrete body of law, mental health law has focused on the conflict between individual autonomy and government intervention designed to provide treatment or protection from risk. This traditional focus is not surprising. Mental health law first emerged in the mid-1960s, when most people with serious mental illnesses were confined to large, often grossly inadequate state psychiatric hospitals. Adopting tactics and arguments first used in the African-American civil rights movement, lawyers argued that mental illness alone should not deprive an individual of his or her civil rights. Federal judges assumed control over state hospitals and ruled that state civil commitment statutes violated constitutional rights to liberty and due process, and in a number of states administrators of public mental health systems engaged in friendly litigation designed to bring more state resources into underfunded public mental health systems. The federal courts were the dominant force in the first two decades of mental health law, and the roles of the legislative and executive branches of government were often secondary.

While the focus on rights remains resilient in policy discussions, particularly in long-standing debates on the use of involuntary civil commitment, mental health law today has a much more expansive reach. For example, the law plays an important and often complex role in the organization, financing, and delivery of mental health services. Examples include legislation such as the Community Mental Health Centers Act and the Americans with Disabilities Act, administration and oversight of Social Security and Medicaid statutes and regulations, and legal issues that have emerged from managed care and health care reform.

This chapter describes the various ways in which the law (not simply the courts) has influenced and even defined mental health services and policy since the mid-1960s. The use of law by policy makers and courts has changed significantly in that time, reflecting changes in judicial philosophy, political ideology, and economic conditions. The role of public mental health systems has also been an important variable in the evolution of mental health law. Legal issues that were dominant when states were primary service providers have receded in importance as the locus of care for most individuals diagnosed with a mental disorder has shifted from state hospitals to the community (Petrila, 1992). The U.S. Constitution is less important in this era than statutory and contractual provisions dealing with access to care.

The chapter has four main sections. The first deals with traditional mental health law, with its emphasis on judicial application of constitutional principles to the lives of people with mental illnesses. It discusses litigation resulting in changes in the relationship between the government and people with mental illnesses, primarily in the areas of civil commitment and the right to refuse psychiatric medications, as well as representative cases in which courts addressed the responsibility of state government as a care provider. The second section covers legislative efforts, both federal and state, to influence mental health policy. The third section addresses legal regulation of the patient–therapist relationship. It focuses on judicial definition of practitioner responsibility through tort litigation and briefly discusses the important issue of confidentiality. The concluding section examines three issues where law and policy continue to be closely intertwined: the antidiscrimination statutes, managed care, and the criminalization of mental illness. The chapter ends with a brief discussion of the implications of mental health law for the organization and delivery of services to people with mental illnesses.

The Constitutional Era of Mental Health Law

In 1960 Morton Birnbaum, a physician and attorney, proposed that individuals confined involuntarily to state psychiatric hospitals had a federal constitutional right to treatment (Birnbaum, 1960). This idea created a conceptual framework for what may fairly be described as the revolution in mental health law that occurred from 1965 to 1982.

Before the 1960s, "mental health" law was confined to a handful of cases alleging negligence in the provision of care or in releasing a patient prematurely, resulting in the patient's death, usually by suicide. Administrators of state psychiatric hospitals, where most care was provided for people with serious mental illnesses, had broad discretion over their facilities, and there was no legal basis for litigation against a state mental health system. In addition, involuntary civil commitment was largely unregulated. Involuntary civil commitment is one of the few areas (other than criminal law) where the state may deprive a person of his or her liberty. In 1960 most state civil commitment laws permitted commitment for an indefinite period on the certification of a physician (who often did not have to be a psychiatrist) that the person had a mental illness (Melton et al., 1997).

Change came, beginning in the 1960s. The catalyst was the civil rights movement and in particular the decision by the U.S. Supreme Court in *Brown v. Board of Education* (1954), in which the Court ruled that "separate but equal" segregated schools violated the U.S. Constitution. As a result of this decision and those that followed, the federal courts became the preferred forum for claims by individuals and groups that government had denied them rights. As the African-American civil rights movement strengthened, other rights movements—for prisoners, for women, and for people with serious mental illnesses—gained momentum.

Litigation seeking changes in the manner in which government treated individuals with mental illnesses grew dramatically from the mid-1960s. This litigation sought to (1) make civil commitment more difficult by tightening substantive and procedural standards; (2) provide increased autonomy to people with mental disabilities, focusing principally on the issue of psychiatric medications; and (3) improve conditions in state hospitals and facilities for people with mental retardation and developmental disabilities.

Civil Commitment

In 1955 the number of individuals with psychiatric conditions confined in state and county mental hospitals in the United States peaked at 558,922. By the mid-1960s that number was in sharp decline. However, involuntary civil commitment continued to be used widely, and the decline in the state hospital population was accompanied by an increase in the number of people hospitalized elsewhere, for example in psychiatric units of community hospitals and nursing homes (Kiesler and Sibulkin, 1987).

The Fourteenth Amendment to the U.S. Constitution prohibits the deprivation of an individual's liberty without "due process" of law. Until the mid-1960s, most state civil commitment laws defined commitment as a *medical* rather than a *legal* decision. In challenging civil commitment laws on the ground that they violated the Constitution, patient advocates first had to persuade the court that a constitutional value (here, liberty) was at stake. In accomplishing this task, litigants used three core arguments. First, drawing on the work of Thomas Szasz, a psychiatrist (1961, 1963, 1965), plaintiffs attacked the validity of psychiatric diagnosis, arguing that at best diagnosis was inherently flawed and that at worst it was a political tool used to label and confine those considered undesirable by society. Second, plaintiffs focused on the stigma and loss of rights associated with mental illness; not atypically, an individual committed to a state hospital lost most or all of his or her civil rights as a result. Third, plaintiffs persuaded judges to examine the conditions in the state hospitals to which people were committed. These conditions were often horrific. For example, the West Virginia Supreme Court, ruling that its state commitment statute was unconstitutional, described conditions in the state psychiatric facility as "Dickensian squalor" (*State ex rel. Hawks v. Lazaro*, 1974, p. 120).

These arguments prevailed and nearly every state, either at the direction of a federal court or to avoid litigation, changed its commitment law. As a result, state civil commitment procedures became more legalistic and typically shared a number of characteristics. First, civil commitment had to be based on the finding that the person had a mental illness and as a result posed a danger to self or others. The definition of danger varied among the states, but because commitment deprives constitutionally protected liberty, something more than a diagnosis of mental illness is necessary.

Second, all states require that a judge decide if someone is to be subject to long-term commitment. Although nearly all states permit emergency and short-term commitments (between 2 and 15 days, depending on the state) without a judicial order, a court hearing must precede commitment for longer periods of time. Third, the civil commitment *process* is more legalistic than it was under more medically oriented statutes. State laws not only require a judicial decision maker but also grant an individual a right to call witnesses, a right to trial by jury, and other rights associated previously with criminal proceedings. There are still differences between civil commitment hearings and a formal criminal trial: the U.S. Supreme Court, for example, has ruled that whether a person meets civil commitment standards need be proved only by "clear and convincing evidence" rather than the more demanding "beyond a reasonable doubt" standard used in criminal trials (*Addington v. Texas*, 1979). However, in general, the civil commitment process today is more legalistic than it was before challenges to state civil commitment laws.

It is worth noting that involuntary commitment laws for children were exempt from the legalization of commitment laws, at least in constitutional terms. The U.S. Supreme Court, in *Parham v. J.R.* (1979), ruled that children may be admitted to a state hospital without a judicial hearing on the application of their parents, a guardian, or the state acting as guardian. While this ruling was widely criticized (Perlin, 1981), it created a legal framework for states to adopt much looser commitment standards for children and adolescents. It is possible that these less strict standards may have been a contributing factor in the widespread inappropriate use of hospitalization of many children during the 1980s (Weithorn, 1988).

Since the early 1990s, many states have sought to liberalize commitment standards in two primary ways. First, many states have expanded the "dangerousness" criterion to permit the commitment of individuals who are "gravely disabled" (i.e., unable as a result of mental illness to provide basic needs such as food, shelter, or medical care) (Ridgely et al., 2001). Other states have adopted standards permitting commitment of an individual who, because of mental illness, may deteriorate to the point where he or she meets more traditional inpatient commitment standards; this standard moves civil commitment toward a more medical model.

Second, nearly 40 states have adopted some form of outpatient commitment, by which a court orders an individual to obtain treatment in an outpatient setting (Torrey and Zdanowicz, 2001). States typically use one of three approaches to outpatient commitment (Petrila et al., 2003). First, in some states, conditional release statutes permit a hospital at the point of discharge to impose conditions for treatment in the community. Second, some states provide that a court may order treatment in the community for an individual who otherwise meets inpatient commitment standards. Finally, a number of states have enacted statutes that establish substantive standards for outpatient commitment that differ from those for inpatient commitment. For example, outpatient commitment might be available for an individual who requires mental health care to avoid deterioration of his or her condition when the same state might permit inpatient commitment only if the person is a current danger to self or others.

Some studies of outpatient commitment suffered from a variety of methodological flaws that weakened their reliability (Ridgely et al., 2001). However, another study examining the implementation of the North Carolina outpatient commitment statute found that long-term (over 6 months) outpatient commitment combined with regular treatment reduced hospitalizations and arrests for people diagnosed with major psychoses (Swartz et al., 2001). While a methodologically similar study in New York City did not yield similar results (Steadman et al., 2001), the results in North Carolina have suggested to advocates of outpatient commitment that combining a judicial order with treatment may produce favorable outcomes for at least some individuals.

It is likely that in the future of both of these developments (more medically oriented criteria, outpatient commitment) will continue. At the same time, the principle that commitment deprives persons of constitutionally protected liberty has deep roots. Therefore, it seems unlikely that, at least in the near future, we will see a return to statutes that are completely medically oriented (e.g., a statute that permits commitment solely on the ground of mental illness, with no behavioral component) or that rely on medical rather than judicial decision making for long-term commitment. It is also to be hoped that research into the implementation of new statutes such as that conducted in North Carolina and New York City will be replicated. This will help ensure that civil commitment is understood not as an ideological struggle between individual liberty and governmental authority but rather as one of a number of tools intended to ensure access to services and to protect the individual and the public from harm.

Right to Refuse Treatment and Informed Consent

It is axiomatic that absent an emergency, an adult must give informed consent to proposed treatment before treatment can occur. The New York Court of Appeals articulated this principle in 1914:

> Every human being of adult years and sound mind has a right to determine what shall be done with his [or her] own body; and a surgeon who performs an operation without his patient's consent commits an assault for which he [or she] may be liable in damages.
> (*Schloendorff v. Society of New York Hospital*, p. 93)

When determining whether the person is of sound mind, the term *competency* or *capacity* often is used: the person lacking capacity is incompetent and therefore is unable to make decisions regarding his or her treatment. As a result, such decisions must be made by a surrogate. Although there is no single definition of competency (Berg et al., 2001), the general notion is that the individual must have the cognitive functioning as well as intellectual maturity to understand and act on information regarding the risks and benefits of proposed treatment, of alternative treatments, and of no treatment.

Although the principle that a competent individual reserves the right to make treatment decisions is long-standing, it came comparatively late to psychiatry. This delay, at least in part, may have been attributable to legal rules that assumed that an individual involuntarily committed for treatment was incompetent; stigma and societal assumptions regarding the impact of mental illness on functioning also undoubtedly played a role.

One consequence of the challenge to the legal principles governing the lives of people with mental illnesses was to separate the notion of competency to make decisions from the issue of civil commitment. Competency had to be judged separately; it could no longer be assumed that the existence of mental illness, or the fact that a person was admitted to treatment, necessarily resulted in a loss of legal competency. As a practical matter, this meant that even those admitted involuntarily to treatment retained the legal right to make decisions regarding other aspects of their treatment.

In addition, because of the state's role as custodian and treatment provider, the constitutional right to liberty was implicated by a decision to medicate someone forcibly, just as it was in a decision to commit an individual civilly. Plaintiffs argued, and the courts in general agreed, that the potentially harmful side effects of psychiatric medication warranted regulation of its use and justified a finding that medication could not be forced absent external review, either by a court or in some cases by administrative panels. For example, the New York Court of Appeals, ruling that medication could be forced only in limited circumstances after judicial review, acknowledged that medications had some positive effects but that "numerous side effects are associated with their usage, including extrapyramidal symptoms, akathesia, Parkisonisms, dystonic reactions, akinesia and dyskinesia. The most potentially devastating side effect is tardive dyskinesia" (*Rivers v. Katz*, 1986, p. 76).

Virtually all states now recognize that psychiatric patients who are competent may refuse treatment, including medications. An exception is that treatment may be given against the individual's will if either the patient or another person is in immediate danger. It is interesting to note that because the right to refuse treatment developed as a constitutional right, it developed on a path parallel to the manner in which state law ordinarily addresses informed consent. For example, a state's public health law will invariably note that consent must be obtained before treatment can be administered and then establish a number of mechanisms (guardianship, health surrogates, health proxies) for obtaining consent if the individual is incompetent. However, the debate in mental disability law had more to do with whether consent must be given by judicial or administrative review; therefore, the mechanisms for obtaining surrogate consent in general health care have come late to mental health, at least for those patients still treated in state custody.

New information has also developed suggesting that were the issue argued today, courts might be less willing to embrace a constitutional right to refuse treatment. Newer medications have fewer side effects (see Chapter 17), and to the degree that the very unpleasant and often dangerous side effects of early medications influenced judicial thinking, this issue has receded in importance. At the same time, however, new information supports the notion that people with serious mental illnesses in general are competent most of the time (Grisso and Appelbaum, 1998). These developments suggest that were the issue of treatment refusals being litigated today for the first time, it could be handled comfortably within the framework established by state public health laws rather than being addressed primarily as a matter of constitutional law.

Right to Treatment

As noted earlier, Morton Birnbaum first proposed a right to treatment in 1960.
The federal court of appeals for the District of Columbia in 1965 became the first
court to rule that such a right existed, finding that prisoners in the District had a
statutory right to treatment (*Rouse v. Cameron*, 1966). The first recognition of a
constitutional right to treatment came in *Donaldson v. O'Connor* (1974). A federal
court of appeals, considering the case of a person confined to a psychiatric hospital for years with no treatment, ruled that

> a person involuntarily civilly committed to a state mental hospital has a constitutional
> right to receive such individual treatment as will give him [or her] a reasonable oppor-
> tunity to be cured or to improve his [or her] mental condition.
>
> (p. 520)

The court believed that the state owed people it hospitalized "rehabilitative treatment, or, where rehabilitation is impossible, minimally adequate habilitation and
care, beyond the subsistence level custodial care that would be provided in a pen-
itentiary" (p. 522).

Other courts, appalled at the conditions of many publicly operated state institutions, ordered states to improve conditions and in many instances assumed operational control of state psychiatric (and developmental disabilities) facilities. In
such cases, courts issued orders governing every area of the facility's operation,
from the number and types of staff to the temperature of the water in the show-
ers. The first and in many ways prototypical example was the case of *Wyatt v.
Stickney* (1972), in which a federal judge ordered sweeping changes in Alabama's
psychiatric facilities.

Through the 1970s, federal courts routinely ruled against states in these cases,
and there were also many cases in which states voluntarily entered consent decrees
(an agreement between the parties approved by the court that resolved the case by
committing the defendant to a certain course of action). However, the U.S.
Supreme Court was more wary of the exercise of federal judicial authority in this
arena. In 1982 the Court brought an effective end to the constitutional era of mental health law with its decision in *Youngberg v. Romeo* (1982). In *Youngberg*, which
involved a claim by an individual who had been injured repeatedly while a resident of a Pennsylvania institution for people with developmental disabilities, the
Court ruled that institutionalized persons had a right to safety and to freedom from
unreasonable restraint. The Court went on to say, however, that even this comparatively limited right would be reviewed by the courts against a standard that
presumed the correctness of the judgment of treatment and administrative officials employed by the state: "in determining whether the State has met its obligations in these respects, decisions made by the appropriate professional are entitled
to a presumption of correctness" (p. 324).

The Court's decision in *Youngberg* and its subsequent application have been cri-
tiqued as an unwarranted grant of authority to state officials (Stefan, 1992). As a
practical matter, the decision ended the era of right-to-treatment litigation, at least
as the era was defined by large lawsuits brought against massive state institutions.
While some commentators believe such litigation has at least limited utility in ju-

venile (Dale, 1998) and sexual offender treatment settings (Depugh, 1998; Weeks, 1998), other factors have combined with the retreat of the federal courts to make such litigation less of a factor today than it was previously. First, because of uncertain economic conditions, few state administrators can afford to agree to expansive court orders. Second, many states no longer wish to turn over operational control of institutions to the federal courts; as the monitoring of court decrees stretched out over decades in some cases, states began to look for ways to reassert operational control. Third, and perhaps most significantly, the size of state institutions has been reduced dramatically; most people with serious mental disorders never enter a state hospital.

Therefore, a legal theory that is driven by the fact that the state was the primary care provider for most people with mental illnesses affects far fewer people today than it did in the early 1970s. Rather, the core issue for many people today is obtaining access to community services, an issue that right-to-treatment litigation based on constitutional principles does not reach.

In 1999, the U.S. Supreme Court issued a ruling that some thought might provide a theory that would support right-to-treatment litigation for access to community services. In this case, *Olmstead v. L.C.* (1999), the Court held that inappropriate institutionalization could violate the Americans with Disabilities Act (ADA). The ADA (discussed in more detail below) bars discrimination based on disability. In *Olmstead*, two individuals had been held in a Georgia psychiatric hospital far beyond the time in which their treatment staff considered them ready for community care. They continued to be hospitalized because of a shortage of space in the community programs. The Supreme Court ruled that "unjustified isolation . . . is properly regarded as discrimination based on disability" (p. 597). The Court based its ruling on two factors. First, it stated that institutionalization "perpetuates unwarranted assumptions that persons so isolated are incapable or unworthy of participating in community life" (p. 600). Second, institutionalization "severely diminishes" the ability to engage in a variety of everyday activities, including family relations, social contacts, and work (p. 601).

However, *Olmstead* did not create an unqualified right to be placed in a less restrictive setting. The state in its defense to a challenge to confinement could rely on the judgment of its own professionals; only if the state's treatment staff believed that the person could be treated more appropriately elsewhere would the ADA be implicated. In addition, a patient who did not wish to be placed in the community could not be placed against his or her will. Finally, the state had to be given the opportunity to demonstrate whether providing relief to the plaintiffs in a particular case would inequitably strip resources from others in the state's care. In the Court's view, the state could prevail in a lawsuit if it "were to demonstrate that it had a comprehensive, effectively working plan for placing qualified persons with mental disabilities in less restrictive settings, and a waiting list that moved at a reasonable pace not controlled by the state's endeavors to keep its institutions fully populated" (pp. 605–606).

The practical impact of *Olmstead* is open to question. While the opinion constitutes the Court's most ringing endorsement of the importance of community-based care, some commentators believe that the Court has limited the reach of its own opinion by its insistence on deference to the judgment of state professionals (Bauman, 2000). As noted above, the Supreme Court's articulation of the principle of deference to professional judgment effectively brought to a close the constitutional era of litigation. In addition, the federal courts, led by the Supreme Court, have grown even more cautious regarding the application of federal judicial power and have dramatically circumscribed the authority of Congress to extend civil rights protections to the states (Hart, 2001). Given these constraints and the self-imposed limitations within the *Olmstead* opinion, it seems likely that *Olmstead* will have a limited impact as a legal tool.

Federal and State Legislative Initiatives

Mental health law traditionally has been discussed and studied as judge-made law. However, statutory and regulatory laws, both federal and state, also play a key role in defining mental health policy and establishing a framework for the organization, financing, and creation of priorities for various services. This section focuses principally on congressional efforts over the years to influence mental health policy and also briefly describes areas in which state legislatures play an important role in the development of mental health policy.

Congressional Influence on Mental Health Law

Congressional efforts to shape mental health policy span nearly five decades, beginning in 1955. During that period, there has been no consistent or comprehensive federal policy. Rather, policy shifts, often dramatic, have occurred as new presidents assumed office and as philosophies changed regarding the roles of state and federal government. The one consistent element has been a failure to address mental health policy within a public health framework. This situation has begun to change since the mid-1990s, with the debates over national health care reform and parity for mental health coverage in insurance plans and the issuance of the first Surgeon General's report on mental health (U.S. Department of Health and Human Services, 1999). Although the debate regarding the appropriateness of considering mental health services within a larger public health framework is not new (contrast Kiesler, 1992, with Institute of Medicine, 1988), the fact that mental health and public health have until recently been considered separately has had important consequences.

Congress has enacted legislation affecting mental health policy in six core areas: (*1*) creation of a federal presence to influence mental health policy and research; (*2*) efforts to create and expand service capacity; (*3*) financing of mental health services; (*4*) creation of a set of principles to govern state planning of mental health services; (*5*) legislation to create insurance coverage parity between mental and somatic illnesses; and (*6*) antidiscrimination legislation. This section considers the first five areas, with antidiscrimination legislation considered separately below.

Creation of a Federal Presence

The National Institute of Mental Health (NIMH) has been the agency most closely associated with articulating and implementing federal mental health initiatives, policies, and research in the United States. Nevertheless, significant organizational changes within NIMH over the years have contributed to the lack of integration of somatic health and mental health research, training, and services delivery.

Congress created the NIMH in 1955 with the Mental Health Study Act (U.S. Congress, 1955). As it is the mental health component of the National Institutes of Health (NIH), Congress directed the NIMH to report annually on research into the treatment of mental illness and to educate the public on mental health issues.

The emphasis on community mental health initiatives during the 1960s was one catalyst in the 1967 decision to separate NIMH from NIH in an effort to focus on the broader issues of services research as well as continued emphasis on funding research into the treatment of mental disorders. In July 1992, however, Congress moved the research components of NIMH back under the umbrella of NIH and created a new agency to conduct services research, the Substance Abuse and Mental Health Services Administration (SAMHSA). This agency, in the first decade of its existence, incorporated treatment and prevention services and administered the federal block grant program to the states. However, SAMHSA appears to be moving away from funding research as part of its core mission, leaving research initiatives to NIMH.

Creation of Service Capacity

The federal government, through the Department of Veteran's Affairs, the American Indian Health Service, and the armed services health care system, is a significant provider of health and mental health services. However the bulk of federal efforts to create service capacity have been through legislation designed to create services operated by others.

The most ambitious U.S. mental health legislation in the area of service development was the Community Mental Health Centers (CMHC) Act, enacted in 1963 with numerous subsequent amendments (U.S. Congress, 1963, 1965a, 1967, 1968, 1970a, 1970b, 1973, 1975, 1978). The intent of the act was to stimulate, through federal financing, the creation of a network of community mental health centers. These centers would then be obligated to provide core services that would create the systems delivery structure necessary to shift from state mental hospitals as the primary service provider for people with serious mental illnesses. The goal of the act was to reduce the state psychiatric hospital census by 50% over 20 years (*Message from the President of the United States Relative to Mental Illness and Mental Retardation*, 1963). This act and its implementation have been discussed extensively (Barton and Sanborn, 1975; Bloom, 1984; Grob, 1991; Naierman et al., 1978).

This legislation had the practical effect of creating separate services delivery systems for mental illnesses, with virtually no integration of mental health services with other existing mental health delivery systems (e.g., U.S. military or veterans mental health services or existing state-operated or -funded services) or somatic health care delivery systems (e.g., neighborhood community health centers). Furthermore, major health planning reforms legislatively mandated in 1966 and 1974 failed to integrate somatic and mental health service delivery systems, continuing the isolation of mental health services from somatic health care (U.S. Congress, 1966, 1974).

During the more than 40 years since enactment of the original CMHC legislation, Congress has not embarked on a similar effort to create a national mental health services delivery network, nor has it taken specific steps to integrate mental health systems within general health care systems (although the state of mental health and services delivery in the United States has recently been detailed in *Mental Health: A Report of the Surgeon General* (U.S. DHHS, 1999, and *Interim Report to the President*, 2002). It is not clear that Congress should make this effort, given that local circumstances often dictate the organization of community health care systems, and it is difficult to imagine creating integrated systems through national legislation. However, Congress could take steps (e.g., through financing mechanisms) that could create incentives to integrate; rather, its major legislative initiative in this area, the CMHC legislation, made integration less rather than more likely.

Financing Services

Chapter 2 covers the financing of mental health services. Here we briefly recount the legislation that has shaped financing at a general level.

Federal entitlement programs have been among the most important ways in which the federal government has shaped the treatment of mental disorders. For example, in 1960 Congress enacted the Medical Assistance for the Aged Act (U.S. Congress, 1960). This statute increased financial assistance for certain types of medical programs for the aged and was the first step toward creating a financial base for the care outside of state mental hospitals of elderly people with mental disorders.

In 1965 Congress amended the Social Security Act with the passage of Titles XVIII and XIX, establishing the Medicare and Medicaid programs (U.S. Congress, 1965b). Congress did not permit federal participation in financing psychiatric services in free-standing psychiatric hospitals on the ground that the states had historically been responsible for paying for long-term psychiatric hospitalization. However, federal reimbursement was made available for individuals aged 65, regardless of the location of treatment, and in 1972 Congress amended the Medicaid laws, permitting federal reimbursement for psychiatric services to individuals under the age of 22 whether those services were provided in a free-standing psychiatric hospital or in a psychiatric unit of a general hospital (U.S. Congress, 1972). Psychiatric services delivered to individuals aged 22 to 64 were reimbursed by the federal government only if delivered in a psychiatric unit of a general hospital. Free-standing psychiatric hospitals were considered *institutions for mental disease* (IMDs) and were generally ineligible for federal financial reimbursement. In recent years, there have been calls for the repeal of the IMD exclusion on the ground that it is anachronistic, given the many changes in financing and delivery of care through the 1990s (Geller, 2000).

Congress also affected the financing of mental health services in 1981 when it enacted changes in the distribution of money to be used for mental health and substance abuse services. Part of the 1981 Omnibus Reconciliation Act (U.S. Congress, 1981), this statute consolidated 57 existing federal aid programs and created nine block grants by which states obtained funding that could be used to create or supplement services. The block grant legislation was part of a broader federal agenda during the first term of the Reagan administration to give more authority to the states while divesting the federal government of the responsibility to shape a national mental health policy.

The Reagan legislation also repealed the Mental Health Systems Act, enacted by Congress at the request of President Jimmy Carter (U.S. Congress, 1980). This statute had provided for continuing funding of CMHCs, with financial support for these centers to provide services for a variety of underserved populations, including individuals with chronic mental disorders as well as children, adolescents, women, minorities, and elderly people with mental disorders. Despite its repeal shortly after enactment, Goldman and Koyanagi (1991) have argued that many of its provisions, in fact, have been implemented as federal policy through subsequent discrete legislative initiatives.

In 1983, Congress changed reimbursement in the Medicare program from cost-based, retroactive payment to a prospective payment system in which Diagnostic Related Groups (DRGs) were used as the basis for payment (U.S. Congress, 1983). Payment was to be made to hospitals based on a schedule of established lengths of stay for discrete diagnostic categories. However, mental health services were exempted from the general DRG system based on research that persuaded Congress that mental health treatment was too varied to be subject to the DRG system because of variations in practice and the unpredictable course of illness for people who might fall into the same diagnostic category (Scherl et al., 1988). Although the decision to exempt mental health services may have made sense empirically, it provides another example of the manner in which Congress has often differentiated between somatic health and mental health.

Congress has enacted other statutes affecting financing. For example, through the McKinney Act (U.S. Congress, 1987a), Congress made available considerable financial support for states to create housing for people who are homeless and mentally ill. Finally, it should be noted that that Social Security Act has played a significant role in financing mental health services. The act provides financial support for individuals who are unable to work because of mental or physical disability. Income generated by this act often provides a way for individuals to defray the cost of housing in particular. This form of financial assistance has been a source of controversy since the 1970s, when the federal government first engaged in a concerted effort to remove people from the Social Security rolls if they had qualified for assistance because of a mental disability. Advocacy groups challenged these practices as arbitrary and discriminatory, and ultimately the U.S. Supreme Court ruled that the Department of Health and Human Services (DHSS) had acted illegally in aggressively removing people with mental disabilities from eligibility (*Bowen v. City of New York*, 1986).

Planning Requirements

Congress has also used its control over financing to impose planning requirements on the states. These planning requirements may express a preference for certain types of services. For example, as part of the block grant legislation, Congress required states to use 20% of the alcohol and drug abuse portion of the block grant for prevention and early treatment programs (U.S. Congress, 1981). Legislation in 1984 and 1985 directed states to set aside 5% of the total mental health and substance abuse block grant for new or expanded alcohol and drug abuse services for women and to use 10% of mental health services allocations for new or expanded community mental health services for underserved populations, particularly children and adolescents with severe emotional disturbances (U.S. Congress, 1984, 1985).

In 1986, dissatisfied with state planning, Congress enacted the Comprehensive State Mental Health Planning Act (U.S. Congress, 1986), which established specific planning requirements for the states, including (*1*) creating objectives for providing mental health prevention and treatment services; (*2*) describing the resources needed to implement the plan; (*3*) providing case management services for each person with a severe mental illness; (*4*) establishing and implementing an outreach program of specialized services for people who are homeless and severely mentally ill; and (*5*) providing for the delivery of services in community mental health centers.

Parity Legislation

Advocacy organizations for people with mental illnesses have adopted as a major goal the enactment of legislation by Congress and the states that would provide parity, or equality, in insurance coverage of mental and physical illnesses. Historically, mental illnesses have received less coverage for a variety of reasons, including stigma and a belief in some quarters that mental illnesses were not real illnesses but rather reflected individual weaknesses or failings. There has also been concern regarding the potential cost of increasing coverage for mental illnesses. The parity issue is discussed in more detail in Chapter 1, and the financing of mental health care is discussed in more detail in Chapter 2. At this point, we provide a brief overview of congressional and state legislative efforts to ensure parity.

In 1996 Congress enacted the Mental Health Parity Act (U.S. Congress, 1996a). The act did not require full parity in coverage but did attempt to redress differences in aggregate lifetime and annual benefits available to plan enrollees. However, the act did not mandate that group health plans offer mental health benefits; alcohol and substance abuse benefits are not affected; and other terms and coverages of health plans, for example, cost sharing, limits on patient visits or days, and prior authorization processes are largely unaffected. Small companies (with 2 to 50 employees) are not covered, and plans that can show that compliance with the act increases plan costs 1% or more are exempt from coverage (Morrison, 2000). Efforts to enact full parity by Congress have been unsuccessful to date, and the death of Senator Paul Wellstone in the 2002 congressional campaigns may impede passage given his status as one of parity's primary advocates.

Currently, 33 states have enacted some type of parity legislation. However, because of federal legislation prohibiting states from certain types of regulation of insurance, states cannot legislate full parity for all citizens. On the other hand, the successful introduction of some type of parity legislation in numerous states clearly suggests that mental illnesses are viewed increasingly as illnesses similar to physical illnesses. While this trend may not foreshadow the end of stigma and discrimination, it does suggest that, incrementally, coverage for mental illnesses may continue to expand.

It appears from a number of studies conducted to date that parity does not increase costs appreciably (Sturm, 1997; Varmus, 1998). In addition, the manner in which parity works may differ in a managed care environment (but not in a manner that increases costs), a topic discussed in greater detail by Frank and McGuire (1998). Given the empirical evidence, arguments against parity based on cost appear unpersuasive (also see Chapters 1, 2, 11, and 13 in this volume).

State Legislative Initiatives

State law also has an obvious impact on mental health policy and services. State law plays a significant role in a number of areas, including (*1*) financing, (*2*) professional licensure laws, (*3*) certificate of need laws, and (*4*) the use of law to shape governance of the mental health system and to develop service capacity.

Financing

The most obvious way in which state law affects mental health systems is through the state budget, which is both a political and a legal document. When public mental health systems consisted largely of state–operated mental health facilities, the majority of revenues allocated to mental health went to the operation of state hospitals. However, the percentage of overall expenditures committed to state hospitals has declined, though in many instances, savings from hospital closures or downsizing were not reinvested in community mental health services. In addition, state expenditures on mental health as a percentage of overall expenditures on human services declined through the 1990s (see Chapter 4).

State laws and executive branch decisions also play an important role in determining expenditures under the Medicaid program. This has been true particularly since the early 1990s with the emergence of managed care as a central feature in many states (Hanson and Huskamp, 2001).

Professional Licensing Laws

States also have primary responsibility for creating and enforcing professional licensure standards. All states have statutorily created standards that individuals must meet before they are licensed to practice. Few quarrel with the need for such laws, but their enforcement has been a long-standing issue, primarily because of concerns that licensure boards are lax in pursuing practitioners who deviate from professional norms (Miller, 1997). Similar concerns have been raised about the efficacy of licensing standards for attorneys (Krause, 2000), and there have been calls for increased oversight of alternative medicine practitioners as well (Van Hemel, 2001).

In partial response, Congress in 1986 created a National Data Bank, requiring providers to report any action taken against the licensing or privileging status of health care professionals (Health Care Quality Improvement Act, 1986). In addition, employers must query the Data Bank for information regarding prospective employees before hiring them and regarding current employees on an annual basis.

Certificate of Need Laws

In 1974 the federal government required that states establish a "certificate of need" process (U.S. Congress, 1974). Enacted during an era in which it was assumed that government regulation was the most effective tool for containing inflation in health care costs, certificate of need laws required any provider wishing to establish a new service to demonstrate to the government that a need for that service existed. In 1986 the federal government repealed this requirement, though a number of states retain a certificate of need process. Such laws have been criticized on a number of grounds, including arguments that they were ineffective at controlling costs; imposed undue cost and administrative burdens on prospective service providers; were often influenced by political considerations; and favored existing providers, with the result that they were actually anticompetitive (Wolfson, 2001). In addition, it has been argued that certificate of need laws are irrelevant in an era of managed care (McGinley, 1995). Others argued that the laws were an important check on the development of services that were superfluous or met comparatively insignificant needs (or in some cases created an artificial need; Timmons, 1994). Today, debate continues, though the trend in the past two decades has been away from reliance on the certificate of need as a significant tool in addressing problems in the health care system.

Governance and Service Issues

In the past two decades, there has been a trend toward eliminating the state mental health agency as an independent agency and placing it in a larger umbrella agency (e.g., a state health department or state human services department). This trend may reflect the continuing decline of the state psychiatric hospital as a locus of care; many state mental health agencies initially were established to oversee large state hospital budgets. As the role of those hospitals changed and diminished, the necessity of maintaining an independent state mental health agency may have seemed less evident to governors and legislators. In addition, managed care, which focused on Medicaid in most states, shifted (at least informal) authority for planning and designing mental health systems away from the state mental health agency to the state agency responsible for Medicaid (Hogan, 2002). Finally, government organization goes through trends, from consolidation of authority in fewer locations in some eras to decentralizing it in other eras. During the past two decades, mental health has been an area subject (in many places) to consolidation.

Some states have also created statutory preferences for the allocation of public funds. For example, Ohio and other states enacted statutes giving priority to the needs of people with serious mental illnesses. The process by which services are planned and delivered may also be affected. Ohio vested authority in local boards to organize and plan services and allocated funds through these boards, which in turn purchased services.

It is likely that state mental health agencies will continue to struggle to define their role and status within state government. States are unlikely to expand their responsibilities as service providers, certainly not to earlier levels, and so the appropriate size and functions of the state mental health agency will continue to be debated. New skills, for example in contract negotiation and oversight, will be increasingly valuable, while those skills necessary to operate large systems may be much less valuable (Glover and Petrila, 1994).

Regulation of the Patient–Therapist Relationship

A third major area of mental health law is concerned with regulating the relationship between patient and therapist. This takes a variety of forms. Some have been alluded to earlier (i.e., informed consent requirements, licensure). This section focuses on two key issues: malpractice and confidentiality.

Purpose and Elements of Malpractice

While malpractice lawsuits against psychiatrists and other mental health professionals have increased over the years (as have malpractice lawsuits in general), mental health professionals face malpractice claims much less frequently than many of their colleagues. A review of malpractice claims received by a major insurer of psychiatrists found that the most frequent types of claims were as follows (Simon, 1998):

Suicide or attempted suicide (33% of all claims)

Incorrect diagnosis (11%)

Improper civil commitment (5%)

Breach of confidentiality (4%)

Unnecessary hospitalization (4%)

Undue familiarity (3%)

Libel/slander (2%)

Other (improper use of electroconvulsive therapy, abandonment of the therapeutic relationship, etc.) (4%).

While malpractice claims may be a comparatively rare event for most mental health professionals, it is useful to understand the elements that must be proved for a plaintiff to prevail. These include (1) the existence of a duty on the part of the professional to the person claiming harm; (2) a breach of that duty; and (3) damages (4) caused by the breach.

Duty

The general duty of a mental health professional is to practice in accordance with professionally accepted standards. Professionals do not owe a duty to every person with a mental health problem; rather, a duty is not established until a patient–therapist relationship is established. However, there are exceptions to this rule. For example, federal law requires that emergency room staff must evaluate anyone admitted to an emergency room even though a patient–therapist relationship has not been established (Stalker, 2001).

In specific cases, the duty may be articulated more precisely and new duties may be imposed as circumstances warrant. For example, historically, mental health professionals had no obligation to protect third parties if a patient presented a potential danger to the other person. Most clinicians assumed that confidentiality would prevent such disclosures. However, this situation changed as the result of *Tarasoff v. Regents of University of California* (1976), in which the California Supreme Court ruled that a therapist had a duty to protect identifiable third parties who might be potential victims of a patient. Although application of this principle varies from state to state (Truscott, 1993), the case illustrates both the changing nature of clinical duties and the interrelationship between such duties and other ethical and legal principles.

Breach of Duty

Once a duty is established, a plaintiff must demonstrate that the defendant has breached the duty. For example, if a plaintiff claims that he or she was released inappropriately from hospitalization and as a result attempted suicide, the plaintiff must show that staff was negligent in deciding to discharge the patient or that the arrangements for follow-up care were inadequate. Whether a duty has been breached may become a matter of debate between expert witnesses, with the jury (or judge where there is no jury) acting as the ultimate decision maker.

Causation

The plaintiff, having established breach of a duty by the defendant, must show that the breach caused damage. The disciplines of law and psychology tend to use different paradigms of causation. The law has a more linear view, attempting to isolate the event or decision that, more than other events or decisions, caused the negative outcome. In specific cases, this view has resulted in troubling outcomes. For example, in one case, a psychiatrist was held liable for an automobile accident caused by a person discharged from a hospital 6 months earlier. The discharge was viewed as the causative event (*Naidu v. Laird*, 1988). Cases like this (fortunately rare) appear simplistic to many mental health professionals. They also appear to make professionals the insurers of public safety for actions taken by former patients even if those actions are at a time far beyond the time of the patient–therapist relationship (Pettis and Gutheil, 1993).

Damages

Finally, the plaintiff must show that he or she has been damaged by the defendant's breach of duty. Some types of damage are comparatively easy to demonstrate, such as medical bills for care made necessary by the defendant's actions; losses from time away from work; and anticipated financial losses of income if the injury has caused a permanent disability. Other types of damage are more difficult to quantify but are often compensable nonetheless—for example, damages for pain and suffering and in some cases for emotional injury.

Although psychiatrists and other mental health professionals are sued comparatively less frequently than other medical professionals, malpractice can be an obvious concern. Some areas of practice may appear to be more vulnerable than others to litigation after the fact; an example is a lawsuit for negligent release in the event of a suicide. As a result, some commentators have attempted to establish risk management principles for mental health providers (see, e.g., Monahan, 1993; Poythress, 1990; Simon, 1998). Such material can provide invaluable assistance to administrators and clinicians struggling to incorporate clinically and legally sound practices. Second, there have been efforts to develop *practice standards* within some areas of medicine, including psychiatry. For example, the NIH has used *consensus panels* to develop standardized processes for certain types of medical procedures (National Guideline Clearinghouse, 2002). The American Psychiatric Association has used similar processes to develop practice standards in psychiatry (American Psychiatric Association, 2000).

In addition, some states have enacted legislation that attempts to ensure the creation of practice standards in a number of specialties. This legislation, if enacted as part of malpractice reform, permits a practitioner charged with malpractice to introduce as evidence of good practice adherence to a practice standard. At the same time, a failure to adhere to practice standards is generally inadmissible as evidence of malpractice. This creates incentives to follow practice standards without converting them into a cookbook that must be followed in all cases in order to avoid liability.

Confidentiality

Confidentiality is a core ethical and legal principle. As a general rule, communications between therapist and patient are confidential, including any records of treatment. Historically, confidentiality and limits to it were defined by state law. However, the federal government, pursuant to the Health Insurance Portability and Accountability Act of 1996 (HIPAA) (U.S. Congress, 1996a), has now established a minimum national standard for protecting the confidentiality of protected health information. The HIPAA is discussed in more detail below.

Confidentiality, as a principle, depends on three values: creating trust in the therapeutic relationship, reducing the impact of stigma, and protecting privacy. The U.S. Supreme Court has endorsed the idea that trust is critical to mental health treatment. In a decision creating a psychotherapist privilege (i.e., enabling a psychotherapist to decline to disclose confidential information in a legal proceeding), the Court wrote:

> Effective psychotherapy . . . depends upon an atmosphere of confidence and trust in which the patient is willing to make a frank and complete disclosure of facts, emotions, memories, and fears. Because of the sensitive nature of the problems for which individuals consult psychotherapists, disclosure of confidential communications made during counseling sessions may cause embarrassment or disgrace. For this reason, the mere possibility of disclosure may impede development of the confidential relationship necessary for successful treatment.
>
> (*Jaffee v. Redmond*, 1996)

Confidentiality also exists to reduce the possible effects of the stigma that might be associated with the treatment of individuals with mental disorders. While many of the legal rules that reinforced discrimination against people suffering from mental illnesses have been removed, public attitudes regarding mental illness continue to suggest wariness, antipathy, and fear in some cases (Link et al., 1999). Finally, confidentiality protects individual privacy; privacy is considered essential in enabling individuals to exercise autonomy in seeking health care.

Research supports the notion that the perception of privacy may affect an individual's decision to seek mental health care (Alpert, 1998; Howland, 1995; Kremer and Gesten, 1998; Norman and Rosvall, 1994). Yet, confidentiality is not an absolute value. Clinicians may breach confidentiality without client consent in a variety of circumstances: during an emergency; during the process of civil commitment; in states that require or permit disclosure to protect a third party (see the discussion of *Tarasoff* above); when conforming to child and elder abuse reporting requirements; or when discussing a case with supervisors or other clinicians involved in the patient's treatment. In addition, state law may permit other disclosures without consent, for example to researchers, public health officials, or payers of health care costs.

The federal government issued HIPAA regulations in final form in 2002 (45 CFR 160 and 164). These regulations were issued after much debate and after Congress failed to enact legislation creating a national standard. The regulations are complex and lengthy. They are designed to protect "identifiable health information" and to ensure the security and privacy of electronic recording and transmission of health information. Although a discussion of HIPAA is beyond the scope of this chapter, it is worth noting that it is designed to create minimum standards for protecting confidentiality; a state may impose stricter rules to govern confidentiality. For example, HIPAA permits a provider of health care to disclose to another provider of health care information regarding a patient without the patient's consent if the provider will be furnishing care to the patient. Many state laws require patients to consent to such disclosures. In that case, the state rule would apply because it is more protective of privacy. In addition, federal laws regarding the privacy of information that would or could identify a person as someone who has obtained alcohol or substance abuse treatment remain in place (42 USC 290dd; 42 CFR, Part II). The mental health professional or administrator must be cognizant of these rules as well.

As noted above, in addition to confidentiality, the law uses the concept of *privilege* to insulate from disclosure in legal proceedings communications made as part of the therapeutic relationship. The privilege belongs to the client, and accordingly, it is for the client to decide whether to waive it. At the same time, the therapist may assert the privilege on behalf of the patient. However, there are circumstances in which privilege does not apply and otherwise confidential information may be disclosed in a legal proceeding. Examples include situations where the person has undergone a court-ordered examination of his or her mental status, legal proceedings where the patient places his or her mental status at issue (e.g., in a malpractice claim against a therapist), civil commitment proceedings, and to some degree custody disputes where the fitness of a parent may be at issue (Weiner and Wettstein, 1993).

Additional Issues in Mental Health Law and Policy

Mental health law began in part as an effort to reduce the use of coercion as a tool to cause people to receive mental health services. In contrast, the major issue today is obtaining access to services, social supports, and entitlements. Antidiscrimination statutes, such as the ADA, attempt to eliminate the barrier of discrimination for people with mental illnesses. In addition, much of the debate regarding managed care has centered on whether people can obtain redress when access to care is denied. Finally, the emerging debate about the *criminalization* of mental illness represents in part an effort to design strategies that will provide access to care without first going through the criminal justice system. These issues are discussed below.

Antidiscrimination Statutes

Congress has enacted two important civil rights laws that bar discrimination on the basis of mental or physical disability. These statues are the Fair Housing Amendments Act (FHAA) of 1988 (U.S. Congress, 1988) and the Americans with Disabilities Act (ADA) (U.S. Congress, 1990). The FHAA bars discrimination in housing; the ADA bars discrimination in employment, public accommodations, telecommunications, and transportation.

The statutes bar disability broadly. The term *disability* includes (*1*) a physical or mental impairment that substantially limits one or more of the major life activities of an individual; (*2*) a record of having such an impairment; or (*3*) being regarded as having such an impairment. In enacting the ADA, Congress estimated that approximately 43 million Americans would meet the statutory definition of disability. In addition, the statutes incorporate the idea of *reasonable accommodation*. For example, an employer may violate the ADA by not offering a reasonable accommodation to an employee who, with the accommodation, would be able to meet the qualifications for a job.

The FHAA has been used to eliminate a number of restrictions in housing for people with mental disabilities. For example, courts have invalidated state and municipal requirements that public hearings be held before a permit is granted for the creation of such housing (*Potomac Group Home Corporation v. Montgomery County*, 1993). Other restrictions (e.g., the use of rules for construction that assume that people with a mental disability are inherently dangerous to themselves) have been ruled invalid as well (*Marbrunak, Inc. v. City of Stow*, 1992).

The ADA has become a source of a volume of litigation, particularly though not exclusively in the area of employment. For example, as noted above, the U.S. Supreme Court in its *Olmstead* decision ruled that inappropriate institutionalization could violate the ADA. The Supreme Court also ruled that the ADA applies to prisoners with mental disabilities (*Pennsylvania Department of Corrections v. Yeskey*, 1998) and that individuals with asymptomatic human immunodeficiency virus have a disability under the ADA because of the potential impact on the major life activity of reproduction (*Bragdon v. Abbott*, 1998).

While these holdings might suggest a general tendency on the part of the Supreme Court to look sympathetically on claims made under the ADA, more recent cases suggest a tendency on the part of the Court to narrow its applicability. These cases include rulings that whether a person is disabled must be considered *after* the person has taken steps to correct the impact of the disability on functioning (*Sutton v. United Airlines*, 1999), as well as a ruling that an employee's disability must affect his or her ability to engage in activities of daily living regardless of the impact on his or her ability to perform a job (*Toyota Motor Manufacturing, Kentucky, Inc. v. Williams*, 2002). These rulings have the practical consequence of making claims of disability more difficult for individuals to pursue (Petrila, 2002; Petrila and Brink, 2001). Even before the Supreme Court began narrowing application of the ADA, individuals with mental disability claims had less success in obtaining relief in the workplace than did those with physical disability claims (Moss et al., 1999; Stefan, 1998). These latest rulings may place added barriers before such claims.

Despite a trend in the courts toward a more conservative reading of the ADA, antidiscrimination statutes will continue to be a source of rights for individuals with mental illnesses seeking to eradicate barriers to those rights most citizens take for granted.

Health Care Reform and Managed Care

The emergence in the 1990s of managed care as a leading set of strategies to control behavioral health costs raised a number of legal issues. While managed care continues to exert enormous influence today, the concept of *managing* health and mental health care has been operational, in one form or another, for almost a century. Whether structured through regulatory initiatives, incentive reimbursement policies, or health care market reform, the focus of these efforts has been on approaches that attempt to create checks and balances in the use of health care resources, cost containment, and quality enhancement. Managed care monitors the intensity and duration of treatment and the setting in which health care is provided, but also affords the opportunity to third parties (which manage and pay for most treatment) to join with providers and consumers in directly controlling the treatment process.

Moreover, managed care strategies have included an evolving array of health care review and service coordination mechanisms that ultimately attempt to control (i.e., reduce) health services use (e.g., through use management techniques including prior authorization review for both hospital and ambulatory treatment; concurrent use review encompassing discharge planning and postdischarge management; retrospective use review; case management; provider profiling; on-site audits; and second opinion programs) and cost controls (e.g., through capitation financing, prospective payment, negotiated fee-for-service payments, and use of alternative settings and service providers).

Although numerous organizational models are categorized under the rubric "managed care" [e.g., preferred provider organizations (PPOs), employee assistance organizations, exclusive provider organizations, point-of-service health plans, behavioral managed care firms], many of the service delivery and financing systems [e.g., health maintenance organizations (HMOs)] were modeled on the prepaid group practice and individual practice plans developed during the 1920s and 1930s. Despite their heterogeneity in organizational structure (Levin and Levin, 1986), these alternative health care financing and delivery systems had certain common characteristics, which included assuming contractual responsibility to provide an integrated and comprehensive range of health and mental health services to a voluntarily enrolled population on a prepaid contractual basis. Additionally, these organizations (and their service providers) contained service costs, as they assumed financial risk if the costs of services exceeded member premiums (for additional discussion of insuring mental health in managed care, see Chapter 2).

The emergence of managed care and the debate over health care reform nationally and within individual states raise a number of interesting legal and financial issues. For example, whether a managed care provider is subject to some types of state regulation may depend on whether the provider is in the *business of insurance*, that is, whether the provider is at financial risk for coverage of subscribers. If a provider is in the business of insurance, it may become subject to state laws that require the establishment of financial reserves, as well as other regulatory requirements (Becker et al., 1992). Similarly, the organizational structure of the provider may determine whether the managed care entity is subject to laws governing HMOs.

At a practice level, the more interesting questions have to do with the distribution of legal responsibility between the payer of care and the treater for any adverse consequences arising from decisions regarding care, including denying it. For example, a basic ethical and legal principle holds that a physician or other health care professional is obligated to prescribe the care most appropriate to his or her patient's needs. Managed care creates stress on the traditional patient–therapist relationship by making cost and limitations on reimbursement issues that increasingly must be considered in the context of the individual treatment relationship.

Early cases made it clear that the therapist retains the legal duty to provide appropriate care to the patient even in the face of financial limitations that may be imposed by insurers and other payers (*Muse v. Charter Hospital of Winston-Salem, Inc.*, 1995; *Wilson v. Blue Cross*, 1990). In each of these cases, a patient committed suicide after release from psychiatric care; the discharge occurred when insurance was exhausted. The courts ruled that the care provider was ultimately responsible for providing appropriate care despite the lack of reimbursement. In addition, many managed care plans were exempt from lawsuits brought in state court because of the Employee Retirement Income Security Act (ERISA) of 1974, which created a federal standard for the governance of qualified health care plans. Because of this statute, most litigation against a managed care plan had to be brought in federal court, and damages available to the plaintiff in such cases were very limited by the statute. However, states increasingly have enacted legislation that permits a managed care company to be sued in state court in some circumstances (principally when the managed care entity also provides or arranges directly for the provision of care), and the courts have upheld the legality of such legislation (*Corporate Health Insurance, Inc. v. Texas Department of Insurance*, 2000).

At the same time, the U.S. Supreme Court has made it clear that it is not for the courts to determine whether specific provisions of managed care plans designed to control costs violate ethical or legal norms. The Court reached this ruling in a case that asked the courts to declare that certain financial incentives that a physician-operated HMO used were illegal. The Supreme Court found such issues more suited to a legislative forum because of their inherent complexity (*Pegram v. Herdrich*, 2000).

The ebb and flow of efforts to regulate cost in the health care system will continue. The legal system, whether legislative or judicial, has established general principles, for example, that the needs of the patient trump a health care professional's financial concerns. However, beyond the establishment of such general parameters, the shaping of health care cost containment efforts occurs in other places, for example, in labor negotiations over health care benefits or in contract negotiations between a state Medicaid agency and an HMO.

The Criminalization of Mental Illness

Perhaps the most significant issue to have emerged in recent years in mental health law and policy is the *criminalization* of mental illness. There are approximately 11 million arrests in the United States each year. The most conservative estimates of the prevalence of mental disorders and substance use disorders among those arrested is between 6% and 15% of all jail inmates. In addition, 10% to 15% of all prison inmates have a severe mental illness. When all mental and substance use disorders are considered, the prevalence estimates run as high as 70% (Lamb and Weinberger, 1998; U.S. Department of Justice, 1997). Prevalence estimates in the juvenile justice system are even higher (Teplin et al., 2002).

Many of those who are most ill have been arrested for nonviolent misdemeanors and may be arrested repeatedly, creating a cycle of arrest, brief incarceration in jail, release without services, and eventual rearrest. As a result, there have been a variety of efforts to divert these individuals, in particular, from the criminal justice system into treatment. One focus has been on training police to enable them to identify an individual with a mental illness more readily and to divert that person into treatment rather than perform an arrest. Perhaps the best-known model for this practice originated in Memphis and is called *crisis intervention training* (or CIT for police). This training is usually offered as a 40-hour course (usually to officers with an interest in and aptitude for such work) and has been offered in many jurisdictions across the United States. The decision to attempt to influence decision making by police recognizes that the police are often the primary decision maker when a judgment must be made whether particular behavior is the product of a mental disorder. Such training was also made possible by the rise of community policing, a philosophy of policing that seeks to align police more closely with communities (Meares, 2002).

Another strategy to minimize the time spent in the criminal justice system by individuals with mental disorders has been the use of special jurisdiction courts. The two most popular special jurisdiction courts relevant to this issue are drug courts and mental health courts. Such courts have several common characteristics (Petrila et al., 2001). For example, both drug and mental health courts attempt to divert their target population (typically first-time felony offenders in drug court; typically nonviolent misdemeanants in mental health court) to treatment. Each court consolidates all eligible cases before a single judge. This is done to enable a judge with special expertise to handle these cases and to reduce the caseloads of the other judges who otherwise would have to hear such cases.

These courts also attempt to solve nonlegal problems. For example, a drug court may have as a goal in a particular case that the person achieve sobriety (Denckla, 2000). In addition, these courts monitor defendants to ensure compliance with treatment; oversight may include urinalysis and drawing of blood samples in drug courts and the use of status hearings, where the defendant's progress in treatment is presented in both drug and mental health courts. There are also differences between the courts. For example, drug courts routinely use punishment if the defendant is noncompliant with treatment, while the use of punishment in mental health courts is less frequent and varies from court to court (Griffin et al., 2002).

The development of such courts has been rapid. The first drug court was established in 1989, and today it is estimated that there are nearly 800 drug courts in place or being planned (Belekno, 2000). The first mental health court was established in 1997, and at the time of writing there are approximately 30 such courts (Griffin et al., 2002). The use of such courts represents not only a changed role for judges, but also the embrace of a philosophy in which courts attempt to use their interventions explicitly for therapeutic purposes (Hora et al., 1999). Called *therapeutic jurisprudence* (Wexler and Winick, 1992), this philosophy holds that the legal system should look specifically at the extent to which substantive rules and legal procedures, as well as the roles adopted by judges and lawyers, produce either therapeutic or antitherapeutic effects.

A literature is beginning to emerge that suggests that these courts are effective. Drug courts appear to reduce recidivism, primarily by ensuring that people stay in treatment (Maxwell, 2000). Less data are available for mental health courts because they are a more recent innovation. However, a study of the Broward County Mental Health Court suggests that individuals who enter the court perceive it as a noncoercive intervention (Poythress et al., 2002). In addition, it appears that individuals are more likely to enter treatment through the mental health court than through a comparison misdemeanor court, and that individuals already in treatment when arrested are more likely to stay in treatment if referred by the mental health court

(Boothroyd et al., 2003). Additional evaluations of other mental health courts will reveal whether these apparent successes are replicable in other jurisdictions.

The issue of criminalization will continue to be a major law and policy issue for the mental health, criminal justice, and social welfare systems. The volume of arrests in the United States, the prevalence figures noted above, and the lack of an integrated mental health system in many communities make this almost inevitable. The question is whether interventions such as those described here can have enough impact to become part of a more permanent solution to such problems or whether the resolution of these issues must await the development of more effective community-based care systems (for additional discussion of issues related to mental health and the criminal justice system, see Chapter 14).

Implications for Mental Health Services

Mental health law emerged from the civil rights movement and, as a result, concerned itself initially with questions of liberty and civil rights. While such issues have continuing importance, today mental health law embraces many more topics. It includes legislative and regulatory law at both the state and federal levels, as well as questions of financing, service delivery, and the elimination of discrimination. Today, mental health law often focuses on questions of access to services and entitlements; this focus differs from that of early mental health litigation, which often attempted to create barriers to the use of state-operated services. As most people with mental illnesses began receiving services in the community and, in most cases, never entered a state hospital, mental health law became much more closely aligned with general health law.

In the future, the law will continue to influence the direction and shape of mental health services. There will be continued concern with questions of access and discrimination, as well as with the issue of parity. Many of these debates will be resolved by legislation, by regulation, or by the courts. Yet coercion, perhaps the core concern of mental disability law throughout the years, will continue to be an important subject, particularly as it becomes more evident that coercion is exercised in a variety of ways in providing services, not simply through civil commitment (Monahan et al., 2001).

The key question in mental health law in the future will be whether it is used successfully to eliminate the historical barriers of access to services. If the law can be used in this manner, perhaps society's readiness to resort to coercion can be significantly diminished, if not eliminated.

REFERENCES

Addington v. Texas, 441 U.S. 418, 1979.
Alpert S. Health care information: access, confidentiality, and good practice. In: Goodman KW (ed). *Ethics, Computing, and Medicine: Informatics and the Transformation of Health Care*. Cambridge: Cambridge University Press, pp. 75–101, 1998.

American Psychiatric Association. *Practice Guidelines for the Treatment of Psychiatric Disorders.* Washington, DC: American Psychiatric Association, 2000.

Barton WT, Sanborn CF (eds). *An Assessment of the Community Mental Health Movement.* Lexington, MA: Health, 1975.

Bauman RL. Needless institutionalization of individuals with mental disabilities as discrimination under the ADA—*Olmstead v. L.C. New Mexico Law Review,* 30:287–306, 2000.

Becker, J, Tiano L, Marshall S. Legal issues in managed mental health. In: Feldman JL, Fitzpatrick RJ (eds). *Managed Mental Health Care: Administrative and Clinical Issues.* Washington, DC: American Psychiatric Association, pp. 159–184, 1992.

Belenko S. The challenges of integrating drug treatment into the criminal justice process. *Albany Law Review,* 63:833–876, 2000.

Berg JW, Appelbaum PS, Parker LS, et al. *Informed Consent: Legal Theory and Clinical Practice.* London: Oxford University Press, 2001.

Birnbaum M. The right to treatment. *American Bar Association Journal,* 46:499, 1960.

Bloom BL. *Community Mental Health: A General Introduction,* 2nd ed. Monterey, CA: Brooks/Cole, 1984.

Boothroyd RA, Poythress NG, McGaha A, et al. The Broward County Mental Health Court: process, outcomes and service utilization. *International Journal of Law and Psychiatry,* 26(1):55–71, 2003.

Bowen v. City of New York, 476 U.S. 467, 1986.

Bragdon v. Abbott, 524 U.S. 624, 1998.

Brown v. Board of Education, 347 U.S. 483, 1954.

Corporate Health Insurance, Inc. v. Texas Department of Insurance, 215 F. 3rd 526, 2000.

Dale MJ. Lawsuits and public policy: the role of litigation in correcting conditions in juvenile detention centers. *University of San Francisco Law Review,* 32:675–733, 1998.

Denckla DA. Essay: forgiveness as a problem-solving tool in the courts: a brief response to the panel on forgiveness in criminal law. *Fordham Urban Law Journal,* 27:1613–1619, 2000.

Depugh D. The right to treatment for involuntarily committed sex offenders in the wake of *Kansas v. Hendricks. Buffalo Public Interest Law Journal,* 17:71–105, 1998.

Donaldson v. O'Connor. 493 F2d 507, 5th Cir., 1974.

Frank RG, McGuire TG. Parity for mental health and substance abuse care under managed care. *The Journal of Mental Health Policy and Economics,* 1:153–159, 1998.

Geller JL. Excluding institutions for mental diseases from federal reimbursement services: Strategy or tragedy? *Psychiatric Services,* 51:1397–1403, 2000.

Glover R, Petrila J. Can the state mental health agency survive health care reform? *Hospital and Community Psychiatry,* 45:911–913, 1994.

Goldman HH, Koyanagi C. The quiet success of the national plan for the chronically mentally ill. *Hospital and Community Psychiatry,* 42:899–905, 1991.

Griffin PA, Steadman, HJ, Petrila J. The use of criminal charges and sanctions in mental health courts. *Psychiatric Services,* 53:1285–1289, 2002.

Grisso T, Appelbaum PS. *Assessing Competence to Consent to Treatment: A Guide for Physicians and Other Health Professionals.* London: Oxford University Press, 1998.

Grob GN. *From Asylum to Community: Mental Health Policy in Modern America.* Princeton, NJ: Princeton University Press, 1991.

Hanson KW, Huskamp HA. State health care reform: behavioral health services under Medicaid managed care: the uncertain implications of state variation. *Psychiatric Services,* 52:447–450, 2001.

Hart M. Symposium. Conflating scope of right with standard of review: the Supreme

Court's "strict scrutiny" of congressional efforts to enforce the fourteenth amendment. *Villanova Law Review*, 46:1091–1110, 2001.

Health Care Quality Improvement Act, 42 U.S.C. 11101-11152, 1986.

Hogan MF. Spending too much on mental illness in all the wrong places. *Psychiatric Services*, 53:1251–1252, 2002.

Howland R. The treatment of persons with dual diagnoses in a rural community. *Psychiatric Quarterly*, 66:33–49, 1995.

Hora PF, Schma WG, Rosenthal JT. Therapeutic jurisprudence and the drug treatment court movement: revolutionizing the criminal justice system's response to drug abuse and crime in America. *Notre Dame Law Review*, 74:439–537, 1999.

Institute of Medicine. *The Future of Public Health*. Washington, DC: Institute of Medicine, 1988.

Interim Report to the President. Washington, DC: The President's New Freedom Commission on Mental Health, 2002.

Jaffee v. Redmond, 518 U.S. 1, 1996.

Kiesler CA. U.S. mental health policy: doomed to fail. *American Psychologist*, 47(9): 1077–1082, 1992.

Kiesler CA, Sibulkin AE. *Mental Hospitalization: Myths and Facts About a National Crisis*. Newbury Park, CA: Sage, 1987.

Krause J. Attorney discipline systems: improving public perception and increasing efficacy. *Marquette Law Review*, 84:273–300, 2000.

Kremer TG, Gesten EL. Confidentiality limits of managed care and clients' willingness to disclose. *Professional Psychology, Research and Practice*, 22:161–170, 1998.

Lamb HR, Weinberger LE. Persons with severe mental illness in jails and prisons: a review. *Psychiatric Services*, 49:483–492, 1998.

Levin BL, Levin JD. Differential HMO organizational structures. *GHAA Journal*, 7(1):43–49, 1986.

Link B, Phelan J, Bresnahan AS, et al. Public conceptions of mental illness: labels, causes, dangerousness and social distance. *American Journal of Public Health*, 89:1328–1333, 1999.

Marbrunak, Inc. v. City of Stow, 1992 West Law 209628, 6th Cir. 1992.

Maxwell S. Sanction threats in court-ordered offender programs: examining their effects on offenders mandated into drug treatment. *Crime and Delinquency*, 46:542–563, 2000.

McGinley PJ. Beyond health care reform: reconsidering certificate of need laws in a "managed competition" system. *Florida State University Law Review*, 23:141–148, 1995.

Meares TL. A colloquium on community policing: praying for community policing. *California Law Review*, 90:1593–1634, 2002.

Melton G, Petrila JP, Poythress N, et al. *Psychological Evaluation for the Courts: A Handbook for Mental Health Professionals and Lawyers*, 2nd ed. New York: Guilford Press, 1997.

Message from the President of the United States Relative to Mental Illness and Mental Retardation. Address by John F. Kennedy to the 88th Congress, U.S. House of Representatives. Document No. 58. Washington, DC: U.S. Government Printing Office, 1963.

Miller FH. Medical malpractice: external influences and controls: Medical discipline in the twenty-first century: are purchasers the answer? *Law and Contemporary Problems*, 60:31–58, 1997.

Monahan J. Limiting therapist exposure to Tarasoff liability. *American Psychologist*, 48:242–250, 1993.

Monahan J, Bonnie RJ, Appelbaum PS, et al. Mandated community treatment: beyond outpatient commitment. *Psychiatric Services*, 52:1198–1205, 2001.

Morrison MA. Changing perceptions of mental illness and the emergence of expansive mental health parity legislation. *South Dakota Law Review*, 45:8–32, 2000.

Moss K, Ullman M, Starrett BE. Outcomes of employment discrimination charges filed under the Americans with Disabilities Act. *Psychiatric Services*, 50:1028–1035, 1999.

Muse v. Charter Hospital of Winston Salem, Inc., 117 N.C. App. 468, 452 S.E.2d 589, *review on add'l issues denied*, 340 N.C. 114, 455 S.E.2d 663, *decision affirmed*, 342 N.C. 403, 464 S.E.2d 44, 1995.

Naidu v. Laird, 539 A. 2d 1064, 1988.

Naierman N, Haskins B, Robinson G. *Community Mental Health Centers: A Decade Later.* Cambridge, MA: Abt Associates, 1978.

National Guideline Clearinghouse. http://www.guideline.gov/body_home.asp (when searched November 23, 2002).

Norman J, Rosvall SB. Help-seeking behavior among mental health practitioners. *Clinical Social Work Journal*, 22:449–460, 1994.

Olmstead v L.C., 527 U.S. 581, 1999.

Parham v. J.R., 442 U.S. 584, 1979.

Pegram v. Herdrich, 530 U.S. 211, 2000.

Pennsylvania Department of Corrections v. Yeskey, 524 U.S. 206, 1998.

Perlin M. An invitation to the dance: an empirical response to Chief Justice Warren Burger's "Time-Consuming Procedural Minuets" theory in *Parham v. J.R. Bulletin of the American Academy of Psychiatry and Law*, 9:149–164, 1981.

Petrila J. Redefining mental health law: thoughts on a new agenda. *Law and Human Behavior*, 16:89–106, 1992.

Petrila J. The U.S. Supreme Court narrows the definition of disability under the Americans with Disabilities Act. *Psychiatric Services*, 53:797–798, 801, 2002.

Petrila J, Brink T. Mental illness and changing definitions of disability under the Americans with Disabilities Act. *Psychiatric Services*, 52:626–630, 2001.

Petrila J, Poythress NG, McGaha A, et al. Preliminary observations from an evaluation of the Broward County Mental Health Court. *Court Review*, 37:14–22, 2001.

Petrila J, Ridgely MS, Borum R. Debating outpatient commitment: controversy, trends, and empirical data. *Crime and Delinquency*, 49:177–192, 2003.

Pettis RW, Gutheil TG. Misapplication of the Tarasoff duty to driving cases: a call for a reframing of theory. *Bulletin of the American Academy of Psychiatry and Law*, 21:263–275, 1993.

Potomac Group Home Corporation v. Montgomery County, 823 F. Supp. 1285, D. Md., 1993.

Poythress NG. Avoiding negligent release: contemporary clinical and risk management strategies. *American Journal of Psychiatry*, 147:994–997, 1990.

Poythress NG, Petrila J, McGaha A, et al. Perceived coercion and procedural justice in the Broward County Mental Health Court. *International Journal of Law and Psychiatry*, 25:517–533, 2002.

Ridgely MS, Borum R, Petrila J. *The Effectiveness of Involuntary Outpatient Commitment: Empirical Evidence and the Experience of Eight States.* Santa Monica, CA: RAND Institute for Civil Justice, 2001.

Rivers v. Katz, 67 New York 2d 485, 495 N.E. 2d 337, 1986.

Rouse v. Cameron, 373 F. 2d 451 (D.C. Cir. 1966).

Scherl DJ, English JT, Sharfstein S (eds). *Prospective Payment and Psychiatric Care.* Washington, DC: American Psychiatric Association, 1988.

Schloendorff v. Society of New York Hospital, 211 N.Y. 2d 125; 105 N.E. 2d 92, 1914.

Simon RI. *A Concise Guide to Psychiatry and Law for Clinicians.* Washington, DC: American Psychiatric Association Press, 1998.

Stalker CJ. How far is too far? EMTALA moves from the emergency room to off-campus entities. *Wake Forest Law Review,* 36:823–843, 2001.

State ex rel. Hawks v. Lazaro, 202 S.E. 2d 109, 1974.

Steadman HJ, Gounis K, Dennis D. Assessing the New York City involuntary outpatient commitment pilot program. *Psychiatric Services,* 52:330–336, 2001.

Stefan S. Leaving civil rights to the "experts": from deference to abdication under the professional judgment standard. *Yale Law Journal,* 102:639–752, 1992.

Stefan S. You'd have to be crazy to work here: worker stress, the abusive workplace, and Title I of the ADA. *Loyola Law Review,* 31:795–845, 1998.

Sturm R. How expensive is unlimited mental health coverage under managed care? *Journal of the American Medical Association,* 278:1533–1539, 1997.

Sutton v. United Airlines, 525 U.S. 1063, 1999.

Swartz MS, Swanson JW, Hiday VA, et al. A randomized controlled trial of outpatient commitment in North Carolina. *Psychiatric Services,* 52:325–329, 2001.

Szasz TS. *The Myth of Mental Illness.* New York: Harper, 1961.

Szasz TS. *Law, Liberty, and Psychiatry: An Inquiry into the Social Uses of Mental Health Practices.* New York: Macmillan, 1963.

Szasz TS. *Psychiatric Justice.* New York: Macmillan, 1965.

Tarasoff v. Regents of University of California, 17 Cal. 3d 425, 551 P. 2d 334, 1976.

Teplin LA, McClelland GM, Dulcan MK, et al. Psychiatric disorders in youth in juvenile detention. *Archives of General Psychiatry,* 59(12):1133–1143, 2002.

Timmons G. Crisis in the mental health care industry: an analysis of the practices of private, for-profit psychiatric hospitals and governmental response. *Houston Law Review,* 31:323–357, 1994.

Torrey EF, Zdanowicz M. Outpatient commitment: what, why, and for whom. *Psychiatric Services,* 52:337–341, 2001.

Toyota Motor Manufacturing, Kentucky, Inc. v. Williams, 534 U.S. 184, 2002.

Truscott D. The psychotherapist's duty to protect: An annotated bibliography. *Journal of Psychiatry and Law,* 21:221–224, 1993.

U.S. Congress. Public Law 94-182. The Mental Health Study Act, 1955.

U.S. Congress. Public Law 86-778. Medical Assistance for the Aged Act, 1960.

U.S. Congress. Public Law 88-164. Mental Retardation Facilities and Community Mental Health Centers Construction Act, 1963.

U.S. Congress. Public Law 89-105. Mental Retardation Facilities and Community Mental Health Centers Construction Act Amendments, 1965a.

U.S. Congress. Public Law 89-97. The Social Security Amendments, 1965b.

U.S. Congress. Public Law 89-749. Comprehensive Health Planning and Public Health Service Amendments Act, 1966.

U.S. Congress. Public Law 90-31. Mental Health Amendments, 1967.

U.S. Congress. Public Law 90-574. Public Health Service Act, 1968.

U.S. Congress. Public Law 91-513. Comprehensive Drug Abuse Prevention and Control Act, 1970a.

U.S. Congress. Public Law 91-211. Community Mental Health Centers Amendments, 1970b.

U.S. Congress. Public Law 92-603. Social Security Act Amendments, 1972.

U.S. Congress. Public Law 93-45. Health Programs Extension Act, 1973.

U.S. Congress. Public Law 93-641. National Health Planning and Resources Development Act, 1974.

U.S. Congress. Public Law 94-63. The Community Mental Health Centers Amendments, 1975.

U.S. Congress. Public Law 95-622. Community Mental Health Centers Act, 1978.

U.S. Congress. Public Law 96-398. Mental Health Systems Act, 1980.

U.S. Congress. Public Law 97-35. Omnibus Budget Reconciliation Act, 1981.

U.S. Congress. Public Law 98-21. Social Security Amendments, 1983.

U.S. Congress: Public Law 98-509. Alcohol Abuse, Drug Abuse, and Mental Health Amendments, 1984.

U.S. Congress. Public Law 99-117. Amendments to the Public Health Service Act, 1985.

U.S. Congress. Public Law 99-660. Comprehensive State Mental Health Planning Act, 1986.

U.S. Congress. Public Law 100-77. Stewart B. McKinney Act, 1987a.

U.S. Congress. Public Law 100-203. The Omnibus Budget Reconciliation Act, 1987b.

U.S. Congress. Public Law 100-430. Fair Housing Amendments Act, 1988.

U.S. Congress. Public Law 101-336. Americans with Disabilities Act, 1990.

U.S. Congress. Public Law 104-204. Mental Health Parity Act, 1996a.

U.S. Congress. Public Law 104-191. Health Insurance Accountability and Portability Act, 1996b.

U.S. Department of Health and Human Services. *Mental Health: A Report of the Surgeon General*. Rockville, MD: Substance Abuse and Mental Health Services Administration, National Institute of Mental Health, 1999.

U.S. Department of Justice. *Correctional Populations in the United States 1997*. Washington, DC: United States Department of Justice, Office of Justice Programs, Bureau of Justice Statistics, 1997.

Van Hemel PJ. A way out of the maze: federal agency preemption of state licensing and regulation of complementary and alternative medicine practitioners. *American Journal of Law and Medicine*, 27:329–344, 2001.

Varmus HE. *Parity in Financing Mental Health Services: Managed Care Effects on Cost Access and Quality: An Interim Report to Congress by the National Advisory Mental Health Council*. Washington, DC: U.S. Department of Health and Human Services, 1998.

Weeks E. Note. The newly found compassion for sexually violent predators: civil commitment and the right to treatment in the wake of *Kansas v. Hendricks*. *Georgia Law Review*, 32:1261–1300, 1998.

Weiner BA, Wettstein RM. *Legal Issues in Mental Health Care*. New York: Plenum, 1993.

Weithorn LA. Mental hospitalization of troublesome youth: an analysis of sky rocketing admission rates. *Stanford Law Review*, 40:773–838, 1988.

Wexler D, Winick B. *Essays in Therapeutic Jurisprudence*. Durham, NC: Carolina Academic Press, 1992.

Wilson v. Blue Cross of Southern California, 271 Cal. Rptr. 876, 222 Cal. App. 3d 660, 1990.

Wolfson, LH. State regulation of health facility planning: the economic theory and political realities of certificate of need. *DePaul Journal of Health Care*, 4:261–315, 2001.

Wyatt v. Stickney, 344 F. Supp. 373, M.D. Ala., 1972.

Youngberg v. Romeo, 457 U.S. 307, 1982.

4

Public Mental Health Systems: Structures, Goals, and Constraints

JENIFER URFF

This chapter provides an overview of public mental health services in the United States, including a brief history of public mental health and the evolving roles of the federal and state governments, a description of the structure of public mental health systems today, and a discussion of factors that constrain public mental health systems and drive systems change.

Perhaps the biggest misnomer in public health today is the frequent reference to the *public mental health system*. In fact, there is no single public mental health system in the United States. Rather, there is a patchwork of 59 state and territorial mental health systems, each interacting with thousands of county and municipal mental health agencies, private providers, and not-for-profit agencies that have become an integral part of the overall system of public mental health care.

Each state mental health system is driven by its own mission, policy priorities, and treatment philosophy. States are constrained, however, in the pursuit of their goals and objectives by several factors, including (*1*) financing, (*2*) fragmented service delivery systems, and (*3*) politics.

A Brief History of Public Mental Health in America

Although caring for people with mental illnesses in colonial America was generally considered to be the responsibility of families, local governments often assumed a role consistent with the general principle that communities had an obligation to assist the poor and dependent. Thus, various municipal codes dating as far back as the 1600s included some protections and obligations to provide for "lunatics" and "distracted persons." (Much of the background in this section was drawn from the historical perspectives provided by Grob, 1994, and Grob, 2001.) Since the focus of concern was on social and economic problems rather than medical problems, communities generally assumed responsibility for the physical maintenance of certain individuals in the same way that they supported other destitute and desperate citizens.

Thus, when Dorothea Dix began her famous crusade during the 1840s and 1850s on behalf of people with mental illness in the United States, she found most of them housed inhumanely with families ill equipped to care for them or locked away in prisons and almshouses. By then, the concepts of treatment and recovery from mental illness had been introduced in the United States and were implemented, with varying degrees of success, in the small number of asylums that existed.

Dix's advocacy was enormously successful. By the end of the nineteenth century, all but a handful of states had at least one state asylum for people with mental illnesses. However, identifying asylums as a panacea for the societal problem of mental illness led to several unanticipated consequences that contributed greatly to the rise of institutions.

First, the establishment of asylums led to enormous demand and, arguably, to overuse of their services. When given an option for institutional care, families that traditionally may have cared for an individual in their home chose the security of an institution in far greater numbers than had been anticipated. In addition, over time asylums became the answer to a range of perceived societal maladies, ranging from homosexuality to public drunkenness. As a result, many state asylums grew at an enormous pace, developing massive campuses with dozens of buildings and often housing thousands of patients.

Second, most states assumed that an asylum located in the center of the state would be most accessible to citizens of the entire state. Where treatment and recovery also were goals of the asylum, many people believed that rural, bucolic settings were more conducive to effective treatment, providing opportunities for both contemplation and work. Thus began a tradition of locating asylums in generally rural areas, which came to rely on the mental institution economically and even as a source of civic pride.

Third, the demand for labor to care for patients in a stigmatized institutional environment led to a close-knit culture of staff that often included many members of the same family and, at some hospitals, long tenures of employment (Moore, 1994). Many campuses encouraged employees to live communally in dormitories on the institution's campus, reinforcing economic dependence, institutional entrenchment, and segregation of staff from the general population that may have contributed to unchecked patient abuse and deep resistance to change in later years.

The establishment of state asylums coincided with an expanding role for state governments in a range of policy arenas and an expanding economy, and Dix's advocacy capitalized on these social trends. However, Dix also envisioned a significant national role in financing care for people with mental illnesses. In 1854, both chambers of Congress passed legislation initiated by Dix to grant 10 million acres of land to the states, which could use the proceeds to build asylums. President Franklin Pierce vetoed the legislation, however, warning that assuming financial responsibility for states' obligations to their own citizens would set a dangerous precedent:

> . . . and the several States, instead of bestowing their own means on the social wants of their own people, may themselves, through the strong temptation . . . become humble supplicants for the bounty of the Federal Government, reversing their true relation to this Union.
>
> (Pierce, cited in Grob, 1994, p. 97)

Thus, until the middle of the twentieth century, the states, along with a few of the nation's largest counties and communities, were essentially the only players in the development and delivery of mental health services in the United States.

Several social movements began to erode the absolute dominance of state control over the mental health system during the twentieth century. Perhaps the most important was the rise of psychiatry as a legitimate field of private practice in medicine. Although psychiatry began to come into its own in the United States during the second half of the nineteenth century, the nation's most important researchers and physicians were associated with great institutional hospitals, and the vision of effective treatment for people with mental illnesses was largely shaped by these researchers, providers, and administrators. The popular attention given to the theories of Sigmund Freud in the 1930s and the growing belief in the post–World War II era that people with mental illnesses could be treated and even cured, rather than just cared for, caused many medical researchers, scholars, and clinicians to choose to work outside large state institutional settings and expanded options for treatment outside public hospitals.

The idea that people with mental illnesses can and do recover also contributed to the federal government's first major foray into the field of public mental health. By the 1950s, state psychiatric hospitals were huge, sprawling campuses, housing nearly 560,000 patients at their peak in 1955. Along with this significant role for state hospitals came public allegations of abuse and neglect, as well as nagging questions about tolerance for deviant behavior within society. Coupled with the advent of new antipsychotic drugs and the rise of a consumer advocacy movement, many professionals, consumers, and others in the field began to see state hospitals as part of the larger problem rather than as part of the solution. In 1963, President John F. Kennedy signed into law the Community Mental Health Centers Construction (CMHC) Act, which provided grants to states to assist in the construction of community mental health centers based on the philosophy that small communities of caring individuals could better serve people with mental illnesses than could mammoth bureaucratic structures. Most grantees were private, not-for-profit agencies, although numerous county and local governments also received grants to establish community programs. States were not barred from receiving grants, but CMHCs were not permitted to be affiliated with state hospital systems.

The modest support provided under the CMHC Act diminished over time, converted in 1981 to a block grant that today, known as the Community Mental Health Services Performance Partnership Block Grant, funds less than 2% of state mental health agency expenditures on community services (Lutterman et al., 2003). However, the impetus of the CMHC Act permanently changed the face of public mental health in the United States. Aided by political and ideological shifts in

American society and favorable legal decisions, the CMHC Act became part of a long trend toward deinstitutionalization, decreasing by almost 90%—to about 65,000 today—the number of resident patients in psychiatric hospitals (Lutterman, 2000). Some CMHCs have disappeared as federal funding has withered, but most have adapted to the economic realities of third-party reimbursement, managed care, and small revenue streams from public and private grants and contracts.

Although financial support under the CMHC Act diminished, the federal government secured a permanent role in the development and framing of public mental health systems with the passage in 1965 of the Medicaid and Supplemental Security Income (SSI) programs. Ironically, the federal government intentionally tried to minimize this role because of concern that the Medicaid program would simply replace state and local financing for mental health services. In an effort to preserve the state and local roles, the federal government specifically prohibits states from using Medicaid to finance services in institutions for mental disease (IMDs).[1] Despite the IMD Exclusion, however, Medicaid became an important source of revenue for providing community-based mental health services and may even have contributed to the rapid transition from reliance on state hospitals to providing services in community-based settings. The impact of Medicaid on public mental health systems is discussed more fully below.

The federal government also provides some support for the public mental health system through Medicare. However, Medicare coverage of mental health services in both the public and private sectors is subject to significant restrictions, including limitations on the number of psychiatric inpatient days and the number of outpatient visits eligible for reimbursement and higher copayments for outpatient visits. As a result, Medicare represents a relatively small share, about 21% in 1997, of public behavioral health expenditures in the United States (Coffey et al., 2000, Fig. 2.8) and less than 2% of revenues to state mental health agencies (Lutterman et al., 2003). In contrast, Medicare accounts for about 44% of all public health expenditures in the United States (Coffey et al., 2000, Fig. 2.8).

Other significant federal support is provided through nonhealth programs, such as housing assistance; food assistance; vocational rehabilitation and other employment assistance; and income support through SSI, Social Security Disability Insurance (SSDI), and Temporary Assistance to Needy Families (TANF). As described below, these programs are critical to meeting the broad range of needs that people with mental illnesses have when they receive services in community settings. In fact, the availability of both Medicaid and other community supports described here was significant in driving deinstitutionalization. However, because these programs generally are not specifically designed to serve people with mental illnesses, they often contribute to fragmentation of the service delivery system.

The Structure of Public Mental Health Systems

As the provider of last resort for people needing mental health services who cannot access them through privately reimbursed providers, states remain the critical player in the development and maintenance of the public mental health system. In fact, mental health, more than any other public health or medical discipline, is singled out for exclusion and discrimination in many federal programs because it is considered to be the principal domain of the states.[2]

Today, most states' mental health systems are administered by a state mental health agency. These agencies may be a department within state government with a cabinet-level agency administrator, but more often are lower-level agencies that fall within another department in state government (usually the department responsible for either health or human services). About half of the states combine mental health and substance abuse services in a single agency (Lutterman and Shaw, 2000). About one-third combine mental health and services for people with mental retardation or developmental disabilities in the same agency (Lutterman and Shaw, 2000).

Almost all state mental health agencies administer state-owned psychiatric hospitals.[3] In addition, many state mental health agencies are responsible for licensing private and other nonstate community service providers and monitoring their performance. All state mental health agencies provide financial support to community service providers. In some states, these providers are state entities administered by staff employed by the state mental health agency. In other states, private entities—both nonprofit and for-profit providers—are supported through reimbursement for specific services, grants and contracts for special programs, or formula grants to community providers or local mental health agencies.

It is important to recognize that the dividing lines between the public and private delivery systems are becoming increasingly blurred and imprecise. Most providers of community-based services are not administered by the state, but these private, nonprofit, and for-profit organizations and hospitals have become an increasingly integral part of the de facto public mental health system as states continue to downsize and close public psychiatric hospitals. In addition, many people who once would have been clients of the public mental health system now receive services from private providers, who bill public insurers (such as Medicaid or Medicare) for reimbursement and may not even have a direct relationship with the state mental health agency.

Some state mental health agencies are responsible for administering mental health benefits under the state's Medicaid plan, especially in those states that have adopted Medicaid managed care approaches that carve out some or all behavioral health services.

The missions of most state mental health agencies focus resources on people with the most severe and persistent mental illnesses, such as schizophrenia, bipolar disorder (manic-depressive illness), and major depression. In part, this is an extension of the historical role state mental institutions played, but it is also a reflection of the medicalization of mental illness and growing bodies of research regarding biological bases for mental disorders (see, e.g., U.S. DHHS, *Mental Health: A Report of the Surgeon General*, 1999, esp. pp. 52–54)

At the same time, a growing consumer movement with considerable influence and lingering traces of the community psychiatry movement of the 1960s and 1970s has helped lead some state mental health agencies to emphasize a broader range of priority populations and issues. This movement identifies environmental factors, such as violence and poverty, both as causes of mental disorders and as barriers to recovery that must be addressed. In particular, children, people with co-occurring substance abuse disorders or medical comorbidities such as acquired immune deficiency syndrome, and older adults are receiving increasing specialized attention. While most agencies continue to focus on treatment and services, a few are exploring approaches to early intervention and prevention.

In addition, new political priorities, including welfare reform and criminal justice, have prompted some state mental health agencies to expand their missions to include initiatives related to these important issues. For example, a growing number of states are collaborating with state and local corrections agencies to deliver mental health services in jails and prisons and, in some cases, to divert people with mental illnesses from the criminal justice system. Other states have arranged with local educational authorities to provide mental health services, especially related to post-traumatic stress, in school settings.

The considerable variation in the structure and role of state mental health agencies has caused many observers to quip: "When you've seen one state mental health system, you've seen one state mental health system." An important advantage of this state-by-state approach is that states and communities are able to tailor their programs to meet the unique needs and environments of the people they serve. However, the lack of a national mental health system has also resulted in crucial disparities, including dramatic state-by-state differences in the pace of deinstitutionalization, the types and quality of services provided, and the identification of priority services and populations.

Although research into the design and implementation of public mental health systems is far from complete, there is a growing consensus among public mental health professionals and consumers about many promising practices and key components of an ideal system. For example, an ideal public mental health system would deemphasize inpatient services for adults with serious mental illnesses and would provide comprehensive, coordinated treatment in community settings. That treatment would be consumer-centered and would include housing, employment, peer support, and opportunities for social interaction and the development of friendships and other adult relationships. Co-occurring disorders, especially substance abuse disorders, would be identified, and consumers would receive integrated treatment in a single setting from a team of cross-trained providers. The public mental health system would work alongside criminal justice systems to identify offenders with mental illnesses and divert them into the mental health system. Consumers would be involved in the development of their own treatment plans, and the public mental health system would use aggressive outreach by interdisciplinary teams of trained professionals to facilitate compliance. An effective service delivery system would minimize, perhaps even eliminate, the need for more coercive measures—such as civil commitment orders—to ensure compliance with treatment (especially medication) regimens. To the extent possible, treatment plans would focus on the many services for which there is a solid base of scientific evidence demonstrating their effectiveness. Children's mental health needs would be identified early and would be addressed through *systems of care* that integrated a comprehensive set of mental health services and other health, education, and community supports. Perhaps most important, everyone who needed treatment would have access to appropriate services.

The reality, of course, is that even states with the most advanced public mental health systems do not come close to the ideal vision that their own mental health agencies have articulated. States are constrained in implementing that vision by many factors, including financing, fragmented delivery systems, and political concerns. As a result, many state mental health administrators have referred to their own systems as "in crisis," and many others acknowledge a significant disconnect between the values and priorities of state mental health agencies and the structure and practices of the current service delivery system.

Financing

As noted earlier, state mental health agencies are funded principally by the states themselves, with about 53% of expenditures derived from state general revenue fund dollars and another 14% from state contributions under Medicaid for programs administered by the state mental health agency (Lutterman et al., 2003)

These data do not reflect the revenues and expenditures of other state agencies that play a critical role in providing services to people with mental illnesses. Although there are no comprehensive data regarding overall revenues and expenditures in the public mental health system, Buck (2001) estimates that approximately half of all expenditures for state and locally administered mental health programs are derived from Medicaid (both federal and state contributions), eclipsing all other sources of revenue for these programs. State child welfare agencies, education agencies, vocational rehabilitation agencies, and corrections agencies also are important sources of revenue for mental health services.

The important role played by state agencies other than state mental health agencies and by federal programs in financing mental health services has increased significantly in recent years. For example, in 1987 Medicaid expenditures for mental health were $5.7 billion, about 29% of overall estimated public expenditures for mental health services in that year (Coffey et al., 2000, p. D-10). By 1997, Medicaid expenditures for mental health services had increased to more than $14.4 billion, about 36% of overall estimated public expenditures in that year.

Therefore, although state mental health agencies continue to define and administer public mental health programs, their roles have become less significant as other agencies have assumed responsibility for financing mental health services and community supports. During the 1980s and 1990s, state mental health agencies experienced gradual but steady erosion of funding, from 2.09% of total state government expenditures in 1981 to 1.81% in 1997 (Lutterman et al., 1999). When adjusted for inflation, per capita expenditures by state mental health agencies decreased more than 8% from 1981 to 2001 (Lutterman et al., 2003).

An important consequence of the declining role of state mental health agencies in financing mental health services is that public mental health systems and individual providers must piece together funding from dozens of disparate and uncoordinated funding streams, including Medicaid, Medicare, and private health insurance, federal, state, and local grants and contracts, and support from private foundations. Many of these funding streams are categorical and include restrictions on the blending of funds, complicating efforts to develop comprehensive, flexible service delivery systems that can be tailored to meet the individualized and varied needs of people with mental illnesses. In addition, many funding options, such as Medicare and private insurance plans, favor institution-based settings over community-based services and include significant limits on reimbursement for both inpatient and outpatient mental health care.

There is no consensus on whether a diminished role for state mental health agencies caused the erosion in funding or whether the lack of resources for state mental health agencies caused community service providers to tailor their services to attract funding support from other state, federal, and private sources. Some scholars and administrators have suggested that funding erosion for state mental health agencies not only coincided with but also was, in fact, caused by successful mental health reform and the declining role of state hospitals (Hogan, 1992; Schinnar, 1992). As fixed state expenses associated with maintaining state hospitals disappeared from state budgets, they argue, legislators also divested themselves of direct responsibility for the care of people with mental illnesses. Others suggest that the erosion of funding is simply the result of lingering stigma about mental illness and the failure of mental health administrators and advocates to "market" mental health services successfully to state policy makers (see, e.g., David L. Bazelon Center for Mental Health Law, 2001, p. 15, observing that, in 2001, only seven states ranked mental health as a top health priority; also see Little Hoover Commission, 2000, esp. pp. 29–36).

Often, the funding streams available to public mental health systems and individual providers drive program development and systems design. For example, the increasing importance of Medicaid as a financing vehicle may result in state mental health dollars being diverted from state mental health agency budgets to draw down federal Medicaid matching dollars. While maximizing federal revenues is, on its face, a good budgeting practice, it also means that public mental health programs must focus on providing specific services reimbursable by Medicaid to populations eligible to receive Medicaid services, rather than focusing on priority services and populations identified by the state mental health agency. To the extent that the public mental health system traditionally and currently serves principally individuals without Medicaid or other insurance coverage, fewer resources are available to serve this population. In addition, fewer dollars are available to provide comprehensive community supports that are not reimbursable under Medicaid.

Partly as a result of this trend, many state mental health agencies are significantly limited in their ability to articulate a vision for their systems or to implement that vision. For example, although almost all states have articulated a preference for community-based treatment over institutional care whenever possible, that preference generally assumes the availability of adequate housing, comprehensive treatment and rehabilitation programs, and other economic and social supports, all services that are often provided and financed by agencies other than the state mental health agency and that may not be prioritized within those agencies.

Within Medicaid, the IMD Exclusion, in particular, has had enormous implications for the public mental health system. In addition to prohibiting reimbursement under Medicaid for institutional care, the IMD Exclusion has had the practical effect of barring states from receiving Home- and Community-Based Services (HCBS) waivers under Medicaid. These waivers, which permit states to use Medicaid flexibly to provide a comprehensive set of community services for priority populations, are available only to states that can demonstrate that the cost to the Medicaid program of providing these services will be offset by savings in institutional care. Because Medicaid does not reimburse for care in IMDs, states generally are unable to demonstrate the required cost savings. The HCBS waivers are the principal means of financing community-based services for almost every other disability group, and the lack of access to this revenue stream contributes significantly to a community-based service delivery system that is widely considered to be fragmented and underfunded.

Beginning in the 1970s, many states began to understand the important role that financing design could play in facilitating change within their own public mental health systems. For example, some states restructured their systems of funding community care, establishing regional or county-based mental health agencies and creating systems of fiscal incentives and disincentives to encourage treatment in community rather than institutional settings. This approach generally resulted in fewer admissions to state hospitals and empowered local agencies to coordinate a comprehensive array of needed community services. This approach also resulted in the devolution of decision making from state to regional or local authorities and, may, ironically, have contributed to a diminished role for state mental health agencies.

Fragmented Service Delivery System

Despite waning resources and, perhaps, the influence of state mental health agencies, these agencies remain, in most states, the focal point of mental health policy development and implementation. However, the reality of evolving responsibilities within state government and a growing role for federal programs such as Medicaid impose important constraints on their ability to implement a vision for comprehensive and effective community-based services. Another important constraint is the fragmentation of services within the public mental health system.

With the decline of state psychiatric institutions and the rise of community-based services, states lost the ability to control all aspects of an individual's care and treatment in a single setting. State hospitals provided not only treatment, but also housing, food, clothing, education, social interaction, and, in some cases, even employment opportunities and small amounts of spending money. As people with mental illnesses began the transition to community settings, they were forced to rely on separate delivery systems, each with its own bureaucracy and special interests and frequently located in multiple settings, to meet these basic human needs.

Ironically, the most important and expensive components of community mental health care, including housing, education, and income support, often have nothing to do with mental health at all. These and other nontreatment components of community services were designed and are administered to meet the needs of very different target populations—people who are indigent, widowed mothers, and people with physical disabilities, for example. As a result, many of these programs are designed in a way that does not fit with the cyclic nature of mental illness, the behavioral symptoms of the illnesses (which sometimes contradict assumptions about the "deserving poor" built into many social service systems), and the comprehensive medical and community support needs of people with mental illnesses.

Equally important, many of these critical community services are delivered not by state-operated providers but by a network of private agencies and providers. Many of these providers are not-for-profits—established for research, philanthropic, or other purposes—while others are for-profit providers that have identified a service need and stepped in to fill it. Although some are designed specifically to serve people with mental illnesses, most are driven not only by their own missions but also by the goals and demands of the public bureaucracies that fund them.

The interaction between the design of service delivery systems and their funding is important in understanding both the shortcomings and the successes of state mental health systems. While fragmented service delivery systems likely were the inescapable result of rapid deinstitutionalization as a result of the social movements of the 1960s, the perpetuation of complicated and uncoordinated funding streams guarantees continued fragmentation.

Politics

As is the case with all public policy, states are constrained in the development of public mental health systems by political issues and interests. In particular, three important issues drive mental health policy in part: (*1*) public safety, (*2*) economics, and (*3*) competing priorities among mental health stakeholders.

Public Safety and Violence

Concerns about public safety and violence intersect with almost all aspects of state mental health policy. Although the missions of state mental health agencies generally focus on the needs of people with serious mental illnesses, state government has a broader range of responsibilities that includes public safety and protection of citizens from violence.

A highly publicized incident in early 1999 provides a poignant example of the importance of addressing public safety concerns in mental health policy. In January 1999, Andrew Goldstein pushed Kendra Webdale, a 32-year-old aspiring writer, into the path of a subway train in New York City. Webdale died. Goldstein, 29, had been diagnosed with schizophrenia and had received treatment in the public mental health system at least six times prior to the incident. In the months immediately preceding the incident, he had repeatedly appeared in hospital emergency rooms requesting treatment but was turned away.

The tragic circumstances of Webdale's death and the public mental health system's failure to anticipate and prevent the threat presented by Goldstein underscored critical political and social questions that have dogged the public mental health system for decades.

In particular, Kendra Webdale's death reopened the decades'-old debate about the appropriateness and consequences of deinstitutionalization. As described earlier, deinstitutionalization was the culmination of several precipitating factors, including new medications that enabled people with serious mental illnesses to live outside institutions and growing awareness of neglect and patient abuse in state hospitals. Although the movement was closely linked to a vision of a strong network of comprehensive community-based services, the existence of those services was not a prerequisite for closing or downsizing hospitals.

There is widespread agreement in the mental health field that the goal of comprehensive community-based mental health services envisioned by advocates, consumers, and professionals has not materialized. At least partly as a result, people with mental illnesses constitute as much as one-fourth of the nation's homeless population (National Coalition for the Homeless, 1999) and 16% of the nation's jail and prison population (Ditton, 1999).

However, there remains significant disagreement about the most effective solutions to these problems. Many citizens and policy makers have concluded that deinstitutionalization has been a failure (e.g., see Julien, 2000; "State of neglect," *San Francisco Chronicle*, February 18, 2001; Torrey and Zdanowicz, 2000). Although few support a return to the days of massive institutions and lengthy hospital stays, many advocate for more flexible commitment criteria and more coercive measures to encourage individuals in the community to comply with their treatment plans. These coercive measures may include outpatient commitment or requiring compliance with medication regimens as a condition of receiving housing, income support, or other public benefits.

Most experts and consumers within the mental health community, however, observe that the failures of the community-based mental health system do not justify the repeal of decades of policy designed to support consumer choice, civil rights, and self-determination. They argue that a more effective, responsive community mental health service system would facilitate treatment compliance, and they tout system reform and an investment of resources as more appropriate solutions (see, e.g., Sudders, 2002).

Many states have sought a policy position that attempts to straddle both perspectives. For example, in response to Kendra Webdale's death, New York passed Kendra's Law, an expansion of outpatient commitment laws accompanied by significant increases in resources for community-based services.

The policy issues inherent in the intersection of mental illness and violence are complicated by the legal and philosophical questions posed by involuntary commitment and institutional treatment. These issues are explored in more depth in Chapter 3.

Economics

In addition to the financing issues discussed earlier in this chapter, states are constrained in their development of mental health systems by several economic factors that, because of political implications, often drive policy development.

As discussed above, deinstitutionalization was the product of several coinciding social factors. An additional factor may be the economic advantages of serving individuals in community-based rather than inpatient settings. It is generally accepted that it is less expensive, on average, to provide community-based services than inpatient hospital services.[4] There is no evidence that cost is a principal motivation for states in moving individuals from state hospitals to community settings. However, it is enough of an incentive that, in the landmark case *L.C. v. Olmstead* (1999), which held that the Americans with Disabilities Act (ADA) may require the delivery of services in community rather than in institutional settings, the U.S. Supreme Court specifically stated that the ADA could not be used to force individuals to leave state hospitals for community-based treatment against their will.[5]

Despite dramatic declines in the number of people residing in state psychiatric hospitals over the past four decades, more than 240 state hospitals remain in the United States (Lutterman, 2000). The National Association of State Mental Health Program Directors Research Institute reports that more hospitals, 44 in total, closed during the 1990s than in the previous two decades combined. Although significant, the rate of hospital closings (about 60 since 1970) represents a decrease in the total number of state hospitals of only about 20%—significantly less than the 85% decline in the number of public inpatient and residential treatment beds during approximately that same period (Lutterman, 2000; Manderscheid et al., 2001, p. 138).

There are many reasons that states have successfully downsized their hospital systems but have not been as effective in closing facilities. Some states have only one hospital and are unlikely to eliminate completely their state-operated inpatient capacity. Other, geographically large states believe that they need several hospitals, albeit with smaller numbers of beds, to serve large regions within the state. Still other states, for the reasons related to deinstitutionalization described above, are reluctant to close facilities until their community-based service delivery infrastructure is in place.

Also important is the significant role that state hospitals historically have played in local economies. In many states, psychiatric hospitals are a principal source of jobs and income in small towns and rural areas, and elected officials oppose closings because of the anticipated negative economic impact on the communities. In addition, unions representing state employees have historically been influential in galvanizing opposition to hospital closings that could result in the loss of state jobs.[6]

Finally, the public mental health system is subject to the same economic and political forces as any other discretionary state-funded program. Competing priorities for funding often crowd out other worthy projects with less political appeal. During the 1990s, only Medicaid and corrections agencies accounted for a larger share of states' overall budgets at the end of the decade than they did at the beginning (Buck, 2001) (for more information on mental health financing, see Chapter 2).

Competing Priorities Among Mental Health Stakeholders

States are, of course, influenced in policy making by the multiple stakeholders within the mental health community, including consumers, families, and mental health professionals. Although most advocates and other stakeholders generally support broad consumer access to mental health services, the similarities in their perspectives often end there. Stakeholders differ with respect to what services they believe are most effective, how involved they believe consumers can and should be in treatment planning, how noncompliance with treatment regimens should be approached, and which settings are most appropriate for serving individuals with mental illnesses of varied severity. These issues are discussed in more depth in Chapter 5.

Implications for Mental Health Services

State mental health agencies remain the dominant player in setting mental health priorities and policy, designing and financing public mental health systems, and articulating a vision for the future of public mental health. However, the growing importance of Medicaid and other funding sources, the continuing fragmentation of mental health financing and service delivery, and a range of political and policy issues all contribute to the development of public mental health delivery systems.

In particular, the expanding role of Medicaid has significant implications for the delivery of public mental health services. As states continue their efforts to maximize federal contributions, public mental health systems will have fewer resources to provide services not reimbursable under Medicaid or to serve populations not eligible for Medicaid reimbursement. Equally important, as Medicaid and other state agencies shoulder more of the burden of funding public mental health services, the ability of traditional mental health policy makers—especially state mental health agencies—to define and implement mental health policy may be further eroded.

In June 2002, a new National Commission on Mental Health began a 1-year study of mental health service delivery in the United States, including problems related to the lack of coordination among federal agencies and policies affecting people with mental illnesses, fragmented financing and service delivery systems, and the consequences of failing to adopt evidence-based ideal systems of comprehensive community care. Although the commission is unlikely to significantly affect the state-by-state structure of public mental health service delivery in the United States, observers hope that federal leadership will drive systems improvement across the country and, in light of the increasing role of a broad range of federal programs (especially Medicaid) in financing and providing mental health services, will help to reform those programs to make them more relevant to meeting the needs of people with mental illnesses.

ACKNOWLEDGMENTS

The author is indebted to Robert Glover, Gerald Grob, Andrew Hyman, Theodore Lutterman, and Jon Western, each of whom provided valuable insights. In particular, Haiden Huskamp reviewed several drafts and made significant contributions to the development of this chapter.

NOTES

1. An IMD is a hospital, nursing facility, or other institution with more than 16 beds that is primarily engaged in providing diagnosis, treatment, or care for individuals with mental diseases, including medical attention, nursing care, and related services (42 CFR 435.1009).

2. We note that federal perspectives on what constitutes a matter that is better left to the states have evolved in many ways but remain principally static with respect to people with mental illnesses. For example, while the care of people who are mentally retarded or developmentally disabled was once almost universally considered to be the domain of the states and was originally excluded from reimbursement under the Medicaid program, Medicaid was subsequently amended to permit reimbursement for services to this population both in institutions and, through specially designed waiver programs, in community settings. By 2000, Medicaid accounted for 75% of all spending for services to people who are mentally retarded or developmentally disabled. (Braddock et al., 2002) As a result, federal priorities regarding appropriate treatment and service settings often drive policy and programming for this population.

3. In a few states, hospitals are administered by a department overseeing a range of state institutions, including state prisons, schools for the blind, and other large public institutions. One state, Rhode Island, does not have a state psychiatric hospital but maintains a psychiatric inpatient capacity at a state general hospital.

4. We note that, despite the general rule that community-based services are less expensive than inpatient services, this is not always the case. If an individual has intensive medical or security needs, for example, it may be less expensive to provide care in an inpatient setting. Also, although the per-patient cost of providing services may be less in community-based settings, states must continue to absorb the costs of maintaining hospitals and units they keep open. Therefore, the overall costs to a state of maintaining a hospital unit with low bed use while, at the same time, providing a greater number of community-based services may well be higher than the costs of serving all individuals in the inpatient setting.

5. The *Olmstead* case involved two women with co-occurring mental illnesses and developmental disabilities who were inpatients in a Georgia state hospital. The women were considered by the hospital's own experts to be appropriate for discharge to a community program, but they remained confined in state institutions pending the availability of such a placement. The U.S. Supreme Court held that the ADA generally entitles individuals with disabilities to receive public services in the most integrated setting appropriate for their needs. A more complete discussion of this case is included in Chapter 3.

6. Increases in spending for community-based services have roughly kept pace with decreases in the number of inpatient beds over the past two decades. When adjusted for in-

flation, state mental health agency-controlled expenditures for community-based services increased by about 60% during the period 1981–97 (Lutterman et al., 1999); during a roughly comparable period (1980–98), the number of state and county inpatient and residential beds decreased by about 60% (Manderscheid et al., 2001, p. 138). However, this does not mean that community-based expenditures have increased by the same amount as inpatient expenditures have decreased; to the contrary, expenditures by state mental health agencies decreased by 7% during the period 1981–97 (Lutterman et al., 1999).

REFERENCES

Braddock D, Hemp R, Rizzolo M, et al. *The State of the States in Developmental Disabilities: 2002 Study Summary*. Boulder: Coleman Institute for Cognitive Disabilities and Department of Psychiatry, University of Colorado, 2002.

Buck J. Spending for state mental health care. *Psychiatric Services*, 52(10):1294, 2001.

Coffey R, Mark T, King E, et al. *National Expenditures for Mental Health and Substance Abuse Treatment 1997*. SAMHSA Pub. No. (SMA) 00-3499. Rockville, MD: Center for Substance Abuse Treatment and Center for Mental Health Services, Substance Abuse and Mental Health Services Administration, 2000.

David L. Bazelon Center for Mental Health Law. *Disintegrating Systems: The State of States' Public Mental Health Systems*. Washington, DC: David L. Bazelon Center for Mental Health Law, 2001.

Ditton P. *Mental Health and Treatment of Inmates and Probationers*. Bureau of Justice Statistics Special Report, Pub. NCJ 174463. Washington, DC: Office of Justice Programs, U.S. Department of Justice, 1999.

Grob G. *The Mad Among Us: A History of the Care of America's Mentally Ill*. New York: Free Press, 1994.

Grob G. Mental health policy in 20th-century America. In: Manderscheid R, Henderson M (eds). *Mental Health, United States, 2000*. DHHS Pub. No. (SMA) 01-3537. Rockville, MD: Center for Mental Health Services, Substance Abuse and Mental Health Services Administration, 2001, pp. 3–14, 2001.

Hogan M. Commentary on Schinnar et al. paper. *Administration and Policy in Mental Health*, 19(4):251–254, 1992.

Julien A. Psychiatric services plan raises fears; state's mentally ill will be put on streets, critics say. *The Hartford Courant*, February 16, 2000, p. A1.

L.C. v. Olmstead, 527 U.S. 1999.

Little Hoover Commission. *Being There: Making a Commitment to Mental Health*. Report No. 157. Sacramento, CA: Little Hoover Commission, 2000.

Lutterman T. *Closing and Reorganizing State Hospitals*. Alexandria, VA: National Association of State Mental Health Program Directors Research Institute, 2000.

Lutterman T, Hirad A, Poindexter B. *Funding Sources and Expenditures of State Mental Health Agencies: Fiscal Year 1997*. Alexandria, VA: National Association of State Mental Health Program Directors Research Institute, 1999.

Lutterman T, Hollen V, Shaw R. *Funding Sources and Expenditures of State Mental Health Agencies: Fiscal Year 2001*. Alexandria, VA: National Association of State Mental Health Program Directors Research Institute, 2003.

Lutterman T, Shaw R. *1999 State Mental Health Agency Profile Reports*. Alexandria, VA: National Association of State Mental Health Program Directors Research Institute, 2000.

Manderscheid R, Atay J, Hernandez-Cartagena M, et al. Highlights of organized mental health services in 1998 and major national and state trends. In: *Mental Health, United States, 2000.* DHHS Pub. No. (SMA) 01-3537. Rockville, MD: Center for Mental Health Services, Substance Abuse and Mental Health Services Administration, pp. 135–171, 2001.

Moore JM. *The Life and Death of Northampton State Hospital.* Northampton, MA: Historic Northampton, 1994.

National Coalition for the Homeless. *Fact Sheet No. 3.* Washington, DC: National Coalition for the Homeless, 1999.

Schinnar A, Rothbard A, Yin D, et al. Public choice and organizational determinants of state mental health expenditure patterns. *Administration and Policy in Mental Health,* 19(4):235–250, 1992.

State of neglect; California's 30-year failure to confront mental illness. Editorial, *The San Francisco Chronicle,* February 18, 2001, p. A22.

Sudders M. Commitment law won't help the mentally ill. *Boston Globe,* June 12, 2002, p. A23.

Torrey EF, Zdanowicz M. State's failure to protect its own. *Baltimore Sun,* March 16, 2000, p. 17A.

U.S. Department of Health and Human Services. *Mental Health: A Report of the Surgeon General.* Rockville, MD: Center for Mental Health Services, Substance Abuse and Mental Health Services Administration, National Institute of Mental Health, National Institutes of Health, 1999.

5

The Recovery Movement: Consumers, Families, and the Mental Health System

SHARON GREEN-HENNESSY
KEVIN D. HENNESSY

In the United States approximately 9% of adults, and a comparable number of children and adolescents, are estimated to have a mental illness with accompanying functional impairment (U.S. Department of Health and Human Services [HHS], 1999). While the direct and indirect financial costs of these illnesses to society are considerable (Kessler and Frank, 1997; HHS, 1999), the emotional costs to the persons so diagnosed and to their family and friends can be overwhelming (Druss et al., 2000; Felker et al., 1996; Harrison et al., 2001; Marsh and Johnson, 1997; Tennakoon et al., 2000). Unfortunately, the psychiatric symptoms experienced by individuals with mental illness represent only part of their difficulties. They also face a society that often reacts to these symptoms with fear and discrimination, a culture that traditionally has not respected their rights and has limited their opportunities, and a mental health system that at times has undermined the very healing it attempts to promote (Chamberlin, 1990; Link et al., 1999; Marsh, 2000; Wahl, 1999).

To meet these challenges, the concept of *recovery* has assumed increasing relevance and force. This began with the writings of consumers and "survivors" of mental health treatment (Anonymous, 1989; Deegan, 1988; Houghton, 1982; Leete, 1989). Anthony (1993, p. 15) described recovery as "a way of living a satisfying, hopeful, and contributing life even with the limitations caused by illness" and wrote that recovery "involves the development of new meaning and purpose in one's life as one grows beyond the catastrophic effects of mental illness" (p. 15). While the concept of recovery has been difficult to define and to measure (Ralph et al., 2002), it has provided a simple yet powerful vision and framework that consumers and other stakeholders have used to begin the process of transforming mental health systems in the United States.

The shared vision of recovery has led to the development of a *recovery movement* that raises awareness about the potential of those with mental illness and the ways in which current attitudes and treatment practices may inhibit this potential. The recovery movement has set as its defining goal nothing less than the ability to profoundly alter the lives of those touched by mental illness. In order to achieve this objective, a transformation of how those with mental disorders, their families, mental health professionals, and society view mental illness is required. By changing views toward mental illness, movement supporters are seeking parallel changes in treatments and in personal and professional opportunities for those with these disorders. Although the recovery movement has made significant progress toward these goals, a lack of consensus on key issues among numerous stakeholders (consumers, advocates, family, mental health professionals, governmental agencies, etc.) has hindered it (Fischer et al., 2002; Jacobson and Greenley, 2001; McLean, 1995). This chapter provides an overview of how the recovery movement has evolved, and discusses the challenges that must be addressed if the movement is to succeed in transforming both the lives of those with mental illnesses and their families, and the system that attempts to address their varied needs and aspirations.

Background

Factors Leading to the Recovery Movement

Several aspects of both the societal and treatment environments appeared to have been an impetus in the formation of the recovery movement. On a societal level, the role of stigma has been dominant, with the mentally ill having been portrayed as violent, ineffective, or the object of ridicule (Bryne, 1997, 2000; HHS, 1999; Link et al., 1999). The impact of such depictions has been significant, with denial of employment, housing, insurance, and educational opportunities having been reported by those with mental illness (Wahl, 1999). Additionally, internalization of such negative views has the potential to alter self-concept, perhaps shedding light on the associations of such stigma with decreased self-esteem (Link et al., 2001) and increased avoidance and isolation (Perlick et al., 2001).

Aspects of the treatment system itself have been attributed as giving rise to consumers' wish for reform. A history of physical and human rights abuses necessitated a variety of legal mandates to provide minimum levels of protection to individuals in psychiatric hospitals (Welsh and Deahl, 2002). Additionally, the relative dominance of the medical model was seen by some to increase patient passivity, given its emphasis on the provider as the "expert" who determines the treatment course and patient as recipient of the professional's direction (Kent and Read, 1998; McCubbin and Cohen, 1996). Disparity between patients' and provider's goals created tension, most notably in cases where the professional perceived the individual's logical capacity to act in his or her best interest had been compromised.

This hierarchical treatment approach has been characterized by some of its recepients in terms ranging from benevolent paternalism to abusive (Munetz and
Frese, 2001; Pellegrino, 1994; Rubenstein, 1986; Stricker, 2000).

Lastly, consumers reacted to the prognoses attached to certain disorders, and
the treatment courses those beliefs implied. Historically, the dominant clinical doc-
trine for schizophrenia was that of an invariably negative course and an extremely
limited ability to lead a meaningful and fulfilling life (Basserman, 1997; Frese and
Walker, 1997). Although not well supported by research at the time, such clinical
"truths" served as the basis for well-meaning advice to patients to lower their expectations, accept their limitations, and avoid challenges for fear of relapse (Anthony, 2000; Glass and Arnkoff, 2000; Marsh, 2000; Mead and Copeland, 2000;
Wahl, 1999). Although mental health professionals were often motivated by a desire to protect the patient from more hurt and harm, individuals with mental illness report that they often experienced such efforts as patronizing, limiting, and
unduly bleak (Wahl, 1999).

Early Efforts Promoting Recovery

In response to these perceptions and limitations, organizations emerged to advocate for and protect persons with mental illness. The forerunner of these groups,
created in 1909, was the National Mental Health Association (NMHA). This organization's constituency and efforts have been broad, but with a special emphasis on primary prevention and garnering additional resources for mental health
(Havel, 1992; HHS, 1999; Lefley, 1996). However, although NMHA played a crucial role in early reform, the recovery movement developed primarily in the past
50 years, when several emerging factors provided an opportunity for more extensive change.

In the second half of the twentieth century, groups previously without a voice
(e.g., African Americans and women) were able to advance their quest for basic
human rights and increased opportunities (Rubenstein, 1986). In parallel with these
groups, individuals with mental illness reacted against their status as second-class
citizens and against the marked abuses of the mental health system. Like the other
societal movements, this protest spawned various militant groups, such as the Mental Patients' Liberation Project and the Insane Liberation Front (Lefley, 1996), as
well as legal challenges to the system. With respect to the latter, the Mental Health
Law Project was formed in 1972 to decrease abuses in institutions and provide disabled children access to the educational system (Lefley, 1996).

The quest for self-determination among individuals with mental illness gained
momentum in other ways as well. Medications were now able to provide better
symptom control and enhance functionality (Grob, 2001; HHS, 1999). Outcome
data on what had been considered progressively incapacitating mental illnesses indicated that such an unconditionally negative prognosis was not justified (Harding et al., 1987). It became clear that it is possible to function well despite having
a mental illness—a realization echoed in the increasing number of first-person
accounts of individuals with satisfying and successful lives despite their illnesses
(Anthony, 2000; Deegan, 1988; Leete, 1989). This knowledge, together with de-

institutionalization's promise of an opportunity to start anew in the community, produced a sense of hopefulness about the future among persons with mental illness (Havel, 1992).

Deinstitutionalization has fueled the recovery movement in other ways as well. By failing to ensure widespread adequate community supports and programs necessary for successful community reintegration, it left many families as primary caregivers of their ill relative (Solomon, 1996). The need for assistance and support among these overburdened families spurred the development in 1979 of the National Alliance for the Mentally Ill (NAMI), an influential advocacy and support group founded by families with a mentally ill member (Havel, 1992). Moreover, the scarcity of organized community-based treatment led consumers to seek alternative sources of care such as self-help groups, some of which later became advocates for their members (Havel, 1992; Lefley, 1996). Self-help groups not only supplemented limited mental health resources, but also provided support for individuals who were confronted by the increased social stigma that accompanied their influx into communities (Arens, 1993; Havel, 1992).

More recently, the advent of managed care has altered the traditional provider–patient relationship, leading to greater input by recipients of treatment and their families. First, some have speculated that changing the financial availability of services also has increased the use of self-help groups (Murray, 1996), so that those with mental illness are not solely dependent on mental health professionals for support. Second, with its emphasis on utilization review, managed care exerts an influence on treatment goals and strategies, thereby increasing the influence that non-providers have in treatment decisions. Third managed care favors the use of varied providers from different disciplines, some of which are perceived by service recepients and their families as being more receptive to their input (Hammond et al., 1999; Sturm et al., 1996; Tessler et al., 1991). These different trends have allowed service recipients and families increasingly to voice their views and preferences about treatment.

At present, the recovery movement may be characterized as evolving. The continued growth of mental health consumer and family organizations such as NMHA and NAMI has fostered greater attention to a range of mental health advocacy issues, including the general principles and goals of recovery. In addition, the emergence of associations representing specific disorders, such as the Anxiety Disorders Association of America and the National Depressive and Manic-Depressive Association, has helped individuals with these illnesses to confront stigmatizing attitudes and discriminatory behaviors and policies that inhibit recovery. Moreover, support for recovery, and greater consumer participation and involvement in all facets of mental health policy and service delivery, have led to a variety of recent advances, including the creation of mental health consumer affairs offices within both federal and state governments; the expansion of community-based treatments and other services that promote engagement and recovery; government support for consumer self-help technical assistance centers and other consumer-directed and peer-support services; and development of a wide range of publications and other resource materials that facilitates both individual and system efforts to achieve and sustain recovery from mental illness (Center for Mental Health

Services, 2002). Nevertheless, despite this progress, relevant stakeholders continue to disagree about the purpose and goals of the recovery movement.

Elements of Recovery and Contrasting Visions of Reform

As previously noted, a central goal of the recovery movement is to transform the lives of the mentally ill. On this goal, all stakeholders are in agreement. There is also consensus that for this goal to be achieved, societal and professional perspectives, policies, and programs must change. However, there is substantial disagreement about *what* changes should be made to these perspectives, policies, and programs and *how* best to go about making them. Although concordance among the relevant groups is theoretically possible, it has not been achieved (Salzer et al., 2001).

Arguably, a better understanding of where the groups depart from one another is a prerequisite to attempts to promote greater unification. Hence, we now turn our attention to the *what* and *how* of reform.

Recovery

The term *recovery* has various meanings because it represents different things to different people (Blanch et al., 1993; HHS, 1999; Jacobson and Greenley, 2001). Nevertheless, virtually all definitions agree that recovery is not synonymous with *cure*. Whereas cure implies the remission of symptoms and a return to normal functioning, recovery is not defined by symptom levels or adherence to the norm, but rather represents a broad view of the whole person. Jacobson and Greenley (2001) have presented a model of what they believe to be the crucial elements in recovery. A number of these key concepts are echoed by others in the recovery movement (Blanch et al., 1993; Davidson and Strauss, 1992; Frese and Davis, 1997; Mead and Copeland, 2000)

Hope

Hope is defined as the belief that it is possible to achieve a fulfilling, meaningful life despite having mental illness (Jacobson and Greenley, 2001). It is an optimistic, strength-based belief that emphasizes the ability of individuals to determine their own life course (Jacobson and Greenley, 2001; Marsh, 2000). Many believe it to be the most crucial factor in recovery (Blanch et al., 1993; Leete, 1989; Marsh, 2000), as it is the lens through which all else is viewed, as well as being "what sustains during periods of relapse and creates possibilities" (Jacobson and Greenley, 2001, p. 483).

As Jacobson and Greenley (2001) suggest, hope fuels an individual's wishes and expectations about what might be possible. That people with mental illness should have aspirations appears not to be in dispute; however, how high those aspirations should be is controversial. How much hope is beneficial, and at what point does it devolve into unrealistic expectations?

Some in the recovery movement contend that "A vision of hope includes *no lim-its*" (Mead and Copeland, 2000, p. 317). This attitude can be perceived as a response to the negative prognoses given to some individuals by providers (Bassman, 1997; Frese and Walker, 1997). Others continue to advance the long-standing argument that such unmitigated optimism is tantamount to "setting up" the person with mental illness in that a failure to achieve extraordinarily ambitious goals will constitute a major setback (Caldwell and Jorm, 2001). It is interesting that this current conflict mirrors somewhat Grob's (2001) description of a pattern of alternating between fatalistic pessimism and unbridled optimism that has characterized mental health treatment in the United States during the past two centuries.

The issue of living independently provides an example of the schism between consumers and other system stakeholders about aspirations. One aspiration of many persons with mental illness is to live more independently (Davidson and Hoge, 1996; Fischer et al., 202; Tanzman, 1993). Studies have indicated that consumers and their family members do not have this same optimistic goal, with family members preferring more restrictive housing alternatives for consumers than either those desired or those representing the current norm (Friedrich et al., 1999; Rogers et al., 1994). In sum, other relevant stakeholders do not always share the vision of hope with no limits.

A Positive Culture of Healing

Managed care, patients' rights legislation and lawsuits, consumer and family advocacy, and diminished adherence to the medical model have all altered the provider–service recipient relationship. The recovery movement believes that such changes may eventually result in "a positive culture of healing" (Jacobson and Greenley, 2001, p. 484) involving a respectful, collaborative relationship between providers and care recipients (Chinman et al., 1999). Research indicating that greater input from service recipients is associated with positive mental health outcomes (Roth and Crane-Ross, 2002) supports this concept. Mead and Copeland (2000) state that consumers "need a caring environment without feeling the need to be taken care of" (p. 317). They believe that to create such a therapeutic environment, mental health providers must be willing to question the assumptions learned in their training.

In general, current clinical training teaches providers that they *are* responsible for using their unique knowledge and skills to serve the best interests of those they treat—in essence, to practice by the principle of beneficence (McCubbin and Cohen, 1996; Pellegrino, 1994). However, an important distinction must be made between beneficence and paternalism. A desire to act in the patient's best interest does not mean assuming what those best interests are (Pellegrino, 1994). By and large, providers work to help individuals with mental illness to increase their self-determination in various aspects of life, both within and outside the treatment setting (Pellegrino, 1994). In fact, the majority of service recipients and their families are satisfied with the services provided by mental health professionals and report that they have a say in how their treatment is structured (Moutoussis et al., 2000; Stengard et al., 2000).

In several circumstances, however, the clinical relationship may inhibit autonomy. The first of these can occur when providers exercise too much control in the therapeutic relationship and impose their own values by unilaterally acting in what they believe to be the patient's best interests. This assumes that the provider can discern what is in the patient's best interest, a task that may be particularly difficult without seeking the patient's direct input (McCubbin and Cohen, 1996).

The second circumstance is more pervasive and likely includes the first. Despite increased awareness of service recipients' autonomy and rights, vestiges of the earlier hierarchical, even autocratic, treatment system remain (Kent and Read, 1998). As noted by Blanche et al. (1993, p. 17), "In the field of medicine, discussion between doctors and patients on how they can best collaborate in dealing with a particular illness has not generally been the norm."

The third issue is the thorniest. In certain cases, the patient's choices are not honored because of concerns regarding competency. A conflict appears to arise between the patient's self-determination and the provider's responsibility to practice in accordance with the principle of beneficence.

Many within the recovery movement contend that an individual has the right to make his or her own choices unless they directly conflict with the law (Chamberlin, 1998). They argue that self-determination is a right that individuals with mental illness should not be denied (Chamberlin, 1998). Moreover, autonomy is seen as a positive, even fundamental, element in the ability to recover (Bassman, 1997; Nelson and Berkovec, 1989; Roth and Crane-Ross, 2002). Self-determination can increase self-efficacy, as well as responsibility and accompanying self-awareness regarding one's decision (Davidson and Strauss, 1992; Jacobson and Greenley, 2001). Hence, in terms of both human rights and therapeutic implications, some in the recovery movement believe that the patient's choices must be respected, even if a provider feels that they are contrary to the patient's best interests (Jacobson and Greenley, 2001). From this perspective, the provider is never justified in substituting his or her judgment for that of the patient.

In contrast, other clinicians argue that what limits a person's self-determination is not the provider's actions but the illness itself. The external restraints (e.g., involuntary hospitalization) the mental health professional imposes are designed to restore the individual's autonomy, allowing for choices that reflect the person and not the illness (Peyser, 2001). From this perspective, to let an individual with markedly impaired competency make choices with potentially significant negative repercussions is tantamount to professional abandonment (Munetz and Freese, 2001). To allow that person to choose a potentially dangerous course of action is to provide autonomy in name but not in spirit (Pellegrino, 1994).

A third perspective between these two extremes has emerged. Munetz and Frese (2001) argue that while not all individuals with mental illness should be assumed incapable of making their own decisions, some are in fact significantly impaired. The authors contend that treatment should be provided in these latter cases, even against the individual's wishes. However, they also believe that control over the treatment process should be returned to the individual with mental illness as that person recovers. They also maintain that a number of safeguards should be put in place to facilitate this transition, including appointing a recovering consumer as a guardian and having a regular capacity review panel composed of a consumer, a family member, and a mental health professional.

Stigma/Self-Definition

The recovery movement's mission includes the reduction of stigma and its effects (Chamberlin, 1997; Link et al., 2001; Perlick et al., 2001; Struening et al., 2001; Wahl, 1999). Efforts to increase the public's knowledge and understanding, as well as decrease insensitivity and discrimination, are perceived as fundamental to altering the day-to-day reality of those with mental illness and their families. There appears to be a consensus on the goal of increasing public understanding of mental illness through an awareness of its causes. However, the controversy centers on *what* view of the etiology of mental illness is to be advanced, with the answer to this question having broader implications.

One view, espoused by organized psychiatry and NAMI, is that mental illnesses are physical disorders of the brain. As such, they are no different from other physical disorders (e.g., cancer, diabetes), and therefore etiological attributions of "bad parenting" or "bringing it on oneself" do not apply (Corrigan et al., 2000). Although promoting this biological view of mental illness has increased funding for mental illness and facilitated efforts to secure parity in insurance coverage (NAMI, 2002), there are those in the recovery movement who strongly feel that the negative effects of emphasizing the biological causes of mental illness outweigh the benefits of this approach.

Some consumers and professionals who examine the sociology of stigma maintain that a strong emphasis on the biological origins of mental illness damages consumers' self concept, diminishes hope, impairs their ability to have a collaborative relationship with providers, and actually increases stigma (Donahue, 2000; Kent and Read, 1998; Phelan, 2002; Read and Law, 1999). These authors argue that emphasizing the biological origins of mental illness labels the person with mental illness as defective, implying that the person can do little to remedy the situation and must rely on medical professionals to do so (Kent and Read, 1998; McCubbin and Cohen, 1996; Phelan, 2002). Blanch et al. (1993, p. 19) describes "a patient who stated: 'I've learned that I have a biological disease and until you [the psychiatrist] find a cure, I'm not going anywhere.'" Phelan (2002) further contends that an emphasis on the biological/genetic etiology of mental illness actually increases some forms of stigma for both consumers and their families. She suggests that a public focus on the biological/genetic causes of mental illness might result in family members, by virtue of their genetic association with their ill relative, being perceived as "carriers" of the illness. These so-called carriers might face problems regarding insurability, and (given the biological nature of the disorder) their potential partners might hesitate to have children (Phelan, 2002).

Self-Help Groups

Self-help groups provide an opportunity to operationalize the recovery movements' goal of providing a sense of connectedness while altering consumers' self-

perception, allowing them to see themselves as providers of help, not just as recipients of help (Jacobson and Greenley, 2001; Mead and Copeland, 2000). Self-
help groups have assisted those with mental illness to reach this goal. These groups
have been shown to improve psychosocial adjustment (Roberts et al., 1999), foster treatment gains (Gould and Clum, 1993), and increase empowerment (Segal
and Silverman, 2002), as well as improve coping among family members who participate in support groups for relatives (Solomon and Draine, 1995). Concerns have
been raised about whether some self-help groups (e.g., Alcoholics Anonymous)
discourage compliance with medication regimens, but these concerns appear to be
largely unfounded (Lewis, 2000; Magura et al., 2002; Meissen et al., 1999).

What remains a concern is the role of self-help groups in the treatment process.
It has been argued that these groups have been largely ignored by clinicians because
of a lack of awareness and an inherent bias toward the services offered by professionals (Davison et al., 2000; Salzer et al., 1999). In fact, some have gone so far as
to say that mental health professionals do not consider self-help to be "serious"
treatment, but rather "as mere inexpensive, naïve adjuncts to therapy—hand-hold-
ing, morale-boosting, do-no-harm meetings of fellow suffers" (Jacobs and Goodman, 1989, p. 536). This may explain in part why relatively few self-help group
participants report learning about the group from a mental health provider, and
among those who do, there is a significant delay before receiving this information
from providers (Lewis, 2000; Looper et al., 1998; Powell et al., 2000).

Many individuals access both self-help and professional interventions. Segal and
colleagues (2002) found that 55% of new users of self-help programs were concurrently receiving care through community mental health agencies. Both crisis
management and stabilization services were emphasized in the mental health agencies, which provided interventions for individuals with acute symptoms. In contrast, self-help programs focused on long-term maintenance and socialization services, reflecting their members' greater self-efficacy and hopefulness about the
future. These results suggest that individuals regularly access both types of care,
as each option addresses unique needs and, further, that self-help groups are a necessary component of the larger array of available services.

Whereas self-help groups emphasize mutual benefit among members, consumer-
provided services are more unidirectional, with consumers themselves providing
treatment (e.g., as a direct provider or manager of program operations). Although
less research exists on this service provision model (HHS, 1999; Solomon and
Draine, 2001), its legitimate place among treatment options has been the focus of
debate (Dixon et al., 1994; Fox and Hilton, 1994; Haiman, 1995; Solomon, 1994;
Stephens and Belisle, 1993).

Family

Marsh and Johnson (1997) have articulated the profound impact of mental illness
on family members, ranging from its emotional toll to its increased objective burden. The need for families to receive psychoeducational and supportive services
has been well documented (Lehman and Steinwachs, 1998). Nevertheless, family

members report dissatisfaction with the psychoeducation/support services typically available to them, as well as the extent to which they are integrated into the patient's care.

Interventions for family members of an individual with mental illness help to avoid rehospitalization, reduce symptoms, decrease the burden on relatives, and improve family functioning (Cuijpers, 1999; Dyck et al., 2000; Falloon et al., 1985; Hogarty et al., 1986; Leff et al., 2000; Mueser et al., 2001). Yet despite their effectiveness, few relatives receive such services (Dixon et al., 1999b). Family members' concerns regarding the benefit they will derive from the programs, in light of potential transportation and scheduling problems, have been cited as a partial explanation (Dixon et al., 2001; Gasque-Carter and Curlee, 1999). However, the reaction of other stakeholders appears equally if not more influential in the accessibility of family services. Consumer concerns regarding treatment autonomy, as well as high provider caseloads and nonsystemic psychopathology models, appear to reduce the frequency of family interventions. In addition, a lack of funding for and reimbursement of professional family interventions can lead mental health professionals to conceptualize family-oriented services as a "luxury" (Dixon et al., 1999a, 2001; Wright, 1997). Even when offered services, relatives often find that they provide little emotional support and practical information (Solomon et al., 1998). Hence, an intervention for one group of stakeholders has not been prioritized by others.

A related issue is the integration of family members into the relative's treatment. Family members often have difficulty receiving specific information relevant to care. This difficulty appears to stem in part from consumers' concerns regarding confidentiality and treatment autonomy (Dixon et al., 2001; Philips, 1998). Family members also feel somewhat constrained by mental health professionals in this regard (Biegel et al., 1995; Marshall and Solomon, 2000; Solomon and Marcenko, 1992). In a survey of community mental health clinicians treating persons with serious mental illness, 60% of therapists reported contact with a family member in the previous year. The majority of providers felt satisfied with their level of contact with family members, which typically consisted of brief telephone contacts primarily during times of crisis (Dixon et al., 2000). Although clinicians may feel satisfied with the level of contact, family members do not (Bernheim and Switalski, 1988; Marsh and Johnson, 1997; Marshall and Solomon, 2000). Their quest for additional information often creates a dilemma for clinicians who wish to respect the consumer's autonomy and abide by confidentiality statutes (Bogart and Solomon, 1999). Families have increasingly advocated for clarity about confidentiality laws, challenged providers' interpretation of such laws as being excessively rigid, and suggested alternative means of sharing information (e.g., providers having consumers sign release of information forms, identifying a member of the professional staff to serve as a liason with relatives). These efforts have loosely been termed making services more *family-friendly* (Bogart and Solomon, 1999; DiRienzo-Callahan, 1998; Mannion et al., 2001; Marsh and Johnson, 1997; Mueser and Fox, 2000). Tension appears to have emerged among all stakeholders because the legitimate goals of each conflict with one another.

Empowerment/Advocacy

Nowhere is the lack of consensus within the recovery movement greater than in the realm of empowerment and advocacy. The lack of agreement on such basics as what terminology to use appears to be due to the fundamental issue of who speaks for whom and, perhaps even more broadly, who speaks for the recovery movement.

To begin, the term *empowerment* has different meanings for the various members of the recovery movement. Although most acknowledge that it "connotes a process by which individuals of lesser power gain control over their lives" (Segal et al., 1995, p. 215), the complexity of the concept leads to discrepant interpretations of what this process entails. One conceptualization emphasizes self-determination, a second prioritizes enacting fundamental change at organizational and political levels, and a third focuses on providing skills to enable specific persons to achieve a variety of goals, in essence improving their self-efficacy (McLean, 1995; Rappaport, 1985; Segal et al., 1995). Each definition suggests a different course of action be used to attain the goal of empowerment.

Family members of those with mental illness, whose efforts are organized through such organizations as NAMI, have enacted a form of empowerment that focuses on political change. In contrast, mental health practitioners have largely seen their role as providing the skills and opportunities to help individuals exercise control over life decisions (McLean, 1995). Thus, the provider perspective is largely consistent with the third definition of empowerment noted above, while the family perspective exemplifies the second definition.

Individuals with mental illness have emphasized the first definition of empowerment, equating it with control over one's destiny. However, even within this group, differing notions of self-determination and how best to obtain it are crucial, and have led to schisms among individuals with mental illness. Individuals who identify themselves as *consumers* often focus on increasing their choices, and the majority have chosen to work for change within the current mental health system. This contrasts to the approaches used by both ex-patients and survivors. *Ex-patients* refer to themselves as such because they maintain that the term *consumer* implies a level of choice in interactions with the mental health system that contradicts their own experiences, whereas *survivors* describe themselves as having persevered despite victimization by the mental health system (Stricker, 2000). Ex-patients and survivors state that empowerment cannot be transmitted from provider to patient through some form of intervention; rather, empowerment requires commitment and effort by individuals with mental illness to design and implement what they need to promote their own healing (Segal et al., 1995; Zimmerman and Warschausky, 1998). As such, survivors and ex-patients do not seek to work within the established mental health system; instead, they emphasize the desire and ability to make changes at a larger systems or societal level.

Such differences in the conceptualization of empowerment, underscore the multifaceted goals of the recovery movement and dissonant methods employed to achieve them. Is the problem that individuals with mental illness do not have enough control over their own treatment and lives? Or does the ability to make good choices need to be addressed first, so that self-determination becomes realistic and feasible? Where does change need to occur—in society, in the mental health system, and/or within the stakeholders themselves? Is it possible to modify preexisting institutions or do fundamental flaws exist that necessitate abolition of these institutions and creation of new ones? The answers to these questions appear to differ among various stakeholders within the recovery movement.

Fischer and colleagues (2002) conducted a survey of 60 stakeholder sets. A *set* was defined as consisting of a person with mental illness and both a family member and a treatment provider for that person. A *stakeholder* refers to all members of a given class (e.g., all family members). The authors found low rates of agreement among members of a set when asked to rank outcomes and service priorities. More important was their finding that agreement was greater among *types* of stakeholders than it was among members within a given *set*. For example, a provider's priorities corresponded more closely to those held by other providers for *different cases* than they did to the priorities of the service recipient and his or her family member. The same pattern held for family members and individuals with mental illness. In essence, one's viewpoint corresponds closely to one's own stakeholder group, and not to other stakeholder groups who are also ostensibly working to advance recovery. The ability of the recovery movement to influence key issues such as those previously noted may depend primarily on the degree to which various stakeholders can reach greater consensus regarding the *what* and *how* of reform (Emmet, 1998).

Implications for Mental Health Services

The concept of recovery and the movement to advance recovery principles as an organizing vision and framework for mental health systems have taken root with remarkable speed. In many respects, Anthony's (1993) assertion that the 1990s would represent the "decade of recovery" has largely been confirmed. Increasingly, both public and private mental health systems have begun to organize financing and service delivery activities in ways that are consistent with a vision of recovery (Anthony, 2000; Ralph et al., 2002). In fact, virtually all state mental health authorities now provide some funding for recovery-based services, and many target resources specifically to consumer-operated and peer-support services (National Association of State Mental Health Program Director's Research Institute, 2002). Perhaps most notably, whereas two decades ago the concept of recovery was barely identified in the professional literature, validation of the recovery vision and support for recovery-based services are fully evident in both the Surgeon General's *Mental Health* report (U.S. DHHS, 1999) and the *Final Report* of the President's New Freedom Mental Health Commission (2003), arguably the two most important and influential mental health documents produced in recent years.

Despite this recognition and progress, a great deal of work remains if the recovery movement is to succeed in transforming the lives of individuals with mental illness. Continued efforts to combat stigma and increase access to treatment are necessary to facilitate recovery. In addition, more attention must be devoted to identifying and measuring fundamental elements of recovery so that best practices for promoting hope and healing among those with mental illness can be developed and advanced. But perhaps most important, various stakeholders must agree to engage with one another in achieving greater consensus on the *what* and *how* of reform to ensure that the initial gains made by the recovery movement become lasting and indelible features that guide mental health services and systems of the future.

REFERENCES

Anonymous. How I've managed chronic mental illness. *Schizophrenia Bulletin,* 15:635–640, 1989.

Anthony WA. Recovery from mental illness: the guiding vision of the mental health service system in the 1990s. *Psychosocial Rehabilitation Journal,* 16(4):11–23, 1993.

Anthony WA. A recovery-oriented service system: setting some system level standards. *Psychiatric Rehabilitation Journal,* 24(2):159–168, 2000.

Arens DA. What do the neighbors think now? Community residences on Long Island, New York. *Community Mental Health Journal,* 29(3):235–245, 1993.

Bassman R. The mental health system: experiences from both sides of the locked doors. *Professional Psychology: Research and Practice,* 28(3):238–242, 1997.

Bernheim KF, Switalski T. Mental health staff and patient's relatives: how they view each other. *Hospital and Community Psychiatry,* 39(1):63–68, 1988.

Biegel DE, Song L, Milligan SE. A comparative analysis of family caregivers' perceived relationships with mental health professions. *Psychiatric Services,* 46(5):477–482, 1995.

Blanche A, Fisher D, Tucker W, et al. Consumer-practitioners and psychiatrists share insights about recovery and coping. *Disability Studies Quarterly,* 13(2):17–20, 1993.

Bogart T, Solomon P. Procedures to share treatment information among mental health providers, consumers, and families. *Psychiatric Services,* 50(10):1321–1325, 1999.

Bryne P. Psychiatric stigma: past, passing and to come. *Journal of the Royal Society of Medicine,* 90:618–620, 1997.

Bryne P. Stigma of mental illness and ways of diminishing it. *Advances in Psychiatric Treatment,* 6(1):65–72, 2000.

Caldwell TM, Jorm AF. Mental health nurses beliefs about likely outcomes for people with schizophrenia or depression: a comparison with the public and other healthcare professionals. *Austrailian and New Zealand Journal of Mental Health Nursing,* 10:42–54, 2001.

Center for Mental Health Services. *Featured Publications.* Available at: www.mental-health.org/consumersurvivor/publications.asp Accessed November 19, 2002.

Chamberlin J. The ex-patients' movement: where we've been and where we're going. *The Journal of Mind and Behavior,* 11(3):323–336, 1990.

Chamberlin J. A working definition of empowerment. *Psychiatric Rehabilitation Journal,* 20(4):43–46, 1997.

Chamberlin J. Citizenship rights and psychiatric disability. *Psychiatric Rehabilitation Journal,* 21(4):405–408, 1998.

Chinman MJ, Allende M, Weingarten R et al. On the road to collaborative treatment planning: Consumers and providers perspectives. *Journal of Behavioral Health Services & Research,* 26(2):211–218, 1999.

Corrigan PW, Philip RL, Lundin RK, et al. Stigmatizing attributions about mental illness. *Journal of Community Psychology*, 28(1):91–102, 2000.

Cuijpers P. The effects of family interventions on relatives' burden: a meta-analysis. *Journal of Mental Health*, 8(3):275–285, 1999.

Davidson L, Hoge MA. Hospital or community living? Examining consumer perspectives on deinstitutionalization. *Psychiatric Rehabilitation Journal*, 19(3):49–57, 1996.

Davidson L, Strauss JS. Sense of self in recovery from severe mental illness. *British Journal of Medical Psychology*, 65:131–145, 1992.

Davison KP, Pennebaker JW, Dickerson SS. Who talks? The social psychology of illness support groups. *American Psychologist*, 55(2):205–217, 2000.

Deegan PE. Recovery: the lived experience of rehabilitation. *Psychosocial Rehabilitation Journal*, 11(4):11–19, 1988.

DiRienzo-Callahan C. Family caregivers and confidentiality. *Psychiatric Services*, 49(2):244–245, 1998.

Dixon L, Krauss N, Lehman A. Consumers as service providers: the promise and challenge. *Community Mental Health Journal*, 30(6):615–625, 1994.

Dixon L, Lucksted A, Stewart B, et al. Therapists' contacts with family members of persons with severe mental illness in a community treatment program. *Psychiatric Services*, 51(11):1449–1451, 2000.

Dixon L, Goldman H, Hirad A. State policy and funding of services to families of adults with serious and persistent mental illness. *Psychiatric Services*, 50(4):551–553, 1999a.

Dixon L, Lyles A, Scott J, et al. Services to families of adults with schizophrenia: from treatment recommendations to dissemination. *Psychiatric Services*, 50(2):233–238, 1999b.

Dixon L, McFarlane WR, Lefley H, et al. Evidence-based practices for services to families of people with psychiatric disabilities. *Psychiatric Services*, 52(7):903–910, 2001.

Donahue AB. Riding the mental health pendulum: mixed messages in the era of neurobiology and self-help movements. *Social Work*, 45(5):427–438, 2000.

Druss BG, Marcus SC, Rosenheck RA, et al. Understanding disability in mental and general medical conditions. *American Journal of Psychiatry*, 157(9):1485–1491, 2000.

Dyck DG, Short RA, Hendryx MS, et al. Management of negative symptoms among patients with schizophrenia attending multiple-family groups. *Psychiatric Services*, 51(4):513–519, 2000.

Emmet W. A family advocate's reply: why consumers and family advocates must work together. *Psychiatric Services*, 49(6):764–765, 1998.

Falloon JR, Boyd JL, McGill CW, et al. Family management in the prevention of of morbidity of schizophrenia: Clinical outcome of a two-year longitudinal study. *Archives of General Psychiatry*, 42(9):887–896, 1985.

Felker B, Yazel JJ, Short D. Mortality and medical comorbidity among psychiatric patients. *Psychiatric Services*, 47(12):1356–1363, 1996.

Fischer EP, Shumway M, Owen RR. Priorities of consumers, providers, and family members in the treatment of schizophrenia. *Psychiatric Services*, 53(6):724–729, 2002.

Fox L, Hilton D. Response to "Consumers as service providers: the promise and challenge." *Community Mental Health Journal*, 30(6):627–629, 1994.

Frese FJ, Davis WW. The consumer-survivor movement, recovery, and consumer professionals. *Professional Psychology: Research and Practice*, 28(3):243–245, 1997.

Friedrich RM, Hollingsworth B, Hradek E, et al. Family and client perspectives on alternative residential settings for persons with severe mental illness. *Psychiatric Services*, 50(4):509–514, 1999.

Gasque-Carter KO, Curlee MB. The educational needs of families of mentally ill adults: the South Carolina experience. *Psychiatric Services*, 50(4):520–524, 1999.

Glass CR, Arnkoff DB. Consumers' perspectives on helpful and hindering factors in mental health treatment. *JCLP/In Session: Psychotherapy in Practice*, 56(11):1467–1480, 2000.

Gould RA, Clum GA. A meta-analysis of self-help treatment approaches. *Clinical Psychology Review*, 13(2):169–186, 1993.

Grob GN. Mental health policy in 20th-century America. In: Manderscheid RW, Henderson MJ (eds). *Mental Health, United States, 2000*. DHHS Pub. No. (SMA) 01-3537. Washington, DC: Superintendent of Documents, U.S. Government Printing Office, pp. 3–14, 2001.

Haiman S. Dilemmas in professional collaboration with consumers. *Psychiatric Services*, 46(5):443–445, 1995.

Hammond K, Bandak A, Williams M. Nurse, physician, and consumer role responsibility perceived by health care providers. *Holistic Nursing Practice*, 13(2):28–37, 1999.

Harding CM, Brooks GW, Ashikaga T, et al. The Vermont longitudinal study of persons with severe mental illness. I. Methodology, study sample, and overall status 32 years later. *American Journal of Psychiatry*, 144(6):718–726, 1987.

Harrison G, Hopper K, Craig T et al. Recovery from psychotic illness: a 15- and 25-year international follow-up study. *British Journal of Psychiatry*, 178:506–517, 2001.

Havel JT. Associations and public interest groups as advocates. *Administration and Policy in Mental Health*, 20(1):27–44, 1992.

Hogarty GE, Anderson CM, Reiss DJ, et al. Family psychoeducation, social skills training, and maintenance chemotherapy in the aftercare of treatment of schizophrenia. I. One-year effects of a controlled study on relapse and expressed emotion. *Archives of General Psychiatry*, 43(7):633–642, 1986.

Houghton JF. Maintaining mental health in a turbulent world. *Schizophrenia Bulletin*, 8(3):548–552, 1982.

Achieving the Promise: Transforming Mental Health Care in America. Washington, DC: Final Report of the President's New Freedom Commission on Mental Health, July 2003.

Jacobs MK, Goodman G. Psychology and self-help groups. Predictions on a partnership. *American Psychologist*, 44(3):536–545, 1989.

Jacobson N, Greenley D. What is recovery? A conceptual model of recovery. *Psychiatric Services*, 52(4):482–485, 2001.

Kent H, Read J. Measuring consumer participation in mental health services: are attitudes related to professional orientation? *International Journal of Social Psychiatry*, 44(4):295–310, 1998.

Kessler RC, Frank RG. The impact of psychiatric disorder on work loss days. *Psychological Medicine*, 27(4):861–873, 1997.

Leete E. How I perceive and manage my illness. *Schizophrenia Bulletin*, 15(2):197–200, 1989.

Leff J, Vearnals S, Brewin CR, et al. The London Depression Intervention Trial: randomized controlled trial of antidepressants vs. couple therapy in the treatment and maintenance of people with depression living with a partner: clinical outcomes and costs. *British Journal of Psychiatry*, 177:95–100, 2000.

Lefley HP. Impact of consumer and family advocacy movements on mental health services. In: Levin BL, Petrila J (eds). *Mental Health Services: A Public Health Perspective*. New York: Oxford University Press, pp. 81–96, 1996.

Lehman AF, Steinwachs DM. Translating research into practice: the Schizophrenia Outcomes Research Team (PORT) treatment recommendations. *Schizophrenia Bulletin*, 24(1):1–10, 1998.

Lewis L. A consumer perspective concerning the diagnosis and treatment of bipolar disorder. *Biological Psychiatry*, 48(6):442–444, 2000.

Link BG, Phelan JC, Bresnahan M et al. Public conceptions of mental illness: labels, causes, dangerousness, and social distance. *American Journal of Public Health*, 89(9):1328–1333, 1999.

Link BG, Struening EL, Neese-Todd S, et al. Stigma as a barrier to recovery: the consequences of stigma for the self-esteem of people with mental illness. *Psychiatric Services*, 52(12):1621–1626, 2001.

Looper K, Fielding A, Latimer E, et al. Improving access to family support organizations: a member survey of the AMI-Quebec Alliance for the Mentally Ill. *Psychiatric Services*, 49(11):1491–1492, 1998.

Magura S, Laudet AB, Mahmood D, et al. Adherence to medication regimens and participation in dual-focus self-help groups. *Psychiatric Services*, 53(3):310–316, 2002.

Mannion E, Solomon P, Steber SA. Implementing family-friendly services. *Psychiatric Services*, 52(3):386–387, 2001.

Marsh DT. Personal accounts of consumer/survivors: insights and implications. *JCLP/In Session: Psychotherapy in Practice*, 56(11):1447–1457, 2000.

Marsh DT, Johnson DL. The family experience of mental illness: implications for treatment. *Professional Psychology: Research and Practice*, 28(3):229–237, 1997.

Marshall TB, Solomon P. Releasing information to families of persons with severe mental illness: a survey of NAMI members. *Psychiatric Services*, 51(8):1006–1011, 2000.

McCubbin M, Cohen D. Extremely unbalanced: interest divergence and power disparities between clients and psychiatry. *International Journal of Law and Psychiatry*, 19(1):1–25, 1996.

McLean A. Empowerment and the psychiatric consumer/ex-patient movement in the United States: contradictions, crisis, and change. *Social Science Medicine*, 40(8):1053–1071, 1995.

Mead S, Copeland ME. What recovery means to us: consumers' perspectives. *Community Mental Health Journal*, 36(3):315–328, 2000.

Meissen G, Powell TJ, Wituk SA, et al. Attitudes of AA contact persons towards group participation by persons with a mental illness. *Psychiatric Services*, 50(8):1079–1081, 1999.

Moutoussis M, Gilmour F, Barker D et al. Quality of care in psychiatric out-patient department. *Journal of Mental Health*, 9(4):409–420, 2000.

Mueser KT, Fox L. Family-friendly services: a modest proposal. *Psychiatric Services*, 51(11):1452, 2000.

Mueser KT, Sengupta A, Schooler NR, et al. Family treatment and medication dosage reduction in schizophrenia: effects on patient social functioning, family attitudes, and burden. *Journal of Consulting and Clinical Psychology*, 69(1):3–12, 2001.

Munetz MR, Frese FJ. Getting ready for recovery: Reconciling mandatory treatment with the recovery vision. *Psychiatric Rehabilitation Journal*, 25(1):35–42, 2001.

Murray P. Recovery, Inc. as an adjunct to treatment in the era of managed care. *Psychiatric Services*, 47(12):1378–1381, 1996.

National Alliance for the Mentally Ill. *Where We Stand*. Available at: www.nami.org/update/wherewestand.html/ Accessed November 19, 2002.

National Association of State Mental Health Program Director's (NASMHPD) Research Institute. *State Profile Reports 2001*. Available at: http://nri.rdmc.org/Profiles01.cfm/ Accessed November 15, 2002.

Nelson RA, Borkovec TD. Relationship of client participation to psychotherapy. *Journal of Behavior Therapy and Experimental Psychiatry*, 20(2):155–162, 1989.

Pellegrino ED. Patient and physician autonomy: conflicting rights and obligations in the physician-patient relationship. *Journal of Contemporary Health and Law Policy*, 10:47–68, 1994.

Perlick DA, Rosenheck RA, Clarkin JF, et al. Stigma as a barrier to recovery: adverse effects of perceived stigma on social adaptation of persons diagnosed with bipolar affective disorder. *Psychiatric Services*, 52(12):1627–1632, 2001.

Peyser H. Commentary: What is recovery? A commentary. *Psychiatric Services*, 52(4):486–487, 2001.

Phelan JC. Genetic bases of mental illness—a cure for stigma? *Trends in Neurosciences*, 25(8):430–431, 2002.

Phillips E. Letter: family advocacy. *Psychiatric Services*, 49(10):1360, 1998.

Powell TJ, Silk KR, Albeck JH. Psychiatrists' referrals to self-help groups for people with mood disorders. *Psychiatric Services*, 51(6):809–811, 2000.

Ralph RO, Lambert D, Kidder KA. *The Recovery Perspective and Evidence-Based Practice for People with Serious Mental Illness*. A guideline developed for the Behavioral Health Recovery Management Project, June 2002.

Rappaport J. The power of empowerment language. *Social Policy*, 16:15–21, 1985.

Read J, Law A. The relationship between causal beliefs and contact with users of mental health services to attitudes to the "mentally ill." *International Journal of Social Psychiatry*, 45(3):216–229, 1999.

Roberts LJ, Salem D, Rappaport J, et al. Giving and receiving help: interpersonal transactions in mutual-help meetings and psychosocial adjustment of members. *American Journal of Community Psychology*, 27(6):841–868, 1999.

Rogers ES, Danely KS, Anthony WA, et al. The residential needs and preferences of persons with serious mental illness: a comparison of consumers and family members. *Journal of Mental Health Administration*, 21(1):42–51, 1994.

Roth D, Crane-Ross D. Impact of services, met needs, and service empowerment on consumer outcomes. *Mental Health Services Research*, 4(1):43–56, 2002.

Rubenstein JD. Treatment of the mentally ill: legal advocacy enters the second generation. *American Journal of Psychiatry*, 143(10):1264–1269, 1986.

Salzer MS, Blank M, Rothbard A, et al. Adult mental health services in the 21st century. In: Manderscheid RW, Henderson MJ (eds). *Mental Health, United States, 2000*. DHHS Pub. No. (SMA) 01-3537. Washington, DC: Superintendent of Documents, U.S. Government Printing Office, pp. 99–112, 2001.

Salzer MS, Rappaport J, Segre L. Professional appraisal of professionally led and self-help groups. *American Journal of Orthopsychiatry*, 69(4):536–540, 1999.

Schlesinger M, Dorwart RA, Epstein SS. Managed care constraints on psychiatrists' hospital practices: bargaining power and professional autonomy. *American Journal of Psychiatry*, 153(2):256–260, 1996.

Segal SP, Hardiman ER, Hodges JQ. Characteristics of new clints at self-help and community mental health agencies in geographical proximity. *Psychiatric Services*, 53(9):1145–1152, 2002

Segal SP, Silverman C. Determinants of client outcomes in self-help agencies. *Psychiatric Services*, 53(3):304–309, 2002.

Segal SP, Silverman C, Temkin T. Measuring empowerment in client-run self-help agencies. *Community Mental Health Journal*, 31(3):215–227, 1995.

Solomon P. Response to "Consumers as service providers: the promise and challenge." *Community Mental Health Journal*, 30(6):631–634, 1994.

Solomon P. Moving from psychoeducation to family education for families of adults with serious mental illness. *Psychiatric Services*, 47(12):1364–1370, 1996.

Solomon P, Draine J. Adaptive coping among family members of person with serious mental illness. *Psychiatric Services,* 46(11):1156–1160, 1995.

Solomon P, Draine J. The state of knowledge of the effectiveness of consumer provided services. *Psychiatric Rehabilitation Journal,* 25(1):20–27, 2001.

Solomon P, Draine J, Mannion E, et al. Increased contact with community mental health resources as a potential benefit of family education. *Psychiatric Services,* 49(3):333–339, 1998.

Solomon P, Marcenko M. Families of adults with severe mental illness: their satisfaction with inpatient and outpatient treatment. *Psychosocial Rehabilitation Journal,* 16(1):121–134, 1992.

Stengard E, Honkonen T, Koivisto AM, et al. Satisfaction of caregivers of patients with schizophrenia in Finland. *Psychiatric Services,* 51(8):1034–1039, 2000.

Stephens CL, Belisle KC. The "consumer-as-provider" initiative. *Journal of Mental Health Administration,* 20(2):178–182, 1993.

Stricker G. Introduction. Listening to the voice of the c/s/x: consumer/survivor/ex-patient. JCLP/In Session: *Psychotherapy in Practice,* 56(11):1389–1394, 2000.

Struening EL, Perlick DA, Link BG, et al. Stigma as a barrier to recovery: the extent to which caregivers believe most people devalue consumers and their families. *Psychiatric Services,* 52(12):1633–1638, 2001.

Sturm R, Meredith LS, Wells KB. Provider choice and continuity for the treatment of depression. *Medical Care,* 34(7):723–734, 1996.

Tanzman B. An overview of surveys of mental health consumers' preferences for housing and support services. *Hospital and Community Psychiatry,* 44(5):450–455, 1993.

Tennakoon L, Fannon D, Doku V, et al. Experience of caregiving: relative of people experiencing a first episode of psychosis. *British Journal of Psychiatry,* 177:529–533, 2000.

Tessler RC, Gamacho GM, Fisher GA. Patterns of contact of patients' families with mental health professionals. *Hospital and Community Psychiatry,* 42(9):929–935, 1991.

U.S. Department of Health and Human Services. *Mental Health: A Report of the Surgeon General.* Rockville, MD: U.S. Department of Health and Human Services, Substance Abuse and Mental Health Services Administration, Center for Mental Health Services, National Institutes of Health, National Institute of Mental Health, 1999.

Wahl OF. Mental health consumers' experience of stigma. *Schizophrenia Bulletin,* 25(3):467–478, 1999.

Welsh S, Deahl MP. Modern psychiatric ethics. *Lancet,* 359:253–255, 2002.

Wright ER. The impact of organizational factors on mental health professionals' involvement with families. *Psychiatric Services,* 48(7):921–927, 1997.

Zimmerman MA, Warschausky S. Empowerment theory for rehabilitation research: conceptual and methodological issues. *Rehabilitation Psychology,* 43(1):3–16, 1998.

Part II

SELECTED POPULATIONS AT RISK

Section A
Children and Adolescents

6

Prevalence of Psychiatric Disorders in Childhood and Adolescence

E. JANE COSTELLO
SARAH MUSTILLO
GORDON KEELER
ADRIAN ANGOLD

From a public health perspective, epidemiologists focus on a number of important questions about diseases, including these: How important is a particular disease? Which group in the population is at highest risk for specific diseases? Are there characteristics of certain environments that increase the risk of particular diseases? What are the most effective methods of preventing or controlling the spread of specific diseases? Encompassed within these central questions are numerous other issues related to prevalence (i.e., how many people have a particular disease at any one time), incidence (i.e., how many new cases of this disease will occur during a defined period), and overall burden to society in terms of mortality, morbidity, economic costs, functional impairments, and need for treatment.

Applied to psychiatric disorders of children and adolescents, each of these questions could be the topic of a separate book. In this chapter, we concentrate on the question that people associate most clearly with epidemiology: How many people have this disease? That is, what is the *prevalence*, or proportion of the population that has the disease during a specific period of time? Where possible, we will also discuss more recent data that address questions regarding incidence, trends, and burden of disease.

There are still big gaps in our picture of the prevalence of psychiatric disorders in childhood and adolescence. For example, the United States has yet to conduct a study of a truly representative population sample of children and adolescents, along the lines of the recent Office for National Statistics study in the United Kingdom (Meltzer et al., 1999) or the Australian National Survey of

Mental Health and Well-Being (Sawyer et al., 2002), or the population studies of adults in the United States. Researchers are just beginning to develop the tools needed to assess the emotional and behavioral problems of infancy and early childhood. So now, just as for the first edition of this book, the prevalence of child and adolescent psychiatric disorder has to be pieced together from a number of smaller-scale studies using different methods and time frames. In this chapter we bring up-to-date the information on the prevalence of child and adolescent psychiatric disorders in developed countries from the data available since Cohen and colleagues wrote their chapter for the first edition of this book (Cohen et al., 1996).

Questions about *incidence*, the number of new cases occurring during a given period, or about whether a disease is increasing or decreasing, can only be answered by longitudinal studies that survey the population at regular intervals and count the number of new cases arising since the previous survey. Incidence studies are still very rare. This means that we can say little about increases or decreases in the incidence of any child and adolescent psychiatric disorders, with the exception of drug use and abuse, on which regular surveys are conducted by the Substance Abuse and Mental Health Services Administration (SAMHSA). Studies of the *cost* of child and adolescent mental illness are only now beginning to appear, and often these concentrate on the cost of treatment, ignoring the cost of failure to treat or the opportunity costs to families and schools of having to devote their resources to mentally ill children. However, we are beginning to learn something about the burden to families of having a mentally ill child, an important aspect of the cost of mental illness.

Questions about who is most at risk and what environments increase the risk of disease are beginning to be addressed by researchers under the general heading of *developmental psychopathology*, a fairly new disciplinary framework that supports the collaborative work of psychologists, psychiatrists, geneticists, epidemiologists, and others to understand the origins and course of child and adolescent mental illness (Cicchetti, 1984; Cicchetti and Cohen, 1995; Sroufe and Rutter, 1984). Even more recent is the effort to set this work in an epidemiologic context under the heading of *developmental epidemiology* (Costello and Angold, 1995; Kellam and Werthamer-Larsson, 1986). The goal is to examine what is known about the development of psychiatric disorders in childhood and adolescence from the public health viewpoint.

It is worth noting at the outset that *psychiatric disorders in childhood and adolescence* is not the same as *child and adolescent psychiatric disorders*. The *Diagnostic and Statistical Manual* of the American Psychiatric Association (1994) specifies certain disorders as characteristic of the early years of life, but many others occurring throughout life may begin in childhood. Indeed, one of the most dramatic and disturbing findings of recent years has been the steady drop in the estimates of onset age for a range of chronic conditions, so that many are now seen as beginning in adolescence or even earlier (Christie et al., 1988). Given the surge of evidence for the role of genes in liability to psychiatric disorders, there is also growing interest in developmental precursors of the onset of illness—signs and symptoms that might alert us to a child's vulnerability to, for example, schizophrenia (Poulton et al., 2000) or depression (Jaffee et al., 2002).

The Prevalence of Psychiatric Disorders of Childhood and Adolescence

In the first edition of this volume, Cohen et al. published prevalence rates from the 8 or 10 studies done since the 1980s that addressed the prevalence of the major disorders (disruptive behavior disorders, depression, anxiety, and substance abuse/dependence). They then presented a table listing the few studies that permitted prevalence estimates to be made for relatively rare disorders such as psychoses, eating disorders, and obsessive-compulsive disorder. The latest papers cited in those tables were published in 1993.

Table 6.1 lists the studies that provide data on prevalence available since 1993. Some of the data come from newly published studies, some from later waves of longitudinal studies, and some are previously unpublished analyses from the 15-to-17-year-olds from the National Comorbidity Study (NCS) and from our own data sets [Great Smoky Mountains Study (GSMS) and Caring for Children in the Community (CCC)]. Studies were included if they used DSM-IIIR, DSM-IV, ICD-9, or ICD-10 criteria, and if the diagnostic process involved something more than a questionnaire.

The first thing to note is that the amount of information on the prevalence of child and adolescent psychiatric disorders has grown rapidly since the publication of the first edition. Cohen's chapter drew on fewer than 10,000 observations spread across eight studies from the previous decade. Now we can draw on close to 40,000 observations from 21 studies. Many of these are longitudinal studies covering the developmental transitions from childhood to adolescence and from adolescence to young adulthood. We can began to develop a sense of how prevalence rates rise and fall developmentally, which in turn may provide estimates of incidence and clues to causes. Ten of the studies have representative population samples of 1000 or more subjects—a big improvement on earlier years, when small sample sizes and consequently wide confidence limits around estimates made it hard to have much confidence in estimates of the size of the problem.

Most contemporary studies have collected information on service use as well as on psychiatric disorders. This is important from the public health viewpoint. Information on service use permits calculations of the gap between service needs and service use. Using attention-deficit/hyperactivity disorder (ADHD) as an example, if we know how many children have ADHD and how many of them have been given any treatment, and if we also know (as we do quite well for ADHD) what constitutes the most effective treatment and how much it costs, then we can calculate how much effort (and money) is needed to provide adequate treatment for ADHD nationally. We can also look at whether, for example, the extent of unmet need is higher in some parts of the country or in some ethnic or other socio-demographic groups. It has been much more common in the past few years for studies to collect information on the level of functioning of children with psychiatric disorders at home, at school, and in the community, another factor of considerable importance for public health planning.

Table 6.2 provides a summary of the prevalence data provided by the studies listed in Table 6.1. For each diagnosis, it lists the number of studies that provide information about prevalence, the range of estimates, and the median estimate. The data from Table 6.2 are illustrated in Figure 6.1.

Table 6.1 Informative Studies on Prevalence of Psychiatric Disorders in Childhood and Adolescence Published Since 1993: Study Details

Study	Location	No. of Subjects*	No. of Data Waves	Total No. of Observations	Age Range	Interviews Used	Informants	Diagnostic System
Canadian National Population Health Survey (Cairney, 1998)	Canada	1847	1	1847	12–14	UM-CIDI	Child	DSM-IIIR
Caring for Children in the Community (Angold et al., 2002)	North Carolina, United States	4950/920	1	920	9–17	CAPA	Parent, child	DSM-I
Chartres Study (Fombonne, 1994)	Eure-et-Loire, France	2158/217	1	217	8–11	Rutter	Parent	ICD-9
Christchurch Study (Fergusson and Horwood, 2001)	Christchurch, New Zealand	1265	1	961–986	15, 18	DISC, DIS, Questionnaires	Child, parent	DSM-IIIR
Dutch Adolescent Study (Verhulst et al., 1997)	The Netherlands	853/274	1	274	13–18	DISC 2.3	Child, parent	DSM-IIIR
Dunedin Study (Douglass et al, 1995; Newman et al., 1996)	Dunedin, New Zealand	1139/993	8	993	18	DIS	Child	DSM-IIIR
Early Development Stages of Psychopathology (Oldehinkel et al., 1999; Perkonigg and Wittchen, 1999; Perkonigg et al., 1998)	Munich, Germany	1345,1228	2	2573	14–17	M-CIDI	Child	DSM-IV
Finnish birth cohort (Almqvist et al, 1999)	Finland	5813/435	1	435	8–9	Isle of Wight	Parent	DSM-IIIR
Great Smoky Mountains Study (Costello et al., 1996)	North Carolina, United States	1420	8	6674	9–16	CAPA	Child, parent	DSM-IV

Study	Location	N	Sites	N	Age	Instrument	Informant	Criteria
HMO study (Costello et al., 1999a)	Pennsylvania, United States	789/278	1	278	12–17	DISC 2.1	Child, parent	DSM-IIIR
Limburg Study (Kroes et al., 2001)	Limburg, the Netherlands	1317/403	1	403	6–9	ADIKA	Parent	DSM-IIIR
Methods for the Epidemiology Studies of Child and Adolescent Mental Disorders (MECA) (Narrow et al., 1998; Rapoport et al., 2000)	Four sites, United States	1285	1	285	9–18	DISC 2.3	Child, parent	DSM-IIIR
Kaiser Permanente Northwest Study (Debar et al., 2001)	Northwestern United States	80,848	1	80,848	3–17	Clinical	Medical records	ICD-9-CM
National Comorbidity Study (Kessler et al., 1994)	United States	479	1	479	15–17	CIDI	Child	DSM-IIIR
National Finnish Health Care Survey (Haarasitla et al., 2001)	Finland	509	1	509	15–19	UM-CIDI	Child	DSM-IIIR
National Survey of Mental Health and Well-Being (Sawyer et al., 2002)	Australia	4509	1	4509	4–17	DISC-IV	Parent	DSM-IV
Northern Plains Indians (Beals et al., 1997)	Northern Plains, United States	109	1	109	15.6 (mean)	DISC 2.1	Child	DSM-IIIR
Oregon Adolescent Depression Project (Lewinsohn et al., 1995, 1998a, 1998b, 2000)	Oregon, USA	1709, 1507	2	3216	14–19	K-SADS, LIFE	Child	DSM-IIIR
Office of National Statistics Study (Fombonne et al., 2001; Heyman et al., 2001; Meltzer et al., 1999)	Great Britain	10,438	1	10,438	5–15	DAWBA	5–10 child, teacher 11–15 parent, child, teacher	ICD-10

(continued)

Table 6.1 Informative Studies on Prevalence of Psychiatric Disorders in Childhood and Adolescence Published Since 1993: Study Details (*Continued*)

Study	Location	No. of Subjects*	No. of Data Waves	Total No. of Observations	Age Range	Interviews Used	Informants	Diagnostic System
Canadian National	Canada	1847	1	1847	12–14	UM-CIDI	Child	DSM-IIIR
Quebec Longitudinal Study (Romano et al., 2001)	Quebec, Canada	1201	1	1201	14–17	DISC 2.25	Child, parent	DSM-IIIR
Quebec Child Mental Heath Study (Bergeron et al., 1992)	Quebec, Canada	139	1	139	6–14	DISC 2.25	Child, parent	DSM-IIIR
Simmons Longitudinal Study (Giaconia et al., 1994; Reinherz et al., 1999)	Boston, United States	386	1	386	18	DIS	Child	DSM-IIIR
South Carolina Study (Cuffe et al., 1998; Milne et al., 1995)	South Carolina, United States	490	1	490	15–19	K-SADS	Child, parent	DSM-IV
Valencia study (Andrés et al., 1999; Gomez-Beneyto et al., 1994)	Valencia, Spain	1200/320	1	320	8, 11, 15	K-SADS	Child, parent	DSM-IIIR
Virginia Twin Study of Adolescent Behavioral Development (Simonoff et al., 1997)	Virginia, United States	2762	1	2762	8–16	CAPA	Child, parent	DSM-IIIR

*If a multistage design was used, the numbers at each stage are separated by a slash. If a multiwave study was used, the numbers at each wave are separated by a comma.
ADIKA, Amsterdam Diagnostic Interview for Children and Adolescents; CAPA, Child and Adolescent Psychiatric Assessment; DAWBA, Development and Well-Being Assessment; DIS, Diagnostic Interview Schedule; DISC, Diagnostic Interview Schedule for Children; DSM, Diagnostic and Statistical Manual of the American Psychiatric Association, editions III, III (Revised), and IV; ICD, International Classification of Diseases, versions 9 and 10; K-SADS, Schedule for Affective Disorders and Schizophrenia, Kiddie version; LIFE, Longitudinal Interval Follow-up Evaluation; M-CIDI Munich Composite International Diagnostic Inventory; UM-CIDI, University of Michigan Composite International Diagnostic Inventory.

Table 6.2   Psychiatric Disorders in Childhood and Adolescence: Number of Studies, Range of Estimates, and Median Estimates

Diagnosis	No. of Studies	Lowest Estimate (%)	Highest Estimate (%)	Median Estimate (%)
Any psychiatric disorder	18	8.2	42.0	25.3, 26.0
Serious emotional disturbance	9	3.0	18.7	11.3
Conduct disorder	12	1.1	10.6	3.0, 3.7
Oppositional defiant disorder	12	1.3	7.4	3.5, 3.7
Attention-deficit/hyperactivity disorder	15	0.3	11.3	2.7
Any disruptive behavior disorder	13	4.6	13.8	6.2
Drug or alcohol abuse or dependence	9	0.8	24.0	4.5
Major depressive disorder	18	0.2	12.9	4.6, 4.7
Bipolar disorder	6	0.0	0.9	0.0, 0.0
Any depressive disorder	18	0.2	18.2	3.8, 4.7
Simple phobia	14	0.1	21.2	2.4, 2.5
Social phobia	11	0.2	12.0	2.0
Separation anxiety disorder	13	0.2	11.0	2.4
Generalized anxiety disorder (DSM-IV)	6	0.4	4.7	1.3, 2.4
Overanxious disorder	10	0.6	14.0	3.1, 3.2
Agoraphobia	9	0.2	4.0	1.1
Panic disorder	8	0.05	3.0	0.3, 0.3
Posttraumatic stress disorder	8	0.0	6.7	0.5, 1.2
Obsessive-compulsive disorder	10	0.1	4.4	0.5, 0.6
Any anxiety disorder	14	1.9	23.8	5.5, 8.1
Bulimia	7	0.0	0.8	0.3
Anorexia nervosa	7	0.0	0.5	0.0
Psychotic disorders	4	0.0	0.05	0.0, 0.01
Autism				

Table 6.2 confirms the conclusions of several earlier reviews, including the chapter by Cohen et al.: in any 3- to 6-month period, approximately one child in four will have a psychiatric disorder. This makes psychiatric disorder one of the most prevalent types of illness affecting children and adolescents, a conclusion that public health policy has ignored for too long.

Among the wide range of disorders included in taxonomies such as the *Diagnostic and Statistical Manual* of the American Psychiatric Association (1994), the most common disorders affecting children and adolescents fall into the broad categories of disruptive behavior disorders, substance abuse and dependence, depressive disorders, and anxiety disorders. There is also a large number of rare conditions, such as tic disorders, eating and elimination disorders, psychotic disorders, autism, and pervasive developmental disorders, on which there is still very little population-based information. Where we could find at least three studies that included a diagnosis, it is included in the tables and figures. Estimates based solely on other types of data collection, such as reviews of school records, are excluded.

Disruptive Behavior Disorders

Disruptive behavior disorders (conduct disorder, oppositional disorder, ADHD) are some of the most common psychiatric disorders of childhood. The 3- to 6-

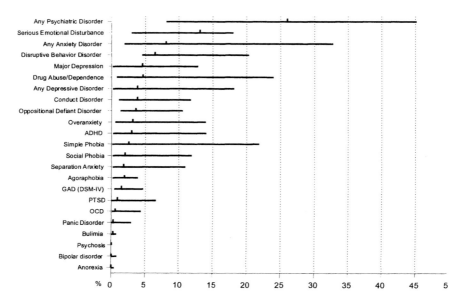

Figure 6.1 Summary of results of prevalence studies since 1993: highest, lowest, and median estimates for age. ADHD: attention-deficit/hyperactivity disorder; GAD: generalized anxiety disorder; OCD: obsessive-compulsive disorder; PTSD: posttraumatic stress disorder.

month prevalence falls between 4% and 20%, with lower rates in younger samples (e.g., 4.6% in the British national sample's 5- to 10-year-olds, and 4.7% in Almqvist's 8- to 9-year-olds) and the median at around 6%. Behind this general picture are very different developmental patterns for different disruptive behavior disorders. Survival curves modeled on the GSMS longitudinal data show a linear onset of new cases of conduct and oppositional disorder through age 13, after which oppositional disorder continues in a linear fashion, while there is an increase in the rate at which new cases of conduct disorders appear. At the level of individual symptoms, the onset of the earliest symptoms of oppositional disorder occurs in boys on average in the earliest grade school years, while the symptoms of conduct disorder begin to appear a couple of years later (see Fig. 6.2). The picture for girls is somewhat different; onset is later for most symptoms, and oppositional symptoms do not all precede conduct symptoms, as they do in boys.

This picture for ADHD is very different. In prospective studies, almost all cases begin by age 12, even if they continue into the teens. Thus, it is likely that the prevalence of ADHD seen in some studies of adolescents refers to cases that had their onset several years earlier. (DSM-IV requires at least some symptoms to have been "present before age 7 years"; (American Psychiatric Association, 1994, p. 84.) All of the disruptive behavior disorders are more common in boys than in girls, but ADHD shows the most extreme disparity (in GSMS the male:female ratio is 6.2:1), followed by conduct disorder (3.2:1) and oppositional disorder (1.8:1).

Depressive Disorders

Most studies measured only major depressive disorder or combined major depression with dysthymia, minor depression, and bipolar disorder under the general heading of "any depressive disorder." There are not enough published studies to permit an estimate of dysthymia. The five estimates of bipolar disorder available generate estimates ranging from no cases to 9 cases per 1000 adolescents. The median estimate was no cases. Clearly, much larger samples are needed to produce a reliable estimate for bipolar disorder.

Major depression, with an overall prevalence of around 4% to 5%, is interesting in showing a marked sex-by-age difference. A review of studies published in the past 20 years (Costello et al., 2002) showed that the median prevalence of depression before age 13 is less than 2% in both boys and girls. After that age, it rises markedly in adolescent girls but not in boys. This change is reflected in Figure 6.1, where the breadth of the range of estimates is caused in part by the difference in the age of study participants; from 5 to 10 years in the study with the lowest estimate to 15 to 17 years in the study with the highest estimate.

There has been some discussion of whether there has been an "epidemic of depression" (Klerman and Weissman, 1989) during the twentieth century that has caused an increasing prevalence in each succeeding generation. If true, this would be of major public health concern. However, much of the evidence comes from asking people to recall episodes from their earliest years; the lower prevalence in older people may thus be caused by the difficulty of recalling over longer periods of time (Warshaw et al., 1991). A review of studies of children born since the mid-1960s and assessed during childhood and adolescence (i.e., not relying on recall over different periods of time) showed no evidence of increasing age-adjusted rates of depression in children born in 1975–86 compared with children born in 1965–74 (Costello et al., 2002). Thus, the epidemic, if there has been one, appears not to have expanded its reach during the last third of the twentieth century.

Anxiety Disorders

It is clear from Figure 6.1 that anxiety disorders show the widest variation in prevalence estimates across studies. A closer examination shows that this is due chiefly to estimates of simple phobia, which range from 0.1% to 21.9%; that is, the highest estimate is more than 200 time the lowest estimate. This range is not attributable to sample characteristics in the way that some of the difference in depression estimates was; studies with similar age and sex distributions provided both low and high estimates. It is more likely to be an artifact of how simple phobia was assessed, specifically, whether the study assessed the extent to which a phobia (e.g., of snakes, heights, or blood) was accompanied by some form of functional impairment. For example, requiring significant levels of impairment before making the diagnosis of a specific phobia in the Methodological Epidemiological Catchment Area (MECA) study reduced the 6-month prevalence from 10% to 2% (Narrow et al., 1998).

Among the anxiety disorders, some are characteristic of early childhood (e.g., separation anxiety), while others are extremely rare before adolescence (panic disorder, agoraphobia). Some (panic disorder, social phobia, overanxious disorder, and generalized anxiety disorder) occur more often in girls, whereas there is little difference between the sexes in the prevalence of separation anxiety, agoraphobia, or simple phobias. There is also only a modest excess of girls with posttraumatic stress disorder and obsessive-compulsive disorder, which are classed with the anxiety disorders in some studies.

Substance Abuse Disorders

Drug abuse or dependence is rare before adolescence, but thereafter it rises rapidly. For example, SAMHSA's National Household Survey on Drug Abuse estimated that in 2000, 17.8% of 16- to 17-year-olds had used one or more illicit drugs (marijuana, psychotherapeutics, cocaine, hallucinogens, or inhalants) in the past month, compared with 10.9% of 14- to 15-year-olds and 3.8% of 12- to 13-year-olds (http://www. samhsa.gov/oas/nhsda/2k1nhsda/vol1/chapter2.htm#2.age). The range of estimates of drug abuse or dependence shown in Figure 6.1 reflects the age difference of the subjects, from 0.8% of the 9- to 12-year-old children in the GSMS study to 24% of the 18-year-olds in the Christchurch study. Even more important from the public health standpoint is the increasing functional impairment that accompanies substance use with age; in GSMS, 4% of 13-year-olds who used drugs or alcohol showed functional impairment. By age 14 it was 11%; by 15, 17%; and by 16, 20%. This increase in impairment is caused at least in part by the well-established trajectory from alcohol to cigarettes, then marijuana, then cocaine and heroin (Kandel, 1975), with use of the last two drugs leading more often to impaired functioning.

Evidence is emerging that comorbid psychiatric disorders affect the age at which adolescents begin to use various drugs. Thus, in GSMS, girls (but not boys) with conduct or oppositional disorders began smoking 18 months earlier than others (Costello et al., 1999b). On the other hand, adolescents with separation anxiety were less likely than other youth to have started drinking by age 16, whereas those with generalized anxiety disorder were more likely to have started by then (Kaplow et al., 2001).

Other Disorders

Of the other psychiatric disorders, only anorexia nervosa, bulimia, and psychosis were reported three times or more in epidemiologic studies of psychiatric disorders in general. The reasons for not taking this approach to estimating the prevalence of very rare disorders is clear: cases are so rare that huge samples are needed to provide accurate estimates. Also, many of the most severe and disabling disorders are (fortunately) the rare ones, and a high proportion of cases may be living outside of their homes in special residential settings, which are often excluded from population-based studies. For example, studies of autism, a rare but disabling condition, have tended to use case-finding methods based on record reviews of special schools or state and national bodies that maintain financial or clinical records

(Bristol et al., 1996) or studies that have looked only for autism and autism-spectrum disorders (Kadesjö et al., 1999) increasing the risk of false positives.

The British Office of National Statistics Study (Meltzer et al., 1999), a national probability sample of 5- to 15-year-olds, estimated the prevalence of pervasive developmental disorder (PDD) at 26.1 per 10,000 and that of Rett syndrome at 3.5 per 10,000 (Fombonne et al., 2001). A smaller study of 15,500 children aged 2.5 to 6.5 in one county in England identified PDD at a rate of 45.8 per 10,000 and autism at 16.8 per 10,000 (Chakrabarti and Fombonne, 2001). Studies using official records have found autism at rates of 5.3 per 10,000 in France (Fombonne et al., 1997), 6.1 per 10,000 in Finland (Kielinen et al., 2000), 16 per 10,000 in Texas (Sturmey and Vernon, 2001), 21.1 per 10,000 in Japan (Honda et al., 1996), and 40 per 10,000 in New Jersey . On the whole, the higher rates are seen in younger children. This has fueled a debate about a possible link between autism and infant immunizations such as the mumps, measles, and rubella vaccine (MMR) (Wakefield, 1999). Studies have failed to find the temporal relationship between the two that would support this hypothesis (Kaye et al., 2001; Taylor et al., 1999), but the debate still rages.

Comorbidity

Comorbidity is one of the most notable characteristics of psychiatric disorders of childhood and adolescence. Figure 6.2 shows the results of a meta-analysis of some 20 studies that provide data from which to calculate the extent to which children with a given disorder are also likely to have another psychiatric disorder. The paper from which this figure was drawn discusses in detail possible methodological and substantive reasons for this high level of comorbidity. The paper concludes that, despite methodological problems with the definition and measurement of psychopathology, there is no question that children with some disorders are at increased risk for others (Angold et al., 1999). Conduct disorders and ADHD are most highly comorbid (odds ratio [OR] 14.8), followed by depression and anxiety (OR 12.0). But conduct disorders and depression, which come from opposite sides of the *internalizing–externalizing* or *emotional–behavioral* divide (Achenbach and Edelbrock, 1981), are also highly comorbid (OR 11.0).

Figure 6.3 shows the results of similar analyses conducted to assess the comorbidity of substance abuse and/or dependence with psychiatric disorders. It shows that there is significant comorbidity (i.e., OR > 2) between substance abuse/dependence and each type of psychiatric disorder (white columns) and that any substance use (with or without abuse) is significantly more common in youth with each type of psychiatric disorder except anxiety disorders.

From a public health viewpoint, comorbidity is a serious issue. Children with comorbid disorders are more likely to have associated functional impairment (80% vs. 40% in GSMS). They are twice as likely to use mental health services as are children with a single disorder and to use twice as many different types of service settings. They are also more likely to be arrested, be expelled or drop out of school, or get pregnant (GSMS data, unpublished). Comorbidity is almost as common in girls as in boys, particularly in adolescents, and its association with impairment is as common in girls as in boys.

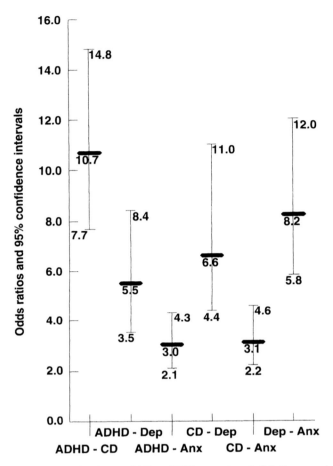

Figure 6.2 Meta-analysis of comorbidity. ADH: attention-deficit/hyperactivity disorder; Anx: anxiety; CD: compulsive disorder; Dep: depression.

Prevalence of Serious Emotional Disturbance

Serious emotional disturbance (SED) is a term introduced by the federal government in 1993 to describe psychiatric conditions severe enough to warrant public intervention through block grants to states, family income supplements via the Social Security Administration, or other public support mechanisms (U.S. Government, 1993). This term was expected to serve the same purpose as the term *serious mental illness* (SMI) for adults (Kessler et al., 1996). Because of its importance as the key to access state and federal services in the United States, the prevalence of SED deserves consideration in a chapter on epidemiology and public health.

According to review of seven data sets published in 1998 (Costello et al., 1998), between 4% and 7%, or 3 to 4 million children in the United States, have a SED, that is, a psychiatric disorder accompanied by significant functional impairment.

Odds Ratio and 95% confidence interval

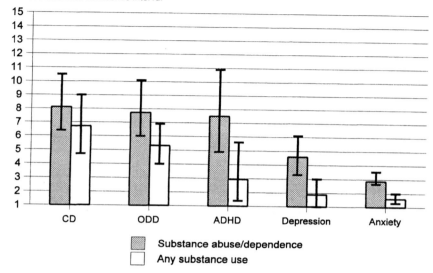

Figure 6.3   Comorbidity with any substance use (*n* = 8) and substance abuse/dependence (*n* = 13): meta-analysis of published studies.

For example, major depression would be classified as a SED only if it is accompanied by a significant reduction in the child's ability to function at the usual level in school, in the family, or with peers. A review by Friedman et al. (1996) put the figure closer to 9%–12%. The median value for the studies listed in Table 6.2 is around 13%. Most studies show no great variation by age, sex, or race/ethnicity, but poverty may be related to the risk of SED. The extent to which psychiatric disorder causes impairment varies from study to study and from disorder to disorder. It results most commonly from drug abuse/dependence, ADHD, and conduct disorder and is least likely to occur in children with simple phobia.

By any standards, children with impairing psychiatric disorders should receive treatment. In the studies that have examined this issue, only one child in four with SED had received any professional mental health care during the most recent period of SED, and only half of them had *ever* received services (Costello et al., 1996a, 1998).

The Burden of Psychiatric Disorders in Childhood and Adolescence

Another way to look at the public health problem of child and adolescent mental illness is in terms of the *burden of disease*. In the past few years, this concept has been given an operational definition in terms of disability-adjusted life years (DALYs), a measure of "the burden of premature mortality and non-fatal health outcomes" (Murray and Lopez, 1996, p. 8). International estimates of the burden of different diseases, sponsored by the World Bank and the World Health Organization, list the diseases that contribute most to the global burden of disease in different parts of the world and for different age groups (Murray and Lopez, 1996). Unfortunately, no table is provided for the 4-to-14 age group. But for the 15-to-44 age group, the 10 leading causes of disability in the developed world include 9 that are either psychiatric disorders or closely linked to psychopathology: major depression, alcohol use, road traffic accidents, schizophrenia, self-inflicted injuries, bipolar disorder, drug use, obsessive-compulsive disorders, and violence (the only exception is osteoarthritis). It is highly likely that many of the same diseases would occur in a similar list restricted to children and adolescents. In fact, since younger people are likely to live longer with disabling but nonfatal disorders, the associated burden of disease, calculated in DALYs, is likely to be even higher. This points to the extraordinary importance of psychiatric disorders and their associated disabilities in contributing to the global burden of disease affecting young people.

Conclusions and Implications for Mental Health Services

At the beginning of this chapter, we presented questions that public health epidemiologists should be able to answer about psychiatric disorders in childhood and adolescence. It is unfortunately still true, as it was when the first edition of this book was published, that we are a long way from knowing the answers to most of those questions. Even when we limit our review to prevalence, as we have in this chapter, it is clear that a great deal remains unknown. But we have learned two things that are very important for the planning of mental health services. First, at any given time, one child in four or five has a psychiatric disorder, and one in seven or eight has a significantly impairing disorder (SED). Second, many adults with severe mental illnesses have their first symptoms in childhood or adolescence.

Paradoxically, while public investment in studies of the epidemiology of adult psychiatric disorders has greatly exceeded that for disorders in childhood and adolescence, the latter is a much more expensive and labor-intensive undertaking. This is because the rapid developmental changes of childhood create the need for (*1*) *different assessment measures* for infancy, early childhood, later childhood, and adolescence; (*2*) *longitudinal studies* to monitor the impact of developmental changes such as puberty on psychiatric disorders; (*3*) *frequent* assessments, so that the onset of disorders can be accurately mapped; and (*4*) *multiple informants*: at least a parent and the index child, and preferably both parents, siblings, and teachers. Thus, developing the information base necessary for understanding the need for child and adolescent behavioral health services will be a resource-intensive undertaking. On the other hand, it is likely to yield a great deal that can help to improve the health and quality of life of children and their families.

ACKNOWLEDGMENTS

This chapter was completed in part with support from a National Institutes of Health Independent Scientist Award to the first author and from the Center for Developmental Epidemiology (Director, Adrian Angold).

REFERENCES

Achenbach TM, Edelbrock CS. Behavorial problems and competencies reported by parents of normal and disturbed children aged four through sixteen. *Monographs of the Society for Research in Child Development*, 46:1–82, 1981.

Almqvist F, Puura K, Kumpulainen K, et al. Psychiatric disorders in 8–9-year-old children based on a diagnostic interview with the parents. *European Child and Adolescent Psychiatry*, 8:IV/17–IV/28, 1999.

American Psychiatric Association. *Diagnostic and Statistical Manual of Mental Disorders*, 4th ed. Washington, DC: American Psychiatric Press, 1994.

Andrés M, Catalá M, Gómez-Beneyto M. Prevalence, comorbidity, risk factors and service utilization of disruptive behavior disorders in a community sample of children in Valencia (Spain). *Social Psychiatry and Psychiatric Epidemiology*, 34:175–179, 1999.

Angold A, Costello E, Erkanli, A. Comorbidity. *Journal of Child Psychology and Psychiatry*, 40:57–87, 1999.

Angold A, Erkanli A, Farmer E, et al. Psychiatric disorder, impairment, and service use in rural African American and white youth. *Archives of General Psychiatry*, 59:893–901, 2002.

Beals J, Piasecki J, Nelson S, et al. Psychiatric disorder among American Indian adolescents: prevalence in northern plains youth. *Journal of the American Academy of Child and Adolescent Psychiatry*, 36:1252–1259, 1997.

Bergeron L, Valla JP, Breton JJ. Pilot study for the Quebec Child Mental Health Survey: part I. Measurement of prevalence estimates among six to 14 year olds. *Canadian Journal of Psychiatry*, 37:374–405, 1992.

Bertrand J, Mars A, Boyle C, et al. Prevalence of autism in a United States population: the Brick Township, New Jersey, investigation. *Pediatrics*, 108:1155–1161, 2001.

Bristol MM, Cohen DJ, Costello EJ, et al. State of the science in autism: report to the National Institutes of Health. *Journal of Autism and Developmental Disorders*, 26:121–155, 1996.

Cairney J. Gender differences in the prevalence of depression among Canadian adolescents. *Canadian Journal of Public Health*, 89:181–182, 1998.

Chakrabarti S, Fombonne E. Pervasive developmental disorders in preschool children. *Journal of the American Medical Association*, 285:3093–3099, 2001.

Christie KA, Burke JD, Regier DA, et al. Epidemiologic evidence for early onset of mental disorders and higher risk of drug abuse in young adults. *American Journal of Psychiatry*, 145:971–975, 1988.

Cicchetti D. The emergence of developmental psychopathology. *Child Development*, 55:1–7, 1984.

Cicchetti D, Cohen DJ. Perspectives on developmental psychopathology. In: Cicchetti D, Cohen DJ (eds). *Developmental Psychopathology, Volume 1: Theory and Methods*. New York: Wiley, pp. 3–20, 1995.

Cohen P, Provet AG, Jones M. Prevalence of emotional behavior disorders during childhood and adolescence. In: Levin BL, Petrila J (eds). *Mental Health Services: A Public Health Perspective*. New York: Oxford University Press, pp. 193–209, 1996.

Costello EJ, Angold A. Developmental epidemiology. In: Cicchetti D, Cohen D (eds). *Developmental Psychopathology, Volume 1: Theory and Methods*. New York: Wiley, pp. 23–56, 1995.

Costello EJ, Angold A, Burns BJ, et al. The Great Smoky Mountains Study of youth: functional impairment and severe emotional disturbance. *Archives of General Psychiatry*, 53:1137–1143, 1996a.

Costello EJ, Angold A, Burns BJ, et al. The Great Smoky Mountains Study of youth: goals, designs, methods, and the prevalence of DSM-III-R disorders. *Archives of General Psychiatry*, 53:1129–1136, 1996b.

Costello EJ, Angold A, Keeler GP. Adolescent outcomes of childhood disorders: the consequences of severity and impairment. *Journal of the American Academy of Child and Adolescent Psychiatry*, 38:121–128, 1999a.

Costello EJ, Erkanli A, Federman E, et al. Development of psychiatric comorbidity with substance abuse in adolescents: effects of timing and sex. *Journal of Clinical Child Psychology*, 28:298–311, 1999b.

Costello EJ, Messer SC, Reinherz HZ, et al. The prevalence of serious emotional disturbance: a re-analysis of community studies. *Journal of Child and Family Studies*, 7:411–432, 1998.

Costello EJ, Pine DS, Hammen C, et al. Development and natural history of mood disorders. *Biological Psychiatry*, 52:529–542, 2002.

Cuffe SP, Addy CL, Garrison CZ, et al. Prevalence of PTSD in a community sample of older adolescents. *Journal of the American Academy of Child and Adolescent Psychiatry*, 37:147–154, 1998.

Debar L, Clarke G, O'Connor E, et al. Treated prevalence, incidence, and pharmacotherapy of child and adolescent mood disorders in an HMO. *Mental Health Services Research*, 3:73–89, 2001.

Douglass HM, Moffitt TE, Dar R, et al. Obsessive compulsive disorder in a birth cohort of 18-year-olds: prevalence and predictors. *Journal of the American Academy of Child and Adolescent Psychiatry*, 34:1424–1431, 1995.

Fergusson D, Horwood L. The Christchurch Health and Development Study: review of findings on child and adolescent mental health. *Australian and New Zealand Journal of Psychiatry*, 35:287–296, 2001.

Fombonne E. The Chartres Study: I. Prevalence of psychiatric disorders among French school-aged children. *British Journal of Psychiatry*, 164:69–79, 1994.

Fombonne E, Du Mazabrun C, Cans C, et al. Autism and associated medical disorders in a French epidemiological survey. *Journal of the American Academy of Child and Adolescent Psychiatry*, 36:1561–1569, 1997.

Fombonne E, Simmons H, Ford T, et al. Prevalance of pervasive developmental disorders in the British nationwide survey of child mental health. *Journal of the American Academy of Child and Adolescent Psychiatry*, 40:820–827, 2001.

Friedman RM, Katz-Leavy JW, Manderscheid RW, et al. Prevalence of serious emotional disturbance in children and adolescents. In: Manderscheid RW, Sonnenschein MA (eds). *Mental Health, United States, 1996*. Rockville, MD: Center for Mental Health Services, pp. 71–89, 1996.

Giaconia RM, Reinherz HZ, Silverman AB, et al. Ages of onset of psychiatric disorders in a community population of older adolescents. *Journal of the American Academy of Child and Adolescent Psychiatry*, 33:706–717, 1994.

Gomez-Beneyto M, Bonet A, Catala MA, et al. Prevalence of mental disorders among children in Valencia, Spain. *Acta Psychiatrica Scandinavica*, 89:352–257, 1994.

Haarasitla L, Marttunen M, Kaprio J, et al. The 12-month prevalence and characteristics of major depressive episode in a representative nationwide sample of adolescents and young adults. *Psychological Medicine*, 31:1169–1179, 2001.

Heyman I, Fombonne E, Simmons H, et al. Prevalence of obsessive-compulsive disorder in the British nationwide survey of child mental health. *British Journal of Psychiatry*, 179:324–329, 2001.

Honda H, Shimizu Y, Misumi K, et al. Cumulative incidence and prevalence of childhood autism in children in Japan. *British Journal of Psychiatry*, 169:228–235, 1996.

Jaffee SR, Moffitt TE, Caspi A, et al. Differences in early childhood risk factors for juvenile onset and adult-onset depression. *Archives of General Psychiatry*, 59:215–222, 2002.

Kadesjö B, Gillberg C, Hagberg B. Autism and Asperger syndrome in seven-year-old children: a total population study. *Journal of Autism and Developmental Disorders*, 29:327–331, 1999.

Kandel DB. Stages in adolescent involvement in drug use. *Science*, 190:912–914, 1975.

Kaplow JB, Curran PJ, Angold A, et al. The prospective relation between dimensions of anxiety and the initiation of adolescent alcohol use. *Journal of Clinical Child Psychology*, 30:316–326, 2001.

Kaye J, Melero-Montes del mar M, Hershel J. Mumps, measles, and rubella vaccine and the incidence of autism recorded by general practitioners: a time trend analysis. *British Medical Journal*, 322:460–463, 2001.

Kellam SG, Werthamer-Larsson L. Developmental epidemiology: a basis for prevention. In: Kessler M, Goldston SE (eds). *A Decade of Progress in Primary Prevention*. Hanover, NH: University Press of New England, pp. 154–180, 1986.

Kessler RC, Berglund PA, Leaf PJ, et al. The 12-month prevalence and correlates of serious mental illness (SMI). In: Manderscheid RW, Sonnenschein MA (eds). *Mental Health, United States, 1996*. DHHS Pub. No. (SMA) 96-3098, Rockville, MD: Center for Mental Health Services, pp. 59–70, 1996.

Kessler RC, McGonagle KA, Zhao S, et al. Lifetime and 12-month prevalence of DSM-III-R psychiatric disorders in the United States: results from the National Comorbidity Study. *Archives of General Psychiatry*, 51:8–19, 1994.

Kielinen M, Linna S, Moilanen I. Autism in Northern Finland. *European Child and Adolescent Psychiatry*, 9:162–167, 2000.

Klerman GL, Weissman MM. Increasing rates of depression. *Journal of the American Medical Association*, 261:2229–2235, 1989.

Kroes M, Kalff A, Kessels A, et al. Child psychiatric diagnoses in a population of Dutch schoolchildren aged 6 to 8 years. *Journal of the American Academy of Child and Adolescent Psychiatry*, 40:1401–1409, 2001.

Lewinsohn PM, Klein DN, Seeley JR. Bipolar disorders in a community sample of older adolescents: prevalence, phenomenology, comorbidity, and course. *Journal of the American Academy of Child and Adolescent Psychiatry*, 34:454–463, 1995.

Lewinsohn PM, Klein DN, Seeley JR. Bipolar disorder during adolescence and young adulthood in a community sample. *Bipolar Disorders*, 2:281–293, 2000.

Lewinsohn PM, Lewinsohn M, Gotlib IH, et al. Gender differences in anxiety disorders and anxiety symptoms in adolescents. *Journal of Abnormal Psychology*, 107:109–117, 1998a.

Lewinsohn PM, Rohde P, Seeley JR Major depressive disorder in older adolescents: prevalence, risk factors, and clinical implications. *Clinical Psychology Review*, 18:765–794, 1998b.

Meltzer H, Gatward R, Goodman R, et al. *The Mental Health of Children and Adolescents in Great Britain*. London: Office for National Statistics, 1999.

Milne JM, Garrison CZ, Addy CL, et al. Frequency of phobic disorder in a community sample of young adolescents. *Journal of the American Academy of Child and Adolescent Psychiatry*, 34:1202–1211, 1995.

Murray CJL, Lopez AD. *The Global Burden of Disease*. Geneva: World Health Organization, 1996.

Narrow WE, Regier DA, Goodman SH, et al. A comparison of federal definitions of severe mental illness among children and adolescents in four communities. *Psychiatric Services*, 49:1601–1608, 1998.

Newman DL, Moffitt TE, Silva PA, et al. Psychiatric disorder in a birth cohort of young adults: prevalence, comorbidity, clinical significance, and new case incidence from ages 11 to 21. *Journal of Consulting and Clinical Psychology*, 64:552–562, 1996.

Oldehinkel AJ, Wittchen HU, Schuster P. Prevalence, 20-month incidence and outcome of unipolar depressive disorders in a community sample of adolescents. *Psychological Medicine*, 29:655–668, 1999.

Perkonigg A, Lieb R, Wittchen HU. Prevalence of use, abuse and dependence of illicit drugs among adolescents and young adults in a community sample. *European Addiction Research*, 4:58–66, 1998.

Perkonigg A, Wittchen HU. Prevalence and comorbidity of traumatic events and post-traumatic stress disorder in adolescents and young adults. In: Maercker A, Schützwohl M, Solomon Z (eds). *Post-Traumatic Stress Disorder: A Lifespan Developmental Perspective*. Seattle: Hogrefe & Huber, pp. 113–133, 1999.

Poulton R, Caspi A, Moffitt T, et al. Children's self-reported psychotic symptoms and adult schizophreniform disorder. *Archives of General Psychiatry*, 57:1053–1058, 2000.

Rapoport J, Inoff-Germain G, Weissman M, et al. Childhood obsessive-compulsive disorder in the NIMH MECA study: parent versus child identification of cases. *Journal of Anxiety Disorders*, 14:535–548, 2000.

Reinherz HZ, Giaconia R, Wasserman MS. Coming of age in the 90's: influences of contemporary stressors on major depression in young adults. In: Cohen P, Robins LN (eds). *Where and When: Historical and Geographical Effects on Aspects of Psychopathology*. Mahway, NJ: Erlbaum, pp. 141–161, 1999.

Robins LN, Helzer J, Croughan J, et al. The NIMH epidemiologic catchment area study. *Archives of General Psychiatry*, 38:381–389, 1981.

Romano E, Tremblay RE, Vitaro F, et al. Prevalence of psychiatric diagnoses and the role of perceived impairment: findings from an adolescent community sample. *Journal of Child Psychology and Psychiatry*, 42:451–461, 2001.

Sawyer M, Arney P, Baghurst J, et al. The mental health of young people in Australia: key findings from the child and adolescent component of the national survey of mental health and well-being. *Australian and New Zealand Journal of Psychiatry*, 35:806–814, 2002.

Simonoff E, Pickles A, Meyer JM, et al. The Virginia Twin Study of adolescent behavioral development: influences of age, sex and impairment on rates of disorder. *Archives of General Psychiatry*, 54:801–808, 1997.

Sroufe LA, Rutter M. The domain of developmental psychopathology. *Child Development*, 55:17–29, 1984.

Sturmey P, Vernon J. Administrative prevalence of autism in the Texas school system. *Journal of the American Academy of Child and Adolescent Psychiatry*, 40:621, 2001.

Taylor B, Miller E, Farrington C, et al. Autisim and measels, mumps, and rubella vaccine: no epidemiological evidence for a causal association. *Lancet*, 353:2026–2029, 1999.

U.S. Government. *Federal Register*, 58:29425, 1993.

Verhulst FC, van der Ende J, Ferdinand RF, et al. The prevalence of DSM-III-R diagnoses in a national sample of Dutch adolescents. *Archives of General Psychiatry*, 54:329–336, 1997.

Wakefield A. MMR vaccination and autism. *Lancet*, 354:949–950, 1999.

Warshaw MG, Klerman GL, Lavori PW. Are secular trends in major depression an artifact of recall? *Journal of Psychiatric Research*, 25:141–151, 1991.

7

Child Mental Health Policy

ROBERT M. FRIEDMAN
KATHERINE A. BEST
MARY I. ARMSTRONG
ALBERT J. DUCHNOWSKI
MARY E. EVANS
MARIO HERNANDEZ
SHARON HODGES
KRISTA B. KUTASH

This chapter reviews child mental health policy and identifies key policy issues at a time when greater attention is being paid to children's mental health than ever before. This reflects both an increasing recognition of the severity of the problem of emotional, behavioral, and mental disorders in children and adolescents and the inadequacy of present attempts to address these disorders. Former Surgeon General David Satcher, under whose leadership the first Surgeon General's report on mental health was published (U.S. Department of Health and Human Services, 1999) and the first Surgeon General's Conference on Children's Mental Health was conducted, proclaimed that "Growing numbers of children are suffering needlessly because their emotional, behavioral, and developmental needs are not being met by those very institutions which were explicitly created to take care of them" (Satcher, 2000, p. 1).

The National Institute of Mental Health (NIMH) convened a workgroup on child and adolescent mental health research and concluded that "no other illnesses damage so many children so seriously" (National Advisory Mental Health Council's Workgroup on Child and Adolescent Mental Health Intervention Development and Deployment, 2001, p. 1). The Executive Director of the Bazelon Center for Mental Health Law, a national mental health advocacy organization, assessed the U.S. response to mental health issues and concluded that while the adult system was in great need of improvement, "the situation is particularly desperate in children's services" (Bernstein, 2001).

Most recently, President George W. Bush established the President's New Freedom Commission on Mental Health in April 2002. In its interim report, this Commission described America's mental health service delivery system as being "in shambles" (Hogan, 2002). As problematic as the overall system is, the Commission indicated that "the 'mental health maze' is more complex and more inadequate for children" (p. 5).

Given these assessments of the seriousness of the problem, this chapter will first put child mental health policy in context by briefly reviewing its history and discussing the prevalence and seriousness of the problem. We will then look at the major policy and system responses to the needs of children and their families, and finally, we will examine a series of important policy and system development issues.

Public policies have been defined as "authoritative decisions that are made in the legislative, executive, or judicial branches of government" (Longest, 1998, p. 4) to influence the actions, behaviors, or decisions of others. The major reason for studying policy is because of its relationship to service delivery and, ultimately, to outcomes for children and families. One model for depicting this relationship comes from the work of Usher and his colleagues (1995). In this model, which was developed in the context of child welfare services and has been adapted for use here, public policy serves as the beginning point for understanding the structure of a service delivery system. The formal public policy context includes legislation and regulations. The legislation and regulations that affect children's mental health are each based on values and principles, and on theories of change, which may or may not be explicitly stated and may or may not be in conflict with one another. The legislation and regulations in turn affect the program's management and structure, which in turn affect program's operations and, ultimately, program impact. There has been very little study of the policy development and implementation process in children's mental health, although a model has been formulated to identify key variables in the effectiveness of policy in achieving its intended outcomes (Friedman, 2003).

A Brief History of Child Mental Health Policy

The first major national report on mental health was issued by the Joint Commission on Mental Illness and Health (1961), created by the U.S. Congress in 1955. The Commission was created because of increased concern about mental health, brought about partly by the large number of individuals either rejected for service during World War II for mental health reasons or returning from war in need of services and partly by deplorable conditions existing in mental hospitals around the country (Joint Commission, 1961). This Commission focused primarily on the needs of adults, although as part of its special reports, it did include a volume specifically on schools and mental health. The strongest recommendation concerning children is that

[P]sychiatric clinics providing intensive psychotherapy for children, plus appropriate medical or social treatment procedures, should be fostered and, where they exist, expanded. Of all categories of psychiatrists, child psychiatrists are in shortest supply—children being especially trying to work with and requiring the close cooperation of the parents and infinite patience on the part of the therapist. The present State aid program is insufficient to provide for the needs in this area. It should be expanded.

(Joint Commission, 1961, p. 262)

Reflecting the prevailing professional view about parents at the time, the report further indicates that treatment of the child will "ordinarily involve an intensive type of psychotherapy centered in the child, plus management of the family and environment" (Joint Commission, 1961, p. 262).

The work of the Joint Commission contributed to the passage of landmark legislation to construct and staff community mental health centers in 1963 and 1965. While this was an important step forward for the mental health field, attention was still focused largely on adults, leading to the creation of the Joint Commission on the Mental Health of Children (1969).

After an extensive study of the children's mental health system, this Commission concluded that services for children were seriously inadequate. They found that only a fraction of children in need of service were receiving any services. This Commission called for the establishment of a child advocacy movement to improve conditions for children and the development of a range of coordinated services for children. The Joint Commission further suggested the establishment of a unit in which all children's programs would be housed and coordinated in the U.S. Department of Health, Education, and Welfare. It also recommended similar coordinated approaches to the needs of children at the state and local levels. The federal response to the Joint Commission has been characterized as "disappointing" (Lourie et al., 1996) since legislation to implement the recommendations was defeated in both 1973 and 1974. Still, the recommendations of the Joint Commission stand as a major influence in the children's mental health field and are largely still relevant.

As Meyers (1985) points out, there were several other short-lived federal efforts to address the mental health needs of children after the Joint Commission report was published. These include the Part F Program, created as an added provision to the Community Mental Health Center Act in 1972 to provide staff grants specifically focused on children, and the Most in Need Program, which operated between 1979 and 1983.

During the Carter administration (1976–80) there was a major emphasis on mental health, including the establishment of the President's Commission on Mental Health and the passage of the Mental Health Systems Act in 1981. The act identified children with serious mental and emotional disturbances as being one of several underserved populations and recommended an approach to serving such children that involved the child welfare, juvenile justice, and education systems in addition to mental health (Lourie et al., 1996). However, after the Reagan administration took office in 1981, the Mental Health Systems Act was repealed before it ever took effect.

As part of President Reagan's "New Federalism" approach, which affected many health and social service areas, federal funding for services related to mental health, alcoholism, and drug abuse was reduced and consolidated into a state-administered block grant. Although this had the positive effect of strengthening the states' role in planning and administering mental health services, it was accompanied by a budget cut and did not directly address children. In future years, the block grant mechanism was used to try to improve services for children with serious emotional disturbances and their families by requiring that states *set aside* a portion of their block grant funds to specifically target this population. However, this was a modest amount of money and had minimal impact.

In 1982, Jane Knitzer published a monograph entitled *Unclaimed Children* on behalf of the Children's Defense Fund. This monograph, based on a survey of states, pointed out that children were an underserved population; that they were frequently shuffled from one service sector to another, with no sector accepting responsibility for them; and that there were only the most modest beginnings within states of the development of a continuum of care. As Lourie and Hernandez (2003, p. 7) point out, "child advocates of the day utilized Knitzer's findings to push for a new child mental health policy based on the findings of the Joint Commission, 15 years earlier." This led to the development of the Child and Adolescent Service System Program (CASSP) within NIMH, an effort to improve the capacity of states to develop systems to serve children with serious emotional disturbances and their families.

Systems of Care

Working within the framework offered by the Joint Commission, federal, state, and local leaders developed a *system of care* model (Stroul and Friedman, 1986) that emphasized the importance of developing a range of services and building partnerships between parents and professionals, and between the different service sectors, and providing of individualized, comprehensive, and culturally competent services. The system was to be designed at the local level based both on a set of values and principles and the best available research evidence.

Elmore (1979–80) has identified four primary policy implementation tools: mandates, inducements, capacity building, and system change. The Child and Adolescent Service System Program focused on both capacity building and system change efforts and provided states with an opportunity to receive $150,000 per year for 5 years to create a system specifically for children with the most serious emotional disturbances and their families, based on the values and principles of a system of care (Stroul and Friedman, 1986).

This effort was influenced as well by lessons learned from states and communities around the country. In particular, in North Carolina a class action lawsuit, *Willie M. et al. v. James B. Hunt, Jr. et al.*, was filed in 1979, maintaining that four minors as well as others had been denied appropriate treatment and education that were rightfully theirs under a series of federal and state statutes (Behar, 1985). The State of North Carolina negotiated a settlement by which children and adolescents who were seriously emotionally disturbed, had accompanying violent or assaultive behavior, received services inappropriate to their needs, and were at risk of being involuntarily institutionalized would be entitled to treatment in the least restrictive, most appropriate environment. Under the leadership of the Division of Mental Health, Mental Retardation, and Substance Abuse Services, the state proceeded to develop an extensive system of services for these children and their families, including intensive case management that was defined as the "cohesive element in a system of services" (Behar, 1985, p. 195). North Carolina implemented a *no eject/no reject policy*, ensuring that all eligible children would be admitted to the system, and that they would not be ejected from the system because of their behavior or lack of response to treatment. This created a need for the system to develop individualized responses to the strengths and requirements of each child and provided important lessons for the entire children's mental health field.

On the other side of the country, in Ventura County, California (Jordan and Hernandez, 1990), a multisector system of care was developed in a medium-sized county north of Los Angeles to serve those children who were in out-of-home placement or at risk for such placement. The system involved close partnerships between mental health, special education, child welfare, and juvenile justice and demonstrated a large reduction in the use of out-of-home placements. The critical element in this model was not the particular services that were offered but the careful planning that was conducted, including defining the population of concern clearly, identifying and engaging collaborative partners, deciding together on actions to be taken, and gathering ongoing data to evaluate success and provide a basis for making change as needed.

Private foundations began to attend to the mental health needs of children as well. In 1988, the Robert Wood Johnson Foundation initiated its Mental Health Services Program for Youth, which provided funding to eight communities to support them in their effort to build systems of care (Cole and Poe, 1993). In 1992, the Annie E. Casey Foundation launched its Urban Child Mental Health Initiative (Gutierrez-Mayka et al., 2000). This initiative specifically targeted children and families in four inner-city communities. It differed from other efforts in that it focused on all children, not just those with serious emotional disturbances.

The State of North Carolina, with funding from the U.S. Department of Defense, initiated a major demonstration project for military dependents at Fort Bragg in the early 1990s. Unlike other efforts to improve outcomes for children with serious emotional disorders, the Fort Bragg project included a large-scale evaluation that included a comparison between youngsters served at Fort Bragg and youngsters served at two other military installations (Bickman et al., 1995). The interpretation of the results of the evaluation generated strong disagreements in the field (Bickman, 1996; Friedman and Burns, 1996). Overall, the results were mixed. Parents at Fort Bragg were more satisfied with the services provided than were parents in the comparison military communities, more children were served at Fort Bragg, and there was less use of inpatient hospitalization, better continuity of care, and more use of intermediate services. However, the cost of care was greater at Fort Bragg, and no differences in clinical outcomes were found. The extra cost and the failure to obtain differences in clinical outcomes is the main message that has been received about the Fort Bragg project. Alternative interpretations of the findings, however, have highlighted that Fort Bragg was not really a multiagency system of care but rather a single-sector effort with participants of moderate need, that service implementation was greatly hampered by an unexpectedly high demand, that financing

procedures contributed to the excessive cost, and that youngsters with serious emotional disturbance served at Fort Bragg did have better outcomes on measures of
functional impairment than youngsters in the comparison group.

Part of the result of the Fort Bragg evaluation and a second evaluation by the
same team (Bickman et al., 1999) that also failed to find significant differences in
clinical outcomes has been to balance the focus on system infrastructure with an
increased emphasis on the actual interaction between the child and family, on the
one hand, and service providers, on the other. Systems of care have always emphasized the delivery of individualized, comprehensive, and culturally competent
interventions based on the strengths and needs of the child and family, and have
been developed in partnership with the family, but at times this focus was not as
strong as the focus on building a strong infrastructure for service delivery at the
system level (Hernandez and Hodges, 2003).

The effort to create systems of care that began in 1984 with CASSP grants continues today. While CASSP grants were essentially capacity building, the federal
government (after reorganization, the relevant federal agency became the Center
for Mental Health Services within the Substance Abuse and Mental Health Services Administration) funded direct service grants to enable communities to establish systems of care that provide the services needed by children with serious
emotional disturbances and their families. By 2002, 67 such grants had been given
out. These grants were for 5 years and totaled over $5 million each, with grant
recipients being required to provide matching funds that increased as the grant
progressed.

Financing of Services

The 1990s saw two important developments in the financing of services. First, the
Medicaid program, established in 1965 to provide health care to the indigent and
the disabled, grew in size and importance. Medicaid is a federal–state partnership
in which there are certain services that the federal government requires and others that are optional and up to the state. The federal government matches state expenditures, with the matching ratio varying as a function of the socioeconomic status of the states. High-income states, for example, get 50 cents from the federal
government for every 50 cents that they spend. In low-income states, for every 20
cents of state expenditure the federal government provides 80 cents.

Since all states, regardless of their income status, could leverage their money
through the Medicaid program, states began to use their general revenue funds to
bring in additional revenue through Medicaid, even though this included restrictions that were not otherwise present on state general revenue programs. In Florida,
for example, in 1989–90, general revenue expenditures on children's mental health
exceeded Medicaid expenditures by over $40 million. By 1998–99, Medicaid ex-
penditures had risen so dramatically that they exceeded general revenue expenditures by over $50 million (Florida Commission on Mental Health and Substance
Abuse, 2001).

Second, the rapid increase in Medicaid expenditures across the country, not just
in mental health but in all areas of health, led to an enormous increase in the use

of managed care strategies to contain costs in the 1990s (Pires et al., 1999; Stroul et al., 1997). A similar move to managed care took place in the private insurance sector. While managed care procedures have contributed to a cost savings in children's mental health, particularly through large reductions in the use of inpatient psychiatric hospitalization, they have not supported as well as had been hoped the development of the broad range of services advocated by proponents of systems of care.

Policy in Education

Another major part of the policy context has to do with federal education law. In 1975, the Education for All Handicapped Children Act went into effect, promoting the right of all children identified with a handicap to a free and appropriate public education based on an individualized education plan. This act stipulated that school systems would be responsible for all services that children identified as handicapped needed to benefit from education. This act, intended to be an enormous advance for children with disabilities, created a large special education system that often seemed to run separately from the regular education system. Further, since federal funds to serve children with disabilities were inadequate to meet the needs of many of the children, the act unintentionally created a fiscal disincentive for school districts to identify children as disabled, because then they would be responsible for paying for what could be expensive educational and related services. This was particularly problematic for the category of children with *serious emotional disturbance,* since school systems worried about being responsible for expensive therapies of unlimited duration, including possibly residential treatment. This has resulted in only about 1% of children nationally being identified as having a serious emotional disturbance (a total of about 500,000 per year), a percentage that is far lower than national prevalence rates. Some school districts rarely identify a child as having a serious emotional disturbance, thereby escaping the fiscal liability for providing educational and related services.

The Education for All Handicapped Children Act was renamed the Individuals with Disabilities Act (IDEA) in 1990 and was again strengthened in 1997. This act embraces many of the same features as the original act while going beyond the access and compliance provisions of the original legislation. It stresses the importance of parent participation and includes an increased emphasis on inclusion of children with disabilities in regular education. However, the federal government still fails to provide adequate funding to meet the needs of children with disabilities.

In 2001, President Bush established the President's Commission on Excellence in Special Education. This Commission, in its report, indicates that "what we found was a system in need of fundamental re-thinking, a shift in priorities, and a new commitment to individual needs. What we saw was a need for reforms that promise to transform and reach the life of every child with a disability as well as empower every parent" (2002, p. 3). The report further indicates that educators and policy makers think about the special education and general education system as separate, "creating incentives for misidentification and academic isolation."

The No Child Left Behind Act, signed into law by President Bush on January 8, 2002, is a statement of current education policy. It emphasizes accountability, particularly for academic achievement, while allowing states flexibility in the methods they choose to use to achieve their academic goals. Emphasis is placed on the increased use of scientifically based programs and teaching methods, as well as full information and options for parents. A section of the act specifically stresses the need to ensure "student access to quality mental health care by developing innovative programs to link local school systems with the local mental health system."

Current innovations in mental health services in schools focus on trying to balance the need to deliver not only prevention services, but also early intervention and intensive interventions and supports with the same school. In developing schoolwide models of support, Adelman and Taylor (2000) indicate that schools have historically operated only two components: an instructional component to directly facilitate learning and a management component for governance and resource management. They propose that a third component, called the *enabling component*, is needed for students who do not come to school ready to learn or have special challenges. The enabling component is a comprehensive multifaceted approach for addressing barriers to learning, and includes an array of activities for schools to use to promote healthy development for all students.

State and Local Roles in Policy

It should be noted that as with education, the major responsibility for mental health policy in this country is at the state and local levels. As noted earlier, however, federal legislation passed in the 1960s to promote community mental health services provided funding directly to local communities, essentially bypassing states and resulting in very uneven distribution of resources and services within states. The block grant approach taken by the Reagan administration changed this situation, sending money for direct services to the states to distribute. This was then reinforced by CASSP, which was essentially designed to build state capacities to develop and implement effective systems of care for children with serious emotional disturbances and their families, and which gave its grants directly to states. With the ending of CASSP in the early 1990s, however, and the initiation of direct service grants from the federal government to local communities, the strong link that had been established between federal policy makers in children's mental health and state policy makers began to weaken.

A recent review of state statutes (Evans and Armstrong, 2003) indicates that most states have statutes supporting the development of community-based systems of care that embrace the principles of CASSP. Of 39 states that responded to a survey, only 5 indicated that they did not have a system of care or submitted materials that were judged as not demonstrating the establishment of a system based on the principles of systems of care (Stroul and Friedman, 1986). Of the 34 states that responded to the survey indicating that their policy was to develop systems of care, 82% had legislation to support this, 15% used inducements, 41% used capacity-building mechanisms, and 44% used other methods to try to bring about system change. While the precise mechanisms that states have chosen to use to try to implement such systems is quite variable, as is the effectiveness of the policy, there is substantial agreement on a general child mental health policy direction and a set of values and principles.

Between June 1997 and October 2001, commissions in 13 separate states issued reports on the status of the mental health system in their states. Three of these states devoted almost their entire report to issues related to adult mental health, but all other states had a heavy focus on children. Despite the fact that each of the reports identifies some areas of substantial progress, the most important and most consistent conclusion drawn from a summary of the reports is serious dissatisfaction with the adequacy of the existing system to meet the mental health needs of children, adolescents, and their families (Friedman, 2002). The recommendations from this report are discussed further later in this chapter.

Seriousness of the Problem

A discussion of policy issues in children's mental health must be placed in the context of the seriousness of the problem. A beginning point for examining seriousness is a review of the prevalence of the problem. A federal task force convened by the Center for Mental Health Services reviewed the research on prevalence and concluded that about 1 in 5 children have a diagnosable mental disorder, and about 1 in 10 children have a serious emotional disturbance (Friedman et al., 1996a, 1998). A child with a serious emotional disturbance not only has a diagnosable disorder but also demonstrates substantial impairment in functioning at home, in school, or in the community because of the disorder. A more recent review of the literature also indicates that the prevalence of diagnosable disorders is approximately 20% (Roberts et al., 1998). Although there is less information about prevalence in young children than there is about prevalence in children between 9 and 17 years of age, the research that is available indicates that the prevalence rate is not very different than it is for older children (Lavigne et al., 1996).

Although serious emotional disturbance, is not a diagnosis, it has become the primary focus of children's mental health policy across the country. This focus was initially selected by CASSP in 1984 after the publication by Knitzer of *Unclaimed Children* (1982) and was supported widely by states in the early to mid-1980s. It has provided direction for public sector mental health activities in children's mental health. It has also created an emphasis that goes beyond the question of diagnosis to the domain of functioning and/or impairment in important community environments.

Another key issue in determining the seriousness of the problem is the duration of emotional disturbances in children. Research has indicated that while many of the milder disorders are short-term in nature and do not have a major effect on functioning in school, at home, or in the community, the serious disorders tend to be more long-lasting and have an effect on functioning (Friedman et al., 1996b; Kessler et al., 1995, 1997). They tend not only to persist as disorders but also to affect educational, vocational, and social outcomes in adults (Kessler et al., 1995, 1997). A recent report by the Institute of Medicine that focuses not specifically on mental disorders but rather on the overall well-being of young people puts this issue in perspective. It indicates that "at least 25 percent of adolescents in the United States are at serious risk of not achieving 'productive adulthood'" (National Research Council and Institute of Medicine, 2002, p. 2).

At their most extreme, mental disorders in young people can contribute to suicide. Suicide is the third leading cause of death in young people between the ages of 15 and 24, and in 87% of the cases it is associated with a diagnosable disorder (Flynn et al., 2002). Between 1980 and 1994, the rate of suicide in young people between the ages of 15 and 19 increased by 30.6%, and the rate for ages 10 to 14 increased by 120% (Metha et al., 1998).

Who Are These Children and What Are Their Needs?

The development of policy should begin with a thorough understanding of the population of concern, their needs, and the system that has been set up to serve them. It should be noted first that mental health problems affect children of any age, socioeconomic status, or racial or ethnic background. While this is the case, the prevalence of disorders is greatest in children from low-income backgrounds (Friedman et al., 1996a). The most common diagnoses applied to children are anxiety and depressive disorders, attention–deficit/hyperactivity disorders, oppositional disorder, and conduct disorder. A review of the research describing youngsters with emotional disorders indicates that they frequently have more than one diagnosis and typically have significant problems in more than one domain (Friedman et al., 1996b). In addition to the emotional and behavioral domains, these youngsters often have difficulty in educational performance and social behavior. This is a reflection of the fact that the causes of children's problems are multiple and complex, often including biological, psychological, and social factors. Those children with the most serious problems are often being served in special systems, such as special education, child welfare, or juvenile justice systems, creating the need to move beyond a focus on any single categorical system.

The children are part of families who have the major responsibility for their care. A common characteristic of these families is the high level of stress under which they live. Also, many of the families have low incomes, adding to the stress, and often have only a single parent. The combination of child and family factors results in a very heterogeneous group, creating a special challenge for policy makers and planners and requiring a broad range of services and supports.

The special problem affecting children and adults from racial and ethnic minority groups was highlighted in the Surgeon General's Report on Mental Health (U.S. Department of Health and Human Services, 1999) and in a special supplement to that report that dealt specifically with issues related to culture, race, and ethnicity (U.S. Department of Health and Human Services, 2001). This supplemental report emphasizes that, compared with whites, minorities have less access to mental health services, are less likely to receive needed services, and often receive poorer-quality service. The report indicates that mistrust of mental health services is an important deterrent to seeking services by individuals of color.

In recent years, there has been increased recognition of the importance of assessing strengths, risk and protective factors, and capacity for resilience as well as needs (Davis, 2002; Matsen and Coatsworth, 1998; Waller, 2001; Wolin and Wolin, 1993). This emphasis on strengths and resilience is very helpful in engaging families and, most important, can serve a very valuable role in the development of interventions. Since the prevailing systems in which children are served are deficit-oriented, and since funding mechanisms are largely based on identification of problems, a challenge is to adjust these systems and mechanisms so that they can support strength-based interventions.

It is also important to recognize that the ability of any child or family to function effectively is a function not only of their own strengths and needs, but also of the availability of natural and special supports in their communities. A child with anxiety disorder or attention-deficit/hyperactivity disorder, for example, will be more or less disabled, depending on the quality of the educational and family supports that he or she receives. Likewise, when parents receive important supports, like assistance with the daily responsibilities of caring for a child who presents special challenges or information to help them understand the problem, they are better able to provide the care that their child requires. A simple parallel in the field of physical disabilities, for example, is that individuals in wheelchairs have become less disabled in our society as we have provided appropriate ramps to promote their physical access within a community. The challenge, therefore, in children's mental health is not just to develop treatments for the child, but to help develop the supports needed by the family and in the community to improve functioning and reduce impairment and stress.

Service Utilization

Given the complexity and severity of many of the emotional disturbances of children, how successful are we in providing services that might help them? This issue is partly reflected in a recent study (Ringel and Sturm, 2001) on the degree of unmet need for mental health services. Using data from the National Health Interview Study, Ringel and Sturm (2001) estimate that about 80% of children with identified mental health needs do not receive services in the specialty mental health sector. This is an extremely high percentage overall, and there is an especially large gap between need and use among African American and Latino children. Jensen et al. (2002) recently completed an analysis of data from several community epidemiological studies and found that even children who demonstrated what were clearly believed to be serious problems, such as making suicide attempts, were unlikely to receive any mental health services.

Two other studies that combined epidemiological data and service use data illustrate the issue. Leaf and colleagues (1996) examined the use of services in the Methodological Epidemiological Catchment Area (MECA) study. Their sample consisted of 1285 youngsters between the ages of 9 and 17 from four different communities. They found that while the prevalence rate of a diagnosable disorder in the sample was 32.3%, only 14.9% of the youngsters had received mental health services in the prior 12 months. Further, of the total sample, 8.1% received services in the specialty mental health sector, 8.1% in the schools, 2.9% in the medical sector, 1.6% from a social services agency, 1.2% from clergy, and 0.7% from other sources.

The Great Smoky Mountain Study is a community epidemiological study done in western North Carolina (Burns et al., 1995). The sample consisted of 1015 youngsters approximately equally divided among 9-, 11-, and 13-year-olds. About one-fifth of the sample received a diagnosis based on a structured diagnostic interview, and in the 3 months preceding participation in the study, 16% received mental health services. However, of those who received mental health services, 75% received them through the school, whereas only 4% received them from the specialty mental health sector. This finding led to the conclusion that "the major player in the de facto system of care was the education sector" (Burns et al., 1995).

Schools are clearly one of the major providers of mental health services for children. Recent research indicates that 4.4% of adolescents receive some type of mental health counseling service in the school during the course of a year, compared to 8.8% who receive service outside of the school (Slade, 2002). Services in the school can be provided by a school-based health clinic, mental health professionals from an outside agency who consult within the school, or school staff such as psychologists, social workers, and counselors. Although not much detailed information is available about the specific services provided within schools, it is clear that schools can be an effective mechanism for increasing access to care. This is illustrated by the research of Catron and Weiss (1994), who randomly assigned students identified as needing mental health services either to school-based treatment or to treatment in the community. Of those for whom services were offered in the school, almost all entered the service and almost all completed treatment. Of those whose families were referred for community treatment, even though they were encouraged and even assisted to get such services, only about one-fifth received them.

In recent years, there has been an enormous increase in the application of positive behavior support (PBS) approaches within the schools (Horner and Carr, 1997; Scott, 2001). Positive behavior support is a team-based, comprehensive, proactive data-based system for facilitating and maintaining positive student behavior across settings. At first, this approach focused specifically on children with significant challenges. It has now developed interventions for three groups of children. The first group is the 75%–80% of children who are estimated to be functioning adequately in school, the second group is the 15%–20% who are considered to be at risk for serious problems, and the third is the 1%–7% who already show serious problems.

The context, therefore, for examining approaches to improving access to care and effectiveness of care is as follows: the prevalence of emotional problems is high and the nature of the problems is very heterogeneous; these problems affect many life domains and service sectors and are often long-lasting; families are under great stress and in need of supports; and only a small percentage of children in need of care are receiving it.

As already indicated, the primary policy approach of the federal and state governments to this situation since the mid-1980s has been to promote the development of community-based systems of care (Stroul and Friedman, 1986, 1996). A *system of care* was defined as "a comprehensive spectrum of mental health and other necessary services which are organized into a coordinated network to meet the multiple and changing needs of severely emotionally disturbed children and adolescents" (1986, p. 3). The system-of-care concept did not represent a specific model but rather a philosophy that was to be based on a core set of values and principles and the best available research. The core values have emphasized the importance of individualized, culturally competent, strength-based, and comprehensive services developed and implemented in partnership with families.

In addition to office-based outpatient treatment and inpatient care, the system-of-care model emphasized the importance of home-based services and supports, day treatment, case management, crisis services, and various types of out-of-home care, including care provided in specialized therapeutic foster homes, therapeutic group homes, and residential treatment centers. In recent years, services such as respite care, mentoring, and tutoring have become very common, and the range of services originally described by Stroul and Friedman (1986) has been greatly expanded. The system-of-care concept also emphasized the importance of collaboration across service sectors since many youngsters with emotional disturbances were found in sectors other than mental health, and many youngsters required the services of more than one sector. This created the challenge of developing effective interagency collaborations across service sectors with different mandates and cultures.

One of the most important parts of the system-of-care movement has been its emphasis on redefining the role of parents. While traditional approaches have frequently viewed parents as the cause of their child's problem and have omitted them from active participation in their child's treatment, the system-of-care movement has emphasized that parents are the most important resource for their child, have the right to be involved in every step of care, and must be involved if interventions are to be successful. The involvement of families in efforts to develop policy and overall systems was also emphasized and has resulted in an enormous increase in family participation around the country, the development of a national family advocacy organization (the Federation of Families for Children's Mental Health), and the development of state and local family organizations.

Another important part of the system-of-care movement has been a strong focus on providing services and developing systems that are responsive to the needs and perspectives of individuals from varying racial and ethnic backgrounds. This focus on *cultural competence* (Cross et al., 1989; Hernandez and Isaacs, 1998) is supported by the recent Surgeon General's special report on services for diverse populations (U.S. Department of Health and Human Services, 2001) and is designed to increase both access to care and effectiveness of care. It builds on the recognition that culture affects help-seeking behavior, the way in which emotional or behavioral challenges are interpreted, the level of trust of mental health approaches, and the willingness to seek out mental health care and participate in it.

In their early days, systems of care succeeded in expanding the range of service options from what had been primarily office-based outpatient care or some form of residential/inpatient care to a broader range of services. However, each of these new services was categorically funded, making it difficult to individualize services for children and families. A critical policy and programmatic development, based on the diversity of the population of children with emotional disturbances and their families, and the philosophy of individualized care, was the development of pools of *flexible* money that could be used to purchase whatever reasonable support or service was needed for a child and family. If a mentor was needed, for example, and such a program did not exist, then the flexible funds could be used to purchase the services. If extra support was needed in the home, this could be purchased, or a new tire could be bought for a car so that a poor family could get to work, or a child could be enrolled in a community class or club that built on his or her special strength and interest.

Initially, these flexible funds were restricted to small numbers of youngsters with the most serious problems. In recent years, however, there has been a tendency to expand their use and to reduce the amount of money that is committed to a specified service. A national leader in this regard has been the Wraparound Milwaukee system of care (Kamradt, 2000), which serves youngsters with serious emotional disturbance who are referred by the court and are also in either the child welfare or juvenile justice system. This system of care, instead of contracting with a few providers, as is traditional, has built a provider network of over 200 individuals and agencies and has developed over 80 different services. This makes it possible for families and treatment teams to have genuine choice, both of services to be provided and the actual provider. Wraparound Milwaukee itself is a care management organization that receives a case rate for each youngster it services. It was able to build this system by taking money, obtained as part of a case rate agreement with the courts, that previously would have been used to contract with specified providers for a guaranteed amount of service, and using it to contract with many more providers who are paid on a fee-for-service basis with no guaranteed volume of service. The amount of service they receive depends on the need, as determined by case managers, treatment teams, and, most important, families. It is also dependent on the value of the service to families, because families provide regular feedback to Wraparound Milwaukee on their satisfaction with services. In addition, a comprehensive quality assurance system is used. This approach, identified in the interim report of the President's New Freedom Commission as a promising approach, has combined the features of flexible funds, an expanded provider network, an expanded range of services, individualized care, family choice and participation at all levels, accountability at the level of individual providers, and the creation of a structure to manage it all. Several other communities have developed similar models as the concept of system of care, and the values that it represents, continue to evolve.

Recommendations from the Surgeon General's Conference and State Mental Health Commission Reports

The Surgeon General's Conference on Children's Mental Health, held on September 18–19, 2000, developed eight general goals for the children's mental health field. These goals essentially represent policy directions for the field. They are:

- Promote public awareness of children's mental health issues and reduce the stigma associated with mental illness;
- Continue to develop, disseminate, and implement scientifically proven prevention and treatment services in the field of children's mental health;
- Improve the assessment and recognition of mental health needs in children;
- Eliminate racial/ethnic and socioeconomic disparities in access to mental health care services;
- Improve the infrastructure for children's mental health services, including support for scientifically proven interventions across professions;
- Increase access to and coordination of quality mental health care services;
- Train front-line providers to recognize and manage mental health care issues, and educate mental health providers about scientifically proven prevention and treatment services;
- Monitor the access to and coordination of quality mental health care services.

A similar but somewhat different list was generated in a review (Friedman, 2002) of recommendations from special commissions created within states to study mental health services. Between June 1997 and October 2001, commissions in 13 states issued reports on the status of mental health in their state. Of these, 10 states included significant recommendations regarding children (California, Connecticut, Florida, Kentucky, Montana, Nevada, Ohio, Tennessee, West Virginia, and Wisconsin). As reported earlier, the most important general conclusion in these reports is a serious dissatisfaction with the adequacy of efforts to address the mental health needs of children and adolescents and their families. Since the major responsibility for policy development and implementation in mental health is at the state and local levels, a review of the recommendations from these reports is presented here in some detail. It essentially presents a policy agenda for the field, based on deliberations of numerous concerned individuals across the country.

The first recommendation is that there be *a continued focus on the values and principles of systems of care,* including collaboration across service sectors, the support of a strong role for families, and the provision of individualized, comprehensive, and culturally competent services. Although it was recognized that the development of effective systems of care was a challenging developmental process, and although there was some dissatisfaction with the pace at which this process had proceeded, there was strong support for the continued efforts. This included very clear recognition that unless the mental health agency had effective partnerships with other child-serving sectors, progress in assisting children and families would be limited.

These key values and principles, while widely agreed on, represent major changes in the children's mental health field, and other fields as well, and create a major policy challenge. The increased involvement of families at the policy level as well as the treatment level, the development of training and financing mechanisms to change practice by supporting individualized and culturally competent care, and the crumbling of walls that divide different service sectors are all complex and difficult undertakings that require much time and well-thought-out strategies.

The second recommendation is that there be *an increased emphasis on prevention and early intervention.* As indicated earlier, with the development of CASSP at the federal level in 1984, the policy focus at the federal, state, and local levels all shifted to children with serious emotional disturbances and their families as the primary population of concern. The reports from the various commissions consistently recognize the importance of this population. However, they emphasize that unless there is a parallel focus on prevention and early intervention, it is unlikely that there will be significant progress in the long run. The need for such a focus is supported by the high prevalence rates reported earlier, as well as the information on the duration of emotional problems and their relationship to functioning in many important life domains.

This recommendation implies that a broad population-based public health approach be taken to improve the overall mental health status of our children. Such an approach might include such steps as identifying risk and protective factors for mental health problems in children; developing, evaluating, and implementing preventive interventions that strengthen protective factors and reduce risk factors; tracking on a regular basis, through systematic data collection, the mental health status of our population; reviewing public policy to determine its effect on the mental health status of children; increasing public awareness of the problem; and continuing to strengthen the knowledge base about effective preventive and intervention strategies.

The focus on protective factors is particularly consistent with the strength-based approach emphasized within systems of care, and with general community development and positive youth development efforts. The National Research Council and Institute of Medicine (2002), for example, concludes that "adolescents who spend time in communities that are rich in developmental opportunities for them experience less risk and show evidence of higher rates of positive development. A diversity of program opportunities in each community is more likely to support broad adolescent development and attract the interest of and meet the needs of a greater number of youth" (pp. 10–11). In addition to the field of resilience, with its emphasis on risk and protective factors, the fields of positive youth development, family support, and community development appear to have much to offer children's mental health in its effort to prevent the development of emotional problems and improve the mental health status of children.

The third recommendation from the commissions is that there be *a reexamination of funding policies* with an intent to create more flexibility in funding, to reduce categorical funding, and to expand the coverage offered under Medicaid. This policy recommendation is based on the characteristics of children with mental health needs. As indicated earlier, they are a diverse group from every perspective, often with co-occurring conditions, and are found in many systems other than the specialty mental health sector. This requires flexible funding so that individualized and comprehensive care can be provided; reduction of categorical funding so that the various sectors involved in children's lives can work together; and availability of a broad range of services to meet the multiple needs of children and their families. It should be noted that the commissions also frequently identified the need for increased funding as a priority.

The fourth recommendation was that there be *greater attention to planning, accountability, and responsibility*. Several of the commissions pointed out that while multiple public and private entities had important roles to play in meeting the mental health needs of children and families, there was an absence of overall comprehensive planning, accountability was fragmented, and as a consequence, there was a sense that nobody was responsible at the system level. Under the federal CASSP initiative, states had some resources and encouragement to convene diverse groups of stakeholders to develop plans to meet the mental health needs of children with serious emotional disturbances and their families. Since the end of these grants in the early 1990s, however, there appears to be a decreased emphasis on such planning.

Consistent with this focus, a fifth recommendation was that there be *a review of governmental structures, with the intent of creating a strong, coordinated voice* for the needs of children and families. The Florida report, for example, called for the creation of a statewide "Coordinating Council for Mental Health and Substance Abuse," and the California reported recommended the appointment of a state "Secretary of Children's Services" as well as the establishment of county-level "Child and Family Service Boards." The Connecticut report called for a prevention budget that cut across department lines.

This concern about diffuse responsibility for children's services overall, and particularly for children's mental health, was very common in the commission reports. Sometimes it focused on prevention issues specifically, more often on children's mental health in its totality, and occasionally on children's issues overall. The California report, prepared by the Little Hoover Commission (2001), an independent oversight group that had also completed in recent years studies of other childserving systems, was the most dramatic in its criticism of the present system and radical in its recommendation. It concluded that "the present system fails more children than it serves. It is broken to the point of needing replacement. A new categorical program—an infusion of more money alone—will not cure this system" (p. 75). The policy issue of how to establish governmental structures that are accountable and responsible for planning and oversight is critical for government at all levels; for stakeholders interested in specific issues related to children, such as their mental health; and for those interested in the overall well-being of children.

The sixth recommendation that had consistent and strong support from the commissions called for *the creation of closer partnerships between the schools and mental health professionals*. This recommendation builds on the earlier emphasis on the need for collaboration across service sectors. It recognizes, however, that schools play an especially critical role in the lives of children from many perspectives. For one, through schools, children in need of care can be identified and those in need can then be provided easier access to care, thereby at least partially addressing a problem of great importance. Also, the overall school environment and culture can have an important impact on social and emotional development, as well as academic achievement (Hoagwood and Johnson, 2003).

Two special populations at opposite ends of the developmental spectrum received special mention. At the older age range, four states specifically identified a need for increased attention to helping older adolescents with emotional problems make the transition to adulthood and the increasing responsibilities that it brings (Clark and Davis, 2000). In response to this need, the Center for Mental Health Services has just initiated a national demonstration program on the transition to adulthood for adolescents with emotional problems.

At the younger age range, there is increased recognition of the importance of early childhood for laying the foundation for healthy social and emotional development. The report of the National Research Council and the Institute of Medicine on early childhood (2000) summarized research indicating that early experiences affect the development of the brain and lay the foundation for intelligence, emotional health, and moral development, and healthy early development depends on nurturing, dependable relationships. Many young children already demonstrate significant mental health problems. The Florida report indicates that "mental health professionals historically have ignored the needs of young children. It has become increasingly apparent in recent years, however, that young children are very vulnerable and are significantly affected by such things as disruptions in key relationships, exposure to violence, and exposure to drugs in utero. Many children already demonstrate serious problems in their early years while others are at a critical junction for the development of such problems" (2001, p. 9). The relationship of social and emotional development in young children to their readiness to success in school is being increasingly recognized as well, linking a mental health outcome to an important educational policy objective.

The next recommendation calls for a focus on *the improvement of quality of services and increased attention to professional training*. The issue of quality and effectiveness of services was related by the commissions to the establishment of professional standards for both organizations and individuals, and to the implementation of continuous quality improvement procedures within systems, organizations, and programs. A strong call has been made in recent years for the careful development of theories of change to guide system and program development, and then the institution of internal accountability procedures that are based on the theory of change and that are used not to prove or disprove the effectiveness of what is happening, but rather to improve it (Hernandez and Hodges, 2001).

Another important part of the focus on quality of services is the development of a large, diverse, and competent workforce that is able to implement the principles of a system of care. It is recognized that this calls for a partnership between mental health systems and universities at both the preservice and inservice training levels. Currently, most university-based training is single-discipline, office-based, and deficit-based, has an inadequate focus on cultural competence and family perspectives, and does not offer a comprehensive approach to understanding the needs of children and families and the development of strengths-based, individualized treatment plans in partnership with families to meet those needs. Any major policy effort to try to change the preparation of professionals is likely to require not only the involvement of universities but also of professional associations and licensing entities in states.

One approach to dealing with the workforce issue has been to try to expand provider networks and increase accountability at the provider level. For example, the Wraparound Milwaukee program, discussed earlier (Kamradt, 2000), has developed a provider network of over 200 individuals and organizations. They have done this essentially by shifting from primarily contracting with large mental health centers for guaranteed volumes of particular services to opening the contracting process to other organizations and individuals, each of whom is paid on a fee-for-service basis for each unit of service provided but is not guaranteed a minimum volume. As a result of this, there may now be 5 or 10 individuals or organizations approved by Wraparound Milwaukee at the same rate of pay to provide treatment for trauma, or mentoring, or home-based therapy, for example. Families in need of such services now have a choice of provider; the families provide feedback to the organization on their satisfaction with the services that were provided; and providers know that the number of referrals they receive is not guaranteed by a contract but instead is dependent on satisfaction with their service and need. Also, experienced practitioners, who previously would not work with mental health organizations, are now more likely to agree to provide services as individual consultants who are paid on a fee-for-service basis. This is one creative approach to addressing the workforce issue that is also consistent with system-of-care values in providing choice to families and keeping resources flexible so that individualized, comprehensive services can be provided.

Another approach to improving the quality and effectiveness of services is to develop, evaluate, and disseminate evidence-based practices. Evidence-based practices are interventions that have met particular scientific criteria for effectiveness. The State of Hawaii has been a leader in trying to strengthen the quality and effectiveness of its services through the use of evidence-based practices (Chorpita et al., 2002).

Interestingly, although there has been great emphasis on evidence-based practices in the published literature in recent years (Hoagwood, 2002, has pointed out an increase in the use of the term *evidence-based* in the published literature, based on a Medline search, from zero prior to 1990 to 86 times between 1990 and 1995 and almost 6000 times between 1995 and 2002), and in the Surgeon General's Conference on Children's Mental Health (U.S. Public Health Service, 2000), there was only minimal mention of it in the reports of the state commissions. This may be due to several factors. Several of the reports were prepared before the increase in the discussion of evidence-based practices began to peak. Also, within systems of care, there has always been an emphasis on using effective practices, although the term *evidence-based practice* has not been formally used (Friedman et al., 1989; Stroul and Friedman, 1986). Also, public mental health systems serve diverse populations of youngsters, often with multiple needs, and much of the research on evidence-based practices has focused on more restricted populations of children served under conditions that differ from those in most communities (Friedman, 2001; Shirk, 2001). Finally, many of the stakeholders serving on or testifying before state commissions, including family members, are strongly concerned about adherence to system-of-care values such as family partnerships in the development of treatment plans and the development of individualized, culturally competent treatment plans.

Burns et al. (1999) have identified interventions such as case management, multisystemic therapy, and therapeutic foster care as particularly promising. However, overall, there are significant limits on the number of interventions that have proven to be effective, particularly with the populations served in the public sector. Therefore, while the movement to identify evidence-based interventions is clearly positive, much of what passes for research on evidence-based practice might more aptly be described as clinical treatment efficacy research, and treatments that have been validated in efficacy studies cannot be assumed to be effective when implemented under routine practice conditions, as Hoagwood et al. (2001) have pointed out. Further, there is still much to be learned about the processes of dissemination and implementation. It is potentially a great leap from the development of an effective intervention by one team of researchers/clinicians to the effective dissemination and implementation of that intervention in other communities, by other teams, and with other populations of children and families. The major challenges, therefore, appear to be to support the preliminary work needed to develop effective practices, particularly those practices targeted at children with multiple and serious problems, and to support research on dissemination and implementation practices.

The final recommendation that appears consistently in the commission reports is that *greater public education efforts* be undertaken both to reduce stigma and to increase support for and understanding of child and adolescent mental health issues. The Surgeon General's Conference on Children's Mental Health (U.S. Public Health Service, 2000) emphasized this same need and called for a partnership between mental health and the media, youth, public health systems, communities, health professionals, and advocacy groups.

Implications for Mental Health Services

This chapter provided background for understanding child mental health policy, including historical information on the development of policy and a discussion of the role of various levels of government, as well as information on the seriousness of the problem of children's mental health needs. It then examined and discussed the primary policy issues confronting the children's mental health field, using two recent reports as the primary sources. In some instances, examples of innovative approaches to addressing some of the issues were presented.

The policy issues are large and complex, and can largely be summarized in three key policy questions:

1. How can we improve access to care for children with mental health needs and their families, and particularly reduce any disparities related to race, ethnicity, or socioeconomic status?
2. How can we improve the quality and effectiveness of services that are provided?
3. Perhaps most important in the long run, how can we improve the overall mental health status of the entire population of children?

The first question calls for a multifaceted approach including greater education of the public and of professionals in key positions, such as pediatricians, child care staff, and educators about how to identify a need for mental health services, and building trust about the value and safety of mental health services, particularly in poor and minority communities. It also includes providing increased screening for mental health needs in key systems, such as primary health care, child care, education, child welfare, and juvenile justice, with linkages to full assessments and treatment as needed. It further involves increasing the ease of obtaining services through such mechanisms as easy and responsive points of access. Finally, it includes eliminating fiscal barriers through adequate funding in public systems and increased coverage by private and public insurance.

The second question, dealing with the quality and effectiveness of services, also calls for many varied efforts, based on the characteristics of children in need of services and their families, and research on the functioning of systems and the effectiveness of present services. This requires such efforts as additional research to develop effective interventions at the practice and systems levels, further efforts to disseminate existing knowledge about the effectiveness of various interventions, strengthening of the workforce through preservice and inservice training, creating stronger collaborations between all of the systems involved in the lives of children and families, the addition of continuous quality improvement and internal accountability procedures, the expansion of the workforce and of provider networks, increased accessibility to a comprehensive range of individualized and culturally competent services, strengthening family voice and choice at both the treatment level and the system/policy level, and establishing empirically based treatment guidelines and standards.

To address the third question, dealing with the overall mental health status of all children, it is essential to move beyond the strong clinical model that has dominated the mental health field and to implement more of a public health approach. This would include a strong epidemiological focus on the prevalence of disorders, the development of disorders, and risk and protective factors as a basis both for determining how well children are doing and for developing preventive interventions. It would further include public education efforts, the increased development and implementation of preventive interventions, systematic screening efforts to identify children in need of services and to intervene early in the development of the problems, ongoing analysis of public policies to promote those policies that support healthy social and emotional development in children, evaluation of existing policies, systems, programs, and treatments to determine their effectiveness, and ongoing efforts to strengthen the workforce and increase access to care.

Given the prevalence of mental disorders in children and adolescents, and given their impact on functioning in many important life domains over many years, substantial progress will ultimately require not only improved access to care and treatment but also a shift toward a public health model that will promote health and reduce the incidence of mental disorders. Such an approach appears to have the greatest likelihood of significantly improving the social and emotional well-being of our children and their ability to contribute to our country.

REFERENCES

Adelman HS, Taylor L. Looking at school health and school reform policy through the lens of addressing barriers to learning. Children's services. *Social Policy, Research, and Practice*, 3(2):117–132, 2000.

Behar L. Changing patterns of state responsibility: a case study of North Carolina. *Journal of Clinical Child Psychology*, 14(3):188–195, 1985.

Bernstein R. Foreword. In: Bernstein R, Koyanagi C (eds). *Disintegrating Systems: The State of States' Public Mental Health Systems*. Washington, DC: Bazelon Center for Mental Health Law, 2001.

Bickman L. A continuum of care: more is not always better. *American Psychologist*, 51:689–701, 1996.

Bickman L, Guthrie PR, Foster EM, et al. *Evaluating Managed Mental Health Services: The Fort Bragg Experiment*. New York: Plenum Press, 1995.

Bickman L, Noser K, Summerfelt WT. Long-term effects of a system of care on children and adolescents. *The Journal of Behavioral Health Services and Research*, 26:185–202, 1999.

Burns BJ, Costello EJ, Angold A, et al. Children's mental health service use across service sectors. *Health Affairs*, 14(3):148–159, 1995.

Burns BJ, Hoagwood K, Mrazek P. Effective treatment for mental disorders in children and adolescents. *Clinical Child and Family Psychology Review*, 2:199–254, 1999.

Catron T, Weiss B. The Vanderbilt school-based counseling program. *Journal of Emotional and Behavioral Disorders*, 2:247–253, 1994.

Chorpita BF, Yim LM, Donkervoet JC, et al. Toward large-scale implementation of empirically supported treatments for children: a review and observations by the Hawaii Empirical Basis to Services Task Force. *Clinical Psychology*, 9(2):165–190, 2002.

Clark HB, Davis M (eds). *Transition to Adulthood: A Resource for Assisting Young People with Emotional or Behavioral Difficulties*. Baltimore: Paul H. Brookes, 2000.

Cole RF, Poe S. *Partnerships for Care; Systems of Care for Children with Serious Emotional Disturbances and their Families*. Washington, DC: Washington Business Group on Health, 1993.

Cross TL, Bazron BJ, Dennis KW, et al. *Towards a Culturally Competent System of Care: Volume I. A Monograph on Effective Services for Minority Children Who Are Severely Emotionally Disturbed*. Washington, DC: Georgetown University Child Development Center, 1989.

Davis NJ. The promotion of mental health and the prevention of mental and behavioral disorders: surely the time is right. *International Journal of Emergency Mental Health*, 4(1):3–30, 2002.

Elmore RF. Backward mapping: implementation research and policy decisions. *Political Science Quarterly*, 94:601–616, 1979–80.

Evans ME, Armstrong MI. *Understanding Collaboration in Systems of Care*. Presentation at the 16th Annual Research Conference—A System of Care for Children's Mental Health: Expanding the Research Base, Research and Training Center for Children's Mental Health, Florida Mental Health Institute, University of South Florida, Tampa, 2003.

Florida Commission on Mental Health and Substance Abuse. *Children's Workgroup Report*. Tampa: University of South Florida, 2001.

Flynn L, McGuire L, Crandall D. *Columbia TeenScreen Program*. New York: Carmel Hill Center for Early Diagnosis and Treatment at the Division of Child and Adolescent Psychiatry, Columbia University, 2002.

Friedman RM. The practice of psychology with children, adolescents, and their families: a look to the future. In: Hughes JN, La Greca AM, Conoley JC (eds). *Handbook of Psychological Services for Children and Adolescents*. New York: Oxford University Press, pp. 3–22, 2001.

Friedman RM. *Child and Adolescent Mental Health: Recommendations for Improvement by State Mental Health Commissions*. Tampa: University of South Florida, 2002.

Friedman RM. A conceptual framework for developing and implementing effective policy in children's mental health. *Journal of Emotional and Behavioral Disorders,* 11(1):11–19, 2003.

Friedman RM, Burns BJ. The evaluation of the Fort Bragg Demonstration Project: an alternative interpretation of the findings. *Journal of Mental Health Administration,* 23:128–136, 1996.

Friedman RM, Duchnowski AJ, Henderson, EL. *Advocacy on Behalf of Children with Serious Emotional Problems.* Springfield, IL: Charles C. Thomas, 1989.

Friedman RM, Katz-Leavy JW, Manderscheid RW, et al. Prevalence of serious emotional disturbance in children and adolescents. In: Manderscheid RW, Sonnenschein MA (eds). *Mental Health, United States, 1996.* Rockville, MD: Substance Abuse and Mental Health Services Administration, pp. 71–89, 1996a.

Friedman RM, Katz-Leavy JW, Manderscheid, RW, et al. Prevalence of serious emotional disturbance: an update. In: Manderscheid RW, Henderson MJ (eds). *Mental Health, United States, 1998.* Rockville, MD: Substance Abuse and Mental Health Services Administration, pp. 110–112, 1998.

Friedman RM, Kutash K, Duchnowski AJ. The population of concern: defining the issues. In: Stroul BA (ed). *Children's Mental Health: Creating Systems of Care in a Changing Society.* Baltimore: Paul H. Brookes, pp. 69–96, 1996b.

Gutierrez-Mayka M, Joseph R, Sengova J, et al. *Evaluation of Systems Reform in the Annie E. Casey Foundation Mental Health Initiative for Urban Children: Summary of Findings and Lessons Learned.* Tampa: University of South Florida, 2000.

Hernandez M, Hodges S. Theory-based accountability. In: Hernandez M, Hodges S (eds). *Developing Outcome Strategies in Children's Mental Health.* Baltimore: Paul H. Brookes, pp. 21–40, 2001.

Hernandez M, Hodges S. Building upon the theory of change for systems of care. *Journal of Emotional and Behavioral Disorders,* 11(1):19–27, 2003.

Hernandez M, Isaacs MR. *Promoting Cultural Competence in Children's Mental Health Services,* Baltimore: Paul H. Brookes, 1998.

Hoagwood K. Implementation and dissemination research in children's mental health services: The question of fit. Paper presented at the National Association of State Mental Health Program Directors' meeting on "Building Evidence-Based Practices for Children: Moving from Science to Service," Tampa, FL, December 2002.

Hoagwood K, Burns BJ, Kiser L, et al. Evidence-based practice in child and adolescent mental health services. *Psychiatric Services,* 52(9):1179–1189, 2001.

Hoagwood K, Johnson J. School psychology: a public health framework. I. From evidence-based practices to evidence-based policies. *Journal of School Psychology,* 41(1):3–21, 2003.

Hogan M. Foreword, *Interim Report to the President.* Washington, DC: President's New Freedom Commission on Mental Health, 2002.

Horner RH, Carr EG. Behavioral support for students with severe disabilities: functional assessment and comprehensive intervention. *Journal of Special Education,* 31:84–104, 1997.

Jensen P, Amsel L, Offord D, et al. *Developing Mental Health Indicators for U.S. Children and Adolescents.* Report submitted to the U.S. Center for Mental Health Services, Rockville, MD, 2002.

Joint Commission on Mental Illness and Health. *Action for Mental Health.* New York: John Wiley & Sons, 1961.

Joint Commission on the Mental Health of Children. *Crisis in Child Mental Health: Challenge for the 1970s.* New York: Harper & Row, 1969.

Jordan DD, Hernandez M. The Ventura planning model: a proposal for mental health reform. *Journal of Mental Health Administration*, 17:26–47, 1990.

Kamradt BJ. Wraparound Milwaukee: aiding youth with mental health needs. *Juvenile Justice Journal*, 7(1):19–26, 2000.

Kessler RC, Berglund PA, Foster CL, et al. Social consequences of psychiatric disorders, II. Teenage parenthood. *American Journal of Psychiatry*, 154(10):1405–1411, 1997.

Kessler RC, Foster CL, Saunders WB, et al. Social consequences of psychiatric disorders, I: Educational attainment. *American Journal of Psychiatry*, 152:1026–1032, 1995.

Knitzer J. *Unclaimed Children: The Failure of Public Responsibility to Children and Adolescents in Need of Mental Health Services*, Washington, DC: Children's Defense Fund, 1982.

Lavigne JV, Gibbons RD, Christoffel KK, et al. Prevalence rates and correlates of psychiatric disorders among preschool children. *Journal of the American Academy of Child and Adolescent Psychiatry*, 35:204–214, 1996.

Leaf PJ, Alegria M, Cohen P, et al. Mental health service use in the community and schools: results from the four-community MECA study. *Journal of the American Academy of Child and Adolescent Psychiatry*, 35:889–897, 1996.

Little Hoover Commission. *Young Hearts and Minds: Making a Commitment to Children's Mental Health*, Sacramento, CA: Little Hoover Commission, 2001.

Longest BB. *Health Policymaking in the United States*. Chicago: Health Administration Press, 1998.

Lourie I, Hernandez M. An historical perspective on national child mental health policy. *Journal of Emotional and Behavioral Disorders*, 11(1):5–10, 2003.

Lourie I, Katz-Leavy J, De Carolis G, et al. The role of the federal government. In: Stroul BA (ed). *Children's Mental Health: Creating Systems of Care in a Changing Society*. Baltimore: Paul L. Brookes, pp. 99–114, 1996.

Matsen AS, Coatsworth HD. The development of competence in favorable and unfavorable environments: lessons from research on successful children. *American Psychologist*, 53:205–220, 1998.

Metha A, Weber B, Webb LD. Youth suicide prevention: a survey and analysis of policies and efforts in the 50 states. *Suicide and Life-Threatening Behavior*, 28(2):150–164, 1998.

Meyers JS. Federal efforts to improve mental health services for children: breaking a cycle of failure. *Journal of Clinical Child Psychology*, 14(3):182–187, 1985.

National Advisory Mental Health Council Workgroup on Child and Adolescent Mental Health Intervention Development and Deployment. *Blueprint for Change: Research on Child and Adolescent Mental Health*. Rockville, MD: National Institute of Mental Health, 2001.

National Research Council and Institute of Medicine. *From Neurons to Neighborhoods: The Science of Early Childhood Development*. Washington, DC: National Academy Press, 2000.

National Research Council and Institute of Medicine. *Community Programs to Promote Youth Development*. Washington, DC: National Academy Press, 2002.

Pires S, Stroul BA, Armstrong MI. *Health Care Reform Tracking Project: Tracking State Health Care Reforms as they Affect Children and Adolescents with Behavioral Health Disorders and their Families—1997–98 State Survey*. Tampa: University of South Florida, 1999.

President's Commission on Excellence in Special Education. *A New Era: Revitalizing Special Education for Children and Their Families*. Washington, DC: President's Commission on Excellence in Special Education, 2002.

Ringel JS, Sturm R. National estimates of mental health utilization and expenditures for children in 1998. *Journal of Behavioral Health Services and Research*, 28(3):319–332, 2001.

Roberts RE, Attkisson C, Rosenblatt A. Prevalence of psychopathology among children and adolescents. *American Journal of Psychiatry*, 155:715–725, 1998.

Satcher D. Foreword. *U.S. Public Health Service, Report of the Surgeon General's Conference on Children's Mental Health: A National Action Agenda*. Washington, DC: U.S. Public Health Service, 2000.

Scott TM. A school-wide example of positive behavioral support. *Journal of Positive Behavioral Interventions*, 3:88–94, 2001.

Shirk SR. The road to effective child psychological services: treatment processes and outcome research. In: Hughes JH, La Greca AM, Conoley JC (eds). *Handbook of Psychological Services for Children and Adolescents*. New York: Oxford University Press, pp. 43–59, 2001.

Slade EP. Effects of school-based mental health programs on mental health service use by adolescents at school and in the community. *Mental Health Services Research*, 4(3):151–166, 2002.

Stroul BA, Friedman, RM. *A System of Care for Seriously Emotionally Disturbed Children and Youth*. Washington, DC: Georgetown University Child Development Center, 1986.

Stroul BA, Friedman RM. The system of care concept and philosophy. In: Stroul BA (ed). *Children's Mental Health: Creating Systems of Care in a Changing Society*. Baltimore: Paul H. Brookes, pp. 3–21, 1996.

Stroul BA, Pires S, Roebuck L, et al. State health care reforms: how they affect children and adolescents with emotional disorders and their families. *Journal of Mental Health Services Administration*, 24:585–598, 1997.

U.S. Department of Health and Human Services. *Mental Health: A Report of the Surgeon General*. Rockville, MD: U.S. Public Health Service, 1999.

U.S. Department of Health and Human Services. *Mental Health: Culture, Race, and Ethnicity. A Supplement to Mental Health: A Report of the Surgeon General*. Rockville, MD: U.S. Public Health Service, 2001.

U.S. Public Health Service. *Report of the Surgeon General's Conference on Children's Mental Health: A National Action Agenda*. Washington, DC: U.S. Public Health Service, 2000.

Usher CL, Gibbs DA, Wildfire JB. A framework for planning, implementing, and evaluating child welfare reforms. *Child Welfare*, 74:859–876, 1995.

Waller MA. Resilience in ecosystemic context: evolution of the concept. *American Journal of Orthopsychiatry*, 71(3):290–297, 2001.

Willie M et al. v. James B. Hunt, Jr. et al. Civil No. C-C-79-294-M (W.D.N.C. 1980).

Wolin S, Wolin S. *The Resilient Self: How Survivors of Troubled Families Rise above Adversity*. New York: Villard Books, 1993.

Section B
Adults

8

The Epidemiology of Adult
Mental Disorders

RONALD C. KESSLER
DOREEN KORETZ
KATHLEEN R. MERIKANGAS
PHILIP S. WANG

The most recent generation of psychiatric epidemiology began in the late 1970s
with the development of fully structured research diagnostic interviews. The first
instrument of this type was the Diagnostic Interview Schedule (DIS; Robins et
al., 1981), which was developed with support from the National Institute of Mental Health for use in the Epidemiological Catchment Area (ECA) Study (Robins
and Regier, 1991). The ECA studies, which involved general population samples
of five U.S. communities, were the first community surveys to estimate the prevalence of DSM-III (American Psychiatric Association, 1980) disorders in the United
States. A 1-year follow up of ECA respondents was also conducted.

Several fully structured research diagnostic interview schedules, most of them
based on the DIS, were subsequently developed. The most widely used of these
is the World Health Organization's Composite International Diagnostic Interview
(CIDI; WHO, 1990). The CIDI was the interview used in the U.S. National Comorbidity Survey (NCS), the major community epidemiological survey of mental
disorders carried out in the United States subsequent to the ECA to estimate DSM
disorders (Kessler et al., 1994). Unlike the ECA, the NCS was based on a nationally representative sample of respondents selected from hundreds of different communities throughout the country and used the criteria in the DSM-III-R (American Psychiatric Association, 1987) system to make diagnoses. The baseline NCS

Portions of this chapter have previously appeared in *A Handbook for the Study of Mental Health: Social Contexts, Theories, and Systems* (eds. A.V. Horwitz and T.L. Scheid), Cambridge: Cambridge University Press, 1999; *Advances in Mental Health Research: Implications for Practice* (eds. J.B.W. Williams and K. Ell), Washington DC: National Association of Social Workers Press, 1998.

was carried out in 1990–92. An NCS Replication (NCS-R) survey is currently being carried out a decade after the baseline NCS to gather data on trends in patterns and correlates of mental disorders (Kessler and Walters, 2002).

This chapter presents a selective overview of the results regarding the descriptive epidemiology of mental disorders in the United States based on results from the ECA and the NCS as well as on some preliminary results from the NCS-R. The focus will be on the estimated proportion of a population that have experienced an episode of DSM mental disorders either in their lifetime or over the past 12 months and on patterns of treatment for these disorders.

Lifetime and Recent Prevalence of Axis I *Diagnostic and Statistical Manual* (3rd Ed., Revised) Disorders

We focus first on results from the NCS, as this is the only nationally representative survey in the United States to have assessed the prevalence of a broad range of DSM-III-R disorders. As described in more detail elsewhere (Kessler et al., 1994), the NCS is based on a national household sample of respondents in the age range 15–54. The NCS also includes a supplemental sample of students living in group housing, the largest segment of the population that is not in the household population. The results in Table 8.1 show NCS/DSM-III-R prevalence estimates for the 14 lifetime and 12-month disorders assessed in the core NCS interview. As noted above, lifetime prevalence is the proportion of the sample that have ever experienced a disorder, while 12-month prevalence is the proportion that reported an episode of the disorder in the 12 months prior to the interview. The prevalence estimates in Table 8.1 are presented without exclusions for DSM-III-R hierarchy rules. Standard errors are reported in parentheses.

The most common mental disorders assessed in the NCS are major depression and alcohol dependence. Seventeen percent (17.1%) of respondents reported a history of a major depressive episode in their lifetime, and 10.3% had an episode in the past 12 months. Fourteen percent (14.1%) of respondents had a lifetime history of alcohol dependence, and 7.2% continued to be dependent in the past 12 months. The next most common disorders are social and simple phobias, with lifetime prevalences of 13.3% and 11.3%, respectively, and 12-month prevalences of 7.9% and 8.8%, respectively. Addictive disorders and anxiety disorders are somewhat more prevalent than mood disorders. Approximately one in every four respondents reported a lifetime history of at least one addictive disorder, and a similar number reported a lifetime history of at least one anxiety disorder. Approximately one in every five respondents reported a lifetime history of at least one mood disorder. Anxiety disorders, as a group, are considerably more likely to occur in the 12 months prior to interview (19.3%) than either addictive disorders (11.3%) or mood disorders (11.3%), suggesting that anxiety disorders are more chronic than either addictive disorders or mood disorders. The prevalences of other NCS disorders are much lower. Antisocial personality disorder, which was assessed only on a lifetime basis, was reported by 2.8% of respondents, while schizophrenia and other nonaffective psychoses were found among 0.5% of respondents. It

Table 8.1 Lifetime and 12-Month Prevalence of CIDI/ DSM-III-R Disorders in the NCS

	Male				Female				Total			
	Lifetime		12-Month		Lifetime		12-Month		Lifetime		12-Month	
Disorders	%	(s.e.)	%	(s.e.)	%	(s.e.)	%	(s.e.)	%	(s.e.)	%	(s.e.)
I. Mood disorders												
Major depression	12.7	(0.9)	7.7	(0.8)	21.3	(0.9)	12.9	(0.8)	17.1	(0.7)	10.3	(0.6)
Dysthymia	4.8	(0.4)	2.1	(0.3)	8.0	(0.6)	3.0	(0.4)	6.4	(0.4)	2.5	(0.2)
Mania	1.6	(0.3)	1.4	(0.3)	1.7	(0.3)	1.3	(0.3)	1.6	(0.3)	1.3	(0.2)
Any mood disorder	14.7	(0.8)	8.5	(0.8)	23.9	(0.9)	14.1	(0.9)	19.3	(0.7)	11.3	(0.7)
II. Anxiety disorders												
Generalized anxiety disorder	3.6	(0.5)	2.0	(0.3)	6.6	(0.5)	4.3	(0.4)	5.1	(0.3)	3.1	(0.3)
Panic disorder	2.0	(0.3)	1.3	(0.3)	5.0	(1.4)	3.2	(0.4)	3.5	(0.3)	2.3	(0.3)
Social phobia	11.1	(0.8)	6.6	(0.4)	15.5	(1.0)	9.1	(0.7)	13.3	(0.7)	7.9	(0.4)
Simple phobia	6.7	(0.5)	4.4	(0.5)	15.7	(1.1)	13.2	(0.9)	11.3	(0.6)	8.8	(0.5)
Agoraphobia	3.5	(0.4)	1.7	(0.3)	7.0	(0.6)	3.8	(0.4)	5.3	(0.4)	2.8	(0.3)
Posttraumatic stress disorder	4.8	(0.6)	2.3	(0.3)	10.1	(0.8)	5.4	(0.7)	7.6	(0.5)	3.9	(0.4)
Any anxiety disorder	22.6	(1.2)	13.4	(0.7)	34.3	(1.8)	24.7	(1.5)	28.7	(0.9)	19.3	(0.8)
III. Addictive disorders												
Alcohol abuse	12.5	(0.8)	3.4	(0.4)	6.4	(0.6)	1.6	(0.2)	9.4	(0.5)	2.5	(0.2)
Alcohol dependence	20.1	(1.0)	10.7	(0.9)	8.2	(0.7)	3.7	(0.4)	14.1	(0.7)	7.2	(0.5)
Drug abuse	5.4	(0.5)	1.3	(0.2)	3.5	(0.4)	0.3	(0.1)	4.4	(0.3)	0.8	(0.1)
Drug dependence	9.2	(0.7)	3.8	(0.4)	5.9	(0.5)	1.9	(0.3)	7.5	(0.4)	2.8	(0.3)
Any addictive disorder	35.4	(1.2)	16.1	(0.7)	17.9	(1.1)	6.6	(0.4)	26.6	(1.0)	11.3	(0.5)
IV. Other Disorders												
Antisocial personality	4.8	(0.5)	—		1.0	(0.2)	—		2.8	(0.2)	—	
Nonaffective psychosis*	0.3	(0.1)	0.2	(0.1)	0.7	(0.2)	0.4	(0.1)	0.5	(0.1)	0.3	(0.1)
V. Any NCS disorder	51.2	(1.6)	29.4	(1.0)	48.5	(2.0)	32.3	(1.6)	49.7	(1.2)	30.9	(1.0)

Notes: All disorders are operationalized using DSM-III-R criteria, ignoring diagnostic hierarchy rules. Mania has been redefined based on methodological refinements described by Kessler et al. (1997). The estimated prevalences of agoraphobia are different here from those reported in Kessler et al. (1994). Agoraphobia is defined here without panic, while it was defined with or without panic in Kessler et al. (1994). Posttraumatic stress disorder was not reported in Kessler et al. (1994) because the disorder was assessed only in the Part II NCS sample. Nonaffective psychosis is redefined based on methodological refinements described by Kendler (1996). CIDI: Composite International Diagnostic Interview; DSM-III-R: *Diagnostic and Statistical Manual* (3rd ed., revised); NCS: National Comorbidity Survey; (s.e.): standard error.

*Nonaffective psychosis = schizophrenia, schizophreniform disorder, schizoaffective disorder, delusional disorder, and atypical psychosis.

Source: Adapted from Kessler et al. (1994). Copyright 1994, American Medical Association.

is important to note that the diagnosis of NAP was based on clinical reinterviews rather than on the lay CIDI interviews. As documented elsewhere (Kendler et al., 1996), the prevalence estimates for nonaffective psychoses based on the CIDI were considerably higher but were found to have low validity when judged in comparison to the clinical reappraisals.

As shown in the last row of Table 8.1, 49.7% of the sample reported a lifetime history of at least one NCS/DSM-III-R disorder and 30.9% had one or more disorders in the 12 months prior to the interview. While there is no meaningful sex difference in these overall prevalences, there are sex differences in prevalences of specific disorders. Consistent with previous research (Bourdon et al., 1992; Robins et al., 1981, 1991); men are much more likely to have addictive disorders and antisocial personality disorder than women, while women are much more likely to have mood disorders (with the exception of mania, for which there is no sex difference) and anxiety disorders than men. The data also show, consistent with a trend found in the ECA (Keith et al., 1991), that women in the household population are more likely to have nonaffective psychoses than men.

It is instructive to compare these NCS results with the results of the earlier ECA study. Comparative ECA-NCS analyses have been carried out and show that the NCS estimates are higher than the estimates in the first wave of the ECA survey but that the estimates in the two surveys are much more similar, both in the prevalence of individual disorders and in the overall prevalence of having any disorder, when the results of the two interviews carried out 1 year apart in the ECA are combined and then compared with the results obtained in the single NCS interview (Narrow et al., 2002; Regier et al., 1998). Methodological research suggests that the higher prevalence estimates in the NCS than in the first wave of the ECA are due to a number of innovations included in the NCS aimed at stimulating active memory search and complete reporting (Kessler et al., 1998c).

It is more difficult to compare results in the NCS and NCS-R, as the NCS-R is still in the field and preliminary results are available for only the first half of the cases. To the extent that comparisons can be made, though, it appears that lifetime prevalence estimates in NCS-R are equivalent to those in the baseline NCS, but that 12-month prevalence estimates are somewhat higher in the NCS-R than in the NCS. This means that the same lifetime disorders appear to be more chronic in the new data. This conclusion is based on comparisons of identical disorders assessed in the two surveys. However, NCS-R expanded the assessment of disorders beyond those considered in the baseline NCS in a number of ways. For example, the NCS-R includes assessments of intermittent explosive disorder and pathological gambling, neither of which was included in the baseline NCS. Although high comorbidities of such newly assessed disorders were found with the disorders assessed in the baseline NCS, a meaningful proportion of the people with these disorders appear never to have met criteria for any of the NCS-assessed disorders. As a result, the proportion of the population who are estimated to have met criteria for a mental disorder at some time in their life is higher in the preliminary NCS-R data than in the baseline NCS.

Comorbidity

An important observation about the results in Table 8.1 is that the sum of the individual prevalence estimates across the disorders in each row consistently exceeds the prevalence of having any disorder in the last row. This means that there is a good deal of comorbidity among these disorders. For example, while the 49.7% lifetime prevalence in the total NCS sample means that 50 respondents out of every 100 in the sample reported a lifetime history of at least one disorder, a summation of lifetime prevalence estimates for the separate disorders shows that these 50 individuals reported a total of 102 lifetime disorders (2.0 per person). This comorbidity is quite important for understanding the distribution of psychiatric disorders in the United States (Kessler, 1995). Although a discussion of the many different types of comorbidity that exist in the population is beyond the scope of chapter, some aggregate results are important to review.

The results presented in Table 8.2 document that comorbidity is very important in understanding the distribution of psychiatric disorders among persons aged 15–54 in the United States. These results also provide an empirical rationale for more detailed examination of particular types of comorbidity. The four rows of the table represent the number of lifetime disorders reported by respondents. As the first column shows, 52% of respondents never had any NCS/DSM-III-R disorder, 21% had one, 13% had two, and 14% had three or more disorders. Only 21% of all the lifetime disorders occurred to respondents with a lifetime history of just one disorder. This means that the vast majority of lifetime disorders in this sample (79%) are comorbid disorders. Furthermore, an even greater proportion of 12-month disorders occurred in respondents with a lifetime history of comor-

Table 8.2 Concentration of Lifetime and 12-Month CIDI/DSM-III-R Disorders among People with Lifetime Comorbidity in the NCS

Number of Lifetime Disorders	Proportion of Sample		Proportion of Lifetime Disorders		Proportion of 12-Month Disorders		Proportion of Respondents with Severe 12-Month Disorders*	
	%	(s.e.)	%	(s.e.)	%	(s.e.)	%	(s.e.)
0	52.0	(1.1)	—	—	—	—	—	—
1	21.0	(0.6)	20.6	(0.6)	17.4	(0.8)	2.6	(1.7)
2	13.0	(0.5)	25.5	(1.0)	23.1	(1.0)	7.9	(2.1)
3 or more	14.0	(0.7)	53.9	(2.7)	58.9	(1.8)	89.5	(2.8)

Notes: The 52% with no lifetime disorder is inconsistent with the 51.2% with any disorder reported in Table 8.1 because NCS Part II disorders were excluded from the calculations reported here. CIDI: Composite International Diagnostic Interview; DSM-III-R: *Diagnostic and Statistical Manual* (3rd ed., revised). NCS: National Comorbidity Survey; (s.e.): standard error.

*Severe 12-month disorders = active mania, nonaffective psychoses, or active disorders of other types that either required hospitalization or created severe role impairment.

Source: Kessler et al. (1994). Copyright 1994, American Medical Association.

bidity. It is particularly striking that close to 6 out of every 10 (58.9%) 12-month disorders and nearly 9 out of 10 (89.5%) severe 12-month disorders occurred to the 14% of the sample with a lifetime history of three or more disorders. These results show that while a history of some psychiatric disorder is quite common among persons aged 15–54 in the United States, the major burden of psychiatric disorder in this sector of our society is concentrated in a group of highly comorbid people who constitute about one-sixth of the population.

Severity

The last column in Table 8.2 refers to severe disorders. Severity has assumed increasing importance in the analysis of mental health epidemiological survey data in recent years. This can be traced to the fact that the ECA and NCS studies both found that only about one-third of the people who met criteria for a DSM disorder at some time during the 12 months before the interview received any type of professional treatment for this disorder over the same time interval (Kessler et al., 1999; Regier et al., 1993). This finding created a good deal of concern among some advocates for mental health care reform (Regier et al., 2000). The concern was that these high numbers might discourage makers away from lobbying for parity of mental health treatment in health reform. Severity came into play when the National Institute of Mental Health's National Advisory Mental Health Council proposed that discussions about parity should be limited to the treatment of severe and persistent mental illness (SPMI; National Advisory Mental Health Council, 1993). This illness was defined by the Council as either nonaffective psychosis, mania, dementia, or a major anxiety or mood disorder (major depression or panic disorder) that is so severe that it requires either hospitalization or the use of major psychotropic medications. Parallel analyses of the ECA and NCS data show that only about 3% of the U.S. population meet criteria for SPMI in a given year (Kessler et al., 1996).

Another use of a severity threshold to define the need for treatment can be found in Public Law (PL) 102-321, the ADAMHA Reorganization Act. This law established a block grant for states to fund community mental health services for people with mental illness who are unable to pay for services. However, in order to contain costs for these services, the law stipulated that block grant funds can only be used by adults with serious mental illness (SMI) and children with serious emotional disturbance (SED). In PL 102-321, SMI is defined as a DSM disorder that "substantially interferes" with "one or more major life activities" including not only basic daily living skills such as eating and bathing, but also "instrumental living skills (e.g., maintaining a household, managing money, getting around the community, taking prescribed medication) and functioning in social, family, and vocational/educational contexts." The DSM disorders explicitly excluded from qualifying for a diagnosis of SMI include conditions not attributable to a mental disorder that are a focus of attention or treatment, such as academic problems or malingering, substance use disorders, and developmental disorders. It is further noted in the definition that "adults who would have met functional impairment criteria during the referenced year without the benefit of treatment or other support services are considered to have serious mental illnesses." A Substance Abuse and Mental Health Services Administration (SAMHSA) advisory group established to operationalize these criteria using the ECA and NCS concluded that approximately 6% of the U.S. population meet criteria for SMI in a given year (Kessler et al., 1996).

A group of researchers from the American Psychiatric Association (APA) has recently proposed another set of severity criteria to define what they call *clinically* significant mental disorders (Narrow et al., 2002). Their goal was to help refine the use of diagnoses as a proxy for mental health treatment need. This was done by focusing on the subset of disorders in the ECA and NCS surveys that were either defined by respondents as "interfering a lot" with their life and activities or for which respondents sought treatment (either told a professional about the symptoms or took medication for the symptoms). These restrictions reduced the proportion of respondents in the NCS who were classified as having a 12-month mental disorder from 30.2% to 20.6%. (These calculations were carried out on NCS respondents in the 18–54 age range rather than the 15–54 age range reported in Table 8.1, accounting for the initial prevalence estimate being 30.2% rather than the 30.9% reported in Table 8.1.) The comparable reduction in the ECA 12-month prevalence estimate among respondents aged 18+ was from 28.0% to 22.5%.

It is clear that these different attempts to distinguish levels of severity are to some extent ad hoc and almost certainly flawed. For example, more than one-third of the people defined by Narrow et al. (2002) as having DSM disorders that are not clinically significant reported a history of suicidal ideation. A critic might well argue that suicidality is clinically significant. Even more important is the fact that current severity is not an adequate basis for evaluating treatment need (Kessler, 2000; Spitzer, 1998). One only has to think of those with colon cancer or cervical cancer who are fortunate enough to have their illness detected at an early stage to appreciate this point. Such patients are not denied treatment because their illness is not yet severe. Indeed, quite the contrary. Colon and cervical cancer screening is used to increase early detection based on evidence that it is more cost–effective to invest in early detection and treatment than to wait for detection at a more advanced stage of illness (Eddy, 1990; Frazier et al., 2000). Comparable cost–effectiveness analyses of the long-term consequences of early detection and treatment of mental disorders have not yet been carried out. Once they are, we might discover that early treatment of mental disorders that are not yet severe makes sense. In the absence of such studies, it is difficult to develop rational criteria for defining the need for treatment.

Age of Onset

The concept of early treatment, mentioned in the previous paragraph, raises questions about the age of onset of mental disorders and the time to first treatment. The first of these questions is addressed in this section, and the second question is addressed in the next section. The ECA and NCS studies both collected retrospective data on the ages of first onset of each lifetime disorder. These data were consistent in showing that simple and social phobia have a much earlier age of onset than the other disorders considered in the surveys (Burke et al., 1991; Magee et al., 1996)—with simple phobia often beginning during middle or late childhood and social phobia during late childhood or early adolescence. Substance abuse was found to have a typical age of onset during the late teens or early 20s. A substantial proportion of people with lifetime major depression and dysthymia also reported that their first episode occurred prior to the age of 20. Some other disorders, such as generalized anxiety disorder and mania, had later ages of onset, but the most striking overall observation from the data is that most psychiatric disorders have first onsets quite early in life and certainly prior to the beginning of middle age.

Given the importance of comorbidity, a related question is which disorders in comorbid sets have the earliest self-reported ages of onset. The results in the first column of Table 8.3 show that there is considerable variation across disorders in

Table 8.3 Percentage and Distribution of Temporally Primary NCS/DSM-III-R Disorders

Disorders	Percent Temporally Primary Among Those Having the Disorder		Distribution of Temporally Primary Disorder	
	%	(s.e.)	%	(s.e.)
I. Mood disorders				
Major depression	41.1	(2.7)	13.4	(0.9)
Dysthymia	37.7	(3.1)	4.8	(0.5)
Mania	20.2	(6.0)	0.7	(0.2)
Any mood disorder	43.8	(2.4)	16.4	(0.9)
II. Anxiety disorders				
Generalized anxiety disorder	37.0	(2.9)	3.6	(0.4)
Panic disorder	23.3	(3.2)	1.6	(0.2)
Social phobia	63.1	(2.0)	16.0	(0.9)
Simple phobia	67.6	(2.7)	14.5	(1.0)
Agoraphobia	45.2	(4.0)	5.9	(0.7)
Posttraumatic stress disorder	52.1	(3.0)	7.5	(0.7)
Any anxiety disorder	82.8	(1.3)	45.3	(1.4)
III. Addictive disorders				
Alcohol abuse	57.0	(2.3)	10.2	(0.6)
Alcohol dependence	36.8	(3.1)	9.9	(0.6)
Illicit drug abuse	39.7	(3.0)	3.4	(0.3)
Illicit drug dependence	20.8	(2.5)	3.0	(0.3)
Any addictive disorder	48.1	(1.6)	24.5	(1.0)
IV. Other Disorders				
Conduct disorder	71.1	(2.0)	17.7	1.0
Adult antisocial behavior	14.0	(1.8)	1.4	(0.2)
Nonaffective psychosis	28.8	(5.6)	0.4	(0.1)

Notes: All disorders are operationalized using DSM-III-R criteria ignoring diagnostic hierarchy rules. DSM-III-R: *Diagnostic and Statistical Manual* (3rd ed., revised); NCS: National Comorbidity Survey; (s.e.): standard error.

Source: Kessler RC. (1997). Copyright 1997 John Wiley & Sons, Inc. Reprinted with permission of John Wiley & Sons, Inc.

the probability of being the first lifetime disorder reported. Simple phobia, social phobia, alcohol abuse, and conduct disorder are the disorders most likely to be temporally primary in this way. In general, anxiety disorders are most likely to be temporally primary, with 82.8% of NCS respondents having one or more anxiety disorders reporting that one of these was their first lifetime disorder compared to 71.1% of those with conduct disorder, 43.8% of those with a mood disorder, and 48.1% of those with a substance use disorder. Results in the third column of the table show the percentage of overall respondents who reported each disorder as temporally primary. Once again, we see that anxiety disorders are more likely to be temporally primary (45.3% of all lifetime cases) than either substance use disorders (24.5%), other disorders (19.5%), or mood disorders (16.4%).

Speed of Initial Treatment Contact

It was noted earlier in the chapter that only about one-third of ECA or NCS respondents with a recent DSM disorder reported that they recently received professional treatment for this disorder. Lifetime treatment-to-date rates are also low among ECA and NCS respondents who report ever having had one of the DSM disorders assessed in the surveys (Kessler et al., 1994; Regier et al., 1993). However, another result involving treatment that was examined in the NCS, but not in the ECA, is even more striking: the vast majority of people with a persistent mental illness eventually obtain treatment. This result was first reported by Kessler et al. (1998) based on analysis of responses to disorder-specific questions in the NCS that asked people with specific lifetime disorders to report how old they were when the disorder started, how old they were when they first saw a professional about the disorder, and how old they were the last time they had symptoms of the disorder. The analysis consisted of comparing the length of time between first onset and first seeking treatment using survival analysis to censor cases who were not followed long enough (although the analysis was actually carried out retrospectively) to know whether or not they will ever obtain treatment.

The results of this analysis showed clearly that the vast majority of people with a number of serious and persistent DSM disorders eventually obtain treatment. This is shown clearly in Figure 8.1, which presents the results of the survival analysis for major depression, dysthymia, generalized anxiety disorder, and panic disorder. Similar results were subsequently obtained in independent analyses of data collected in a survey carried out in parallel to the NCS in Ontario, Canada (Olfson et al., 1998) and in a survey of patient advocate group members in 11 countries around the world (Christiana et al., 2000). Although these studies found lower lifetime probabilities of obtaining treatment associated with some other disorders, such as phobias and substance use disorders, the main conclusion from these results is that the low rates of recent treatment found in studies of people with recent mental disorders are due, at least in part, to delays in initial help seeking rather than to never obtaining help.

An analysis of the determinants of delays in initial help seeking for incident mental disorders yielded two important results. First, delays were found to be

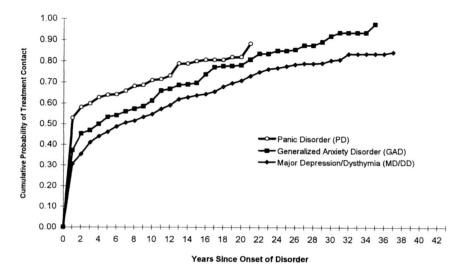

Figure 8.1 Kaplan-Meier speed-of-contact curves of first treatment contact[a] for major depression/dysthymia, generalized anxiety disorder, and panic disorder in the National Comorbidity Survey. (Adapted from Kessler et al., 1998. Copyright 1998, American Psychiatric Association)

much shorter in recent than in earlier cohorts (Kessler et al., 1998a), controlling for intercohort differences in length of recall and other potentially methodological factors that could confound the analysis of cohort effects. Why this is true could not be determined from the NCS analysis. It is almost certainly the case, though, that increasing mass media dissemination of information about mental disorders and effective treatments is responsible for a large part of the decrease in treatment delays. Increases in awareness and recognition of mental disorders have also been fostered by innovations in direct-to-consumer advertisement campaigns and the expansion of employee assistance programs in recent years.

Second, delays in initial treatment seeking were inversely related to age at first onset of the disorders both in the United States and in Ontario (Olfson et al., 1998). This pattern can be seen clearly in Figure 8.2, which presents speed-of-contact curves by cohort for phobia in the NCS. Importantly, this pattern was found consistently across cohorts for all disorders. This means that there continue to be greater delays in seeking treatment for child-onset and adolescent-onset mental disorders than for adult-onset disorders. It is not clear why this pattern exists, but one obvious fact is that children must rely on adults to bring them into contact with the treatment system. It is easy to understand how children who are either silent or unclear about their distress can remain out of treatment even when they have disorders that cause clinically significant distress and impairment unless their parents and teachers are very vigilant or the disorders become so severe that they cannot be missed. Interestingly, the NCS results show that people with early-onset mental disorders are less likely to seek treatment than those with similarly

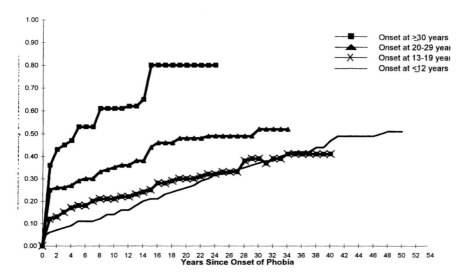

Figure 8.2   Kaplan-Meier speed-of-contact curves of first treatment contact[a] for phobia[b] in subsamples defined by age at onset of phobia for subjects in the National Comorbidity Survey. (Adapted from Kessler et al., 1998. Copyright 1998, American Psychiatric Association)

serious later-onset disorders even when they become adults. This may happen because early onsets can lead to the development of accommodations in living with these disorders that may in turn increase coping capacities and, in this way, reduce the probability of help seeking.

The problem of long treatment delays among people with early-onset mental disorders is of considerable importance in light of evidence that early-onset mental disorders are often more persistent and severe than later-onset disorders and that early-onset disorders have much greater adverse effects than later-onset disorders on critical developmental outcomes such as educational attainment, timing of marriage and first child-bearing, and employment stability (Kessler et al., 1995, 1997a, 1998b). Importantly, referring back to the previous section on severity, early-onset mental disorders are often not seriously impairing at the time they first occur. This is especially true for accretion disorders, such as major depression, which often begin in childhood or adolescence with minor depression or recurrent brief depression and only later develop into full-blown major depressive disorder (Angst and Merikangas, 1997). As noted in the previous section, there is a great need for experimental intervention trials that evaluate the long-term cost–effectiveness of early interventions with children and adolescents by following experimental subjects into adulthood to evaluate effects on the course of primary disorders as well as on the prevention of secondary disorders and secondary difficulties in role functioning. One major effort along these lines is a study of the long-term effects of an intervention to treat generalized social phobia among adolescents on the prevention of secondary anxiety, mood, and substance use disorders (Dierker et al., 2001). The rationale for this intervention is based on the results of analyses carried out in the NCS and other epidemiological surveys (Kessler et al., 2002), as well as in family studies (Merikangas et al., 1998), showing that early-onset social phobia is a powerful predictor of the subsequent onset and course of a wide range of secondary mental and substance use disorders. Other adolescent treatment studies currently underway have the potential for similar assessment of the long-term preventive value of early intervention. Beidel and colleagues (2000) are conducting a 5-year follow-up of a randomized clinical trial of social effectiveness therapy for children with social phobia. In addition to examining the durability of treatment and its effects on functioning, this trial will determine risk factors for relapse and the development of secondary disorders. The Multimodal Treatment Study of children with attention-deficit/hyperactivity disorder (MTA, 1999) is another long-term randomized clinical trial of medication management strategies and/or intensive behavioral treatment. Over the decade-long follow-up period, the MTA Study will identify predictors, mediators, and moderators of long-term outcome in mid-adolescence, including the development of comorbidity and functioning.

Reasons for Not Being in Treatment

The NCS included a series of questions about reasons for not being in treatment. The most commonly reported reason among respondents with a DSM disorder was "I don't have a problem" (Kessler et al., 2001). It is plausible to think that some of the persons who responded in this way are correct. Many mental disorders are self-limiting and do not require treatment. However, it is difficult to make this interpretation of the fact that 54.6% of NCS respondents who met criteria for SMI gave this as their main reason for not seeking treatment, as people with serious mental illness are in need of treatment. An even higher proportion of respondents with less serious mental disorders (83.4%) reported that they did not seek treatment because they did not have a problem. Some unknown proportion of these people have disorders that are sufficiently mild and transient that they would not profit from currently available treatments. For other people, though, the response "I don't have a problem" is a way of saying "I don't want to talk about it."

Among NCS respondents with a disorder who recognized that they had an emotional problem, the most commonly reported reasons for not seeking treatment were the desire to solve the problem on their own (72.1%) and the belief that the problem would improve by itself (60.6%). In addition, situational barriers, financial barriers, and perceived lack of effectiveness of treatment were all reported by sizable minorities of respondents. The modal respondent endorsed four reasons. Very similar patterns and frequencies of reasons for not seeking treatment were reported by those with and without SMI who defined themselves as having a problem that required treatment. The only notable exception is that a significantly higher proportion of respondents with disorders other (37.6%) than those with SMI (24.9%) reported that the problem resolved by itself before they could seek treatment.

Current Treatment of Prevalent Cases

The results reported above regarding patterns of treatment are based on data obtained either in the early 1980s (ECA) or in the early 1990s (NCS). There have been many dramatic changes in mental health treatments and mental health care delivery systems since that time. Newer classes of psychotropic medications with potentially greater tolerability have become widely available. A larger proportion of the U.S. population is now covered under managed care. Primary care clinicians are increasingly being given the responsibility of providing mental health care. Interventions have also been attempted to improve the adequacy of mental health treatment. For example, large-scale community programs have been implemented to promote detection and treatment, such as the annual National Mental Illness Awareness Week, Anxiety Screening Day, Depression Screening Day, Depression/Awareness, Recognition, and Treatment program, and the National Public Education Campaign on Clinical Depression program (Hirschfeld et al., 1997). Evidence-based guidelines for the treatment of depression have been developed for primary care physicians by the federal Agency for Health Care Policy and Research (Agency for Health Care Policy and Research, 1993), while the APA has developed guidelines for psychiatrists for a growing list of disorders (APA, 1993, 1998, 2000). Performance standards are also increasingly being used to improve treatment for mental disorders in health care systems (McGlynn, 1996; National Committee for Quality Assurance, 1996).

The impact of these changes and interventions on the current prevalence and adequacy of treatment for common mental disorders in the United States is largely unknown. As a result, up-to-date data are critically needed. It is also crucial to identify the current reasons why those with mental disorders receive no care or poor-quality mental health care. Many studies of patterns and determinants of receiving mental health treatments are at least a decade old, and others were restricted to specialized study populations (Cooper-Patrick et al., 1994; Horgan, 1986; Johnson and McFarland, 1994; Leaf et al., 1988; Robins and Regier, 1991; Wells et al., 1994). Some possess methodological limitations, including inadequate power and examination of only a narrow range of potential determinants of receiving adequate care. Few have examined the care received by those with the most severe and impairing forms of mental illness or have identified patterns and predictors of treatment within particular sectors both inside and outside of the health care system. These are among the most important reasons we are currently carrying out the NCS-R survey.

Even before the NCS-R was launched, some preliminary data regarding recent care of common mental disorders in the United States were obtained as part of a 1996 survey carried out by the John D. and Catherine T. MacArthur Foundation on Mid-life Development in the United States (MIDUS; Brim et al., 2004). The MIDUS survey was a general-purpose telephone-mail survey that, although it included only a small number of questions about prevalence and treatment of mental disorders, nonetheless yielded striking information about recent patterns and correlates of treatment for three common mental disorders: depression, panic disorder, and generalized anxiety disorder. The analysis of these data also focused on the care received by respondents with the most severe and impairing forms of these three disorders because such patients are often the most vulnerable to changes in treatment availability (Wang et al., 2000).

The MIDUS results were striking in two respects. First, they showed that a much higher proportion of the respondents with at least one of the disorders received some form of treatment at some time during the 12 months before the interview than the proportions found in the ECA or NCS surveys. Second, they showed that fewer than one-third of those who obtained treatment received care that could be considered even minimally consistent with evidence-based treatment recommendations. Even among respondents with the most serious and impairing disorders (SMI), only 25% received guideline-concordant treatment. Factors associated with receiving guideline-consistent care included being white, having more severe mental illness, having health insurance coverage for mental health visits, and being seen by a mental health specialist rather than by a primary care physician.

Implications for Mental Health Services

The results reviewed here show that mental disorders are highly prevalent in the general population. Although no truly comprehensive assessment of all Axis I and Axis II disorders has ever been carried out in a general population sample, such a study would probably find that the majority of the population met criteria for at least one of these disorders at some time in their lives. Although such a result might initially seem remarkable, it is actually quite easy to understand. The DSM classification system is very broad. It includes a number of disorders that are usually self-limiting and not severely impairing. It should be no more surprising to find that half of the population has met criteria for one or more of these disorders in their lives than to find that the vast majority of the population has had the flu or measles or some other common physical malady at some time in their lives.

The more surprising result is that while many people have been touched by mental illness at some time in their lives, the major burden of psychiatric disorder in the population is concentrated in the relatively small subset of people who are highly comorbid. This means that the accumulation of multiple disorders is the most important defining characteristic of serious mental illness, a result that points to the previously underappreciated importance of research on the primary prevention of secondary disorders (Kessler and Price, 1993). It also means that epidemiological information on the prevalence of individual disorders is probably less important than information on the prevalence of functional impairment, comorbidity, and chronicity. This realization, as noted above, has led to a recent interest in severity, which has shown that approximately 3% of the population meet criteria for a severe-persistent mental disorder, 6% meet criteria for SAMHSA's definition of an SMI, and 20% or more of the population have a "clinically significant" mental disorder.

Only a minority of these people receive treatment in a given year even though we know that the vast majority of them, if their symptoms persist long enough, will eventually obtain treatment. The main reason for this low rate of treatment appears to be that many people with mental disorders, even though they have serious mental illness, do not define themselves as having an emotional problem that needs to be treated. This low level of perceived need is a serious problem from a public health perspective.

The central role of perceived need for treatment was an unexpected result in the NCS. As a result, only a superficial assessment of perceived need was included in the survey. In fact, the wording of the NCS question about perceived need was ambiguous, making it unclear whether the people who responded affirmatively meant that (*1*) they did not believe they had an emotional problem, (*2*) they realized that they had a problem but felt that they were able to manage it on their own, or (*3*) they did not believe that treatment would be effective. The implications of the results for the design and implementation of outreach efforts clearly differ, depending on which of these three meanings is applicable. As noted above, NCS-R is including a much more detailed assessment aimed at distinguishing among these different meanings.

Even in the absence of further research, the reasons given by respondents who reportedly recognize that they need help are clear in showing that a number of modifiable factors converge to create barriers to treatment among untreated people with DSM disorders. These include a pervasive desire for self-reliance (wanting to solve the problem on their own) coupled with situational barriers (the most important of which are being unsure where to go and inconvenience), financial barriers, and uncertainties about the likely effectiveness of treatment. Psychological barriers are critical in this mix. For example, either wanting to solve the problem on one's own and/or perceived lack of treatment efficacy characterizes the reason statements of more than 80% of untreated people with SMI. This means that overhauling the existing treatment system to reduce financial and situational barriers is unlikely, by itself, to eliminate unmet needs entirely. The Canadian case clearly illustrates this assertion. A comparative analysis of the NCS and a parallel survey carried out in Ontario found that the proportion of people with serious disorders seeking treatment is no higher in Ontario than in the United States even though provincial health insurance makes free treatment available to all residents of Ontario (Kessler et al., 1997b). This is true because, despite the removal of financial barriers, psychological barriers continue to exist as much in Ontario as in the United States (Katz et al., 1997).

Public education programs such as the National Institute of Mental Health Depression, Awareness, Recognition, and Treatment Program initiative (Regier et al., 1988) hold promise for increasing self-diagnosis and awareness of mental health treatment efficacy. Demand management strategies of the sort developed by health educators also offer hope for reducing barriers to treatment (Carleton et al., 1996; Velicer et al., 1995). However, NCS results show that the psychological barriers to seeking treatment will require more than mere public relations management targeted to the uninformed. This is true because the psychological barriers to treatment most plausibly considered under the control of the treatment system—perceived lack of efficacy and wanting to solve the problem on one's own—were reported more often in the NCS by nonpatients with SMI with a prior treatment history than by those with no prior treatment history. This important finding implies that changes must be made in the way mental health services are delivered in order to reduce these psychological barriers. It is likely that an increase in the patient-centered approach to treatment, which is becoming so important in other areas of medicine (Gerteis et al., 1993), will be needed here. The new SAMHSA Center for Mental Health Services Consumer-Oriented Mental Health Report Card (Substance Abuse and Mental Health Services Administration, 1996) and the new National Committee for Quality Assurance (National Committee for Quality Assurance, 1997) requirement of ongoing patient satisfaction surveys for Health Plan Employer Data and Information Set accreditation are encouraging innovations likely to stimulate development along these lines. In addition, recent evidence that mental disorders are far more costly than most physical health problems in terms of societal burden (Murray and Lopez, 1994, 1996) might create an impetus for further study of the mental health treatment area in ways that will greatly benefit people in need of treatment for serious mental disorders.

The results reported here regarding treatment adequacy are especially important in light of the evidence that it is extremely difficult to get people with mental disorders into treatment. After all that effort to get people into treatment, we cannot afford to have adequate treatments in only a minority of cases. Such findings suggest that interventions are needed not only to improve mental health awareness and treatment seeking in the general population, but also to increase the extent to which the care received conforms with evidence-based recommendations. To properly develop and target quality improvement interventions, it is crucial to understand why treatment so often fails to conform with evidence-based recommendations. The observation that insurance coverage is significantly related to receiving guideline-consistent care in both the general medical and mental health specialty sectors is relevant in the debate over the need for parity between coverage for physical disorders and mental disorders. It might be that broad insurance coverage for mental illness is required to guarantee quality treatment. Even with insurance, though, our data show that treatment adequacy is not assured. There are the enormous challenges in improving the quality of and adherence to treatment, tasks made more difficult by limited health care resources. The epidemiological data provide little guidance on how this challenge can be met, but they show clearly that this is an issue of great importance in the broad agenda of improving the health outcomes of people with mental disorders.

ACKNOWLEDGMENTS

Preparation of this chapter was supported by National Institutes of Health Grants U01-MH60220-03 and R01 DA12058-03 and by grants from the John D. and Catherine T. MacArthur Foundation and the Pfizer Foundation. The authors appreciate the helpful comments of Bedirhan Ustun and Uli Wittchen on an earlier draft.

REFERENCES

Agency for Health Care Policy and Research. *Depression in Primary Care: Volume 2. Treatment of Major Depression.* Rockville, MD: Agency for Health Care Policy and Research, U.S. Department of Health and Human Services, 1993.

American Psychiatric Association. *Diagnostic and Statistical Manual of Mental Disorders.* Washington, DC: American Psychiatric Press, 1980.

American Psychiatric Association. *Diagnostic and Statistical Manual of Mental Disorders, rev. 3rd ed.* Washington, DC: American Psychiatric Press, 1987.

American Psychiatric Association. Practice guideline for major depressive disorder in adults. *American Journal of Psychiatry,* 150(suppl):1–26, 1993.

American Psychiatric Association. *Practice Guideline for the Treatment of Patients with Panic Disorder.* Washington, DC: American Psychiatric Association Press, 1998.

American Psychiatric Association. *Practice Guidelines for the Treatment of Psychiatric Disorders: Compendium 2000.* Washington, DC: American Psychiatric Association Press, 2000.

Angst J, Merikangas K. The Depressive spectrum: diagnostic classification and course. *Journal of Affective Disorders,* 45:31–39, 1997.

Beidel DC, Turner SM, Morris TL. Behavioral treatment of childhood social phobia. *Journal of Consulting and Clinical Psychology,* 68:1072–1080, 2000.

Bourdon KH, Rae DA, Locke BZ, et al. Estimating the prevalence of mental disorders in U.S. adults from the Epidemiologic Catchment Area study. *Public Health Report,* 107:663–668, 1992.

Brim OG, Ryff CD, Kessler RC (eds). *How Healthy Are We?: A National Study of Well-Being at Midlife.* Chicago: University of Chicago Press, 2004.

Burke KC, Burke JD, Rae DS, et al. Comparing age of onset of major depression and other psychiatric disorders by birth cohorts in five U.S. community populations. *Archives of General Psychiatry,* 48:789–795, 1991.

Carleton RA, Bazzarre T, Drake J, et al. Report of the Expert Panel on Awareness and Behavior Change to the Board of Directors. *Circulation,* 93:1768–1772, 1996.

Christiana JM, Gilman SE, Guardino M, et al. Duration between onset and time of obtaining initial treatment among people with anxiety and mood disorders: an international survey of members of mental health patient advocate groups. *Psychological Medicine,* 30:693–703, 2000.

Cooper-Patrick L, Crum RM, Ford DE. Characteristics of patients with major depression who received care in general medical and specialty mental health settings. *Medical Care,* 32:15–24, 1994.

Dierker LD, Albano AM, Clarke GN, et al. Screening for anxiety and depression in early adolescence. *Journal of the American Academy of Child and Adolescent Psychiatry,* 40:929–936, 2001.

Eddy DM. Screening for cervical cancer. *Annals of Internal Medicine,* 113:214–226, 1990.

Frazier AL, Colditz CS, Kuntz KM. Cost-effectiveness of screening for colorectal cancer in the general population. *Journal of the American Medical Association,* 284:1954–1961, 2000.

Gerteis M, Edgman-Levitan S, Delbanco TL. *Through the Patient's Eyes: Understanding and Promoting Patient-Centered Care.* San Francisco: Jossey-Bass, 1993.

Hirschfeld RM, Keller MB, Panico S, et al. The national depressive and manic–depressive association consensus statement on the undertreatment of depression. *Journal of the American Medical Association,* 277:333–340, 1997.

Horgan C. The demand for ambulatory mental services from specialty providers. *Health Services Research,* 21:291–319, 1986.

Johnson RE, McFarland BH. Treated prevalence rates of severe mental illness among HMO members. *Hospital and Community Psychiatry,* 45:919–924, 1994.

Katz SJ, Kessler RC, Frank RG, et al. The use of outpatient mental health services in the United States and Ontario: the Impact of mental morbidity and perceived need for care. *American Journal of Public Health,* 87:1136–1143, 1997.

Keith SJ, Regier DA, Rae DS. Schizophrenic disorders. In: Robins LN, Regier DA (eds). *Psychiatric Disorders in America: the Epidemiologic Catchment Area Study.* New York: Free Press, pp. 33–52, 1991.

Kendler KS, Gallagher TJ, Abelson JM, et al. Lifetime prevalence, demographic risk factors, and diagnostic validity of nonaffective psychosis as assessed in a U.S. community sample: the National Comorbidity Survey. *Archives of General Psychiatry*, 53:1022–1031, 1996.

Kessler RC. The epidemiology of psychiatric comorbidity. In: Tsuang MT, Tohan M, Zahner GEP (eds). *Textbook of Psychiatric Epidemiology.* New York: Wiley, pp. 179–197, 1995.

Kessler RC. The prevalence of psychiatric comorbidity. In: Wetzler S, Sanderson WC (eds). *Treatment Strategies for Patients with Psychiatric Comorbidity.* New York: Wiley, pp. 23–48.

Kessler RC. Some considerations in making resource allocation decisions for the treatment of psychiatric disorder. In: Andrews G (ed). *Unmet Need in Mental Health Service Delivery.* Cambridge: Cambridge University Press, pp. 59–84, 2000.

Kessler RC, Walters EE. The National Comorbidity Survey. In: Tsuang MT, Tohen M, Zahner GEP (eds). *Textbook in Psychiatric Epidemiology, 2nd ed.* New York: Wiley, pp. 343–362, 2002.

Kessler RC, Aguilar-Gaxiola S, Andrade L, et al. Cross-national comparisons of comorbidities between substance use disorders and mental disorders: results from the International Consortium in Psychiatric Epidemiology. In: Bukoski WJ, Sloboda Z (eds). *Handbook for Drug Abuse Prevention Theory, Science, and Practice.* New York: Plenum, pp. 447–472, 2003.

Kessler RC, Berglund PA, Bruce ML, et al. The prevalence and correlates of untreated serious mental illness. *Health Services Research* 36:987–1007, 2001.

Kessler RC, Berglund PA, Foster CL, et al. Social consequences of psychiatric disorders, II: teenage parenthood. *American Journal of Psychiatry*, 154:1405–1411, 1997a.

Kessler RC, Berglund, PA, Zhao, S, et al. The 12-month prevalence and correlates of serious mental illness (SMI). In: Mandersheid RW, Sonnenschein MA (eds). *Mental Health, United States 1996.* Washington, DC: U.S. Government Printing Office, pp. 59–70, 1996.

Kessler RC, Foster CL, Saunders WB, et al. Social consequences of psychiatric disorders, I: educational attainment. *American Journal of Psychiatry*, 152:1026–1032, 1995.

Kessler RC, Frank RG, Edlund M, et al. Differences in the use of psychiatric outpatient services between the United States and Ontario. *New England Journal of Medicine*, 336:551–557, 1997b.

Kessler RC, McGonagle KA, Zhao S, et al. Lifetime and 12-month prevalence of DSM-III-R psychiatric disorders in the United States: results from the National Comorbidity Survey. *Archives of General Psychiatry*, 51:8–19, 1994.

Kessler RC, Olfson M, Berglund PA. Patterns and predictors of treatment contact after first onset of psychiatric disorders. *American Journal of Psychiatry,* 155:62–69, 1998a.

Kessler RC, Price RH. Primary prevention of secondary disorders: a proposal and agenda. *American Journal of Community Psychology*, 21:607–634, 1993.

Kessler RC, Rubinow DR, Holmes C, Abelson JM, Zhao S. The epidemiology of DSM-III-R bipolar I disorder in general population survey. *Psychological Medicine*, 27(5):1079–1089, 1997c.

Kessler RC, Walters EE, Forthofer MS. The social consequences of psychiatric disorders, III: probability of marital stability. *American Journal of Psychiatry*, 155:1092–1096, 1998b.

Kessler RC, Wittchen H-U, Abelson JM, et al. Methodological studies of the Composite International Diagnostic Interview (CIDI) in the U.S. National Comorbidity Survey. *International Journal of Methods in Psychiatric Research*, 7:33–55, 1998c.

Kessler RC, Zhao S, Katz SJ, et al. Past-year use of outpatient services for psychiatric problems in the National Comorbidity Survey. *American Journal of Psychiatry*, 156:115–123, 1999.

Leaf PJ, Bruce ML, Tischler GL, et al. Factors affecting utilization of specialty and general medical mental health services. *Medical Care*, 26:9–26, 1988.

Magee WJ, Eaton WW, Wittchen H-U, et al. Agoraphobia, simple phobia, and social phobia in the National Comorbidity Survey. *Archives of General Psychiatry*, 53:159–168, 1996.

McGlynn EA. Choosing chronic disease measures for HEDIS: conceptual framework and review of seven clinical areas. *Management Care Quarterly*, 4:54–77, 1996.

Merikangas KR, Dierker LC, Szamari P. Psychopathology among off-spring of parents with substance abuse and/or anxiety disorders: a high risk study. *Journal of Child Psychiatry*, 39:337–343, 1998.

MTA Cooperative Group. A 14-month randomized clinical trial of treatment strategies for attention-deficit/hyperactivity disorder. The Multimodal Treatment Study of Children with ASHD. *Archives of General Psychiatry*, 56:1073–1086, 1999.

Murray CJL, Lopez AD. *Global Comparative Assessments in the Health Sector*. Geneva: World Health Organization, 1994.

Murray CJL, Lopez AD. *The Global Burden of Disease: A Comprehensive Projected to 2020*. Cambridge, MA: Harvard University Press, 1996.

Narrow WE, Rae DS, Robins LN, et al. Revised prevalence of mental disorders in the United States using a clinical significance criterion to reconcile 2 surveys estimates. *Archives of General Psychiatry*, 59:115–123, 2002.

National Advisory Mental Health Council. Health care reform for Americans with severe mental illnesses. *American Journal of Psychiatry*, 150:1447–1465, 1993.

National Committee for Quality Assurance. *Health Plan Employer Data and Information Set*. Washington, DC: National Committee for Quality Assurance, 1996.

National Committee for Quality Assurance. *HEDIS 3.0: Narrative: What's In It and Why It Matters*. Washington, DC: National Committee for Quality Assurance, 1997.

Olfson M, Kessler RC, Berglund PA, et al. Psychiatric disorder onset and first treatment contact in the United States and Ontario. *American Journal of Psychiatry*, 155:1415–1422, 1998.

Regier DA, Hirschfeld RMA, Goodwin FK, et al. The NIMH depression, awareness, recognition, and treatment program: structure aims, and scientific basis. *American Journal of Psychiatry*, 145:1351–1357, 1988.

Regier DA, Kaelber CT, Rae DS, et al. Limitations of diagnostic criteria and assessment instruments for mental disorders: implications for research and policy. *Archives of General Psychiatry*, 55:109–115, 1998.

Regier DA, Narrow WE, Rae DS, et al. The de facto U.S. mental and addictive disorders service system: epidemiologic Catchment Area prospective 1-year prevalence rates of disorders and services. *Archives of General Psychiatry*, 50:85–94, 1993.

Regier DA, Narrow WE, Rupp A, et al. The epidemiology of mental disorder treatment need: community estimates of "medical necessity." In: Andrews G, Henderson S (eds). *Unmet Need in Psychiatry: Problems, Resources, Responses*. Cambridge: Cambridge University Press, pp. 41–58, 2000.

Robins LN, Helzer JE, Croughan JL, et al. National Institute of Mental Health Diagnostic Interview Schedule: its history, characteristics and validity. *Archives of General Psychiatry*, 38:381–389, 1981.

Robins LN, Locke BZ, Regier DA. An overview of psychiatric disorders in America. In: Robins LN, Regier DA (eds). *Psychiatric Disorders in America: The Epidemiologic Catchment Area Study*. New York: Free Press, pp. 28–366, 1991.

Robins LN, Regier DA. *Psychiatric Disorders in America: The Epidemiologic Catchment Area Study*. New York: Free Press, 1991.

Spitzer RL: Diagnosis and need for treatment are not the same. *Archives of General Psychiatry*, 55:120, 1998.

Substance Abuse and Mental Health Services Administration. *Consumer-Oriented Mental Health Report Card*. Rockville, MD: Center for Mental Health Services, SAMHSA, 1996.

Velicer WF, Hughes SL, Fava JL, et al. An empirical typology of subjects within stage of change. *Addictive Behaviors*, 20:299–320, 1995.

Wang PS, Berglund PA, Kessler RC. Recent care of common mental disorders in the U.S. population: prevalence and conformance with evidence-based recommendations. *Journal of General Internal Medicine*, 15:284–292, 2000.

Wells KB, Katon W, Rogers B, et al: Use of minor tranquilizers and antidepressant medications by depressed outpatients: results from the Medical Outcomes Study. *American Journal of Psychiatry*, 151:694–700, 1994.

World Health Organization. *Composite International Diagnostic Interview (CIDI, Version 1.0)*. Geneva: World Health Organization, 1990.

9

Services for Adults with Mental Illness

ALEXANDER S. YOUNG
JENNIFER L. MAGNABOSCO

During the past few decades, there have been remarkable advances in mental health treatment. Vague classification schemes have been replaced by structured diagnoses. Basic science research has demonstrated that severe psychiatric disorders are brain-based conditions. Effective treatments for bipolar disorder, major depression, and schizophrenia have been developed and proven to be effective (American Psychiatric Association, 1994, 1997; Depression Guideline Panel, 1993). New, safe medications improve or eliminate psychotic and affective symptoms. Structured psychotherapies, such as interpersonal and cognitive-behavioral therapy, reduce disabling depression and anxiety. Assertive Community Treatment—intensive provision of a comprehensive array of services—allows people with treatment-resistant disorders to live successfully in community settings. Rehabilitation interventions allow many people with chronic psychotic disorders to obtain competitive, paid employment. Finally, helping families and other caregivers, and involving them in treatment, reduces relapse rates.

Overall, outcomes are good when competent clinicians provide state-of-the-art treatments. Unfortunately, effective treatments have not been delivered to many people who would benefit from them. In the United States only one-third of people with serious depression or anxiety receive care (Young et al., 2001). Even with severe, chronic disorders such as schizophrenia and bipolar disorder, only half the sufferers have any contact with a professional during a given year (Wang et al., 2002), and treatment is often intermittent, inadequate, or inappropriate (Lehman, 1999; Unutzer et al., 2000). Certain populations, such as African Americans, men, young adults, and the elderly are particularly unlikely to receive needed treatment (Young et al., 1999, 2001) (for additional discussion of outcomes, see Chapter 15).

Consequently, actual outcomes for persons with mental illness are much worse than would be expected. In state-of-the-art treatment programs for schizophrenia, annual relapse rates are near zero, whereas at typical community clinics, half or more of patients have been found to relapse in a given year (Kissling, 1994). While state governments spend approximately $16 billion a year on adult public mental health services, recent estimates of economic burdens associated with untreated or improperly treated psychiatric problems are severalfold higher (Lutterman et al., 1999; Sederer and Clemens, 2002). Psychiatric disorders are one of the leading causes of disability worldwide, and death rates in people with severe psychiatric disorders are twice those in the general population (Allebeck, 1989). Many cities have substantial populations of homeless persons with untreated psychiatric problems. Many persons with mental illness are institutionalized in jails and prisons, where they receive inadequate or no treatment (Criminal Justice/Mental Health Consensus Project, 2002).

In summary, many people with disabling psychiatric disorders are not receiving effective treatments that would improve their health, well-being and functioning. This is a problem with the *quality* of care. What accounts for it? A wide variety of ideological, social, economic, and political factors have hindered our ability to meet the needs of persons with mental illness (Mechanic, 2001a). We introduce these factors by presenting three critical problems with U.S. mental health policy.

There is no comprehensive health care system. Current mental health delivery is a result of struggles between "conscience and convenience," strongly negative attitudes and discrimination toward indigent groups, countless incremental policies, and marketplace pressures (Bhugra, 1989; Morrissey and Goldman, 1984; Rothman, 1980; Pescosolido et al., 1999). While comprehensive, community-based care has remained a stated national policy goal for over 40 years (National Institute of Mental Health, 1991; President's New Freedom Commission on Mental Health, 2003; President's Commission on Mental Health, 1978), it has never been realized. Mental health services in the United States have not been organized into a coherent system. Rather, a patchwork of policies, laws, contracts, providers and purchasers has evolved into highly complex subsystems of care (Bloche and Cournos, 1990).

There is little policy regarding health care financing. There is little or no policy regarding the appropriate overall level of spending or the allocation of this spending. As a result, health care in the United States is extremely inefficient. The United States spends more than $1 trillion per year, or about 14% of its gross national product, on health care (Blumenthal, 2001). On a per-person basis, this is about twice as much as any other industrialized nation. Despite this, health outcomes in the United States are among the worst of the industrialized nations (Starfield, 2000). Of 13 nations, the United States ranks 13th in infant mortality, 10th in life expectancy at 40 years, and 12th overall. This is presumably because large sums are spent on expensive, high-technology treatments that have little effect on patient outcomes, while many people have poor access to the most basic primary care. Poor access to primary care increases death rates and is a particular problem among the 40 million people in the United States with no insurance and among people with severe psychiatric problems (Cradock-O'Leary et al., 2002; Lurie et al., 1986).

The remarkably high level of U.S. health care expenditures has created strong pressure to cut costs wherever possible. Mental health services have been an attractive target. Because mental health disorders are common and treatable, their treatment is a nontrivial component of health care expenditures. In 1996, about 7% of all U.S. health care expenditures were for the treatment of psychiatric disorders and 1% were for the treatment of addictive disorders (U.S. Surgeon General, 1999). However, the forces advocating for mental health spending are relatively weak. People with severe psychiatric and addictive disorders are often unemployed, have relatively low socioeconomic status, are strongly stigmatized, and can have difficulty advocating for themselves because of cognitive problems. Also, people with generous health care benefits through their employer often pay little attention to their mental health benefit until they try to use it. As a result, over the past few decades there have been large, ongoing reductions in spending for mental health treatment (Frank and McGuire, 1998). Funding for psychiatric hospitals has been dramatically cut, funding for outpatient services has not increased to compensate for this, and many people have been *transinstitutionalized* to nursing homes, locked community facilities, jails, and prisons (for additional information on financing, see Chapter 2).

Little attention has been given to the quality of mental health services. In the 1990s, rising costs and a growing emphasis on total quality management and customer satisfaction spearheaded the need for accountability across the human services fields (Mullen and Magnabosco, 1997). In general health care, there has been substantial work on the quality of care for more than two decades. For instance, systems were developed in the 1970s and 1980s that accurately measure the quality of cardiac surgery (Fitch et al., 2001). These have been implemented in New York State, where they have led to improvement in hospitals' cardiac surgery programs and substantial reductions in death rates (Chassin, 2002). The mental health field has been more reluctant to define which services are appropriate, and only recently has there been broad interest in measuring the quality of routine care. In the mid-1990s, the Schizophrenia Patient Outcomes Research Team became the first prominent national effort to identify evidence-based treatments for schizophrenia (Lehman and Steinwachs, 1998). Researchers have examined routine mental health treatment and have found that a large proportion of patients do not receive these treatments (Drake et al., 2001). Appropriate treatments are often not even offered by public mental health authorities. For instance, a survey of state mental health authorities found that only 1 of 11 evidence-based practices had been implemented across states in 2000 (NASMHPD Research Institute, 2002).

The remainder of this chapter begins with a review of the major adult psychiatric disorders and their treatment, emphasizing severe mental illness. We then provide an overview of the organization and delivery of mental health care in the United States and discuss key problems, including homelessness. We conclude by discussing approaches to improving behavioral health services and policy.

The Major Psychiatric Disorders

Like physical health, mental health exists on a continuum. This continuum extends from no problems, to normal sadness, grief and worrying, to serious psychiatric disorders that acutely or chronically impair functioning and quality of life.

The *Diagnostic and Statistical Manual of Mental Disorders* and the International Classification of Disease are similar, and are the most widely accepted schemes for defining psychiatric problems (American Medical Association, 2001; American Psychiatric Association, 2000). The most common psychiatric illnesses are classified as anxiety disorders, mood disorders, schizophrenia, dementias, and addictive disorders, though there are a wide variety of other important disorders such as personality disorders and eating disorders. During a given year, about 18.5% of adults will have a clinically significant psychiatric disorder (Narrow et al., 2002).

The most common adult mental illnesses in the United States are anxiety disorders (Narrow et al., 2002). Persons with these disorders have serious nervousness, worrying, or fearfulness. There are several types of anxiety disorders (American Psychiatric Association, 2000). Panic disorder consists of repeated episodes of intense fear that emerge without warning. Generalized anxiety disorder consists of ongoing, exaggerated worrying and tension about routine life activities. Obsessive-compulsive disorder consists of repetitive, intrusive thoughts and/or compulsive behaviors that seem impossible to stop or control. Posttraumatic stress disorder consists of symptoms that persist after one experiences a traumatic event. Phobias are overwhelming, disabling, and irrational fears of social or other specific situations or objects.

Clinical depression is the most common mood disorder. As with anxiety disorders, there are different types of depression, including major depressive disorder, bipolar disorder (manic depression), and dysthymia (American Psychiatric Association, 2000). Persons with major depression feel sad most of the time, and cry a great deal, feel worthless, or believe that their life is meaningless. They can have changes in sleep and appetite, trouble concentrating, and are at increased risk for suicide. Depression is often accompanied by serious anxiety. Dysthymia consists of depression that is less severe but occurs daily for 2 years or more. Persons with bipolar disorder have recurrent episodes of both major depressions and mania. While manic, people can feel "high as a kite," have unreal, grandiose ideas, and engage in risky behaviors.

Schizophrenia occurs in about 1% of the population and consists of chronic disorders of thought. People with schizophrenia have psychotic symptoms such as disorganization of thought and behavior, auditory or visual hallucinations, and paranoid and other delusional ideas (Torrey, 2001). Cognitive problems are common and serious. While symptoms of schizophrenia vary widely among individuals, they are often categorized as *positive* or *negative*. Positive psychotic symptoms include hallucinations and delusions. Negative symptoms include blunting of affect, poverty of thought and speech, lack of motivation, and social withdrawal. Schizoaffective disorder is similar to schizophrenia, with predominant mood symptoms in addition to chronic psychosis.

Most psychiatric disorders are caused by a combination of genetic vulnerability and environmental stress. For instance, if one parent has schizophrenia, the likelihood of the child's having the illness increases to about 13%. If both parents have schizophrenia, the child has a 36% chance of having the disorder (Torrey, 2001). Environmental stresses are poorly defined but appear to include, for instance, interpersonal relationship problems for depression and perinatal injuries for schizophrenia.

Severe, persistent mental illness (SPMI) refers to any serious psychiatric disorder that has an ongoing, profound effect on functioning and quality of life. While SPMI most commonly results from schizophrenia and bipolar disorder, it can be caused by numerous other disorders as well. People with SPMI experience major difficulties in multiple areas, such as thought, mood, behavior, physical health, social interactions, or employment. In schizophrenia, for instance, cognitive deficits cause problems with concentration, memory, and social and vocational functioning. Cognitive problems are often not fully corrected by medication, impeding recovery of functioning. A high proportion of people with SPMI do not maintain employment and live in poverty.

Persons with SPMI are at high risk for having co-occurring disorders, such as drug and alcohol abuse or dependence, comorbid depression, or health care problems such as diabetes and cardiovascular disease. People with major depression, bipolar disorder, schizophrenia, and drug and alcohol disorders are at substantially elevated risk for suicide. For instance, more than half of people with schizophrenia make a suicide attempt and 10% die by suicide (Young et al., 1998a). People with schizophrenia also have an increased rate of death from homicide, medical disorders, and accidents (Allebeck, 1989).

The prognosis for people with psychiatric disorders is highly variable. Major depression typically resolves within 1 year without treatment and within a few weeks or months with appropriate treatment. If treatment is provided promptly, disability can be prevented (Wells et al., 2000). Psychotic disorders such as schizophrenia have a more chronic course. Two decades after becoming ill, between a third and a half of people with schizophrenia will have returned to the level of functioning they had before becoming ill (Harding and Zahniser, 1994). However, schizophrenia and bipolar disorder generally require medication for many years, and the first decade of the illness tends to be the most severe.

Treatment of Severe Psychiatric Disorders

Because psychiatric disorders can affect many facets of a person's life, successful treatment requires attention to a range of biological, psychological, and social needs. During the second half of the nineteenth century and the first half of the twentieth century, mental health services were delivered primarily in asylums, such as state mental hospitals and almshouses (Rothman, 1980). These were established as beneficent systems of care for large numbers of indigent groups, including immigrants, the poor, and persons with mental illnesses and other disabilities. At their peak in 1955, out of a total U.S. population of 165 million, 559,000 persons with mental illness were institutionalized in state mental hospitals (Lamb and Bachrach, 2001).

This asylum-oriented approach was reversed starting in the late 1950s by the *deinstitutionalization* movement (Mechanic, 1986). The stated goal of this movement was to implement treatment alternatives in the community to replace round-the-clock care in mental hospitals. It was facilitated by the development of effective psychotropic medications and led by an alliance between civil libertarians and politicians eager to redirect revenues to purposes other than mental health treatment. Throughout the 1960s and 1970s, deinstitutionalization released persons from back wards and chronic care hospitals (Committee on Government Operations, 1988). In 1998, out of a total U.S. population of 275 million, only about 57,000 state mental hospital beds were occupied.

It proved much easier to discharge people from hospitals than to provide appropriate care in community settings. In 1963, the Community Mental Health Facilities Act set in motion national plans for a Community Mental Health Center system that, by 1980, had reached only 40% of its goal (Lerman, 1982). Other efforts to improve community services include the Community Support Program guidelines of the 1970s and follow-up legislation in the 1980s and 1990s (Stroul, 1989). For instance, in 1986, PL 99-660 (the State Comprehensive Mental Health Planning Act) was designed to encourage the establishment of comprehensive state public mental health systems. It focused on people with chronic mental illness or at risk of homelessness, and linked block grant funding to service system requirements such as provision of a core set of services (Stockdill, 1990). In some locales, state-of-the-art services were implemented and people with SPMI benefited from deinstitutionalization (Lamb et al., 2001). However, access to these services has not been broadly provided, and the result has been widespread homelessness, frequent brief rehospitalizations (the *revolving door* syndrome), and transinstitutionalization to squalid board-and-care homes, privately owned chronic care facilities, and jails and prisons (Criminal Justice/Mental Health Consensus Project, 2002).

Comprehensive Care

High-quality care for serious mental health problems begins with a health care system that has a wide variety of available treatment options and can deliver high-quality treatments to each patient. The system must be prepared to attend to a range of needs, such as psychiatric treatment, rehabilitation, medical and dental care, and housing (Vaccaro and Young, 1996). Fortunately, there is now a very large body of science and clinical experience that identifies effective psychiatric treatments. Numerous treatments have been repeatedly and consistently shown to improve outcomes in people with specific mental health problems. In particular, there is a strong consensus regarding appropriate treatments for depression, bipolar disorder, and schizophrenia (American Psychiatric Association Steering Committee, 1996; American Psychiatric Association Steering Committee, 1999; Lehman and Steinwachs, 1998; Schulberg et al., 1998; Veterans Health Administration, 1997). A high-quality health care system would offer these treatments to patients who could benefit from them (Goldman et al., 2001).

However, merely creating evidence-based services somewhere in a health care system is not sufficient. People with depression and anxiety disorders often do not seek psychiatric treatment, and require education and outreach if they are to receive care (Young et al., 2001). In people with SPMI, the problem is even more severe. Individuals with disorders such as schizophrenia can deny that they are ill or in need of treatment, and those who acknowledge a need for help may be unable to seek it due to cognitive deficits that limit their interpersonal effectiveness.

In these circumstances, a specific intervention, Assertive Community Treatment (ACT), is effective (Phillips et al., 2001). This starts with a team of treatment professionals that includes a physician who is a psychiatrist. Clinicians have small caseloads. The team provides care in noninstitutional settings and assertively reaches out to patients to ensure that they have an opportunity to receive effective treatments. Originally, ACT was developed as a "hospital without walls," and has proven to be highly effective in severely ill patients who are homeless or at risk for rehospitalization. It is much more expensive than typical mental health treatment but somewhat less expensive than hospitalization or incarceration. Unfortunately, ACT has been disseminated to only a small fraction of people with SPMI who would benefit from it.

People with SPMI who are less severely ill can be successfully treated without ACT, but they still require comprehensive care. The traditional locus for this care has been the solo clinician or community mental health center, making extensive use of *case management*. Traditional case management is often provided by social workers, and consists of linking patients by phone or referral to various services and coordinating service provision. Caseloads are quite large (100 or more patients per clinician), and the focus tends to be on linking people to benefits and dealing with crises. For instance, people with SPMI often need disability payments, such as Supplemental Security Income (SSI) or Social Security Disability Income (SSDI); public health insurance, such as Medicaid or Medicare; and support for housing costs, such as Section 8 vouchers. Case management is a nearly ubiquitous part of public mental health treatment organizations. Unfortunately, research studies have not consistently found that typical case management improves patient outcomes (Holloway, 1991).

Appropriate care for people with SPMI can require interventions as diverse as vocational rehabilitation, antipsychotic medication, and supportive housing. It is not likely that any one clinician will have the skills to provide all needed treatments. Instead, the best approach is often team-based, with team members specializing while working together to coordinate care (Liberman et al., 2001). An increasingly popular infrastructure for this team-based approach is the psychosocial rehabilitation program (Hughes et al., 1996). These programs use a holistic philosophy that extends beyond symptoms, emphasizing rehabilitation, illness self-management, peer support, patient empowerment, and *recovery* (Mueser et al., 2002). Recovery is a process of individual improvement based on the belief that it is possible to regain purpose and meaning in life while having a serious disability (Anthony, 1993). Psychosocial programs value natural supports and meaningful activities, as opposed to activities designed solely for psychiatric patients. They can include a variety of components, such as clubhouses and drop-in programs, patient-run businesses, housing, money management assistance, assertive outreach, skills training, peer support, and services for comorbid substance abuse.

Treatment Components: Medication and Psychotherapy

Psychiatric treatment begins with, and relies on, an accurate diagnosis. In major depression, dysthymia, and anxiety disorders, treatment starts with a choice of medication and/or psychotherapy. Effective treatments for major depression and dysthymia include antidepressant medications and cognitive-behavioral and interpersonal psychotherapies (Snow et al., 2000). In panic disorder, effective treatments include cognitive-behavioral psychotherapies, some antidepressant medications, and benzodiazepines (Roy-Byrne et al., 1998). Effective treatments for generalized anxiety disorder include antidepressant medications, benzodiazepines, cognitive-behavioral psychotherapies, and probably relaxation and unstructured therapy techniques (Barlow and Lehman, 1996). Obsessive-compulsive disorder improves with antidepressants that block serotonin reuptake and with behavioral psychotherapies (Stein, 2002).

Antidepressant medications were once poorly tolerated, potentially dangerous, and difficult to prescribe (Henry, 1992). This situation changed in the late 1980s with the release of fluoxetine (Prozac) and the subsequent development of numerous other new medications that are typically safe and easy to prescribe. There have also been major advances in our understanding of psychotherapy. Unstructured counseling and psychodynamic psychotherapies may be helpful for some clinicians and patients, but there is little research to support their efficacy. On the other hand, research strongly supports the efficacy of certain structured psychotherapies (Gabbard, 2001). Cognitive therapy involves working with patients to recognize and improve dysfunctional thinking patterns (Beck, 1993). Behavioral therapy focuses on stopping undesired behaviors using approaches such as exposure, desensitization, and response prevention. Interpersonal psychotherapy includes identification and management of stressful social situations (Swartz, 1999).

The appropriate treatment of bipolar disorder almost always begins with an appropriate mood-stabilizing medication (American Psychiatric Association, 1994). Lithium was the first mood stabilizer to be discovered and remains quite effective. It has a high rate of unpleasant side effects and is safe and effective only within a narrow dosage range. Other effective mood stabilizers, such as carbamazepine and valproate, are easier to use. However, with any of these medications, many people continue to have depressions or manias, or suffer significant side effects such as weight gain or sedation. Antipsychotic medications, such as olanzapine, are also effective in bipolar disorder but carry potential side effects of their own, including tardive dyskinesia, a potentially irreversible movement disorder.

Depression during the course of bipolar disorder must be treated carefully, since treatments for depression can cause the patient to switch to mania. Effective treatments for bipolar depression include antidepressant medications, cognitive-behavioral therapy, social rhythm therapy, and interpersonal psychotherapy (Swartz and Frank, 2001). With regard to preventing mania, no psychotherapies have been shown to be effective; however, there is interest in psychoeducational interventions that improve illness self-management skills. Mania is treated with an appropriate level of care (often hospitalization) and with mood-stabilizing and antipsychotic medication.

The appropriate treatment of schizophrenia or schizoaffective disorder almost always includes an antipsychotic medication (Herz and Marder, 2002). The first antipsychotic medications, such as chlorpromazine (Thorazine), were identified and disseminated in the 1950s and 1960s. More than a dozen similar medications were developed over the next two decades. These were effective against positive psychotic symptoms, disorganization, and, to a lesser extent, negative symptoms. However, they had a high rate of very unpleasant side effects—particularly motor side effects such as muscle stiffness, severe restlessness, and tardive dyskinesia.

Fortunately, a number of second-generation antipsychotic medications have been developed that cause fewer unpleasant side effects. The first of these was clozapine. Released in the United States in 1989, it was effective in a large proportion of patients who had previously failed to respond to antipsychotic medications, and was more effective than prior medications against mood and negative symptoms. It caused no motor side effects. Clearly a breakthrough, it also caused a higher than usual rate of seizures and agranulocytosis, a temporary, though dangerous, disorder of the immune system. It has therefore been reserved for treatment-refractory patients. Since the early 1990s, a number of additional second-generation medications have been released (risperidone, olanzapine, quetiapine, ziprasidone, and aripiprazole). While these appear to be no more effective against positive symptoms than older medications, they cause less motor restlessness and muscle stiffness, have a better effect on mood and negative symptoms, and are easier to prescribe (Marder et al., 2002). Also, the older antipsychotic medications cause tardive dyskinesia in about 4% of adults per year, while the second-generation agents cause this side effect at about one tenth this rate. Patients usually prefer the second-generation medications, though they do have important side effects, such as weight gain, sedation, and cardiac conduction problems. Although they typically cost $3000 to $5000 per year, these new medications have captured more than three-quarters of the antipsychotic medication market and represent a major advance in the treatment of psychotic disorders.

Treatment Components: Rehabilitation, Caregivers, and Peer Support

In people with SPMI, treatment often needs to move beyond medication and psychotherapy to include rehabilitation, caregiver services, and services for concurrent disorders such as substance abuse (Young et al., 2000a). A variety of rehabilitation technologies improve outcomes in people with SPMI (Anthony et al., 2002). Just as medication treatment is based on diagnostic assessment, rehabilitation begins with an accurate functional assessment (Vaccaro et al., 1992). Functional assessment includes identification of the patient's preferences regarding education, work, and leisure, as well as his or her sources of motivation, resources, strengths, major problems, and deficits. Goals are identified and rehabilitation plans developed. Illness self-management can be improved using psychoeducational strategies and cognitive-behavioral interventions that target medication compliance, relapse prevention, and coping with symptoms (Mueser et al., 2002). Vocational functioning can be improved using Individual Placement and Support (IPS). In IPS, employment specialists help patients obtain competitive, paid employment and then provide them ongoing support in the workplace (Bond et al., 2001). With IPS, employment rates in people with SPMI have increased from about 10% to between 30% and 60% (Crowther et al., 2001).

Outcomes in patients can also be substantially improved through the use of interventions that target family members and other caregivers. Interventions that educate and involve family members in the treatment process have consistently reduced relapse rates and facilitated recovery in people with these disorders. Interventions vary but generally include education regarding psychiatric illness and its treatment, emotional and peer support, development of problem-solving skills, and assistance with crises (Dixon et al., 2001). Recent research suggests that family services may not need to be highly intensive (Schooler et al., 1997). While these interventions were initially developed for family members of patients with schizophrenia, they also appear to work in bipolar disorder and with other caregivers, such as board-and-care operators (Mueser and Glynn, 1999). There is also a role for caregivers supporting and educating other caregivers. The National Alliance for the Mentally Ill (NAMI; www.nami.org) is a leading national consumer organization focused on people with SPMI and their families. It has disseminated structured *family-to-family* programs involving education and support.

Finally, there is increasing interest in peer support to improve outcomes in people with SPMI. Peer support is a structured process whereby people with SPMI provide assistance to each other (Chinman et al., 2002). It is based on the belief that people with chronic disorders can help themselves and each other achieve better outcomes in their treatment and their lives. Though peer support groups are not widely available, they have been increasing in number. Schizophrenics Anonymous, Recovery Inc., and GROW are peer support organizations with groups operating around the world. In these organizations, persons with psychiatric disabilities meet on a regular basis and discuss, for instance, stigma, employment, interpersonal issues, medication, symptoms and how they are coping with their disorders. This process can provide new information and perspectives while facilitating vicarious learning and enhancement of problem-solving skills (Davidson et al., 1999). Peer support may help individuals make the best use of treatment while creating dense social networks and exposing them to role models who provide hope for recovery.

Mental Health Systems: Organization and Financing in the United States

The Private Sector

As of 1996, mental health treatment costs in the United States were about $66 billion, of which 30% was spent in the private sector, 53% in the public sector, and 17% paid out of pocket (McKusick et al., 1998). In the private sector, health care coverage is generally obtained through one's employer, who contracts with an insurance company and pays most of the premium. The insurance market works relatively well for people who are employed by large organizations. These organizations distribute the risk for high-cost treatment over many individuals and can bargain effectively with health insurance companies. Plans offered by large corporate or governmental organizations are relatively generous and usually include coverage for mental health treatment. On the other hand, the insurance market works poorly for small businesses and for individuals who must purchase their own health insurance. Insurers have little incentive to provide affordable insurance to individuals who have medical problems or to small businesses that have an employee or a dependent with a costly medical problem. As a result, more than 40 million people in the United States have no health insurance, and many more are at risk to lose their insurance should they become ill.

During the 1990s, insurance plans moved to managed care arrangements to control mental health service use (Manderscheid et al., 2001). This shift was led by large corporations seeking to reduce health care expenditures and increase accountability. Funding for mental health care was *carved out* from primary health care insurance and managed by specialty managed behavioral health care organizations (MBHOs). These MBHOs dramatically reduced the cost of mental health insurance for corporations in the 1990s, cutting expenditures by half for some large companies in the first year (HayGroup, 1999). At the same time that costs have been reduced, however, there has been little independent information regarding the effect of MBHOs on treatment quality. Given the large cost savings and the paucity of objective evidence that managed care is harming patients, managed care has been very popular to purchasers. In 1987, fee-for-service plans were the most prevalent mental health plan type for 92% of employers. By 1998, this had dropped to 14% of employers (HayGroup, 1999). In the private sector, managed care is delivered by a relatively small number of for-profit corporations that use similar mechanisms to control care. More than half of the market is controlled by 3 MBHOs, and more than 85% of the market is controlled by the 11 largest MBHOs.

Whatever the insurance arrangement, treatment is usually provided by private and community hospitals, freestanding clinics and health care centers, and independent doctor groups and solo clinicians. While care structures are organized within one's community, the choice of physician, psychiatrist, psychologist, and other clinicians is usually dictated by one's health insurance company. The MBHOs manage treatment use by requiring preapproval for intensive or ongoing treatment, making it time-consuming for clinicians to request more than a small number of treatment visits and steering patients to clinicians who use time-limited and inexpensive treatment modalities. The MBHOs improve access to low-intensity psychiatric treatment by use of toll-free referral numbers, established provider networks, and low deductibles and copayments. They place tight restrictions on the use of psychiatric hospitals, and reduce access to intensive services and services other than individual psychotherapy or medication management. Private insurance often includes relatively low coverage limits and therefore does not function as insurance against severe or prolonged illnesses. People with expensive disorders often must appeal for extra coverage, pay out of pocket, or seek care in the public sector.

The Public Sector

When people do not have private mental health coverage or exhaust their benefits, they must pay for care themselves or receive treatment in the public sector.

Compared to the private sector, the public sector treats a different population of patients and uses different treatment modalities. In general medical care, the public and private health care sectors treat similar illnesses, with the public sector focusing on people without health insurance. In mental health, however, the private sector largely provides treatment for mild or time-limited disorders such as anxiety and depression. Services required by people with severe and persistent mental illness, such as rehabilitation and ACT, are not funded by private insurance. People with SPMI often receive their care in the public sector, even if covered by a health insurance policy. These public mental health services are funded by Medicaid, Medicare, the Department of Veterans Affairs, and state and local governments. Since these resources are usually inadequate, public sector providers focus on people with SPMI and people with less severe disorders can have difficulty receiving public services, even if they are poor or uninsured.

One striking feature of the public sector is its incredible complexity and fragmentation. Care is managed by countless agencies at multiple policy levels and provided by a large array of safety-net hospitals, community mental health clinics, and solo providers. Organizations involved in mental health care can be understood as *subsystems of larger systems* with many interdependencies (Scott, 1983). National surveys conducted by the National Institute of Mental Health (NIMH), the Center for Mental Health Services (CMHS), and the National Association of State Mental Health Program Directors (NASMHPD) have provided the most comparable data on organizations that manage and deliver mental health services. Four sets of national surveys provide data on mental health organizations, staffing, and expenditures for adult services: the periodic Survey of Mental Health Organizations and General Hospital Mental Health Services; the 1997 Client/Patient Sample Survey of demographic, clinical, and service use characteristics in specialty mental health organizations; the biennial State Mental Health Agency (SMHA) Profiling System surveys; and the NASMHPD Research Institute's SMHA Controlled Expenditures and Revenues reports. We report trends from the most recent (1998 and 1994) SMHA surveys (Manderscheid et al., 2001; Milazzo–Sayre et al., 2001).

In 1998, the largest number of organizations in the United States were "all other" mental health organizations or multiservice organizations that "provide services in both 24-hour and less than 24-hour settings . . . such as federally funded community mental health centers . . . and are not classifiable to other organizations such as psychiatric . . . [or] general hospitals" (Manderscheid et al., 2001; p. 318), followed by nonfederal general hospitals, separate psychiatric services, private psychiatric hospitals, state and county mental hospitals, and Department of Veterans Affairs (VA) medical centers. Between 1970 and 1998 the total number of mental health organizations available in the United States almost doubled (from 3005 to 5722), the number of organizations providing services in various treatment settings also increased, and the number of psychiatric beds provided by all mental health organizations decreased by half. By 1998, many patient care episodes had shifted from 24-hour hospital care to less than 24-hour services, and from state mental hospitals to nonfederal general and private psychiatric hospitals and all other organizations.

Unfortunately, current service "systems" are difficult for clinicians and patients to understand, let alone use. For example, people with SPMI who have Medicaid or no insurance typically receive care from state or county mental health systems and local mental health centers. They may receive psychosocial rehabilitation at a nonprofit community agency, medication management from a clinic that will accept Medicaid, employment services from a state vocational rehabilitation agency, substance abuse treatment from a provider funded with a federal block grant, general medical care from a public health clinic, and housing under the federal Section 8 program. People with Medicare are often seen by solo psychiatrists or psychologists, or at a clinic or hospital. Individuals who worked in noncivilian jobs in the military receive care in the military care system or at VA facilities—the largest system of care in the United States. Medication is paid for by Medicaid, a local mental health authority, the VA, the patient, or special programs for indigent people.

One attempt by the federal government to better integrate and target services was the landmark Mental Health Systems Act of 1980. However, this was quickly short-circuited by the 1981 Omnibus Care Act, which implemented a *block grant* policy and changed federal–local grant relationships to federal–state–local arrangements (Logan et al., 1985). State mental authorities were assigned control over the development, implementation, financing, and management of public mental health systems. However, care continued to be financed with the same numerous independent funding mechanisms, and no coordinating entity emerged (Miller, 1996).

During the 1990s, state and local governments began to contract with MBHOs to manage public sector mental health financing. Between 1988 and 1997, the proportion of Medicaid beneficiaries in managed care rose from 9% to 48% (U.S. Surgeon General, 1999). The fastest growth was in the non–SPMI population that qualifies for Medicaid based on enrollment in Temporary Assistance to Needy Families, the income-based program primarily serving children with unemployed parents. People with SPMI generally qualify for Medicaid based on receiving SSI and are less likely to encounter managed care.

However, a number of prominent managed care experiments have occurred in populations with SPMI. The structure of these experiments has varied widely (Hanson and Huskamp, 2001). In some states, such as Iowa, an MBHO managed all Medicaid mental health care. In others, such as Massachusetts, the process was incremental, with a substantial role for the public mental health authority. In Colorado, an MBHO entered into a 50-50 partnership with local provider organizations. In some locales, the MBHO merely pays mental health claims and/or manages hospital use. When public sector managed care programs have been evaluated, the results have been highly variable (Bothroyd et al., 2002; Dickey et al., 1998; Hausman et al., 1998; Lurie et al., 1992, 1998; Sabin and Daniels, 2000; Young et al., 1998c). In some programs, the most severely ill patients may have done worse under managed care. However, in general, some patient outcomes have improved while others have worsened. Certain programs are highly regarded (Dahl and Forquer, 2001), while others have clearly been disasters (Chang et al., 1998). It is becoming increasingly apparent that managed care is a mechanism, not a goal, and that it can improve or worsen patient care, depending on how policy makers use it (Mechanic, 2001b).

Public sector managed care has been attacked by provider organizations concerned about losing revenue and by advocacy organizations that want to see improved services (Hall et al., 1997). When public sector MBHOs have cut costs, governmental agencies often have not used savings to create needed services but instead have cut mental health funding. Also, MBHOs have been held to small profit margins despite the substantial challenges and risks associated with managing care for people with SPMI (Huskamp et al., 2001). As a result, MBHOs have become less interested in public sector contracts and growth in this area has slowed.

Key Problems in Care

Poor Public Information and Stigma

Many, if not most, people in society are poorly informed about mental illness, and stigma pervades all social, political, and economic domains associated with mental health care (Draine et al., 2002; Mechanic, 1986). For instance, press coverage often implies that too many people are taking antidepressants or getting counseling. In reality, while some people may be receiving unnecessary treatment, most people with psychiatric disorders get no treatment at all (Young et al., 2001). Similarly, there is a great deal of publicity when a person with untreated SPMI commits a violent crime. While people with schizophrenia or with a drug and alcohol problem are at somewhat higher risk for violence than the general population, research has consistently demonstrated that the vast majority of people with SPMI are not violent (Arseneault et al., 2000).

Though stigma has decreased in the United States over the past few decades, it remains a severe problem for people with SPMI (U.S. Surgeon General, 1999). Appropriate demand for mental health treatment has been consistently undercut by stigma and pervasive poor public information. For instance, although mental illness is common among all socioeconomic groups, people do not believe they may need psychiatric treatment. Therefore, people do not consider the adequacy of coverage for mental health treatment when they choose their insurance, creating little demand for adequate coverage. A recent national study found that one-third of people with private insurance did not know if they had mental health coverage (Gresenz and Sturm, 1999). In fact, one-quarter of people with a mental health disorder did not know if they had such insurance. A similar information problem exists with schizophrenia and bipolar disorder. People do not understand that they and their children have a nontrivial risk of developing SPMI; hence they do not adequately support private insurance coverage or high-quality public services for these disorders. Campaigns exist to stamp out stigma; however, their reach has been relatively limited (National Alliance for the Mentally Ill, 2002).

Inadequate Attention to Treatment Quality

To improve care, it is necessary to first understand the quality of current treatment services. Fortunately, it is possible to measure the quality of health care reliably and accurately, including mental health treatment (Wells et al., 2000). The Institute of Medicine has defined the quality of care as the extent to which health services "increase the likelihood of desired health outcomes and are consistent with current professional knowledge" (Institute of Medicine, 1999).

Quality is measured in three domains: the structure, the process, and the outcomes of care (Donabedian, 1980). The *structure* of care includes organizational factors such as insurance benefits, staffing, buildings, and hours of operation. For example, is there adequate financing, and are there clinicians who are competent to provide needed services? The *process* of care consists of the services that patients actually receive. For instance, does someone with major depression receive psychotherapy or antidepressant medication? The *outcomes* of care are domains that are inherently important. For instance, does someone's depression improve and how satisfied is the person? How often do people die or remain disabled? Conceptually, the structure of care affects the process of care, which in turn affects the outcomes of care (Wells, 1999). Patient and environmental factors are also very important and directly affect both the process of care and outcomes. In fact, medical care typically has a weaker effect on patient outcomes than do factors such as genetics, severity of illness, and available resources.

It seems appealing, at first, to study only the outcomes of care. For example, over time, do patients at a clinic get better, worse, or stay the same? Unfortunately, while outcomes are inherently important, poor outcomes have many causes. For instance, if patients at a particular clinic have a poor quality of life and improve slowly, this could be because the clinic is particularly good at keeping severely ill patients in care (Young et al., 2000b). In addition, knowing outcomes provides little information about how to improve care. For example, patients at a clinic may have a high rate of psychotic symptoms. Is that because clinicians lack critical competencies, because patients do not receive appropriate medication treatment, or because needed medications are not on formulary? Since a major goal of quality measurement is to inform quality improvement, one must measure processes that strongly affect outcomes and that can be improved. This requires information regarding how often patients are accessing or dropping out of care and information on the details of the encounter between patient and clinician. Given patients' clinical needs, are they receiving the appropriate treatments?

Quality problems have been grouped into three categories: underuse, overuse, and error (Chassin, 1996). Underuse occurs when an individual does not receive a treatment that would be beneficial. This is the most common problem in psychiatric disorders. Overuse occurs when people receive treatments that are expected to provide little or no benefit. Unnecessary procedures tend to be harmful, since they have little potential for benefit, leaving complications and side effects as the predominant outcomes. Overuse is, for instance, a common problem with cardiac procedures and back surgery (Larequi-Lauber et al., 1997; Winslow et al., 1988). Error occurs when a mistake is made. For example, many patients with schizophrenia are receiving the wrong medication treatment and having unnecessary psychosis or side effects (Young et al., 1998b). It is important to note that while cost is often a consideration, it is not a domain of quality. However, it is possible to evaluate both the cost of a given treatment and the extent to which it improves patient outcomes. By examining a *cost–effectiveness* ratio, policy makers can prioritize treatments when resources are limited (Gold et al., 1996; Sabin et al., 1997).

Need for Quality Improvement

In depressive and anxiety disorders, about two-thirds of people with a disorder receive no mental health treatment at all (Young et al., 2001). People are particulary unlikely to access mental health care if they have no insurance or insurance that is not managed (Wells et al., 2002). Only one-fifth of people with a disorder see a mental health specialist. However, 80% of people with a disorder do see a health care professional—usually in primary care, where rates of psychotherapy and medication treatment are low.

Efforts to improve care for depression clearly need to reach out to and identify people with a disorder and increase the likelihood that they will receive treatment. Models exist that do this in primary care. They are feasible and affordable to implement and substantially improve care and outcomes (Wells et al., 2000). These models have not been widely adopted. Even worse, organizations that adopted these care models during special projects have subsequently dropped them, despite evidence that they were improving care. While stigma may contribute to this decision, another problem is that the costs of treating mental illness accrue to practices and plans, while the benefits accrue to patients and families. This leaves health care practices and insurance companies with little incentive to improve mental health care.

In bipolar disorder and schizophrenia, researchers have found different, though no less serious, quality problems. These disorders are usually managed by mental health specialists, often at busy public mental health facilities with modest budgets. The most effective and efficient care is believed to be provided by a team of professionals, including psychologists, social workers, nurses, psychiatrists, other mental health workers, and primary care practitioners. Because efforts have been made to do as much as possible with fewer resources, there has been an impressive loss of clinical professionals from these facilities over the past several decades. Whereas once doctoral staff had prominent roles at public mental health clinics, today the modal staff member is a social worker or "mental health worker" with little clinical training (Young and Clark, 1996).

At the same time, the patient population being served has become progressively sicker, with more treatment-refractory mental health problems, frequent concurrent drug abuse problems, and serious chronic medical conditions. Also, new, highly effective treatments have been developed (e.g., clozapine and ACT) that require highly trained staff who possess specific competencies. *Clinical competencies* have been defined as values, knowledge, and skills that are required to deliver high-quality care (Coursey et al., 2000). National projects have developed sets of core competencies for clinicians caring for people with SPMI and have estimated that these are usually not present in current providers (Young et al., 2000a).

To improve care broadly, it will be necessary to make quality measurement a routine part of mental health care. While this is not yet the case, there has been more progress in general medical care. Nationally, a number of projects have been implemented that evaluate the quality of medical care and provide information to guide health care purchasing, consumer choice, and quality improvement. None of these efforts has been led by the federal government, which has avoided substantial health care policy changes since the demise of the Clinton health care reform effort in the 1990s. Until the late 1990s, the Agency for HealthCare Policy and Research (AHCPR) had funded and led numerous national projects to evaluate and improve the quality of care. However, these efforts ran into strong opposition from powerful political constituencies, such as surgeons and health care provider organizations. Researchers found, for instance, that back surgery was often performed unnecessarily—a finding that was quite unpopular. The AHCPR was almost eliminated by Congress and continued only with greatly reduced funding, a new name (the Agency for Healthcare Research and Quality), and an understandable aversion to studies that would inform national health care policy.

In the absence of federal government leadership, private organizations have sought to evaluate care. The National Council on Quality Assurance (NCQA) is an independent organization with substantial funding from managed care organizations. It has developed a "report card," the Health Plan Employer Data and Information Set (HEDIS), that uses computerized data from health care organizations. This report focuses on measures of quality that can be assessed using computerized data that already exist or that can be readily obtained. For instance, it is possible to use existing data to estimate vaccination rates. A limitation of this approach is that measures must be selected so that when health plans and providers improve their information systems, their HEDIS ratings also improve. As a result, it is difficult to develop measures of poor outcomes that are comparable across health plans. Also, failure to detect a disorder (such as depression) cannot be directly assessed. Even more important, HEDIS reporting is voluntary, and plans with poor performance are less likely to report their HEDIS results (McCormick et al., 2002).

Until recently, HEDIS included only one measure of mental health care: the rate of outpatient follow-up after hospitalization for a mood disorder. The usefulness of this measure appears to be limited (Druss and Rosenheck, 1997). Recently, HEDIS added measures of antidepressant prescribing and follow-up for patients diagnosed with a mood disorder. The value of these measures to improve care will need to be studied. It is possible, for instance, that improving detection of depression could worsen an organization's apparent performance on this measure. Accurate measures of depression care are likely to require better clinical information regarding plan members who have a major mood disorder.

There have also been prominent efforts to measure consumer satisfaction. In general medical care, experience of care and detailed consumer satisfaction have been widely assessed using the Consumer Assessment of Health Plans Survey. The companion project in private sector mental health is the Consumer Assessment of Behavioral Health Survey, which has evolved into the Experience of Care and Health Outcomes (ECHO) survey (Eisen et al., 2001). Designed for managed care, ECHO evaluates, from the patient's perspective, promptness of treatment, communication with clinicians, patient involvement in decision making, information about self-help and treatment options, information regarding medication side effects, and MBHO administrative services (Cubanski et al., 2002). In the public sector and in patients with SPMI, the leading national effort to evaluate satisfaction has been the Mental Health Statistical Improvement Program (MHSIP) (MHSIP, 2000). While MHSIP attempts to improve data broadly, its focus is a survey of satisfaction and subjective experience with care that has been fielded at mental health clinics across the nation.

Both MHSIP and ECHO represent important advances in the routine measurement of mental health care quality, though there are challenges to the use of these instruments. The most important issue pertains to how people are selected to complete these surveys. Access is a major problem in private and public sector care, and one would like to survey all people in need of treatment or, at the very least, the population of people with any provider contact. However, to do this requires substantial extra effort. Especially in the public sector, most surveys focus on a convenient population of patients in regular care, which is not typical of the broader population of interest (Young et al., 2000b). Another challenge is that individuals do not appear to be using satisfaction data when choosing their health plan or provider (Farley et al., 2002). Finally, satisfaction is only one of several important domains of quality. Satisfaction is not strongly correlated with technical quality (whether the right treatment is offered), and there is a pressing need for new methods that monitor whether people are receiving appropriate treatment (Edlund et al., 2003).

Homelessness

Homelessness is a term that has been used to encompass a range of human conditions, from living on the streets every night to living in shelters, hotels, public facilities, vehicles, or with friends and family. It has been estimated that 26 million people in the United States have been homeless at some point in their lives, and 600,000 people are homeless on any given night (Baumohl, 1996). About one-quarter of the homeless living on the streets have a serious mental illness, and two-thirds have a alcohol and/or drug use disorder (Koegel et al., 1999; National Coalition for the Homeless, 1999).

A variety of factors contribute to homelessness (Bianco and Wells, 2001; Sullivan et al., 2000). Individual risk factors include having severe mental illness, a substance abuse disorder, a history of exposure to physical or sexual abuse, poor family relationships, a childhood history of unstable housing, and being poor. People who become homeless often have multiple risk factors—more than, for instance, mental illness. Social factors and lack of comprehensive services also play a strong role. Massive street homelessness as we know it today emerged in the 1980s when federal funding for affordable housing was cut by more than 75% (Lezak and Edgar, 1996). At around that time, there was a loss of low-cost housing options such as single room occupancy (SRO) hotels that provide rooms by the week or month, and small, inexpensive apartments or rooms for rent. Shelters in major cities were eliminated. Housing that remained affordable was typically unsafe, in bad condition, or located far from mental health services and public transportation. Finally, in the 1980s, many people had their disability income terminated by the federal government, and those who remained on SSI and SSDI have had to cope with benefits that, over time, have fallen far below what would be required to obtain decent housing.

Inadequate access to affordable and appropriate housing has become an especially important problem for people with SPMI (Technical Assistance Collaborative, 1999). For years, the disabled have not been part of mainstream housing policy debates, and no one agency has been responsible for the range of services necessary to meet a homeless person's needs (Bianco and Wells, 2001; Lezak et al., 1996). Efforts to create services for the homeless have devolved into debates about civil liberties and "not on my block" opposition (Currie et al., 1989). Within mental health, adequate housing has not consistently been considered part of treatment services (Newman, 2001). As a result, many clinical agencies lack evidence-based housing services, while housing agencies do not manage mental health and substance abuse services. At the same time, state vocational rehabilitation agencies have preferred to focus on people who do not have SPMI because they are easier to return to work.

Evidence-based care for the homeless with SPMI includes support for housing combined with mental health treatment. It begins by creating affordable housing options such as community residential facilities, supervised apartments, halfway homes, and SRO hotels. It also includes outreach to the homeless and assertive provision of mental health services. The ACT model has been successfully used in this population (Lehman et al., 1999). When evidence-based services are provided, outcomes are excellent (Rosenheck, 2000). Unfortunately, high-quality programs for the homeless are usually not available.

There have been many legislative, programmatic, and research activities with the goal of improving care for the homeless. In 1987, the first federal legislation was passed: the Stewart B. McKinney Homeless Assistance Act. The McKinney Act established a variety of programs and services, such as emergency food and shelter programs, the PATH program (Projects for Assistance in Transition from Homelessness), and community-based services for people who had a serious mental illness, a co-occurring disorder, and were at risk for homelessness (Bianco and Wells, 2001). In 1988, the Fair Housing Amendments Act was passed to help decrease stigma and discrimination against persons with mental illness in the housing market.

Although federal government support for affordable housing has been decreasing, during the past two decades the U.S. Department of Housing and Urban Development (HUD) has supported a number of programs to promote a comprehensive housing and mental health community. To receive funds, communities must engage in a strategic planning and grant process called a Consolidated Plan (ConPlan). These are local housing and community development plans that consolidate applications for funds from HUD programs: the HOME and Community Development Block Grants programs to assist with affordable housing, Emergency Shelter Grants to assist the homeless, and Housing Opportunities for People with AIDS. Also, HUD directly subsidizes rents for many people who are poor or disabled with the Section 8 program. However, Section 8 is severely underfunded, and it can take years or be impossible for qualifying individuals to get a housing voucher.

In the 1990s, comprehensive community-based systems of care for persons with mental illness and other disabilities were promoted by a federal Task Force on Homelessness and Severe Mental Illness, by a "Blueprint for a Cooperative Agreement between Public Housing Agencies and Local Mental Health Authorities," and by the U.S. Supreme Court's *Olmstead* decision.[1] While both the Task Force and the Blueprint report focused on persons with mental illness, by the end of 2000, states had not included housing as an element in their *Olmstead*-related plans (Bianco and Wells, 2001). This may have occurred because states were engaged in business as usual: using federal funds already available for treating the homeless or developing housing plans and their own state legislative initiatives.

In the absence of an adequate federal response to the homelessness problem for people with SPMI, state and local officials have employed a variety of prevention and treatment strategies. Examples include providing substance abuse experts on ACT teams in Illinois; developing independent living skills training, support, and service linkages to people in scattered site apartments in Michigan; working with local public defenders in the release of jail inmates at risk for homelessness in Florida; enhancing hospital psychiatric crisis services in New York; developing an integrated community at Los Angeles Men's Place (LAMP); creating a nonprofit housing development corporation in Rhode Island; and providing rent subsidies in Massachusetts. Creating these programs has required concerted efforts to foster working relationships between stakeholders to strategically plan so that resources can be maximized by governments at all levels (Bristol and Greiff, 2002; Culhane et al., 2001; Lowery, 1992; Marcos et al., 1990).

There have been many successful model programs for homelessness. However, these have not generalized more broadly and therefore have served only a small fraction of homeless persons with SPMI. Model programs often have special, limited funding, either from a research grant, a private foundation, or a governmental agency. They are typically designed to meet a defined need, such as demonstrating the effectiveness of a service model or convincing constituents that something is being done about a problem without actually allocating the necessary resources. Often, model programs are not clearly defined or based on empirical work and are not carefully evaluated. A seminal review of the literature in this area found that program evaluations are frequently uncontrolled, pay too little attention to critical contextual factors, and lack adequate research measures or methods. In addition, "no systematic body of knowledge on housing and mental illness has been compiled" (Newman, 2001). As a result, it is not possible to extract critical elements from successful programs. Dissemination of complete model programs is almost always unaffordable with existing resources. It may be possible to improve services by disseminating program components or staff competencies; however, the lack of consistent and careful research in this area has made it difficult to know how to proceed. Bridging the gap between research and practice in homelessness services is likely to require unwavering commitment, major policy changes, and substantially more resources than is usually acknowledged.

Implications For Mental Health Services

The mental health care system in the United States has both serious problems and the potential to provide remarkably good care. When an individual is cared for by competent clinicians and has access to appropriate psychosocial and medical treatments, outcomes are often excellent. Individuals with time-limited or moderately severe disorders can return to a good quality of life and functioning. Whereas many people with SPMI once spent years in state hospitals or back rooms, disabled or with a poor quality of life, they can now live satisfying, productive lives in the community. Unfortunately, positive outcomes remain the exception rather than the rule. As a result, the most pressing mental health challenge in the United States today is to bring effective care to the *majority* of those in need. As Robert Rosenheck has stated, we need to develop a "dissemination science" (Rosenheck, 2001).

Improving mental health care begins by ensuring that individuals have adequate insurance that pays for mental health and support services that are available and accessible. While funding is not sufficient to ensure appropriate care, it is necessary. As David Mechanic has written, "no single initiative would do more . . . than to provide appropriate insurance coverage" (Mechanic, 2001b). Over the past several decades, private insurers and large corporations have increasingly offered benefits for mental health and substance abuse treatment. However, these benefits have been much more limited than benefits for other components of medical care. During recent years, national mental health organizations have tried to get parity legislation enacted that would make copayments, deductibles, and insurance limits comparable with those of general medical care. These efforts have been buttressed by research demonstrating that these changes are affordable under managed care (Sturm, 1997). In the late 1990s, the federal government mandated parity in the federal employees' health benefits program. Legislation was also enacted to mandate parity for private corporations; however, it was quite weak and readily nullified by trivial changes in mental health benefit design (Gitterman et al., 2001). Although federal law exempts the insurance plans of many large corporations from state legislation, numerous states have passed parity legislation that impacts other plans. This appears to have improved coverage in plans that previously had a very limited mental health benefit (Branstrom and Sturm, 2002). However, under managed care it remains too easy to restrict access to effective mental health treatments. Genuine parity will require more substantial changes in insurance and financing (Burnam and Escarce, 1999).

It is not necessary to wait for improvements in funding before improving the quality of services. Public mental health authorities currently spend thousands of dollars per year on care for the average patient. While current funding levels are too low to provide high-quality care to the majority of people in need, important improvements in care are possible within existing budgets. Indeed, these improvements may be a prerequisite to increased funding, since purchasers are often reluctant to increase funding to systems that cannot demonstrate that they are using existing funds efficiently.

Because mental health systems have been plagued by myriad service system integration issues, many have assumed that improving coordination would improve care (Kahn and Kamerman, 1992). Until recently, most funding to improve care went to improve system integration—efforts in this area have included legislation (Miller, 1996), demonstration projects (Bickman, 1997; Rosenheck et al., 2002), and widespread practice changes (Stroul, 1989). Remarkably, when these efforts have been evaluated, it has consistently been found that integrating services does not improve treatment quality. While a number of large research studies support this conclusion, the best example was the 1994 Robert Wood Johnson Foundation Program on Chronic Mental Illness. This project established centralized mental health authorities in nine communities across the United States. It consolidated funding and oversight but did not improve patient care (Lehman et al., 1994).

There is, however, a growing science regarding how to improve care and disseminate effective health care interventions (Donovan et al., 1999; Schoenwald and Hoagwood, 2001). Different approaches have been studied, including those that focus on reorganization of services (Christianson et al., 1997; Khurana, 1999), diffusion of innovations (Pathman et al., 1996; Rogers, 1995), and factors that affect provider behavior (Mittman et al., 1992). In health care, simple educational strategies, such as continuing medical education, have little effect on provider behavior (Davis et al., 1995). A more powerful effect results from interventions that affect the daily activities of clinicians (Rubenstein et al., 2000), empower patients, or change organizational structure at the clinician or practice level (Oxman et al., 1995; Stone et al., 2002).

Since there are multiple barriers to improving care for SPMI, interventions will almost certainly need to be multidimensional to improve outcomes. For instance, it may not be sufficient to implement medication algorithms without attending to organizational factors that limit access to clozapine and psychosocial treatments. It should be possible to learn from projects in primary care and care for depression, where *collaborative care* and *chronic illness management* models have been effective (Bodenheimer et al., 2002; Wells et al., 2000). These models involve activating and educating patients, reorganizing care at the practice level, improving clinical information and decision support systems, and enhancing community supports. Applying these in organizations that care for people with SPMI will be challenging but not impossible. With regard to patient activation, there is an emerging national consumer empowerment movement that focuses on the value of peer support, consumer leaders and providers, and systems that are patient-centered (Corrigan, 2002). Effective patient empowerment models are just starting to be developed, and careful research is needed to define these models and test their effectiveness (Davidson et al., 1999). Similarly, research is needed to develop new care models that better address patient needs and ensure delivery of comprehensive and effective care.

One component of chronic disease management is ready to be implemented in mental health. Many mental health organizations have antiquated information systems or computer systems with little useful clinical information. Improving computerized clinical information can keep clinicians informed regarding their patients, allow monitoring of treatment quality, and identify problems in care that can be addressed. Assertive outreach, regular contact with patients, and reminders are often needed in chronic disease but difficult to manage without good information systems at the practice level. In primary care, information is routinely collected regarding, for instance, blood pressure, glucose, and glycated hemoglobin. Quality measures based on this information are useful in quality improvement efforts, because improving control of hypertension or diabetes clearly improves outcomes. In mental health, good quality indicators would include measures of, for instance, psychotic or depressive symptoms. Unfortunately, current documentation practices are highly inconsistent and medical records typically have little useful clinical information (Cradock et al., 2001). As a result, quality improvement efforts have had to focus on standardizing medication dosages or ensuring at least one outpatient visit after hospitalization, interventions that would be expected to have a limited effect on outcomes.

This lack of clinical information can be addressed by implementing computer systems that obtain information, either directly from patients or from clinicians who have been trained to reliably evaluate the severity of symptoms, side effects and patients' psychosocial needs. Some organizations have started to make progress in this area. The VA has implemented a national, fully electronic medical record and national systems for monitoring use of inpatient care, outpatient services, and medications. These have already been used to identify and remediate problems in access to and overuse of mental health services (Fontana and Rosenheck, 1997; Rosenheck and Cicchetti, 1998).

Efforts to improve care must be studied, since health care organization is highly complex and unintended consequences are very possible. One approach to improving care starts with treatment guidelines, which define effective treatments. Clinical information is collected to identify gaps between actual practice and guideline-concordant care. Interventions use these data to address problems, reach out to patients, and encourage clinicians to improve their care. A complementary approach to improving care begins with the use of competency sets that define the values, knowledge, and skills that clinicians need to provide effective care (Young et al., 2000a). Competency assessment is used to educate clinicians, ensure that all clinicians are competent, and direct patients to the clinicians who are most likely to improve their outcomes. Clinician competency can be assessed by clinical supervisors, using survey instruments, or by tracking the quality of a clinician's care (Chinman et al., 2003). For instance, one private sector MBHO is using a system that monitors patient outcomes over time for each clinician (Brown et al., 2001).

Clinicians and administrators can, of course, engage in continuous quality improvement activities at any point in time to improve the management of care and to monitor treatment processes and outcomes. However, effective management of mental health provider organizations requires standards for administrative practice. The field of mental health needs to develop and implement more systematic continuous quality improvement methods that produce more useful and valid outcome measures (Mullen and Magnabosco, 1997), and in turn, best practices. Research is needed regarding how to disseminate effective care at the policy, organizational, clinician, and patient levels. We need to know more, for instance, regarding how purchasers, mental health authorities, and insurers create incentives that increase the provision of high-quality care.

Improved services for mental illness would produce economic benefits for society, a more productive work force for employers, and reductions in homelessness and incarceration. They would strongly benefit ill individuals and their families, including some of the most vulnerable members of our society. These outcomes are reasonable incentives for change. However, we have only begun to understand how stakeholders can be motivated to support improvements in the quality of care (Etzioni, 1991). Access to appropriate mental health treatment is limited, and the United States is entering a serious health care cost crisis that could make this access even worse. If mental health services are to be provided at adequate levels, the value of existing and improved services will need to be demonstrated and people with mental illness empowered to demand evidence-based care.

ACKNOWLEDGMENTS

This work was supported by the Department of Veterans Affairs and the UCLA RAND NIMH Research Center on Managed Care for Psychiatric Disorders. Opinions expressed are only the authors' and do not necessarily represent the views of any affiliated institutions.

NOTES

1. 1999 landmark decision builds on American Disabilities Act by ruling against "unjustified isolation" or "institutionalization," for persons with disabilities. "In appropriate circumstances . . . the placement of persons with disabilities [should be made] in a community integrated setting whenever possible." Reference: www.whitehouse.gov/news/freedominitiative/freedominitiative.html

REFERENCES

Allebeck P. Schizophrenia: a life-shortening disease. *Schizophrenia Bulletin*, 15(1):81–89, 1989.

American Medical Association. *International Classification of Diseases, 9th Revision, Clinical Modification: Pphysician ICD-9-CM, 2002*. Chicago: American Medical Association Press, 2001.

American Psychiatric Association. Practice guidelines for the treatment of patients with bipolar disorder. *American Journal of Psychiatry*, 151(Suppl 12):S1–S36, 1994.

American Psychiatric Association. Practice guideline for the treatment of patients with schizophrenia. *American Journal of Psychiatry*, 154(Suppl 4):1–63, 1997.

American Psychiatric Association. *Diagnostic and Statistical Manual of Mental Disorders (DSM-IV-TR)*. Washington, DC: American Psychiatric Press, 2000.

American Psychiatric Association Steering Committee. The expert consensus guideline series. Treatment of bipolar disorder. *Journal of Clinical Psychiatry*, 57(Suppl 12A):3–88, 1996.

American Psychiatric Association Steering Committee. The expert consensus guideline series. Treatment of schizophrenia 1999. *Journal of Clinical Psychiatry*, 60(Suppl 11):3–80, 1999.

Anthony WA. Recovery from mental illness: The guiding vision of the mental health service system in the 1990s. *Psychosocial Rehabilitation Journal*, 16(4):11–23, 1993.

Anthony WA, Cohen M, Farkas M, et al. *Psychiatric Rehabilitation*. Boston: Boston University Center for Psychiatric Rehabilitation, 2002.

Arseneault L, Moffitt TE, Caspi A, et al. Mental disorders and violence in a total birth cohort: results from the Dunedin Study. *Archives of General Psychiatry*, 57(10):979–986, 2000.

Barlow DH, Lehman CL. Advances in the psychosocial treatment of anxiety disorders. Implications for national health care. *Archives of General Psychiatry*, 53(8):727–735, 1996.

Baumohl J. National Coalition for the Homeless (U.S.) (eds). *Homelessness in America*. Phoenix, AZ: Oryx Press, 1996.

Beck AT. Cognitive therapy: past, present, and future. *Journal of Consulting and Clinical Psychology*, 61(2):194–198, 1993.

Bhugra D. Attitudes towards mental illness. A review of the literature. *Acta Psychiatrica Scandinavica*, 80(1):1–12, 1989.

Bianco C, Wells SM. *Overcoming Barriers to Community Integration for People with Mental Illnesses*. Advocates for Human Potential. 2001. Available at: www.ahpnet.com/OvercomingBarriers.pdf Accessed October 30, 2002.

Bickman L. Resolving issues raised by the Fort Bragg evaluation: new directions for mental health services research. *American Psychologist*, 52(5):562–565, 1997.

Bloche MG, Cournos F. Mental health policy for the 1990s: tinkering in the interstices. *Journal of Health Politics, Policy and Law*, 15(2):387–411, 1990.

Blumenthal D. Controlling health care expenditures. *New England Journal of Medicine*, 344(10):766–769, 2001.

Bodenheimer T, Wagner EH, Grumbach K. Improving primary care for patients with chronic illness. *Journal of the American Medical Association*, 288(14):1775–1779, 2002.

Bond GR, Becker DR, Drake RE, et al. Implementing supported employment as an evidence-based practice. *Psychiatric Services*, 52(3):313–322, 2001.

Bothroyd RA, Shern DL, Bell NN. The effect of financial risk arrangements on service access and satisfaction among Medicaid beneficiaries. *Psychiatric Services*, 53(3):299–303, 2002.

Branstrom RB, Sturm R. Economic Grand Rounds: an early case study of the effects of California's mental health parity legislation. *Psychiatric Services*, 53(10):1215–1216, 2002.

Bristol K, Greiff D. *Review of Best Practices: The Frequent Users of Health Services Initiative*. California Endowment and California HealthCare Foundation. 2002. Available at: www.csh.org/fuhsi/pdf/FUHSI_BestPractices_final.pdf Accessed October 23, 2002.

Brown GS, Burlingame GM, Lambert MJ, et al. Pushing the quality envelope: a new outcomes management system. *Psychiatric Services*, 52(7):925–934, 2001.

Burnam MA, Escarce JJ. Equity in managed care for mental disorders: benefit parity is not sufficient to ensure equity. *Health Affairs*, 18(5):22–31, 1999.

Chang CF, Kiser LJ, Bailey JE, et al. Tennessee's failed managed care program for mental health and substance abuse services. *Journal of the American Medical Association*, 279(11):864–869, 1998.

Chassin MR. Quality of health care. Part 3: improving the quality of care. *New England Journal of Medicine*, 335(14):1060–1063, 1996.

Chassin MR. Achieving and sustaining improved quality: lessons from New York State and cardiac surgery. *Health Affairs*, 21(4):40–51, 2002.

Chinman MJ, Kloos B, O'Connel M, et al. Service providers' views of psychiatric mutual support groups. *Journal of Community Psychology*, 30:1–18, 2002.

Chinman MJ, Young AS, Rowe M, et al. An instrument to assess competencies of providers treating severe mental illness. *Mental Health Services Research*, 5(2):97–108, 2003.

Christianson JB, Pietz L, Taylor R, et al. Implementing programs for chronic illness management: the case of hypertension services. *Joint Commission Journal on Quality Improvement*, 23(11):593–601, 1997.

Committee on Government Operations. *From Backwards to Back Street: The Failure of the Federal Government in Providing Services for the Mentally Ill.* Rockville, MD: U.S. Government Printing Office, 1988.

Corrigan PW. Empowerment and serious mental illness: treatment partnerships and community opportunities. *Psychiatric Quarterly,* 73(3):217–228, 2002.

Coursey RD, Curtis L, Marsh DT, et al. Competencies for direct service staff members who work with adults with severe mental illnesses in outpatient public mental health/managed care systems. *Psychiatric Rehabilitation Journal,* 23(4):370–377, 2000.

Cradock J, Young AS, Sullivan G. The accuracy of medical record documentation in schizophrenia. *Journal of Behavioral Health Services and Research,* 28(4):456–465, 2001.

Cradock-O'Leary J, Young AS, Yano EM, et al. Use of general medical services by VA patients with psychiatric disorders. *Psychiatric Services,* 53(7):874–878, 2002.

Criminal Justice/Mental Health Consensus Project. *Project Report.* Council of State Governments. 2002. Available at: consensusproject.org Accessed October 30, 2002.

Crowther RE, Marshall M, Bond GR, et al. Helping people with severe mental illness to obtain work: systematic review. *British Medical Journal,* 322:204–208, 2001.

Cubanski J, Shaul JA, Eisen SV, et al. *Experience of Care and Health Outcomes (ECHO) Survey: A Survey to Elicit Consumer Ratings of Their Behavioral Health Treatment and Counseling.* NCQA Committee on Performance Measurement. 2002. Available at: www.ncqa.org/Programs/HEDIS/Part%202.pdf Accessed October 31, 2002.

Culhane DP, Metraux S, Hadley TR. *The Impact of Supportive Housing for Homeless People with Severe Mental Illness on the Utilization of the Public Health, Corrections, and Emergency Shelter Systems.* Fannie Mae Foundation. 2001. Available at: www.knowledgeplex. org/kp/text_document_summary/scholarly_article/relfiles/hpd_1301_culhane.pdf Accessed October 18, 2002.

Currie R, Trute B, Tefft B, et al. Maybe on my street: the politics of community placement of the mentally disabled. *Urban Affairs Quarterly,* 25(2):298–321, 1989.

Dahl PM, Forquer SL. Improved emergency access for Medicaid clients: a Colorado case study. In: Dickey B, Sederer LI (eds). *Improving Mental Health Care: Commitment to Quality.* Washington, DC: American Psychiatric Press, pp. 227–233, 2001.

Davidson L, Chinman ML, Kloos B, et al. Peer support among individuals with severe mental illness: a review of the evidence. *Clinical Psychology: Science and Practice,* 6(2):165–187, 1999.

Davis DA, Thomson MA, Oxman AD, et al. Changing physician performance. A systematic review of the effect of continuing medical education strategies. *Journal of the American Medical Association,* 274(9):700–705, 1995.

Depression Guideline Panel. *Clinical Practice Guideline Number 5: Depression in Primary Care.* AHRQ Pub. No. 93-0551. Rockville, MD: U.S. Department of Health and Human Services, Agency for Health Care Policy and Research, 1993.

Dickey B, Norton EC, Normand S-LT, et al. Managed mental health experience in Massachusetts. In: Mechanic D (ed). *New Directions for Mental Health Services, No. 78: Managed Behavioral Health Care: Current Realities and Future Potential.* San Francisco: Jossey-Bass, pp. 115–122, 1998.

Dixon L, McFarlane WR, Lefley H, et al. Evidence-based practices for services to families of people with psychiatric disabilities. *Psychiatric Services,* 52(7):903–910, 2001.

Donabedian A. *Explorations in Quality Assessment and Monitoring. Volume 1: The Definition of Quality and Approaches to its Assessment.* Ann Arbor, MI: Health Administration Press, 1980.

Donovan S, Bransford JD, Pelligrino JW. *How People Learn: Bridging Research and Practice.* Washington, DC: National Academies Press, 1999.

Draine J, Salzer MS, Culhane DP, et al. Role of social disadvantage in crime, joblessness, and homelessness among persons with serious mental illness. *Psychiatric Services*, 53(5):565–573, 2002.

Drake RE, Goldman HH, Leff HS, et al. Implementing evidence-based practices in routine mental health service settings. *Psychiatric Services*, 52(2):179–182, 2001.

Druss B, Rosenheck R. Evaluation of the HEDIS measure of behavioral health care quality. Health Plan Employer Data and Information Set. *Psychiatric Services*, 48(1):71–75, 1997.

Edlund M, Young AS, Kung FY, et al. Does satisfaction reflect the technical quality of mental health care? *Health Services Research*, 38:631–645, 2003.

Eisen SV, Shaul JA, Leff HS, et al. Toward a national consumer survey: evaluation of the CABHS and MHSIP instruments. *Journal of Behavioral Health Services and Research*, 28(3):347–369, 2001.

Etzioni A. *A Responsive Society: Collected Essays on Guiding Deliberate Social Change*. San Francisco: Jossey-Bass, 1991.

Farley DO, Short PF, Elliott MN, et al. Effects of CAHPS health plan performance information on plan choices by New Jersey Medicaid beneficiaries. *Health Services Research*, 37(4):985–1007, 2002.

Fitch K, Bernstein S, Aguilar MD, et al. *The RAND/UCLA Appropriateness Method User's Manual*. Santa Monica, CA: RAND Corporation, 2001.

Fontana A, Rosenheck R. Effectiveness and cost of the inpatient treatment of posttraumatic stress disorder: comparison of three models of treatment. *American Journal of Psychiatry*, 154(6):758–765, 1997.

Frank RG, McGuire TG. The economics of behavioral health carve-outs. In: Mechanic D (ed). *New Directions for Mental Health Services, No. 78: Managed Behavioral Health Care: Current Realities and Future Potential*. San Francisco: Jossey-Bass, 1998.

Gabbard GO (ed). *Treatments of Psychiatric Disorders*. Washington, DC: American Psychiatric Press, 2001.

Gitterman DP, Sturm R, Scheffler RM. Toward full mental health parity and beyond. *Health Affairs*, 20(4):68–76, 2001.

Gold MR, Siegel JE, Russell LB, et al. (eds). *Cost-Effectiveness in Health and Medicine*. New York: Oxford University Press, 1996.

Goldman HH, Ganju V, Drake RE, et al. Policy implications for implementing evidence-based practices. *Psychiatric Services*, 52(12):1591–1597, 2001.

Gresenz CR, Sturm R. Who knows what: Americans and their health insurance coverage for behavioral health care. Santa Monica, CA: RAND/UCLA Research Center on Managed Care for Psychiatric Disorders, Working Paper H-154, May 1999.

Hall LL, Edgar ER, Flynn LM. *Stand and Deliver: Action Call to a Failing Industry. The NAMI Managed Care Report Card*. Arlington, VA: National Alliance for the Mentally Ill, 1997.

Hanson KW, Huskamp HA. State health care reform: behavioral health services under Medicaid managed care: the uncertain implications of state variation. *Psychiatric Services*, 52(4):447–450, 2001.

Harding CM, Zahniser JH. Empirical correction of seven myths about schizophrenia with implications for treatment. *Acta Psychiatrica Scandinavica, Supplementum*, 90(Suppl 384):140–146, 1994.

Hausman JW, Wallace N, Bloom JR. Managed mental health experience in Colorado. In: Mechanic D (ed). *New Directions for Mental Health Services, No. 78: Managed Behavioral Health Care: Current Realities and Future Potential*. San Francisco: Jossey-Bass, pp. 107–114, 1998.

HayGroup. *Health Care Plan Design and Cost Trends—1988 through 1998.* 1999. Available at: www.naphs.org/News/hay99/hay99.pdf Accessed October 30, 2002.

Henry JA. Toxicity of antidepressants: comparisons with fluoxetine. *International Clinical Psychopharmacology*, 6(Suppl 6):22–27, 1992.

Herz MI, Marder SR. *Schizophrenia: Comprehensive Treatment and Management.* Philadelphia: Lippincott Williams & Wilkins, 2002.

Holloway F. Case management for the mentally ill: looking at the evidence. *International Journal of Social Psychiatry*, 37(1):2–13, 1991.

Hughes RA, Lehman AF, Arthur TE. Psychiatric rehabilitation. In: Breakey WR (ed): *Integrated Mental Health Services: Modern Community Psychiatry.* New York: Oxford University Press, pp. 286–299, 1996.

Huskamp HA, Garnick DW, Hanson KW, et al. The impact of withdrawals by Medicaid managed care plans on behavioral health services. *Psychiatric Services*, 52(5):600–602, 2001.

Institute of Medicine. *Measuring the Quality of Health Care.* Washington, DC: National Academies Press, 1999.

Kahn AJ, Kamerman SB. *Integrating Services Integration: An Overview of Initiatives, Issues, and Possibilities.* New York: National Center for Children, 1992.

Khurana A. Managing complex production processes. *Sloan Management Review*, 40(2):85–97, 1999.

Kissling W. Compliance, quality assurance and standards for relapse prevention in schizophrenia. *Acta Psychiatrica Scandinavica, Supplementum*, 382:16–24, 1994.

Koegel P, Sullivan G, Burnam A, et al. Utilization of mental health and substance abuse services among homeless adults in Los Angeles. *Medical Care*, 37(3):306–317, 1999.

Lamb HR, Bachrach LL. Some perspectives on deinstitutionalization. *Psychiatric Services*, 52(8):1039–1045, 2001.

Larequi-Lauber T, Vader JP, Burnand B, et al. Appropriateness of indications for surgery of lumbar disc hernia and spinal stenosis. *Spine*, 22(2):203–209, 1997.

Lehman AF. Quality of care in mental health: the case of schizophrenia. *Health Affairs*, 18(5):52–65, 1999.

Lehman AF, Dixon L, Hoch JS, et al. Cost-effectiveness of assertive community treatment for homeless persons with severe mental illness. *British Journal of Psychiatry*, 174:346–352, 1999.

Lehman AF, Postrado LT, Roth D, et al. Continuity of care and client outcomes in the Robert Wood Johnson Foundation Program on chronic mental illness. *Milbank Quarterly*, 72(1):105–122, 1994.

Lehman AF, Steinwachs DM. Translating research into practice: the Schizophrenia Patient Outcomes Research Team (PORT) treatment recommendations. *Schizophrenia Bulletin*, 24(1):1–10, 1998.

Lerman P. *Deinstitutionalization and the Welfare State.* Piscataway, NJ: Rutgers University Press, 1982.

Lezak AD, Edgar E. *Preventing Homelessness Among People with Serious Mental Illnesses: A Guide for States.* Policy Research Associates and National Resource Center on Homelessness and Mental Illness. 1996. Available at: www.nrchmi.com/pdfs/publications/Preventing_Homelessness.pdf Accessed October 30, 2002.

Liberman RP, Hilty DM, Drake RE, et al. Requirements for multidisciplinary teamwork in psychiatric rehabilitation. *Psychiatric Services*, 52(10):1331–1342, 2001.

Logan BM, Rochefort DA, Cook EW. Block grants for mental health: elements of the state response. *Journal of Public Health Policy*, 6(4):476–492, 1985.

Lowery M. LAMP in L.A.'s skid row: a model for community-based support services. *New Directions for Mental Health Services*, 56:89–98, 1992.

Lurie N, Christianson JB, Gray DZ, et al. The effect of the Utah Prepaid Mental Health

Plan on structure, process, and outcomes of care. *New Directions for Mental Health Services*, 62(78):99–106, 1998.

Lurie N, Moscovice IS, Finch M, et al. Does capitation affect the health of the chronically mentally ill? Results from a randomized trial. *Journal of the American Medical Association*, 267(24):3300–3304, 1992.

Lurie N, Ward NB, Shapiro MF, et al. Termination of Medi-Cal benefits. A follow-up study one year later. *New England Journal of Medicine*, 314(19):1266–1268, 1986.

Lutterman T, Hirad A, Poindexter B. *Funding Sources and Expenditures of State Mental Health Agencies: Study Results Fiscal Year 1997*. Alexandria, VA: National Association of State Mental Health Program Directors Reseach Institute, 1999.

Manderscheid RW, Atay JE, Hernandez-Cartagena MR, et al. *Highlights of Organized Mental Health Services in 1998 and Major National and State Trends*. Rockville, MD: Center for Mental Health Services and the U.S. Government Printing Office, 2001.

Marcos LR, Cohen NL, Nardacci D, et al. Psychiatry takes to the streets: the New York City initiative for the homeless mentally ill. *American Journal of Psychiatry*, 147(11): 1557–1561, 1990.

Marder SR, Essock SM, Miller AL, et al. The Mount Sinai conference on the pharmacotherapy of schizophrenia. *Schizophrenia Bulletin*, 28(1):5–16, 2002.

McCormick D, Himmelstein DU, Woolhandler S, et al. Relationship between low quality-of-care scores and HMOs' subsequent public disclosure of quality-of-care scores. *Journal of the American Medical Association*, 288(12):1484–1490, 2002.

McKusick D, Mark TL, King E, et al. Spending for Mental Health and Substance Abuse Treatment, 1996: the first comprehensive look at nationwide spending trends in this decade. *Health Affairs*, 17(3), 1998.

Mechanic D. The challenge of chronic mental illness: a retrospective and prospective view. *Hospital and Community Psychiatry*, 37(9):891–896, 1986.

Mechanic D. Closing gaps in mental health care for persons with serious mental illness. *Health Services Research*, 36(6 Pt 1):1009–1017, 2001a.

Mechanic D. The managed care backlash: perceptions and rhetoric in health care policy and the potential for health care reform. *Milbank Quarterly*, 79(1):35–54, 2001b.

MHSIP. *Consumer Survey, Version 1.1*. Mental Health Statistics Improvement Program. 2000. Available at: www.mhsip.org/surveylink.htm Accessed October 31, 2002.

Milazzo-Sayre LJ, Henderson MJ, Manderscheid RW, et al. *Persons Treated in Specialty Mental Health Care Programs, United States, 1997*. Washington, DC: Center for Mental Health Services and the U.S. Government Printing Office, 2001.

Miller E. *The Evolution of Integration: Federal Efforts from the 1960s to Present Day*. Delmar, NY: Policy Research Associates and National Resource Center on Homelessness and Mental Illness, 1996.

Mittman BS, Tonesk X, Jacobson PD. Implementing clinical practice guidelines: social influence strategies and practitioner behavior change. *QRB Quality Review Bulletin*, 18(12):413–422, 1992.

Morrissey JP, Goldman HH. Cycles of reform in the care of the chronically mentally ill. *Hospital and Community Psychiatry*, 35(8):785–793, 1984.

Mueser KT, Corrigan PW, Hilton DW, et al. Illness management and recovery: a review of the research. *Psychiatric Services*, 53(10):1272–1284., 2002.

Mueser KT, Glynn SM. *Behavioral Family Therapy for Psychiatric Disorders*. Oakland, CA: New Harbinger, 1999.

Mullen EJ, Magnabosco JL (eds). *Outcomes Measurement in the Human Services: Cross-Cutting Issues and Methods*. Washington, DC: National Association of Social Workers Press, 1997.

Narrow WE, Rae DS, Robins LN, et al. Revised prevalence estimates of mental disorders in the United States: using a clinical significance criterion to reconcile 2 surveys' estimates. *Archives of General Psychiatry*, 59(2):115–123, 2002.

NASMHPD Research Institute. *Implementation of Evidence-Based Services by State Mental Health Agencies: 2001.* Alexandria, VA: National Association of State Mental Health Program Directors, 2002.

National Alliance for the Mentally Ill. *Stigma Busters Campaign.* 2002. Available at: www.nami.org/campaign/stigmabust.html Accessed October 18, 2002.

National Coalition for the Homeless. *Fact Sheet: How Many People Experience Homelessness?* 1999. Available at: www.nationalhomeless.org/numbers.html Accessed October 21, 2002.

National Institute of Mental Health. *Caring for People with Severe Mental Disorders: A National Plan of Research to Improve Services.* DHHS Pub. No. (ADM) 91-1762. Rockville, MD: National Institute of Mental Health, 1991.

Newman SJ. Housing attributes and serious mental illness: implications for research and practice. *Psychiatric Services*, 52(10):1309–1317, 2001.

Oxman AD, Thomson MA, Davis DA, et al. No magic bullets: a systematic review of 102 trials of interventions to improve professional practice. *Canadian Medical Association Journal*, 153(10):1423–1431, 1995.

Pathman DE, Konrad TR, Freed GL, et al. The awareness-to-adherence model of the steps to clinical guideline compliance: the case of pediatric vaccine recommendations. *Medical Care*, 34(9):873–889, 1996.

Pescosolido BA, Monahan J, Link BG, et al. The public's view of the competence, dangerousness, and need for legal coercion of persons with mental health problems. *American Journal of Public Health*, 89(9):1339–1345, 1999.

Phillips SD, Burns BJ, Edgar ER, et al. Moving assertive community treatment into standard practice. *Psychiatric Services*, 52(6):771–779, 2001.

President's New Freedom Commission on Mental Health. *Achieving the Promise: Transforming Mental Health Care in America. Final Report.* 2003. Available at: http://www.mentalhealthcommission.gov/reports/reports.htm Accessed July 31, 2003.

Rogers EM. *Diffusion of Innovations.* New York: Free Press, 1995.

Rosenheck RA. Cost-effectiveness of services for mentally ill homeless people: the application of research to policy and practice. *American Journal of Psychiatry*, 157(10):1563–1570, 2000.

Rosenheck RA. Organizational process: a missing link between research and practice. *Psychiatric Services*, 52(12):1607–1612, 2001.

Rosenheck RA, Cicchetti D. A mental health program report card: a multidimensional approach to performance monitoring in public sector programs. *Community Mental Health Journal*, 34(1):85–106, 1998.

Rosenheck RA, Lam J, Morrissey JP, et al. Service systems integration and outcomes for mentally ill homeless persons in the ACCESS program. Access to community care and effective services and supports. *Psychiatric Services*, 53(8):958–966, 2002.

Rothman D. *Conscience and Convenience: The Asylum and Its Alternatives in Progressive America.* Boston: Little, Brown, 1980.

Roy-Byrne P, Stein M, Bystrisky A, et al. Pharmacotherapy of panic disorder: proposed guidelines for the family physician. *Journal of the American Board of Family Practice*, 11(4):282–290, 1998.

Rubenstein LV, Mittman BS, Yano EM, et al. From understanding health care provider behavior to improving health care: the QUERI framework for quality improvement. Quality Enhancement Research Initiative. *Medical Care*, 38(6 Suppl 1):I129–141, 2000.

Sabin JE, Daniels N. Setting behavioral health priorities: good news and crucial lessons from the Oregon Health Plan. *Psychiatric Services*, 48(7):883–884, 889, 1997.

Sabin JE, Daniels N. Public-sector managed behavioral health care: V. Redefining "medical necessity"—the Iowa experience. *Psychiatric Services*, 51:445–459, 2000.

Schoenwald SK, Hoagwood K. Effectiveness, transportability, and dissemination of interventions: What matters when? *Psychiatric Services*, 52(9):1190–1197, 2001.

Schooler NR, Keith SJ, Severe JB, et al. Relapse and rehospitalization during maintenance treatment of schizophrenia: the effects of dose reduction and family treatment. *Archives of General Psychiatry*, 54(5):453–463, 1997.

Schulberg HC, Katon W, Simon GE, et al. Treating major depression in primary care practice: an update of the Agency for Health Care Policy and Research Practice Guidelines. *Archives of General Psychiatry*, 55(12):1121–1127, 1998.

Scott RW. Systems within systems: the mental health sector. In: Scott WR, Black BL (eds). *Organizational of Mental Health Services: Societal and Community Systems*. Beverly Hills, CA: Sage, pp. 31–52, 1986.

Sederer LI, Clemens NA. The business case for high-quality mental health care. *Psychiatric Services*, 53(2):143–145, 2002.

Snow V, Lascher S, Mottur-Pilson C. Pharmacologic treatment of acute major depression and dysthymia. *Annals of Internal Medicine*, 132:738–742, 2000.

Starfield B. Is U.S. health really the best in the world? *Journal of the American Medical Association*, 284(4):483–485, 2000.

Stein DJ. Obsessive-compulsive disorder. *Lancet*, 360(9330):397–405, 2002.

Stockdill CN. On the federal scene. *Administration and Policy in Mental Health*, 17(3):193–197, 1990.

Stone EG, Morton SC, Hulscher ME, et al. Interventions that increase use of adult immunization and cancer screening services: a meta-analysis. *Annals of Internal Medicine*, 136:641–651, 2002.

Stroul BA. Community support systems for persons with long-term mental illness: a conceptual framework. *Psychological Rehabilitation Journal*, 12(3):9–39, 1989.

Sturm R. How expensive is unlimited mental health care coverage under managed care? *Journal of the American Medical Association*, 278(18):1533–1537, 1997.

Sullivan G, Burnam A, Koegel P. Pathways to homelessness among the mentally ill. *Social Psychiatry and Psychiatric Epidemiology*, 35(10):444–450, 2000.

Swartz HA. Interpersonal psychotherapy. In: Hersen M, Bellack AS (eds). *Handbook of Comparative Interventions for Adult Disorders* (2nd ed.). New York: Wiley, pp. 139–155, 1999.

Swartz HA, Frank E. Psychotherapy for bipolar depression: a phase-specific treatment strategy? *Bipolar Disorders*, 3(1):11–22, 2001.

Technical Assistance Collaborative. *Seizing the Moment: Using HUD's Consolidated Plan to Identify Affordable Housing Opportunities for Homeless People with Serious Mental Illnesses*. Policy Research Associates and National Resource Center on Homelessness and Mental Illness. 1999. Available at: www.nrchmi.com/pdfs/publications/Seizing_the_Moment. pdf Accessed October 30, 2002.

Torrey EF. *Surviving Schizophrenia: A Manual for Families, Consumers, and Providers*. New York: Quill, 2001.

Unutzer J, Simon G, Pabiniak C, et al. The use of administrative data to assess quality of care for bipolar disorder in a large staff model HMO. *General Hospital Psychiatry*, 22(1):1–10, 2000.

U.S. Surgeon General. *Mental Health: A Report of the Surgeon General*. Rockville, MD: U.S. Department of Health and Human Services, Substance Abuse and Mental Health Services Administration, and the National Institute of Mental Health, 1999.

Vaccaro JV, Pitts DB, Wallace CJ. Functional Assessment. In: Liberman RP (ed). *Handbook of Psychiatric Rehabilitation*. New York: Macmillan, pp. 78–94, 1992.

Vaccaro JV, Young AS. Contemporary treatment of individuals with chronic mental illness. In: Vaccaro JV, Clark GH (eds). *Practicing Psychiatry in the Community: A Manual.* Washington, DC: American Psychiatric Press, pp. 173–189, 1996.

Veterans Health Administration. *Clinical Guideline for Management of Persons with Psychoses, Version 1.0.* Washington, DC: Department of Veterans Affairs, 1997.

Wang PS, Demler O, Kessler RC. Adequacy of treatment for serious mental illness in the United States. *American Journal of Public Health,* 92(1):92–98, 2002.

Wells KB. The design of Partners in Care: evaluating the cost-effectiveness of improving care for depression in primary care. *Social Psychiatry and Psychiatric Epidemiology,* 34(1):20–29, 1999.

Wells KB, Sherbourne C, Schoenbaum M, et al. Impact of disseminating quality improvement programs for depression in managed primary care: a randomized controlled trial. *Journal of the American Medical Association,* 283(2):212–220, 2000.

Wells KB, Sherbourne CD, Sturm R, et al. Alcohol, drug abuse, and mental health care for uninsured and insured adults. *Health Services Research,* 37(4):1055–1066, 2002.

Winslow CM, Kosecoff JB, Chassin M, et al. The appropriateness of performing coronary artery bypass surgery. *Journal of the American Medical Association,* 260(4):505–509, 1988.

Young AS, Clark GH. Guidelines for community psychiatric practice. In: Vaccaro JV, Clark GH (eds). *Practicing Psychiatry in the Community: A Manual.* Washington, DC: American Psychiatric Press, pp. 331–341, 1996.

Young AS, Forquer SL, Tran A, et al. Identifying clinical competencies that support rehabilitation and empowerment in individuals with severe mental illness. *Journal of Behavioral Health Services and Research,* 27(3):321–333, 2000a.

Young AS, Grusky O, Jordan D, et al. Routine outcome monitoring in a public mental health system: the impact of patients who leave care. *Psychiatric Services,* 51(1):85–91, 2000b.

Young AS, Klap R, Sherbourne CD, et al. The quality of care for depressive and anxiety disorders in the United States. *Archives of General Psychiatry,* 58(1):55–61, 2001.

Young AS, Nuechterlein KH, Mintz J, et al. Suicidal ideation and suicide attempts in recent-onset schizophrenia. *Schizophrenia Bulletin,* 24(4):629–634, 1998a.

Young AS, Sullivan G, Burnam MA, et al. Measuring the quality of outpatient treatment for schizophrenia. *Archives of General Psychiatry,* 55(7):611–617, 1998b.

Young AS, Sullivan G, Duan N. Patient, provider, and treatment factors associated with poor-quality care for schizophrenia. *Mental Health Services Research,* 1(4):201–211, 1999.

Young AS, Sullivan G, Murata D, et al. Implementing publicly funded risk contracts with community mental health organizations. *Psychiatric Services,* 49(12):1579–1584, 1998c.

Section C
Older Adults

10

Epidemiology of Mental Disorders in Older Adults

CELIA F. HYBELS
DAN G. BLAZER

Over the past two decades, the United States has seen increases in the number of individuals aged 65 or older and in the proportion of the total population that is in that age group. According to the 2000 United States Census, persons 65 or older made up 13% of the population. About 1.6% were 85 years or older. By the year 2050, the proportion of individuals in the population in the over-85 group is expected to be 5% (Federal Interagency Forum on Aging Related Statistics, 2000). These changing demographics pose special challenges for providers of mental health services to older adults. To understand the potential impact, it is necessary to study the epidemiology of mental disorders in late life. By definition, *epidemiology* is the study of the distribution and determinants of disease frequency in populations (MacMahon and Pugh, 1970).

We begin this chapter by introducing some of the challenges in studying the epidemiology of mental disorders in older adults, including case definition, cohort effects, and comorbidity. We then describe the epidemiology of key disorders in late life: mood disorders, anxiety disorders, dementia, schizophrenia, and alcohol use. For each of these disorders we provide data on both the prevalence, the number of cases present in the population at a particular time, and the incidence, the number of new cases that develop in the population over a specified time period— for their subclinical as well as clinical forms. To shed more light on the determinants of disease frequency, we discuss risk factors and correlates of these mental disorders and syndromes, including comorbidity. We describe findings from longitudinal studies on outcomes associated with mental disorders in late life, including the high risk of suicide in older adults. We conclude with a summary of the implications of these findings for behavioral health services.

Defining Disease—What Is a Case?

The American Psychiatric Association *Diagnostic and Statistical Manual of Mental Disorders* (4th ed.) (DSM-IV) (American Psychiatric Association, 1994) defines case identification by the presentation of specific symptoms. For each disorder, a set of specified symptoms must be present, sometimes within a particular time period, for the individual to meet criteria for the disorder. Compared with younger adults, case definition in older adults is challenging. Older adults often present with symptoms of a potential mental disorder, but it may not be clear whether the symptoms are a result of medication use or comorbid physical illness. Older adults often fail to meet the specific criteria for a disorder because they do not have a sufficient number of symptoms, the symptoms have not been present for the required time interval, or the symptoms have not occurred for the first time before a particular age. And yet these symptoms may be clinically significant and related to impairments in functioning and decreased quality of life. In the sections that follow, we show how recent research suggests that the criteria for some mental disorders may be less applicable to older adults.

The instruments used to determine the presence of symptoms also affect case identification. The past two decades have seen the development of specific instruments, such as the National Institute of Mental Health (NIMH) Diagnostic Interview Schedule (DIS) (Robins et al., 1981) and the Composite International Diagnostic Interview (CIDI) (World Health Organization, 1990), that can be administered by either clinicians or lay persons and from which many DSM diagnoses can be determined. Epidemiological studies of older adults often use screening scales to identify individuals with mental disorder. For example, the Center for Epidemiologic Studies–Depression (CES-D) Scale (Radloff, 1977) is often used to determine if the individual is depressed, and the Mini-Mental State Examination (MMSE) (Folstein et al., 1975) is used to assess cognitive function. Screening instruments such as these are not intended to identify persons who meet specific criteria for mental disorders, but rather to identify individuals with particular symptoms. Therefore, much of the research on mental disorders in older adults includes individuals who do not necessarily meet the diagnostic criteria for a disorder. Yet these epidemiological studies have provided valuable information for understanding mental disorders in late life.

Cohort Effects

In studying the epidemiology of mental disorders in older adults and its implications for planning for health services, it is important to note the potential impact of cohort effects. That is, it is important to examine whether the prevalence of a disorder in adults aged 65 or older will most likely be stable in future samples of older individuals or whether an observed prevalence may be related to the particular characteristics of a given cohort. The burden of mental disorders in younger adults suggests that the prevalence of diagnoses may not remain constant in future cohorts.

Comorbidity of Mental Disorders

As in other age groups, the issue of comorbidity of mental disorders in older adults is important in defining a case. In the following sections, we will address examples of comorbidity of mental disorders in older adults. Comorbidity between mental and physical illnesses in older adults is also important. Because of the high prevalence of chronic diseases in late life compared to earlier periods, it can be difficult to distinguish between symptoms of mental disorders and those due to physical illness.

Prevalence of Mental Disorders in Older Adults

The NIMH Epidemiologic Catchment Area (ECA) Program was established to determine the prevalence and incidence of specific psychiatric disorders in both community and institutional populations (Regier et al., 1984). Although the ECA Program was not based on a national probability sample, data were collected in five U.S. communities: New Haven, Baltimore, St. Louis, Durham (North Carolina), and Los Angeles. While these data were collected more than two decades ago, the ECA Program continues to remain the landmark study in the United States to measure the prevalence of mental disorders in older adults. Psychiatric disorders were determined through the use of the NIMH DIS (Robins et al., 1981).

Among noninstitutionalized adults aged 65 or older, the 1-month prevalence of any DIS disorder was 12.3%, compared to 16.9% in those aged 18–24, 17.3% in those aged 25–44, and 13.3% in those aged 45–64 (Regier et al., 1988). With the exception of severe cognitive impairment, all disorders were less frequent among older adults. The prevalence of severe cognitive impairment was 4.9% in persons aged 65 or older, while the most prevalent disorder in this age group was any anxiety disorder (5.5%), primarily phobic disorder (4.8%). The prevalence of any DIS disorder was 13.6% in women 65 or older and 10.5% in men in the same age group. Alcohol and drug disorders, however, were higher in men than in women.

The National Comorbidity Survey (NCS), a national survey of psychiatric disorders using a representative sample of persons 15–54 years of age, was conducted in 1990–92 (Kessler et al., 1994), but since older adults were not included, NCS data are not discussed here.

Since the time of the ECA studies, numerous community- and clinical-based studies conducted in the past 20 years in the United States and other countries have contributed data to clarify further the prevalence, incidence, correlates, and outcomes of mental disorders in older adults. Table 10.1 presents the results of selected studies of the prevalence of mental disorders in older adults. Disorders presented include mood disorders, anxiety disorders, dementia, schizophrenia, and alcohol use disorders. Each of these disorders is also discussed below.

Table 10.1 Representative Studies of the Prevalence of Mental Disorders in Older Adults

Author(s) and Date of Study	Sample and Instrument Description	Prevalence	Comments
MOOD DISORDERS			
Regier et al. (1988)	ECA Community-dwelling adults 65+ in five U.S. communities DIS (*n* = 5702)	0.7% 1-month prevalence of major depression 0.9% women 0.4% men	
Bland et al. (1988)	Edmonton, Alberta Community-dwelling adults 65+ DIS (*n* = 358)	1.2% 6-month prevalence of major depression	
Beekman et al. (1995)	LASA—The Netherlands Community-dwelling adults 55–85 DIS and CES-D (*n* = 3056)	2.02% major depression 12.9% minor depression	Major depression rooted in vulnerability factors, while minor depression was more often a reaction to stress
Copeland et al. (1987)	Liverpool 1070 community residents 65 or older GMS-AGECAT	11.3% diagnostic cases of depressive illness 7.6% men 13.6% women	
Copeland et al. (1999)	EURODEP Age 65 or greater in nine European countries GMS-AGECAT (*n* = 13,808)	12.3% diagnostic cases of depression 14.1% women 8.6% men	Much variation in prevalence of depression across Europe
Henderson et al. (1993)	Canberra, Australia 825 community residents 43 institutional residents age 70+ DSM-III-R and ICD-10 (draft)	3.3% ICD-10-defined depressive episodes 1.0% DSM-III-R major depressive disorder	Number of depressive symptoms correlated with neuroticism, poor physical health, disability, and history of depressive symptoms
Blazer et al. (1987)	North Carolina ECA Adults 60 or older DIS (*n* = 1,304)	27% depressive symptoms	19% mild dysphoria, 4% symptomatic depression, 2% dysthymia, 1.2% mixed depression-anxiety, and 0.8% major depression
Parmelee et al. (1989)	708 nursing home or congregate housing residents Mean age 84 years GDS and DSM-III checklist	12.4% major depression 30.5% minor depression	
Koenig et al. (1997)	Medically ill hospitalized adults 60 or older (*n* = 460)	Major depression 10%–21% Minor depression 14%–25%	Diagnostic scheme affects reported prevalence

Table 10.1 *(Continued)*

Author(s) and Date of Study	Sample and Instrument Description	Prevalence	Comments
Lyness et al. (1999)	Primary care patients 60 or older HAM-D (*n* = 224)	5.2% minor depression 9.9% subsyndromal depression 6.5% major depression 0.9% Dysthymia	

ANXIETY DISORDERS

Author(s) and Date of Study	Sample and Instrument Description	Prevalence	Comments
Regier et al. (1988)	ECA Community-dwelling adults 65+ in five U.S. cities DIS (*n* = 5702)	5.5% any anxiety disorder 3.6% men 6.8% women 4.8% phobic disorder 0.1% panic disorder	GAD not included in these data
Bland et al. (1988)	Edmonton Community-dwelling adults 65+ DIS (*n* = 358)	3.0% phobic disorder 1.5% obsessive-compulsive disorder	
Blazer et al. (1991b)	North Carolina ECA	2.2% GAD	
Beekman et al. (1998)	The Netherlands LASA Community-dwelling adults 55–85 CES-D and DIS (*n* = 3107)	10.2% any anxiety disorder 7.3% GAD 1.0% panic disorder 3.1% phobic disorder 0.6% obsessive-compulsive disorder	
Lindesay et al. (1989)	London Guy's Age Concern Survey of community-dwelling adults 65+ (*n* = 890)	3.7% GAD 10.0% phobic disorder	Instruments developed by investigator
Forsell and Winblad (1998)	Sweden 966 adults 78+ Structured psychiatric interview	24.4% feelings of anxiety	
Kvaal et al. (2001)	Norway 98 inpatients 70+ STAI	41% of women and 47% of men had significant anxiety symptoms	

DEMENTIA

Author(s) and Date of Study	Sample and Instrument Description	Prevalence	Comments
Regier et al. (1988)	ECA Community-dwelling adults 65+ in five U.S. cities DIS (*n* = 5702)	4.9% severe cognitive impairment 2.9% adults 65–74 6.8% adults 75–84 15.8% adults 85+	

(Continued)

215

Table 10.1 Representative Studies of the Prevalence of Mental Disorders in Older Adults (*Continued*)

Author(s) and Date of Study	Sample and Instrument Description	Prevalence	Comments
Bland et al. (1988)	Edmonton 358 community-dwelling adults 65+ 199 adults 65+ in institutions DIS	68.8% prevalence of cognitive impairment in institutions 3.3% prevalence among community-dwelling elderly	
Copeland et al. (1987)	Liverpool 1070 community-dwelling adults 65+ GMS-AGECAT	5.2% probable dementia	
Copeland et al. (1992)	Liverpool 1070 community-dwelling adults 65+ GMS-AGECAT	3.3% Alzheimer's disease	
Canadian Study of Health and Aging Working Group (1994)	Canada 9008 community-dwelling and 1255 institutionalized adults 65+ Diagnostic clinical examination	8.0% Dementia 5.1% Alzheimer's disease	2:1 female:male ratio of dementia
Evans et al. (1989)	East Boston EPESE Community-dwelling adults 65+ Screening and clinical evaluation (n = 3623)	10.3% probable Alzheimer's disease	3.0% of those 65–74, 18.7% of those 75–84, and 47.2% of those 85+

SCHIZOPHRENIA

Author(s) and Date of Study	Sample and Instrument Description	Prevalence	Comments
Regier et al. (1988)	ECA Community-dwelling adults 65+ in five U.S. cities DIS (n = 5,702)	0.1% schizophrenia	DSM-III used, which did not allow for late-onset disease
Copeland et al. (1998)	Sample of 5222 persons 65+ selected from general practitioner lists GMS-AGECAT	0.12% schizophrenia 0.04% delusional disorder	DSM-III = R criteria used
Christenson and Blazer (1984)	North Carolina 997 community-dwelling adults 65+	4.0% persecutory ideation	
Ostling and Skoog (2002)	347 persons aged 85 living in the community or in institutions in Sweden	10.1% prevalence of any psychotic symptom, 6.9% hallucinations, 5.5% delusions.	
Henderson et al. (1998)	1377 persons 70+	5.7% psychotic symptoms	

Table 10.1   (*Continued*)

Author(s) and Date of Study	*Sample and Instrument Description*	*Prevalence*	*Comments*
Yassa et al. (1993)	288 patients 65+ admitted to a psychogeriatric unit	2.4% of all admissions diagnosed with symptoms of paranoid schizophrenia	
ALCOHOL DISORDERS			
Regier et al. (1988)	ECA Community-dwelling adults 65+ in five U.S. communities DIS (*n* = 5,702)	0.9% alcohol abuse/dependence	
Bland et al. (1988)	Edmonton 358 community-dwelling adults 65+ DIS	1.7% alcohol use/dependence	
Bristow and Clare (1992)	327 male and 323 female medical and geriatric admissions 65+	9% of men drank in excess of recommended limits; an additional 10% had previously drunk heavily	
Adams et al. (1996)	5065 patients 60+ in primary care	15% of men and 12% of women regularly drank in excess	
Saunders et al. (1989)	Liverpool 1070 subjects 65+ GMS-AGECAT	0.09% current drinking problems 19.5% of male regular drinkers and 19.6% of female regular drinkers exceeded recommended limits	

CES-D: Center for Epidemiologic Studies–Depression Scale (Radloff, 1977); DIS: Diagnostic Interview Schedule (Robins et al., 1981); ECA: Epidemiologic Catchment Area Surveys; EPESE: Established Populations for Epidemiologic Studies of the Elderly; GAD: generalized anxiety disorder; GDS: Geriatric Depression Scale (Yesavage et al., 1983); GMS-AGECAT: Geriatric Mental State-Automated Geriatric Examination for Computer Assisted Taxonomy (Copeland et al., 1976); HAM-D: Hamilton Rating Scale for Depression (Williams, 1988); LASA: Longitudinal Aging Study Amsterdam; STAI: State Trait Anxiety Inventory (Speilberger et al., 1983).

Mood Disorders

In the ECA studies, the 1-month prevalence of major depression in persons aged 65 or older was 0.7%, which was considerably lower than the prevalence in other age groups: 2.2% in those aged 18–24, 3.0% in those aged 25–44, and 2.0% in those aged 45–64 (Regier et al., 1988).

The lifetime prevalence in the ECA data of any affective disorder (primarily major depression) was 1.6% in men 65 or older compared to 3.3% in women in the same age group. The lifetime prevalence was 1.5% in white men, 1.9% in African American men, and 4.3% in Hispanic men 65 or older, while the proportion was 3.4% in older white women, 3.4% in African American women, and 2.6% in Hispanic women (Weissman et al., 1991).

As shown in Table 10.1, other community-based studies have reported a similar prevalence of major depression in older adults, ranging from approximately 1% to 3% (Beekman et al., 1995; Bland et al., 1988; Henderson et al., 1993). Other studies have reported a higher prevalence. Steffens et al. (2000) reported that the point prevalence of major depression in a sample of nondemented adults aged 65 to 100 was 4.4% in women and 2.7% in men. An even higher prevalence was reported from the Liverpool and EURODEP studies, as shown in Table 10.1 (Copeland et al., 1987, 1999). The current prevalence of major depression in older adults sampled from inpatient and outpatient clinical settings as well as long-term care facilities is generally higher, with estimates ranging from 6.5% to 21%, as shown in Table 10.1 (Koenig et al., 1997; Lyness et al., 1999; Parmelee et al., 1989).

The incidence or onset of depression in late life has also been reported from several studies. Forsell and Winblad (1999) reported that the incidence of first-onset depression in a sample of 875 persons with a mean age of 85 years was 1.4% per person-year, while an incidence of 133.49 per 1000 person-years was reported among adults 85 or older in a community study in Munich (Meller et al., 1996). Among Australian elders followed for 3 to 6 years, 2.5% of those originally non-depressed developed major depression (Henderson et al., 1997).

The prevalence of subsyndromal/minor depression, or of depressive symptoms not meeting criteria for major depression or dysthymia, is much higher than that of major depression in late life. Among older adults from the North Carolina ECA study, the overall prevalence of depressive symptoms was 27% (Blazer et al., 1987). A similar prevalence of depressive symptoms has been reported from similar community and clinical studies, as shown in Table 10.1 (Beekman et al., 1995; Lyness et al., 1999).

In the Duke Established Populations for Epidemiologic Studies of the Elderly (EPESE) the prevalence of depression, as defined by the CES-D, was 9.0% (Blazer et al., 1991a). In addition, depressive symptoms below the cutpoint of the CES-D in these data were shown to be prevalent in older adults (9.9%) and were associated with impairment in physical functioning, disability days, poorer self-rated health, the use of psychotropic medications, low perceived social support, female gender, and being unmarried (Hybels et al., 2001). In the Duke EPESE, the demographic and social predictors and correlates of subthreshold depression were shown to be similar to those of CES-D depression, suggesting that the overall prevalence of depressive symptoms was over 18%.

Blazer et al. (1991a) examined the association between age and depression in the Duke EPESE and found that depressive symptoms were correlated with increased age, being female, lower income, physical disability, cognitive impairment, and having no close relatives. When these factors were simultaneously controlled, however, the association between depression and age reversed, with the oldest old reporting fewer symptoms. Henderson et al. (1993) also reported that in a sample of adults aged 70 or older, the number of symptoms did not increase with older age.

In the LASA, major depression was associated with being unmarried and having functional limitations, impaired social support, poorer self-rated health, perceived loneliness, and an internal locus of control. Minor depression was associated with, in addition, lower level of education, urban living, chronic physical illness, and mild cognitive impairment (Beekman et al., 1995).

Some studies have shown that disability in older adults can lead to depression (Kennedy et al., 1990), while others have shown that depression can lead to declines in physical functioning (Cronin-Stubbs et al., 2000; Penninx et al., 1999b). Research on whether depressive symptoms are predictive of cognitive decline has also been inconclusive. Henderson et al. (1997) found that depressive symptoms did not predict cognitive decline or dementia in a 3- to 6-year follow-up period, while Yaffe et al. (1999) found evidence that depression can lead to cognitive decline.

Finally, surveys of depression as a risk factor for mortality in older adults have also yielded mixed results. Bruce and Leaf (1989) found a fourfold increase in the risk of death over a 15-month period among adults 55 or older if the individual had experienced a mood disorder at the time of the initial interview. Similar results were reported from Australia (Henderson et al., 1997). Using data from the Duke ECA, however, Fredman et al. (1989) did not find an association between either major depression or depressive symptoms and 2-year mortality in adults 60 or older. Blazer et al. (2001) recently reported that in older adults depression was associated with 3-year mortality through different independent mechanisms such as chronic disease, functional impairment, and social support. Gender differences in the association between depression and mortality have also been noted. Penninx et al. (1999a) reported from the LASA that major depression was associated with mortality for men and women, while minor depression was associated with mortality only for men.

Comorbidity between depression and dementia is not uncommon. Patterson et al. (1990) reported that 18% of Alzheimer's disease patients seen in an outpatient setting had mild to moderate symptoms of depression. Alexopoulas et al. (1993) followed a sample of severely depressed elders and found that some experienced cognitive impairment during their depression.

Anxiety Disorders

In the ECA studies, anxiety disorders were the most common disorders among persons 65 or older, with a 1-month prevalence of 5.5%. The prevalence was lower than that for other age groups (7.7% for those aged 18–24, 8.3% for those aged 25–44, and 6.6% for those aged 45–64) (Regier et al., 1988). These proportions do not include generalized anxiety disorder (GAD), so the actual prevalence of any anxiety disorder in persons 65 or older is likely higher. Generalized anxiety disorder was assessed, however, in three of the five communities of the ECA program. In these studies, a total of 2.2% of individuals 65 and older met criteria for GAD during the year prior to the interview. This disorder was more common in women than in men (Blazer et al., 1991b). In the ECA, both phobic disorder and panic disorder were also more common in older women compared to older men (Eaton et al., 1991).

As shown in Table 10.1, other community-based studies have found a similar prevalence of anxiety disorders (Beekman et al., 1995; Bland et al., 1988), while the prevalence of phobic disorder reported from the Guy's Age Concern Survey was higher (Lindesay et al., 1989).

The prevalence of anxiety symptoms is much higher in older adults than the prevalence of anxiety disorders, and selected studies are presented in Table 10.1. These studies indicate that the prevalence of anxiety symptoms may be as high as 40% (Forsell and Winblad, 1998; Kvaal et al., 2001). Several correlates of and risk factors for anxiety disorders and anxiety symptoms in late life have been noted, including having a history of one or more psychiatric disorders (Forsell and Winblad, 1997, 1998), current psychiatric disturbance, being female, impairment of or dissatisfaction with the social network (Forsell and Winblad, 1998), and impaired activities of daily living (Forsell and Winblad, 1997).

In a 3-year study of individuals 75 or older in Sweden, onset of anxiety symptoms was predicted by a history of depression/anxiety and an impaired social network (no regular visitors) in the baseline study (Forsell, 2000). In the LASA, when respondents were followed for 3 years, hearing and eyesight problems, distress due to life events (especially loss of a spouse), being female, and high neuroticism were associated with becoming anxious. Female gender and neuroticism increased the likelihood of chronicity of anxious symptom, but life events were not related to chronicity (DeBeurs et al., 2000). DeBeurs et al. (2000) also examined changes in anxiety symptoms over 3 years in the LASA and found that of the 1602 subjects without anxiety symptoms at baseline, 310 had symptoms at follow-up.

Chronic anxiety has been associated with an increased risk of mortality. In the Normative Aging Study, the odds of mortality from coronary disease were 3.20 in men who reported significant symptoms of anxiety and the odds of sudden cardiac death were 5.73 in men with anxiety compared to those without it, suggesting an association between anxiety and fatal cardiac disease (Kawachi et al., 1994).

Comorbidity among anxiety disorders and with other psychiatric disorders is not uncommon. In the LASA, 10% of those with a DSM-III diagnosis of an anxiety disorder had two or more anxiety disorders. Other psychiatric factors were also more prevalent among older adults with an anxiety diagnosis. Specifically, DSM-III major depression (13% in those with an anxiety disorder vs. 3% in those without it), chronic somatic diseases (12% vs. 7%), and benzodiazepine use (24% vs. 11%) were more common (van Balkom et al., 2000). Lenze et al. (2000) found that anxiety disorders were prevalent among patients 60 or older with depression seen in primary care and psychiatric settings. A total of 35% of patients with a depressive disorder had at least one lifetime anxiety disorder diagnosis, and 23% had a current anxiety diagnosis. Comorbid anxiety in depressed patients was associated with poorer social functioning and a higher level of somatic symptoms compared to persons with depression without concurrent anxiety. Finally, Beekman et al. (2000) found in the LASA that 47.5% of those with major depression also met criteria for an anxiety disorder.

Dementia

In the ECA studies, the 1-month prevalence of severe cognitive impairment was 4.9% in adults 65 or older. While the prevalence was 4.2% in men aged 65–74 compared to 1.9% in women in the same age group, the gender differences reversed with age. The prevalence of severe cognitive impairment was 8.2% in men 85 or older compared to 19.5% in women 85 or older (Regier et al., 1988).

Similar results were reported from studies in Edmonton and Liverpool (Bland et al., 1988; Copeland et al., 1987). Note that in Table 10.1, the prevalence of cognitive impairment is higher among institutionalized older adults (Bland et al., 1988; Canadian Study of Health and Aging Working Group, 1994). Jorm et al. (1987) reviewed studies of dementia and concluded that its prevalence in older adults doubled every 5.1 years.

The prevalence of Alzheimer's disease is lower than that of dementia. The prevalence of Alzheimer's disease was 5.1% in the Canadian Study of Health and Aging (Canadian Study of Health and Aging Working Group, 1994) and 3.3% in the Liverpool study (Copeland et al., 1992). A higher prevalence was reported from the East Boston site of the EPESE (Evans et al., 1989).

The incidence of dementia also has been shown to increase with age. In the Framingham research, the incidence ranged from 7.0 per 1000 person-years at ages 65 to 69 to 118.0 per 1000 person-years at ages 85 to 89 (Bachman et al., 1993). Similar results were reported from a sample aged 75 or older in the United Kingdom: the incidence of dementia approximately doubled every 5 years (Paykel et al., 1994). Fillenbaum et al. (1998) reported from the Duke EPESE that the 3-year incidence of dementia was 0.058 for blacks and 0.062 for whites. Neither race nor gender differences in incidence were significant.

Christensen et al. (1994) studied the relationship between health status and cognitive performance in an Australian sample of 708 community-dwelling individuals aged 70 or older. Cognitive performance was weakly associated with self-rated health and self-reported physical symptoms but was not associated with blood pressure or many physical conditions. The authors concluded that cognitive function in older adults was not mediated by ill health.

Depression has been shown to be a risk factor for cognitive decline. In a study of 1070 adults 60 or older, depressed mood at baseline was associated with an increased risk of dementia over a 1- to 5-year period (relative risk = 2.94). The effect remained after adjustment for age, gender, education, language of assessment, and both memory and functional activity scores (Devanand et al., 1996). Yaffe et al. (1999) found that depressive symptoms were associated with both poor cognitive function and subsequent cognitive decline in older women.

Lower levels of education have also been shown to predict cognitive decline (Evans et al., 1993; Farmer et al., 1995). Other risk factors for dementia include head trauma (Mortimer et al., 1991) and the E4 allele of apolipoprotein E (Evans et al., 1997; Saunders et al., 1993). Possible protective factors include nonsteroidal anti-inflammatory use (Breitner et al., 1995) and estrogen use (Kawas et al., 1997), although other studies have not found a protective effect of estrogen against cognitive decline related to aging (Fillenbaum et al., 2001).

Cognitive dysfunction has been shown to predict decline in physical functioning. Moritz et al. (1995) found in the Yale EPESE that persistent incident limitations in activities of daily living occurred more frequently in persons with more errors on cognitive function tests 3 years earlier at baseline. Similar findings were reported from Sweden (Aguero-Torres et al., 1998). Finally, cognitive impairment is a risk factor for mortality. Kelman et al. (1994) followed 1855 community residents in New York aged 65 or older for 4 years. The survival probability was .85 for the cognitively unimpaired, .69 for the mildly impaired, and .51 for the severely impaired.

Schizophrenia

The 1-month prevalence of schizophrenia in adults 65 or older reported in the ECA surveys was 0.1%, which was much lower than that of other age groups (0.4% in those aged 45–64, 0.9% in those aged 25–44, and 0.7% in those aged 18–24) (Regier et al., 1988). The lifetime prevalence of schizophrenia or schizophreniform disease (same symptoms but less duration) was 0.3% in those 65 or older in the ECA, again much lower than that in younger age groups (Keith et al., 1991). In the 65+ age group, the 1-month prevalence was higher for black men (0.2%) and black women (0.4%) compared to other ethnic/gender subgroups (Keith et al., 1991). As shown in Table 10.1, Copeland et al. (1998) found a similar prevalence of schizophrenia in their Liverpool study.

The prevalence of paranoid symptoms in older adults is much higher, ranging from 4% to 10% (Blazer et al., 1996; Christenson and Blazer, 1984; Ostling and Skoog, 2002). These studies suggest that, as with other disorders, clinically significant symptoms not meeting criteria for the disorder may be prevalent in older adults. The incidence of schizophrenia among older adults has been estimated to be 3.0 per 100,000 persons per year for new cases and 45.0 for new and relapsed cases (Copeland et al., 1998).

There are several other reasons for the lower prevalence of DSM schizophrenia in older adults. Younger adults with schizophrenia are at risk for mortality and may not survive to older age (Black and Fisher, 1992). A second reason is that DSM-III (American Psychiatric Association, 1980), which was used in the ECA surveys, required onset of symptoms before age 45 to meet criteria for the disorder. Older adults may not recall the age at which the symptoms were first experienced. More important, recent work has focused on late-onset schizophrenia or disease onset after age 45. Yassa et al. (1993) reported that the prevalence of late-onset schizophrenia was 2.4% among patients admitted to a psychogeriatric unit. Castle and Murray (1993) compared patients across all ages of onset and found a later onset of schizophrenia in women. They also found that late-onset patients were more likely than early-onset patients to have good premorbid functioning.

Jeste et al. (1995) compared patients with late-onset schizophrenia to early-onset patients and normal controls and found that those with late-onset disease were similar to those with early-onset disease and were different from controls in terms of clinical and neuropsychological variables. However, the group with late-onset schizophrenia had a higher percentage who had ever married, a better work history, and more patients of the paranoid subtype.

Research examining correlates of schizophrenia in older adults has focused on both older patients with schizophrenia diagnosed when they were younger and older adults who first developed symptoms later in life. Heaton et al. (1994) found that neuropsychological impairment in older schizophrenic patients was unrelated to current age, age at onset, and duration of illness. Patterson et al. (1997) reported that older patients with schizophrenia had more impairments in social functioning than controls. Physical disability has also been found to be more prevalent in older adults with schizophrenia or with subclinical symptoms compared to controls (Blazer et al., 1996; Klapow et al., 1997; Ostling and Skoog, 2002), while lower physical comorbidity among schizophrenic patients has also been reported (Lacro and Jeste, 1994). Jeste et al. (1996) have also reported that while schizophrenic patients may have lower physical comorbidity, their illness tends to be more severe. Blazer et al. (1996) found that in their sample of community-dwelling subjects, psychotic symptoms were more prevalent in African Americans, subjects with lower education and income, subjects who exercised less, and subjects with more depressive symptoms.

Psychiatric comorbidity among patients with delusional symptoms also presents a challenge. Among a sample of 161 elderly inpatients with major depression, 45% reported delusions (Meyers and Greenberg, 1986). Similarly, Wragg and Jeste (1989) reviewed 30 studies of patients with Alzheimer's disease and found that depressive and psychotic symptoms occurred in 30%–40%.

Finally, adverse outcomes associated with schizophrenia in older adults have been noted. Copeland et al. (1998) followed their sample of subjects with schizophrenia from the Liverpool area and found after 2 to 4 years that while none of them had fully recovered, none were deluded. However, most had developed another psychiatric illness. Similarly, Ostling and Skoog (2002) found that their subjects with psychotic symptoms were at increased risk for dementia after 3 years.

Alcohol Use

The 1-month prevalence of alcohol abuse/dependence in adults 65 or older in the ECA was 0.9%. The prevalence of alcohol abuse/dependence in those aged 18–24 was 4.1%, in those aged 25–44 3.6%, and in those aged 45–64 2.1%. Overall, the prevalence was higher in older men than in older women (Regier et al., 1988). As shown in Table 10.1, a similar prevalence was reported from Edmonton (Bland et al., 1988).

In cross-sectional studies, the prevalence of alcohol use has been shown to decline with age. Cahalan and Cisin (1968) reported that among adults 60 or older, 65% of the men and 44% of the women said they drank alcohol at least once a year. The prevalence was lower than that observed in younger groups (84% in men aged 21–29, 86% in men aged 30–39, 70% in women aged 20–29, and 72% in women aged 30–39). More recently, in the National Longitudinal Alcohol Epidemiologic Survey, the 1-year prevalence of alcohol use among persons 55 or older was 29.5%, and there was an inverse relationship between alcohol use and increasing age (Grant, 1997).

There are several reasons why the prevalence of alcohol use is lower in older adults. Selective survival may play a role in that persons who drink may be less likely to survive to older age. Also, there may be a cohort effect; that is, persons who grew up in the era of Prohibition and economic depression in the United States may have had lower alcohol use throughout their lives (Blazer and Penny-backer, 1984). Also, some studies have shown that some elderly persons decrease their alcohol use as they age (Busby et al., 1988).

In spite of a decline with age, the prevalence of alcohol use in adults 65 or older remains high. In the multisite EPESE, the proportion who had used alcohol in the past month ranged from 24.6% in North Carolina to 54.7% in East Boston (Cornoni-Huntley et al., 1986, 1990). The prevalence of heavy use among users is also high. Cahalan and Cisin (1968) reported that 20% of the men 60 or older and 2% of the women in the same age group from their sample were classified as heavy drinkers. As shown in Table 10.1, studies of older adults who use alcohol show that a significant number drink in excess of recommended limits (Adams et al., 1996; Bristow and Clare, 1992; Saunders et al., 1989).

Although the prevalence of alcohol use in older adults may appear low, alcohol consumption at any level may cause problems. Higher peak ethanol concentrations per dose are found in older compared to younger subjects because of decreased lean body mass and a smaller volume of distribution (Vestal et al., 1977).

In a study of 270 men and women 65 or older, alcohol use in late life was positively associated with male gender, income, and amount of education and negatively associated with age (Goodwin et al., 1987). At-risk drinkers among medical inpatients 65 or older were more likely to smoke, not to be married, and to have some impairment in mobility (Bristow and Clare, 1992).

Saunders et al. (1991) found that men 65 or older with a history of heavy drinking had more than a fivefold risk of a current psychiatric diagnosis compared to men without a history of heavy drinking. Finlayson et al. (1988) reported similar findings of comorbid psychiatric diagnoses in patients 65 or older admitted for treatment of alcoholism.

Among older adults who are problem drinkers, two groups emerge—those who have had problems with alcohol most of their lives and those who do not become problem drinkers until later in life. Atkinson et al. (1990) studied age of onset and found that those who began drinking heavily after age 60 had milder problems and greater psychological stability. Brennen and Moos (1991) reported similar results of fewer problems in late-onset drinkers.

Adverse outcomes have been reported for those with a history of alcohol use or current use. Hurt et al. (1988) found that the prevalence of medical disorders was higher among 216 patients 65 or older treated for alcoholism than would be expected for that age group. Alcohol use in the elderly has also been associated with increased hospitalizations (Callahan and Tierney, 1995). In the Canadian Study of

Health and Aging, the occurrence of all types of dementia except probable Alzheimer's disease was higher in those with definite or questionable alcohol abuse (Thomas and Rockwood, 2001).

A higher risk of mortality in older adults who use alcohol has also been reported (Callahan and Tierney, 1995; Thomas and Rockwood, 2001). Hurt et al. (1988) followed 60 of their patients being treated for alcoholism for an average of 5.2 years and found that 32% had died by follow-up; 47% of the deaths could be attributed to the patient's alcoholism.

Finally, some studies have found a protective effect in older adults using alcohol. Scherr et al. (1992), using data from the EPESE, found that low to moderate alcohol consumption was associated with lower 5-year total mortality as well as cardiovascular mortality in East Boston and New Haven, but they did not find a protective effect among the subjects from the Iowa EPESE. Similarly, LaCroix et al. (1993) found a higher risk of losing mobility among subjects who did not consume alcohol compared to those with low to moderate alcohol consumption.

Suicide in Older Adults

In the United States, suicide rates increase with age and are highest among white men over the age of 65. About 20% of suicide deaths occur in older adults, although older adults make up only 13% of the population (Centers for Disease Control, 2000). Among older patients seen in primary care, completed suicides are associated with depressive illness, physical health burden, and functional limitations (Conwell et al., 2000). In the United States from 1980 to 1986, suicide rates for persons 65 or older increased by 21%. The rate increase ranged from 9% in those 65–69 years of age to 38% in those 80–84 years of age (Meehan et al., 1991). Blazer et al. (1986) studied suicide rates in white men in successive cohorts and found that birth cohort was a strong predictor of suicide rates.

Implications for Mental Health Services

It is clear from these studies of the prevalence, incidence, and outcomes of mental disorders in older adults that the burden of psychiatric disorders and their associated subclinical syndromes in this population is significant. While dementia is a major contributor to this burden, other disorders are also represented. Comorbidity among mental disorders as well as with physical illness is a particular problem both in identifying and in treating mental disorders in older adults. Though less apparent in community-based epidemiological studies, in clinical studies of more severe disorders it is evident that comorbid medical and psychiatric symptoms can increase the burden of both medical and psychiatric illnesses. In addition, adverse outcomes such as disability have significant implications for behavioral health services for older adults.

Finally, the proportion and number of older adults are increasing and are projected to continue to increase, especially those of the "oldest old," aged 80 or older.

In addition, the population is dynamic. New cohorts will enter old age with a higher lifetime prevalence of mental disorders than the current cohort of older adults, especially for psychiatric illness such as depression and substance abuse. Given these statistics, the prevalence of psychiatric illness in older adults and the subsequent demand for health services are likewise expected to increase.

REFERENCES

Adams WL, Barry KL, Fleming MF. Screening for problem drinking in older primary care patients. *Journal of the American Medical Association*, 276:1964–1967, 1996.

Aguero-Torres H, Fratiglioni L, Guo Z, et al. Dementia is the major cause of functional dependence in the elderly: 3-year follow-up data from a population based study. *American Journal of Public Health*, 88:1452–1456, 1998.

Alexopoulas GS, Meyers BS, Young RC. The course of geriatric depression with "reversible dementia": a controlled study. *American Journal of Psychiatry*, 150:1693–1699, 1993.

American Psychiatric Association. *Diagnostic and Statistical Manual of Mental Disorders*, 3rd ed. Washington, DC: American Psychiatric Press, 1980.

American Psychiatric Association. *Diagnostic and Statistical Manual of Mental Disorders*, 4th ed. Washington, DC: American Psychiatric Press, 1994.

Atkinson RM, Tolson RL, Turner JA. Late versus early onset problem drinking in older men. *Alcoholism: Clinical and Experimental Research*, 14:574–579, 1990.

Bachman DL, Wolf PA, Linn RT, et al. Incidence of dementia and probable Alzheimer's disease in a general population: the Framingham Study. *Neurology*, 43:515–519, 1993.

Beekman ATF, Bremmer MA, Deeg DJH, et al. Anxiety disorders in later life: a report from the Longitudinal Aging Study Amsterdam. *International Journal of Geriatric Psychiatry*, 13:717–726, 1998.

Beekman ATF, de Beurs E, van Balkom AJLM, et al. Anxiety and depression in later life: co-occurrence and communality of risk factors. *American Journal of Psychiatry*, 157: 89–95, 2000.

Beekman ATF, Deeg DJH, van Tilberg T, et al. Major and minor depression in later life: a study of prevalence and risk factors. *Journal of Affective Disorders*, 36:65–75, 1995.

Black DW, Fisher R. Mortality in DSM-III R schizophrenia. *Schizophrenia Research*, 7:109–116, 1992.

Bland RC, Newman SC, Orn H. Prevalence of psychiatric disorders in the elderly in Edmonton. *Acta Psychiatrica Scandinavica, Supplementum*, 338:57–63, 1988.

Blazer DG, Bachar JR, Manton KG. Suicide in late life. *Journal of the American Geriatrics Society*, 34:519–525, 1986.

Blazer DG, Burchett B, Service C, et al. The association of age and depression among the elderly: an epidemiologic exploration. *Journal of Gerontology A: Biological Sciences and Medical Sciences*, 46:M210–215, 1991a.

Blazer DG, Hays JC, Salive ME. Factors associated with paranoid symptoms in a community sample of older adults. *The Gerontologist*, 36:70–75, 1996.

Blazer D, Hughes DC, George LK. The epidemiology of depression in an elderly community population. *The Gerontologist*, 27:281–287, 1987.

Blazer D, Hughes D, George LK. Generalized anxiety disorder. In: Robins L, Regier D (eds). *Psychiatric Disorders in America: The Epidemiologic Catchment Area Study*. New York: Free Press, pp. 180–203, 1991b.

Blazer DG, Hybels CF, Pieper CF. The association of depression and mortality in elderly persons: a case for multiple, independent pathways. *Journal of Gerontology A: Biological Sciences and Medical Sciences*, 56A:M505–M509, 2001.

Blazer DG, Pennybacker MR. Epidemiology of alcoholism in the elderly. In: Hartford JT, Samorajski T (eds). *Alcoholism in the Elderly*. New York: Raven Press, pp. 25–33, 1984.

Breitner JC, Welsh KA, Hlems MJ, et al. Delayed onset of Alzheimer's disease with nonsteroidal anti-inflammatory and histamine H2 blocking drugs. *Neurobiology of Aging*, 16:523–530, 1995.

Brennen PL, Moos RH. Functioning, life context, and help-seeking among late-onset problem drinkers: comparisons with nonproblem and early-onset problem drinkers. *British Journal of Addiction*, 86:1139–1150, 1991.

Bristow MF, Clare AW. Prevalence and characteristics of at-risk drinkers among elderly acute medical in-patients. *British Journal of Addiction*, 87:291–294, 1992.

Bruce ML, Leaf PJ. Psychiatric disorders and 15-month mortality in a community sample of older adults. *American Journal of Public Health*, 79:727–730, 1989.

Busby WJ, Campbell AJ, Borrie MJ, et al. Alcohol use in a community-based sample of subjects aged 70 years and older. *Journal of the American Geriatrics Society*, 36:301–305, 1988.

Cahalan D, Cisin IH. American drinking practices: summary of findings from a national probability sample. *Quarterly Journal of Studies in Alcohol*, 29:30–151, 1968.

Callahan CM, Tierney WM. Health services use and mortality among older primary care patients with alcoholism. *Journal of the American Geriatrics Society*, 43:1378–1383, 1995.

Canadian Study of Health and Aging Working Group. Canadian Study of Health and Aging: study methods and prevalence of dementia. *Canadian Medical Association Journal*, 150:899–912, 1994.

Castle DJ, Murray RM. The epidemiology of late-onset schizophrenia. *Schizophrenia Bulletin*, 19:691–700, 1993.

Centers for Disease Control, Suicide and Suicidal Behavior. *Fact Book for the Year 2000*. National Center for Injury Prevention and Control, 2000.

Christensen H, Jorm AF, Henderson AS, et al. The relationship between health and cognitive functioning in a sample of elderly people in the community. *Age and Ageing*, 23:204–212, 1994.

Christenson R, Blazer D. Epidemiology of persecutory ideation in an elderly population in the community. *American Journal of Psychiatry*, 141:1088–1091, 1984.

Conwell Y, Lyness JM, Duberstein P, et al. Completed suicide among older patients in primary care practices: a controlled study. *Journal of the American Geriatrics Society*, 48:23–29, 2000.

Copeland JRM, Beekman ATF, Dewey ME, et al. Depression in Europe: geographic distribution among older people. *British Journal of Psychiatry*, 174:312–321, 1999.

Copeland JRM, Davidson IA, Dewey ME, et al. Alzheimer's disease, other dementias, depression, and pseudodementia: prevalence, incidence, and three-year outcome in Liverpool. *British Journal of Psychiatry*, 161:230–239, 1992.

Copeland JRM, Dewey ME, Scott A, et al. Schizophrenia and delusional disorder in older age: community prevalence, incidence, comorbidity, and outcome. *Schizophrenia Bulletin*, 24:153–161, 1998.

Copeland JRM, Dewey ME, Wood N, et al. Range of mental illness among the elderly in the community: prevalence in Liverpool using the GMS-AGECAT package. *British Journal of Psychiatry*, 150:815–823, 1987.

Copeland JRM, Kelleher MJ, Kellett JM, et al. A semi-structured clinical interview for the assessment of diagnosis and mental state in the elderly. *Psychological Medicine*, 6:439–449, 1976.

Cornoni-Huntley J, Blazer DG, Lafferty ME, et al. *Established Populations for Epidemiologic Studies of the Elderly: Resource Data Book Volume II.* Washington, DC: National Institute on Aging, 1990.

Cornoni-Huntley J, Brock D, Ostfeld A, et al. *Established Populations for Epidemiologic Studies of the Elderly: Resource Data Book.* Bethesda, MD: National Institute on Aging, 1986.

Cronin-Stubbs D, Mendes de Leon CF, Beckett LA, et al. Six-year effect of depressive symptoms on the course of physical disability in community-living older adults. *Archives of Internal Medicine,* 160:3074–3080, 2000.

DeBeurs E, Beekman ATF, Deeg DJH, et al. Predictors of change in anxiety symptoms of older persons: results from the Longitudinal Aging Study, Amsterdam. *Psychological Medicine,* 30:515–527, 2000.

Devanand DP, Sano M, Tang M-X, et al. Depressed mood and the incidence of Alzheimer's disease in the elderly living in the community. *Archives of General Psychiatry,* 53:175–182, 1996.

Eaton W, Dryman A, Weissman M. Panic and phobia. In: Robins L, Regier D (eds). *Psychiatric Disorders in America: The Epidemiologic Catchment Area Study.* New York: Free Press, pp. 155–179, 1991.

Evans DA, Beckett LA, Albert MS, et al. Level of education and change in cognitive function in a community population of older persons. *Annals of Epidemiology,* 3:71–77, 1993.

Evans DA, Beckett LA, Field T. Apolipoprotein E e4 and incidence of Alzheimer's disease in a community population of older persons. *Journal of the American Medical Association,* 277:822–824, 1997.

Evans DA, Funkenstein HH, Albert MS, et al. Prevalence of Alzheimer's disease in a community population of older persons: higher than previously reported. *Journal of the American Medical Association,* 262:2551–2556, 1989.

Farmer ME, Kittner SJ, Rae DS, et al. Education and change in cognitive function: the Epidemiologic Catchment Area Study. *Annals of Epidemiology,* 5:1–7, 1995.

Federal Interagency Forum on Aging-Related Statistics. *Older Americans 2000: Key Indicators of Well-Being,* Washington, DC: Federal Interagency Forum on Aging-Related Statistics, 2000.

Fillenbaum GG, Hanlon JT, Landerman LR, et al. Impact of estrogen use on decline in cognitive function in a representative sample of older community-resident women. *American Journal of Epidemiology,* 153:137–144, 2001.

Fillenbaum GG, Heyman A, Huber MS, et al. The prevalence and 3-year incidence of dementia in older Black and White community residents. *Journal of Clinical Epidemiology,* 51:587–595, 1998.

Finlayson RE, Hurt RD, Davis LJ, et al. Alcoholism in elderly persons: a study of the psychiatric and psychosocial features of 216 inpatients. *Mayo Clinic Proceedings,* 63:761–768, 1988.

Folstein MF, Folstein SE, McHugh P. Mini-mental state: a practical method for grading the cognitive state of patients for clinicians. *Journal of Psychiatric Research,* 12:189–198, 1975.

Forsell Y. Predictors for depression, anxiety and psychotic symptoms in a very elderly population: data from a 3-year follow-up study. *Social Psychiatry and Psychiatric Epidemiology,* 35:259–263, 2000.

Forsell Y, Winblad B. Anxiety disorders in non-demented and demented elderly patients: prevalence and correlates. *Journal of Neurology, Neurosurgery, and Psychiatry,* 62:294–295, 1997.

Forsell Y, Winblad B. Feelings of anxiety and associated variables in a very elderly population. *International Journal of Geriatric Psychiatry,* 13:454–458, 1998.

Forsell Y, Winblad B. Incidence of major depression in a very elderly population. *International Journal of Geriatric Psychiatry*, 14:368–372, 1999.

Fredman L, Schoenbach VJ, Kaplan BH, et al. The association between depressive symptoms and mortality among older participants in the Epidemiologic Catchment Area-Piedmont Health Survey. *Journal of Gerontology B: Psychological Sciences and Social Sciences*, 44:S149–156, 1989.

Goodwin JS, Sanchez CJ, Thomas P, et al. Alcohol intake in a healthy elderly population. *American Journal of Public Health*, 77:173–177, 1987.

Grant BF. Prevalence and correlates of alcohol use and DSM-IV alcohol dependence in the United States: results of the National Longitudinal Alcohol Epidemiologic Survey. *Journal of Studies in Alcohol*, 58:464–473, 1997.

Heaton R, Paulsen JS, McAdams LA, et al. Neuropsychological deficits in schizophrenia. *Archives of General Psychiatry*, 51:468–476, 1994.

Henderson AS, Jorm AF, MacKinnon A, et al. The prevalence of depressive disorders and the distribution of depressive symptoms in later life: a survey using Draft ICD-10 and DSM-III-R. *Psychological Medicine*, 23:719–729, 1993.

Henderson AS, Korten AE, Jacomb PA, et al. The course of depression in the elderly: a longitudinal community-based study in Australia. *Psychological Medicine*, 27:119–129, 1997.

Henderson AS, Korten AE, Levings C, et al. Psychotic symptoms in the elderly: a prospective study in a population sample. *International Journal of Geriatric Psychiatry*, 13: 484–492, 1998.

Hurt RD, Finlayson RE, Morse RM, et al. Alcoholism in elderly persons: medical aspects and prognosis of 216 patients. *Mayo Clinic Proceedings*, 63:753–760, 1988.

Hybels CF, Blazer DG, Pieper CF. Toward a threshold for subthreshold depression: an analysis of correlates of depression by severity of symptoms using data from an elderly community sample. *The Gerontologist*, 41:357–365, 2001.

Jeste DV, Gladsjo JA, Lindamer LA, et al. Medical comorbidity in schizophrenia. *Schizophrenia Bulletin*, 22:413–430, 1996.

Jeste DV, Harris MJ, Krull A, et al. Clinical and neuropsychological characteristics of patients with late-onset schizophrenia. *American Journal of Psychiatry*, 152:722–730, 1995.

Jorm AF, Korten AE, Henderson AS. The prevalence of dementia: a quantitative integration of the literature. *Acta Psychiatrica Scandinavica*, 76:465–479, 1987.

Kawachi I, Sparrow D, Vokonas PS, et al. Symptoms of anxiety and risk of coronary heart disease. The Normative Aging Study. *Circulation*, 90:2225–2229, 1994.

Kawas C, Resnick S, Morrison A, et al. A prospective study of estrogen replacement therapy and the risk of developing Alzheimer's disease: the Baltimore Longitudinal Study of Aging. *Neurology*, 48:1517–1521, 1997.

Keith SJ, Regier DA, Rae DS. Schizophrenic disorders. In: Robins L, Regier D (eds). *Psychiatric Disorders in America*. New York: Free Press, pp. 33–52, 1991.

Kelman HR, Thomas C, Kennedy GJ, et al. Cognitive impairment and mortality in older community residents. *American Journal of Public Health*, 84:1255–1260, 1994.

Kennedy GJ, Kelman HR, Thomas C. The emergence of depressive symptoms in late life: the importance of declining health and increasing disability. *Journal of Community Health*, 15:93–103, 1990.

Kessler RC, McGonagle KA, Zhao S, et al. Lifetime and 12-month prevalence of DSM-III-R psychiatric disorders in the United States. *Archives of General Psychiatry*, 51:8–19, 1994.

Klapow JC, Evans J, Patterson TL, et al. Direct assessment of functional status in older patients with schizophrenia. *American Journal of Psychiatry*, 154:1022–1024, 1997.

Koenig HG, George LK, Peterson BL, et al. Depression in medically ill hospitalized older adults: prevalence, characteristics, and course of symptoms according to six diagnostic schemes. *American Journal of Psychiatry*, 154:1376–1383, 1997.

Kvaal K, Macijauskiene J, Engedal K, et al. High prevalence of anxiety symptoms in hospitalized geriatric patients. *International Journal of Geriatric Psychiatry*, 16:690–693, 2001.

Lacro JP, Jeste DV. Physical comorbidity and polypharmacy in older psychiatric patients. *Biological Psychiatry*, 36:146–152, 1994.

LaCroix AZ, Guralnick JM, Berkman LF, et al Maintaining mobility in late life: II. Smoking, alcohol consumption, physical activity, and body mass index. *American Journal of Epidemiology*, 137:858–869, 1993.

Lenze E, Mulsant BH, Shear MK, et al. Comorbid anxiety disorders in depressed elderly patients. *American Journal of Psychiatry*, 157:722–728, 2000.

Lindesay J, Briggs K, Murphy E. The Guy's/Age Concern Survey. Prevalence rates of cognitive impairment, depression and anxiety in an urban elderly community. *British Journal of Psychiatry*, 155:317–329, 1989.

Lyness JM, King DA, Cox C, et al. The importance of subsyndromal depression in older primary care patients: prevalence and associated functional disability. *Journal of the American Geriatrics Society*, 47:647–652, 1999.

MacMahon B, Pugh TF. *Epidemiology: Principles and Methods*, Boston: Little, Brown, 1970.

Meehan PJ, Saltzman LE, Sattin RW. Suicides among older United States residents: epidemiologic characteristics and trends. *American Journal of Public Health*, 81:1198–1200, 1991.

Meller I, Fichter MM, Schroppel H. Incidence of depression in octo- and nonagenerians: results of an epidemiological follow-up community study. *European Archives of Psychiatry and Clinical Neurosciences*, 246:93–99, 1996.

Meyers BS, Greenberg R. Late-life delusional depression. *Journal of Affective Disorders*, 11:133–137, 1986.

Moritz DJ, Kasl SV, Berkman LF. Cognitive functioning and the incidence of limitations in activities of daily living in an elderly community sample. *American Journal of Epidemiology*, 141:41–49, 1995.

Mortimer JA, van Duijn CM, Chandra V, et al. Head trauma as a risk factor for Alzheimer's disease: a collaborative re-analysis of case-control studies. EURODEM Risk Factors Research Group. *International Journal of Epidemiology*, 20(Suppl 2):S28–35, 1991.

Ostling S, Skoog I. Psychotic symptoms and paranoid ideation in a nondemented population-based sample of the very old. *Archives of General Psychiatry*, 59:53–59, 2002.

Parmelee PA, Katz IR, Lawton MP. Depression among institutionalized aged: assessment and prevalence estimation. *Journal of Gerontology A: Biological Sciences and Medical Sciences*, 44:M22–M29, 1989.

Patterson MB, Schnell AH, Martin RJ, et al. Assessment of behavioral and affective symptoms in Alzheimer's disease. *Journal of Geriatric Psychiatry*, 3:21–30, 1990.

Patterson TL, Semple SJ, Shaw WS, et al. Self-reported social functioning among older patients with schizophrenia. *Schizophrenia Research*, 27:199–210, 1997.

Paykel ES, Brayne C, Huppert FA, et al. Incidence of dementia in a population older than 75 years in the United Kingdom. *Archives of General Psychiatry*, 51:325–332, 1994.

Penninx BWJH, Geerlings SW, Deeg DJH, et al. Minor and major depression and the risk of death in older persons. *Archives of General Psychiatry*, 56:889–895, 1999a.

Penninx BWJH, Leveille S, Ferrucci L, et al. Exploring the effect of depression on physical disability: longitudinal evidence from the Established Populations for Epidemiologic Studies of the Elderly. *American Journal of Public Health*, 89:1346–1352, 1999b.

Radloff LS. The CES-D scale: a self-report depression scale for research in the general population. *Applied Psychological Measurement*, 1:385–401, 1977.

Regier DA, Boyd JH, Burke JD, et al. One-month prevalence of mental disorders in the United States. *Archives of General Psychiatry*, 45:977–986, 1988.

Regier DA, Myers JK, Kramer M, et al. The NIMH Epidemiologic Catchment Area Program: historical context, major objectives and study population characteristics. *Archives of General Psychiatry*, 41:934–994, 1984.

Robins LN, Helzer JE, Croughan J, et al. National Institute of Mental Health Diagnostic Interview Schedule: its history, characteristics, and validity. *Archives of General Psychiatry*, 38:381–389, 1981.

Saunders AM, Schmader K, Breitner J. Apolipoprotein E epsilon 4 allele distributions in late-onset Alzheimer's disease and in other amyloid forming disease. *Lancet*, 342:710–711, 1993.

Saunders PA, Copeland JRM, Dewey ME, et al. Heavy drinking as a risk factor for depression and dementia in elderly men: findings from the Liverpool Longitudinal Community Study. *British Journal of Psychiatry*, 159:213–216, 1991.

Saunders PA, Copeland JRM, Dewey ME, et al. Alcohol use and abuse in the elderly: findings from the Liverpool Longitudinal Study of Continuing Health in the Community. *International Journal of Geriatric Psychiatry*, 4:103–108, 1989.

Scherr PA, LaCroix AZ, Wallace RB, et al. Light to moderate alcohol consumption and mortality in the elderly. *Journal of the American Geriatric Society*, 40:651–657, 1992.

Speilberger CD, Gorsuch RL, Lushene R, et al. *Manual for the State-Trait Anxiety Inventory (Form Y)*. Palo Alto, CA: Consulting Psychologists Press, 1983.

Steffens DC, Skoog I, Norton M, et al. Prevalence of depression and its treatment in an elderly population: the Cache County Study. *Archives of General Psychiatry*, 57:601–607, 2000.

Thomas VS, Rockwood KJ. Alcohol abuse, cognitive impairment, and mortality among older people. *Journal of the American Geriatrics Society*, 49:415–420, 2001.

van Balkom AJLM, Beekman ATF, de Beurs E, et al. Comorbidity of the anxiety disorders in a community-based older population in the Netherlands. *Acta Psychiatrica Scandinavica*, 101:37–45, 2000.

Vestal RE, McGuire EA, Tobin JD, et al. Aging and ethanol metabolism. *Clinical Pharmacology and Therapeutics*, 21:343–354, 1977.

Weissman M, Bruce M, Leaf P, et al. Affective disorders. In: Robbins LN, Regier D (eds). *Psychiatric Disorders in America: The Epidemiologic Catchment Area Study*. New York: Free Press, pp. 53–80, 1991.

Williams JBW. A structured interview guide for the Hamilton Depression Rating Scale. *Archives of General Psychiatry*, 45:742–747, 1988.

World Health Organization. *Composite International Diagnostic Interview (CIDI, Version 1.0)*, Geneva: World Health Organization, 1990.

Wragg RE, Jeste DV. Overview of depression and psychosis in Alzheimer's Disease. *American Journal of Psychiatry*, 146:577–587, 1989.

Yaffe K, Blackwell, T, Gore R, et al. Depressive symptoms and cognitive decline in nondemented elderly women. *Archives of General Psychiatry*, 56:425–430, 1999.

Yassa R, Dastoor D, Nastase C, et al. The prevalence of late-onset schizophrenia in a psychogeriatric population. *Journal of Geriatric Psychiatry and Neurology*, 6:120–125, 1993.

Yesavage JA, Brink TL, Rose TL, et al. Development and validation of a geriatric depression screening scale. *Journal of Psychiatric Research*, 17:37–49, 1983.

11

Mental Health Policy and Aging

STEPHEN J. BARTELS
ARICCA R. DUMS
DENNIS G. SHEA

The number of older adults with major psychiatric illnesses will more than double over the coming three decades as the baby boomer cohort ages, increasing from an estimated 7 to 15 million individuals (Jeste et al., 1999). The needs of this rapidly growing population have been neglected in the public policy debate on how best to organize and finance mental health services. In this chapter, we provide an overview of the major issues pertaining to mental health policy and aging including the following: (*1*) the prevalence and impact of geriatric mental disorders; (*2*) service use and costs associated with mental disorders in older persons; (*3*) the mental health service delivery system for older adults; (*4*) financing geriatric mental health services; (*5*) the impact of federal regulatory initiatives; and (*6*) future policy directions and challenges.

Prevalence and Impact of Geriatric Mental Disorders

Nearly one in five adults over the age of 55 experience a mental disorder that is not characteristic of normal aging. Data on prevalence rates of mental disorders in older persons are based on the Epidemiological Catchment Area survey conducted between 1980 and 1985, though rates vary based on diagnostic criteria used to classify disorders. The most common disorders include anxiety (10.6%–11.4%), mood disorders (3.4%–4.4%), and severe cognitive impairment (2.0%–6.6%) (Narrow et al., 2002; Robins et al., 1991). However, several factors suggest that available epidemiological data underestimate the true prevalence of the problem. Mental disorders are frequently underdiagnosed owing to (*1*) misattribution of psychiatric symptoms due to cognitive disorders, medical disorders, or normal aging, (*2*) lack of age-appropriate diagnostic criteria for certain psychiatric problems, and (*3*) underreporting of symptoms by older persons due to increased prevalence of cognitive disorders and stigma associated with psychiatric illness (Jeste et al., 1999). Adjusted estimates suggest that up to one-fourth (26.3%) of older adults have a mental disorder, including 16.3% with a primary psychiatric illness, 3% with dementia complicated by significant psychiatric symptoms, and 7% with uncomplicated dementia (Jeste et al., 1999). Left untreated, late-life mental disorders are associated with impaired functioning, compromised quality of life, poor health outcomes, cognitive impairment, increased disability and mortality, and increased caregiver stress (Bartels et al., 1997c, 2000; Lenze et al., 2001; 1997a; Unützer et al., 1997; USDHHS, 1999).

Service Use and Costs Associated with Geriatric Mental Disorders

Mental disorders in older persons are associated with increased use and costs of health care. For example, depression in older primary care outpatients is associated with increased use and costs of general medical services (Druss et al., 1999; Luber et al., 2001; Unützer et al., 1997, 2000), an association that persists after controlling for physical comorbidity (Unützer et al., 1997). Depressed older adults have 38% more outpatient visits and 61% higher outpatient expenses than older adults without a depressive episode (Callahan et al., 1994). In addition, older primary care patients with alcohol use disorders are hospitalized more often and have a higher risk of death within 2 years than older adults without alcohol use problems (Callahan and Tierney, 1995). Furthermore, economic costs of caring for individuals with cognitive impairment disorders are also considerable. Over 4 million individuals currently are affected by Alzheimer's disease, and approximately 360,000 new cases are expected each year (Brookmeyer et al., 1998). Total costs are estimated to reach $100 billion annually (Alzheimer's Association, 2002). Costs of caring for individuals with Alzheimer's disease or other dementias are heightened in the presence of behavioral symptoms, leading to more hospitalizations and nursing home use (Bartels et al., 2003; O'Donnell et al., 1992) and resulting in higher costs than uncomplicated dementia (Kales et al., 1999).

The Mental Health Service Delivery System for Older Persons

The mental health service delivery system for older adults has been frequently characterized as fragmented, lacking adequate financing and trained professionals, underserving the older mentally ill population, and in need of improved implementation of appropriate and effective interventions (Cohen and Cairl, 1996; Gatz and Smyer, 1992). This system of care is particularly ill equipped to accommodate the growing service needs and preferences of consumers for community-based services outside of intensive, institution-based care settings (Bartels and Colenda, 1998; Bartels et al., 1999). The different types of providers and service delivery settings comprise a complex and often inefficient system of care that is generally poorly coordinated and difficult for consumers to navigate (AoA, 2001). The mental health system for older adults encompasses an array of service providers and service sectors including (*1*) primary care, (*2*) long-term care, (*3*) psychiatric hospitalization, (*4*) specialty outpatient mental health care, (*5*) aging network services, and (*6*) informal or family providers.

Primary Care

The majority of older adults who receive mental health care are treated by primary care physicians (Olfson and Pincus, 1996). As such, primary care providers constitute the de facto mental health system for older persons (Gray et al., 2000). Approximately 12% of older primary care patients have symptoms of depression, and 32% have a major psychiatric disorder (Lyness et al., 1999). In general, older persons are more likely to seek mental health care from their primary care provider as opposed to a mental health specialist due to stigma associated with specialty mental health services and the greater convenience and comfort associated with seeing their own physician (USDHHS, 1999). However, the many demands of primary care present substantial challenges to the delivery of mental health services. Mental disorders in primary care tend to be underdiagnosed and undertreated, and primary care providers have limited training in geriatric psychiatry (USDHHS, 1999) or in geriatrics (Zylstra and Steitz, 2000). Older adults with mental health problems in primary care settings are more at risk to receive inappropriate pharmacological treatment and are less likely to be treated with psychotherapeutic interventions compared to younger patients (Bartels et al., 1997a; Kaplan et al., 1999). Traditional educational programs alone have not shown success in changing physician behavior. However, novel approaches, including decision support systems, academic detailing (brief, one-on-one meetings with an expert addressing specific topics coupled with feedback on treatment practices), and systems change interventions with combinations of physician and patient education, care management, and improved communication and coordination between primary care and mental health care show promise in improving the care of older adults with mental illness (Callahan, 2001; Oxman and Dietrich, 2002).

Long-Term Care

If primary care comprises the current outpatient mental health service delivery system for older adults, then nursing homes have become the de facto system of institution-based mental health care. Almost 1.6 million older adults reside in nursing homes (Jones, 2002) and estimates suggest that significant psychiatric or behavioral problems (including dementia) are experienced by 65% to 91% of residents (Burns and Taube, 1990; Smyer et al., 1994; Tariot et al., 1993). The prevalence of depression among nursing home residents is as high as 22% (Burrows et al., 1995). Finally, the closure and downsizing of state mental hospitals has resulted in *transinstitutionalization* of older persons with schizophrenia and other severe mental illnesses, such that 89% of all older adults with severe mental illness in institution-based care are in nursing homes and only 11% are in hospitals (Burns and Taube, 1990).

Federal nursing home reforms initiated in 1987 required screening of potential nursing home residents to prevent the admission of persons with serious mental illness who did not meet other nursing home criteria. Although the enactment of these procedures has slowed the rate of inappropriate nursing home admissions, the prevalence of psychiatric morbidity within long-term care settings remains high (USDHHS, 1999). (The evolution and impact of these regulatory policies are discussed in more detail later in this chapter.) Despite the high prevalence, nursing homes are generally ill-equipped to serve individuals with chronic mental illness (USDHHS, 1999). Psychiatric services are needed by more than two-fifths of nursing home residents; however, half of nursing home facilities have inadequate access to psychiatric consultation services, and three-quarters are unable to access consultation and educational services for behavioral interventions (Reichman et al., 1998). Inadequate access to specialty mental health services is particularly acute in rural areas (Shea et al., 1994).

Psychiatric Hospitalization

Historically, mental health services for older persons have been substantially biased toward inpatient hospitalization (AoA, 2001). Older adults with severe mental illness are one of the last groups to experience deinstitutionalization from state psychiatric hospitals. However, the last several decades have been associated with progressive and significant decreases in psychiatric hospitalization rates for older persons. For example, the number of elderly state hospital inpatients decreased by 82% from 1972 to 1987 (APA, 1993), followed by a subsequent decrease of 33% from 1986 to 1990 (Atay et al., 1995).

Although there was substantial proliferation of general hospital or free-standing specialized geropsychiatric inpatient units in the late 1980s and early 1990s, subsequent restrictions associated with Medicare Diagnostic Related Groups (DRGs) and the emergence of managed care were associated with overall reductions in inpatient use rates. For example, overall rates of psychiatric hospitalization (including all inpatient psychiatric hospitalizations in the United States) showed a decline of approximately 25% from 1988 to 1994, whereas use of outpatient ambulatory care services increased for people over age 65 by approximately 15% over the same time period (Demmler, 1998). Despite these reforms, inpatient hospitalizations are disproportionately represented in Medicare expenditures for psychiatric services. For example, during 1999, inpatient services accounted for almost half (48%) of all Medicare mental health expenditures (HCFA, 2000a).

Specialty Outpatient Mental Health Care

Over the past decades, there has been a trend toward increased use of specialty outpatient mental health services (Demmler, 1998). Many state and national policies have promoted the use of home- and community-based services following efforts to decrease the number of institutionalized individuals (Demmler, 1998). In addition, home- and community-based services have expanded to accommodate more older adults with chronic care needs (Institute for Health and Aging, 1996). However, current specialty outpatient mental health services are lacking with respect to integrated medical and psychiatric treatment or accommodations for the unique and complex needs of older adults with mental disorders (Colenda et al., 2002). Few older adults (less than 3%) report seeing a mental health professional for treatment, a rate that is lower than that of any other adult age group (Lebowitz et al., 1997).

Aging Network Services

A variety of community-based programs supplement formal mental health services. Adult day centers provide opportunities for social interaction and recreation, and may facilitate rehabilitative and skills training and health maintenance programs for older functionally and cognitively impaired individuals (AoA, 2001). They also help alleviate caregiver burden and may delay institutionalization (USDHHS, 1999). Older adults also often use senior centers, congregate meal sites, and other community services. These settings may facilitate the delivery of community-based mental health services (AoA, 2001). For example, mental health outreach programs, such as the Gatekeeper Program, train individuals in the community (e.g., mail carriers, meter readers, law enforcement officers) to identify and refer older persons who are at risk for cognitive impairment, depression, substance abuse, and other mental health problems (Florio et al., 1998). Finally, support and peer counseling programs offer a less formal approach to accessing support, information, and a broader social network.

Informal Caregivers

Informal caregivers are often neglected in descriptions of the service delivery system for people with mental illness. However, they provide substantial direct and indirect financial and physical support. For example, most of the costs of caring for individuals with dementia are associated with informal caregiving. Costs include not only out-of-pocket expenses, but also lost wages and the cost of caregiving time (Moore et al., 2001). In addition, the burden placed on caregivers has substantial emotional and health consequences. Caregivers who experience emotional strain due to their role are more likely to develop depression (Livingston et al., 1996) and have a 63% higher risk of mortality than noncaregiving controls (Schulz and Beach, 1999).

Financing Geriatric Mental Health Services

The substantial growth in the number of older persons with mental illness represents a major and costly public health problem. This section describes the benefits and drawbacks of current financing of geriatric mental health care. Providing reimbursement for mental health treatment can serve as a major barrier to offering effective interventions.

Fee-for-Service Medicare

Medicare accounts for 38% of public expenditures and 17% of overall spending on health care among all age groups (Levit et al., 2002). Eighty-six percent of Medicare beneficiaries are over age 65, and the remaining beneficiaries are disabled persons under the age of 65 (HCFA, 2000a). Medicare provides health insurance coverage under two programs. Hospital Insurance (Part A) covers inpatient hospital care, home health and hospice care, and 60 days of skilled nursing home care. Supplemental Medical Insurance (Part B) provides reimbursement for physician and outpatient hospital services, as well as an assortment of additional medical services. Enrollment in Medicare Part B is voluntary, and members pay an additional premium. During fiscal year 1999, Medicare benefit spending amounted to almost $212 billion. Most spending was appropriated for inpatient hospital services (48%) and physician services (27%) (HCFA, 2000a). Based on 1999 figures, Medicare spends an average of $5410 per beneficiary. However, a small number of beneficiaries use a disproportionately large amount of services. For instance, over 75% of 1997 Medicare payments were spent on 15% of enrollees with average expenditures of over $10,000 each (HCFA, 2000a).

Medicare coverage has several limitations in serving individuals with mental health and long-term care needs. First, there is a lack of parity between psychiatric and medical services, and Medicare does not have a general outpatient prescription drug coverage plan. Second, the number of reimbursable inpatient psychiatric days and the coverage of essential services such as adult day care, respite care, residential care, and home health care are limited or nonexistent (AoA, 2001; Bartels and Colenda, 1998; Gottlieb, 1996). Finally, despite the well-documented impact of psychiatric disorders on health care, mental health expenditures represent a remarkably small proportion of overall Medicare expenditures. A substantial proportion of these expenditures are for acute inpatient care, leaving $718 million (0.34% of total Medicare expenditures) for outpatient mental health services (OIG, 2001c). In 1998, mental health spending amounted to $1.2 billion, representing only 0.57% of total Medicare expenditures ($211.4 billion) (CMS, 2001).

Fee-for-Service Medicaid

Medicaid provides health care services to individuals who are poor, blind, or disabled (including individuals with severe mental illness). Medicaid is the third largest source of health insurance, following employer coverage and Medicare (HCFA, 2000b). In addition to providing insurance for individuals with disabilities and long-term care for older adults, Medicaid offers supplemental coverage to low-income Medicare recipients for costs partially covered or not covered by Medicare, including outpatient prescription drugs and Medicare premiums and deductibles (HCFA, 2000b). In 1998, approximately 4 million older adults were enrolled in the Medicaid program, representing 12% of the then 32.4 million individuals over age 65 (HCFA, 2000b). Medicaid funds 46% of nursing home expenditures and is the major source of reimbursement for state-funded services for individuals with chronic mental illness. Although relatively few beneficiaries use institutional long-term care, these services represent $44 billion of the total 1998 Medicaid budget ($174 billion) (HCFA, 2000b).

Financing of Medicaid is split between the federal and state governments, with states contributing up to 50% of the cost and retaining the ability to determine eligibility criteria and designate reimbursement policies for health care services. Due to the high degree of state control, Medicaid programs differ across states, territories, and the District of Columbia. States must cover mandatory services but have substantial variability in their decision to provide optional services. As an example, while most Medicaid programs offer prescription drug coverage, many have limitations that affect copayment costs and the number of refills. Some states also require prior authorization for mental health services and restrict the number of visits to providers.

A subset of individuals is eligible for both Medicare and Medicaid funding based primarily on age, financial need, and/or the presence of a debilitating disorder. Approximately 6.4 million beneficiaries are dually eligible, representing 16.5% of the Medicare population and 19% of the total Medicaid population (HCFA, 2000a, 2000b). However, despite accounting for less than one-fifth of the total Medicaid population, this group of dually eligible individuals often requires intensive services and accounts for over one-third of Medicaid expenditures (HCFA, 2000b). Because many dually eligible beneficiaries, by definition, are both over age 65 and have significant disabilities, older persons with SMI are overrepresented in this group.

Managed Medicare

While most Medicare recipients use traditional fee-for-service programs (Parts A and B), increasing Medicare expenditures and cost-containment strategies have led many older adults to enroll in managed Medicare + Choice. The 1990s were marked by an initial growth phase in managed Medicare. In 1993, 1.53 million Medicare beneficiaries were enrolled in managed care plans. Enrollment increased by 30%–40% per year and peaked in 1999, with over 16% or 6.35 million beneficiaries. However, following the introduction of the Balanced Budget Act of 1997, changes in Medicare reimbursement policy and incentives have been associated with a subsequent abandonment of the managed Medicare market by many carriers. By August 2001, withdrawal from the market left only 14% of Medicare beneficiaries enrolled in Medicare + Choice. Projections suggest that 500,000 beneficiaries will be dropped in 2002, leading to a 4-year decline of 2.2 million beneficiaries. These data suggest that managed care is likely to be less of a crucial health policy issue for Medicare than was initially predicted (Berenson, 2001; Gold, 2001).

Managed care has the potential to deliver comprehensive and effective preventive, acute, and chronic care services. However, the managed care system has shown limited ability to care for individuals who require chronic care and intensive services, including mentally impaired or frail elderly individuals (Miller and Luft, 1997). Conventional managed care programs are unlikely to meet the needs of older persons with severe mental illness. Within health maintenance organizations (HMOs), geriatric programs are often inadequate and poorly implemented (Kane et al., 1997; Pacala et al., 1995). There is often minimal use of specialty mental health providers and inadequate pharmacological management within primary care settings (Bartels et al., 1997a). It is unlikely that HMOs can provide the array of community, residential, and rehabilitative services that older adults with mental illness need.

Long-Term Care Financing: Social Health Maintenance Organizations, the Program for All-Inclusive Care of the Elderly, and State Medicaid Waiver Programs

A variety of innovative approaches to organizing and financing services are being developed that limit nursing home expenditures and respond to consumer preferences (Kane, 1998). These home- and community-based initiatives were developed to create alternatives to institutional care. Social health maintenance organizations and the Program for All-Inclusive Care of the Elderly offer integrated acute and long-term care under a single system financed through pooled funding sources (HCFA, 2000b; Kane et al., 1997). In addition, Medicaid waiver programs provide federal funding to develop programmatic initiatives and develop and test novel benefit design and service delivery models (HCFA, 2000b). Many aspects of these programs could be used to help meet the future long-term care needs of older persons with mental illness; however, they currently offer limited mental health coverage (Eng et al., 1997; Kane et al., 1997).

Regulatory Policies and Their Impact on Services

The health care system for older adults with mental illness is largely regulated by federal legislative policies and regulatory initiatives. From the early 1960s to the present, these policies have helped to define appropriate care and medical necessity and to ensure consumer protection.

The 1963 Community Mental Health Centers Act was the first in a series of legislative decisions that attempted to decrease unnecessary institutionalization of individuals with mental illness and to promote community-based care. However, while many individuals with mental illness were effectively shifted from psychiatric institutions to community-based care, older adults were among the last group to participate in this movement. Furthermore, as previously noted, many older patients were not transferred to the community but instead were transinstitutionalized to nursing homes (Burns and Taube, 1990).

At roughly the same time, the Older American's Act (OAA) of 1965 was developed to maintain independent functioning of older adults. The OAA services are targeted at older adults who are at risk of losing their independence due to social and economic needs, as well as individuals with low incomes or minority status (Takamura, 1999). Many home- and community-based services and programs that offer supportive assistance, congregate and home-based nutritional services (meals on wheels), transportation, long-term care ombudsmen, and informational programs on aging are sponsored by the OAA (Takamura, 1999).

The next major legislation to directly impact older adults occurred almost 20 years later. Federal nursing home reforms were instituted under the Omnibus Budget Reconciliation Acts (OBRA) of 1987 and 1989. The OBRA Act of 1987 mandated the use of Preadmission Screening and Resident Review (PASRR) to identify and prevent potential admissions of persons with serious mental illness who did not otherwise meet nursing home criteria. The PASRR procedure was also designed to improve the quality of mental health assessments and care for nursing home residents (USDHHS, 1999). However, while PASRR may have slowed the rate of inappropriate nursing home admissions and reduced the inappropriate use of restraints and overuse of psychotropic medications, its enactment had limited effectiveness in improving quality of care (USDHHS, 1999).

The OBRA Acts of 1987 and 1989 also liberalized Medicare reimbursement for mental health services. The OBRA Act of 1987 raised the reimbursement cap on mental health services from $250 to $1100, set reimbursement for 2 days of partial hospitalization equal to 1 day of inpatient care, and reduced copayments for psychotropic prescription drugs to 20%, aligning it with copayment rates for other prescription coverage. The OBRA Act of 1989 eliminated the cap on outpatient mental health services, gave provider status to psychologists and social workers, and provided full reimbursement for partial hospitalization (Bartels and Colenda, 1998).

Although this health policy was apparently designed to increase access to mental health care by removing caps and expanding the range of eligible providers, subsequent increases in expenditures were met with federal scrutiny and assumptions of fraudulent billing practices. The modest increases in mental health service provision and reimbursement were met by a series of investigations by the Office of the Inspector General (OIG) to identify medically inappropriate services.

The first of these studies, released in 1996, found one-third (32%) of mental health services in nursing homes to be "medically unnecessary," representing $17 million (24%) of all 1993 Medicare payments for mental health services for nursing home residents (OIG, 1996). Unnecessary and questionable services included 62% of mental health services for older (85+) patients, 58% of mental health services for dementia patients, 80% of psychological testing, 75% of group therapy, and 47% of evaluation and individual therapy (OIG, 1996).

A 2001 follow-up study determined that 27% of mental health services in nursing homes are medically unnecessary (OIG, 2001a). Remarkably, the 2001 report specifically cited psychiatric services for individuals with dementia complicated by behavioral and psychiatric symptoms as medically unnecessary. "More than half of all unnecessary services are provided to individuals who have limited cognitive ability and therefore may not benefit from the psychiatric intervention. Services are given to patients with, for example, advanced dementia, severe agitation, delusions, and paranoia" (OIG, 2001a, p. 7). These findings appear to conflict with research supporting the effectiveness of geriatric mental health interventions for psychiatric symptoms in dementia (Doody et al., 2001) and documentation of dramatic unmet need in nursing homes. For example, a recent survey found that 38% of nursing home residents were in need of psychiatric evaluation, but only half of these residents received it (Reichman et al., 1998). Other studies based on Medicare expenditure survey data conclude that one-half of nursing homes experience difficulty obtaining psychiatric services and only one-fifth of nursing home residents with identified psychiatric disorders see a mental health specialist for treatment (Shea et al., 1994; Smyer et al., 1994).

Considerable attention has also focused on inappropriate use of chemical and physical restraints for patients of hospitals and nursing homes. Reforms under OBRA 1987, policies aimed at reducing and reviewing use of antipsychotic medications, and advocacy for *restraint-free* environments in nursing homes have resulted in substantial reductions (Snowden and Roy-Byrne, 1998). For example, rates of physical restraint use were as high as 25% to 85% prior to implementation of OBRA but more recently were reported to be used for 25% to 59% of residents (Snowden and Roy-Byrne, 1998). Similarly, rates of treatment with antipsychotic medications in nursing homes were as high as 34% prior to 1990, yet more recent reviews of antipsychotic medication prescriptions in nursing homes report rates of 16% (Kidder and Kalachnik, 1999). Of note, a recent study by the OIG found little or no evidence that psychotropic drugs were being used inappropriately as chemical restraints in nursing homes (OIG, 2001b).

A ruling by the Supreme Court in June 1999 also defines federal policy regarding appropriate care and consumer protections with a specific focus on addressing unnecessary or inappropriate institutional placement of individuals with disabilities. In the *Olmstead v. L.C.* decision, the Court ruled that maintaining persons with disabilities in restrictive institution-based facilities when they were capable of benefiting from living in a community-based setting was in violation of Title II of the Americans with Disabilities Act (ADA) (Williams, 2000). The ADA prohibits discrimination in the provision of state and local government programs, services, and benefits (Herbert and Young, 1999). To comply with the *Olmstead* ruling, states must evaluate thousands of individuals residing in psychiatric institutions and nursing homes to determine whether they could be receiving care in a less restrictive community-based setting (NCCBH, 2000a). States must also revamp their mental health systems, develop plans to end unnecessary institutionalization, and find new resources to provide opportunities for community living (NCCBH, 2000a).

Future Challenges in Mental Health Policy and Aging

Policy and legislative initiatives enacted over the past three decades have enhanced the quality of care and defined the current financing and delivery system for older adults with mental illness. However, several areas warrant attention. For example, major issues for policy makers include resolving the debate over mental health parity and prescription drug coverage; addressing the need for integrated financing and delivery of mental health and medical care; defining the role of psychiatric services in the treatment of the growing population with Alzheimer's disease; and addressing the treatment needs of a growing number of aging persons with severe mental illness.

Mental Health Parity

In 1996, a limited version of federal mental health parity legislation (Public Law 104-204, the Mental Health Parity Act of 1996) was passed by the U.S. Congress that prohibits insurers serving more than 50 employees from setting lower annual or lifetime dollar caps on mental health benefits than for other health benefits. This legislation recognized mental health care as a component of comprehensive care; however, it did not address limits on the number of mental health visits, co-payments, or deductibles (NCCBH, 2000b). It provided a federal floor for private health plans; states are permitted to enact stronger standards, although another federal law (the Employee Retirement Income Security Act) limits their scope. Despite considerable debate and controversy, experience to date with implementation of mental health parity has found minimal impact on costs, access, or quality of mental health care. Parity laws have raised federal and state health care costs less than 5% (Greenwald, 2000) and have required minimal costs when care is implemented within an existing managed care network (Hennessy and Goldman, 2001; Marwick, 1998; NCCBH, 2000b; Sturm, 1997). Other studies suggest that instituting equal coverage of mental health treatment can even result in decreased total health care costs (Goldman et al., 1998, 1999; Ma and McGuire, 1998). However, the overall impact of the 1996 federal legislation has been modest. Under this reform, parity has had limited impact on consumer access to mental health services (Pacula and Sturm, 2000; Sturm and Pacula, 1999, 2000), and many beneficiaries have seen minimal changes to their health benefits (NCCBH, 2000b). Many employers bypass restrictions on dollar limits by restricting the number of outpatient and hospital visits. In addition, many employers do not fully equalize medical and psychiatric benefits, set annual or lifetime dollar limits on employees' mental health care that are lower than the limits for general medical services, or lower limits on general medical care to align them with existing mental health coverage (Shea, 2002).

The 1996 Mental Health Parity Act was due to expire on December 31, 2001. The federal legislative debate began in March of that year with the introduction of the Mental Health Equitable Treatment Act of 2001 (Senate bill 543). This bill expands the Mental Health Parity Act of 1996 to prohibit a group health plan from treating mental health benefits differently from the coverage of medical and surgical benefits. This bill only applies to group health plans already providing mental health benefits and is modeled on the mental health benefits provided through the Federal Employees Health Benefit Program (which implemented full parity benefits to its 8.7 million beneficiaries as of January 1, 2001). Consideration by the full Senate was slowed by the events of September 11, but the bill passed with only minor changes in October and proceeded to a conference committee, where it was defeated. The committee voted immediately to extend the 1996 Mental Health Parity Act for 1 year.

In 2002, the goal of mental health parity seemed closer than ever. In March, a new House bill, H.R. 4066 (the Mental Health Equitable Treatment Act), almost identical to Senate bill 543, was introduced. As of mid–August, 2002, a majority of both houses of Congress were formal cosponsors of parity legislation. This is the first time that a majority of the House has cosponsored a mental health parity bill. Several bills were also introduced in both the House of Representatives and the Senate in 2001 seeking to achieve parity and modernization of the Medicare mental health benefit. To date, the fate of these bills and the potential for broad-based mental health parity legislation remain uncertain.

Meanwhile, at the state level, as of the summer of 2002, 35 states had enacted parity laws with varying approaches to prohibit discrimination in insurance and managed care coverage of mental disorders. Key differences among these laws related to which illnesses are covered by the legislation and what benefits must be provided at parity with other medical illnesses. During 2002, more than 80 bills were considered in 28 states. However, not all the policy developments are favorable. Rising prescription drug costs, among other factors, resulted in a failure to achieve a prescription drug benefit for Medicare beneficiaries. In addition, while nearly half of the states introduced or expanded pharmaceutical assistance programs for various groups in the population, 35 states increased restrictions on access to prescription drugs (National Conference of State Legislatures, 2002a, 2002b) (for additional discussion of parity, see Chapters 1, 2, 3, and 13).

Prescription Drug Coverage

Pharmaceuticals are among the most rapidly growing costs in health care. For example, mean total drug spending for the elderly rose from $827 in 1997 to $1378 in 2000, an 18.5% annual increase, compared with 2.3% average annual general inflation during this period (Thomas et al., 2001). Despite the growing costs of pharmaceuticals for older adults, Medicare coverage does not include a prescription drug benefit. Less than half of all Medicare beneficiaries are able to afford additional full-year insurance coverage to offset the expense of medications (Stuart et al., 2001), and one-third are unable to afford any coverage for medications (HCFA, 2000a). Many Medicare beneficiaries supplement Medicare benefits with additional insurance, such as Medigap, retiree coverage, and Medicaid. However, a substantial number of Medicare beneficiaries (14%) do not have supplemental coverage (HCFA, 2000a). Medicare recipients who have a mental illness often rely on Medicaid policies to cover the cost of medication prescriptions (Shea, 2002). Yet, sources of prescription drug coverage for older adults with mental illness are limited, and coverage varies over time and across providers (Shea, 2002). For instance, Medicaid finances over 85% of total prescription costs, while Medigap funding covers only a third of prescription costs. Thus, older adults who are eligible for both Medicaid and Medicare have lower out-of-pocket prescription costs. With increasing costs of prescription drugs and reductions in managed Medicare coverage (as well as increasing copayments, additional premiums, and no cap on out-of-pocket expenses), national changes in prescription drug coverage for Medicare beneficiaries are necessary to ensure that older adults with mental illness and dementia are able to access essential medications (Shea, 2002). The debate over prescription drug coverage for Medicare beneficiaries represents a crucial aspect of improving mental health care. Without comprehensive prescription drug coverage, many older adults with mental illness may compromise quality of care by avoiding or stopping drug therapy due to excessive costs.

Integrated Care

Underdiagnosis of mental health problems is common in primary care (Higgins, 1994; Wells et al., 1989); conversely, physical illnesses are often undetected in patients with psychiatric disorders (Koranyi, 1979). Integration of medical and mental health treatment has been proposed as an effective and efficient approach to addressing the gap between psychiatric and general health care (Cummings, 1997). Cost-offset studies in adult populations have identified decreased medical use following mental health treatment (Holder and Blose, 1987; Katzelnick et al., 1997), with the greatest effect associated with inpatient services (Mumford et al., 1984; Strain et al., 1991). Reduction of expensive hospitalizations produces more cost savings than a reduction in the use of less expensive outpatient services. Although this finding is encouraging, it is important to note that research on cost offsets has not consistently demonstrated an association between reduced general medical use and the provision of integrated mental health services in primary care (Simon et al., 1995a, 1995b).

Nonetheless, the jury is out on the effectiveness and costs associated with integrated mental health and medical care for older adults in primary care settings. Several ongoing studies are systematically evaluating mental health intervention models for older persons in primary care settings, including the Prevention of Suicide in Primary Care Elderly Collaborative Trial (PROSPECT) (Coyne et al., 2001), the study on Improving Primary Care for Depression in Late Life (IMPACT) (Unützer et al., 2001), and the Primary Care Research in Substance Abuse and Mental Health for elderly (PRISMe) study (Bartels et al., 2002a). The PROSPECT and IMPACT studies evaluate a manualized pharmacological and psychotherapeutic intervention in primary care compared to usual care, and the PRISMe study compares the effectiveness of an integrated mental health provider and an enhanced referral model. These studies will provide information on recognition and treatment of mental disorders in older primary care patients, allow us to "triangulate" on the effects of usual care versus collaborative care versus specialty referral, and will provide an evidence base for the design of care systems and health policy.

Integrated financing of care has been examined extensively in debates on carved-in and carved-out managed care. Essentially, carved-in care directly integrates medical and mental health care, whereas carved-out care is based on a contractual agreement with a separate specialty mental health care organization. Carved-in organizations are designed to provide more integrated care, increase communication between providers, reduce stigma and medical expenditures, and help avoid misattributions of the origins of medical or psychiatric problems (Mechanic, 1997;

Mollica and Riley, 1996). However, mental health specialty services are often a low priority (Bartels et al., 1997a), and integration of services is not guaranteed. General care providers are often unprepared to provide the array of services needed by older adults with mental illness (Mechanic, 1997). Finally, economic complications include differing mental health care coverage by different providers (Frank et al., 1995), incentives to avoid patients with high service use and costs, and difficulties in adjusting for increased financial risk in payment rates (Frank et al., 1997).

On the other hand, mental health carve-out organizations can provide high-quality specialized mental health treatment. They offer comprehensive services from specialty providers that are committed to serving high-risk populations (Riley et al., 1997). Savings associated with decreased inpatient service use are often reinvested in developing and improving treatments. However, carve-out arrangements may result in misattributions of responsibility and increased fragmentation of medical and mental health care, which tend to increase the risks of misdiagnosis, poor health outcomes, and medication interactions. Fragmented reimbursement sources also complicate the provision of appropriate treatment and the identification of cost-offset effects.

Alzheimer's Disease: Is It a Mental Health Problem?

Alzheimer's disease is a degenerative neuropsychiatric illness that impairs cognitive and functional abilities and has a high comorbidity with psychiatric syndromes (Bartels and Colenda, 1998; Chung and Cummings, 2000). However, advocates and policy makers differ in their beliefs as to whether dementia is a psychiatric or a medical disorder. Advocacy groups wish to avoid the stigma and inferior coverage associated with psychiatric disorders relative to neurological diseases. Meanwhile, policy makers are reluctant to classify dementia as a serious mental illness, as the growing population with dementia is likely to overwhelm funding that is currently set aside for other mental disorders (Cohen and Cairl, 1996). The current classification of Alzheimer's disease as a neurological disorder has improved reimbursement and access to medical treatments. However, it leaves individuals with dementia ineligible for many state-funded services and has resulted in increased federal scrutiny of psychosocial and community support services (Bartels and Colenda, 1998).

Although effective interventions are being developed for dementia (Doody et al., 2001), there are substantial barriers to the provision of adequate mental health services. Dementia with psychiatric and behavioral symptoms is a complex disorder, and quality of care varies widely. Older adults with dementia are more often prescribed anticholinergic agents and more than one drug from the same therapeutic class than cognitively intact individuals (Giron et al., 2001). There is a lack of consensus on the role of mental health services in the treatment of dementia, and it is difficult to determine which services and settings should be reimbursed. However, mental health services must be made available to individuals with dementia complicated by psychiatric symptoms.

Aging Persons with Schizophrenia and Other Severe Mental Illnesses

Older adults with severe mental illness (including schizophrenia, bipolar disorder, and treatment-refractory depression) require intensive institution-based care and are high utilizers of other health care services (Bartels and Miles, 1997b; Mulsant et al., 1993; Semke and Jensen, 1997). However, to date they have received little attention with regard to treatment or policy initiatives. Two-thirds of older adults with severe mental illness (SMI) experience at least one hospitalization or nursing home admission annually, and they are three times more likely to be admitted to a nursing home than older individuals without SMI (Bartels et al., 2000). The high rate of medical co-morbidity among older adults with severe mental illness is associated with worse health status, more severe psychiatric symptoms, and increased morbidity and mortality (Dixon et al., 1999; Jeste et al., 1996). In addition, older adults with SMI are at substantial risk of receiving inadequate or inappropriate health care (Druss et al., 2001).

Mental health policy will need to respond to the demands of an increasingly vocal contingent who view old age as a period in life with new opportunities and activities. To date, psychosocial rehabilitation services for persons with SMI have focused on younger persons, while services for older persons have been marginalized and aimed at providing long-term care (Pratt et al., under review). Skills training and psychotherapeutic interventions such as cognitive-behavioral therapy hold promise for improving symptoms and functioning in older persons with SMI (Granholm et al., 2002). Evidence-based practices for people with SMI, such as vocational rehabilitation and assertive case management, have established benefits for younger persons (Torrey et al., 2001) and should be considered within the range of supported services for older persons with SMI. This paradigm shift toward including rehabilitation within the array of services for older persons will challenge conventional assumptions but may potentially decrease reliance on costly institution-based services.

Bridging the Gap Between Research, Practice and Policy: Evidence-Based Medicine

The need to bridge the gap between research findings on effective treatments and clinical services delivered by health care providers has been highlighted as one of the most important priorities in contemporary health care. The recent Institute of Medicine report *Crossing the Quality Chasm* (Institute of Medicine, 2001) and the National Institute of Mental Health report *Bridging Science and Service* (NIMH, 1999) underscore the gap between the empirical evidence base on treatment effectiveness and health care received by the public. Modern medicine is rallying to address this problem in health care quality by promoting the use of treatments that are clearly supported by systematic evaluations of the research literature under the banner of *evidence-based medicine* (Friedland et al., 1998; Guyatt and Rennie, 2002; Sackett et al., 1996).

Evidence-based medicine follows the principles initially proposed by Cochrane in 1972 suggesting that limited health care resources should be allocated to pro-

viding treatments that have been proven to be effective through rigorously designed evaluation trials, with an emphasis on randomized, controlled trials (The
Cochrane Collaboration, 2002). Although mental health has lagged behind medicine in adopting these principles, research advances in the field of geriatric
psychiatry over the past two decades have begun to define a substantial set of
evidence-based practices (EBPs) with known effectiveness in the treatment of mental disorders in older persons (Bartels et al., 2002b, 2002c, in press). Continued
efforts to establish geriatric mental health EBPs should be a major priority over
the coming decade in order to support informed policy decisions. For example,
definitions of reimbursable services considered to be medically necessary and the
selection of medications covered under Medicaid and private insurance pharmacy
formularies are increasingly being held to these standards of scientific evidence.

Bridging the gap between what we know and what we do in clinical practice will
also require developing effective approaches to knowledge dissemination and actual change in clinical practice. Conventional educational approaches such as continuing medical education conferences and dissemination of guidelines have been
shown to be ineffective in improving the quality of care or actual clinical practice
by providers (Bartels et al., 2002b; Callahan, 2001). Thus, an organized quality
improvement strategy is needed that provides incentives and creates structures that
encourage the systematic implementation and use of treatments with proven effectiveness (Bartels et al., 2002b). An additional challenge involves the translation
of research findings into mental health policy that will affect the organization and
financing of mental health services for older adults. Currently, an information barrier hinders the extrapolation of research findings to policy (Feldman et al., 2001).
Finally, meeting the future needs of a growing aging population will require closing the gap between physical health care and mental health care in order to produce integrated, cost-effective services.

Implications for Mental Health Services

Older adults with mental illness represent a major health policy challenge for the
coming decades due to their burgeoning population growth and age-associated
needs for specialized services and financing. Mental disorders in older persons are
associated with increased use and costs of general health care. Substantial unmet
need persists for mental health services in long-term care institutions, such as nursing homes and assisted living facilities, and in community-based settings. Among
those receiving mental health services, treatment is provided in a fragmented service delivery system consisting of a patchwork of primary care, long-term care, psychiatric hospitals, specialty outpatient mental health clinics, aging network service providers, and assistance from informal caregivers.

The current infrastructure and financing support services for older adults with
mental illness are a result of over 40 years of federal programs and regulations that
have shaped today's system of care. Financing for mental health services largely
consists of fee-for-service Medicare and Medicaid in the absence of a pharmacy
benefit under Medicare and without broad-based parity for mental health. Fed-

eral definitions of appropriate care and medical necessity have evolved from a series of legislative initiatives including the Community Mental Health Center Act,
the OAA, federal nursing home legislation (i.e., OBRA), financing regulations under the Center for Medicare and Medicaid (formerly HCFA), national Medicare
audits and OIG investigations, and the recent *Olmstead* decision interpreting the
implications of the ADA in long-term care.

Key policy challenges and controversies need to be addressed to avert a potential health care crisis associated with the growing number of older persons with
mental disorders. Mental health parity and prescription drug benefits are likely to
significantly improve access to appropriate care of older adults; however, the financing and structure of such programs remain unresolved. As previously mentioned, meeting the future needs of a growing aging population will also require
closing the gap between physical health care and mental health care to produce integrated, and cost-effective services. Though the potential merits of integrated services are widely recognized, there are an array of options for functional and fiscal integration of services and a daunting number of provider groups, settings, needs,
and sources of financing to be considered. Several special populations requiring intensive, high-cost services are likely to present unique challenges for future services. Alzheimer's disease and an aging population of adults with severe, persistent
mental illness have intensive treatment and long-term care needs that will only increase as a proportion of the public sector health care budget. Finally, achieving efficient and effective services for older persons with mental disorders will require
closing the growing gap between research findings and services actually provided
in the community. Systematic efforts to disseminate, implement, and sustain EBPs
hold particular promise for further improving the mental health care of older adults.

REFERENCES

Administration on Aging. *Older Adults and Mental Health: Issues and Opportunities.*
    Rockville, MD: Administration on Aging, Department of Health and Human Services,
    2001.
Alzheimer's Association: *Statistics About Alzheimer's Disease.* Available: http://www.alz.
    org/AboutAD/Statistics.htm Accessed August 21, 2002.
American Psychiatric Association. *State Mental Hospitals and the Elderly: A Task Force Re-
    port of the American Psychiatric Association.* Task Force on Geriatric Psychiatry in the
    Public Health Sector, Washington, DC, 1993.
Atay JE, Witkin MJ, Manderscheid RW. Data highlights on utilization of mental health or-
    ganizations by elderly persons. *Mental Health Statistical Note,* 214:1–7, 1995.
Bartels SJ, Coakley E, Oxman TE, et al. Suicidal and death ideation in older primary care
    patients with depression, anxiety and at-risk alcohol use. *American Journal of Geriatric
    Psychiatry,* 10(4):417–427, 2002a.
Bartels SJ, Colenda CC. Mental health services for Alzheimer's disease. Current trends in
    reimbursement and public policy, and the future under managed care. *American Jour-
    nal of Geriatric Psychiatry,* 6(2 Suppl 1):S85–100, 1998.
Bartels SJ, Dums AR, Oxman TE, et al. Evidence-based practices in geriatric mental health
    care. *Psychiatric Services,* 53(11):1419–1431, 2002b.

Bartels SJ, Dums AR, Oxman TE, et al. The practice of evidence-based geriatric psychiatry. In: Grossberg GT, Sadavoy J, Jarvik LF, et al (eds). *The Comprehensive Review of Geriatric Psychiatry,* 3rd ed. Washington, DC: American Psychiatric Association, in press.

Bartels SJ, Forester B, Miles KM, et al. Mental health service use by elderly patients with bipolar disorder and unipolar major depression. *American Journal of Geriatric Psychiatry,* 8(2):160–166, 2000.

Bartels SJ, Haley WJ, Dums AR. Implementing evidence-based practices in geriatric mental health. *Generations,* 26(1):90–98, 2002c.

Bartels SJ, Horn S, Sharkey P, et al. Treatment of depression in older primary care patients in health maintenance organizations. *International Journal of Psychiatry in Medicine,* 27(3):215–231, 1997a.

Bartels SJ, Horn SD, Smout RJ, et al. Agitation and depression in frail nursing home elderly with dementia: treatment characteristics and service use. *American Journal of Geriatric Psychiatry,* 11(2):231–238, 2003.

Bartels SJ, Levine KJ, Mueser KT. A biopsychosocial approach to treatment of schizophrenia in late life. In Duffy M (ed): *Handbook of Counseling and Psychotherapy with Older Adults.* New York: Wiley, pp. 436–452, 1999.

Bartels SJ, Miles KM. Level of care and mental health service needs of elderly with serious mental illness. Paper presented at the Seventh Annual National Conference on State Mental Health Agency Services Research and Program Evaluation, Arlington, VA, February 1997b.

Bartels SJ, Mueser KT, Miles KM. Functional impairments in elderly patients with schizophrenia and major affective illness in the community: social skills, living skills, and behavior problems. *Behavior Therapy,* 28:43–63, 1997c.

Berenson R. Medicare + Choice: doubling or disappearing. *Health Affairs, Web Exclusive: Nov 28,* W65–W82, 2001.

Brookmeyer R, Gray S, Kawas C. Projections of Alzheimer's disease in the United States and the public health impact of delaying disease onset. *American Journal of Public Health,* 88(9):1337–1342, 1998.

Burns BJ, Taube CA. Mental health services in general medical care and nursing homes. In: Fogel B, Furino A, Gottlieb G (eds). *Mental Health Policy for Older Americans: Protecting Minds at Risk.* Washington, DC: American Psychiatric Press, pp. 63–84, 1990.

Burrows AB, Satlin A, Salzman C, et al. Depression in a long-term care facility: clinical features and discordance between nursing assessment and patient interviews. *Journal of the American Geriatrics Society,* 43:1118–1122, 1995.

Callahan CM. Quality improvement research on late life depression in primary care. *Medical Care,* 39(8), 772–784, 2001.

Callahan CM, Hui SL, Nienaber NA, et al. Longitudinal study of depression and health services use among elderly primary care patients. *Journal of the American Geriatrics Society,* 42:833–838, 1994.

Callahan CM, Tierney WM. Health services use and mortality among older primary care patients with alcoholism. *Journal of the American Geriatrics Society,* 43(12):1378–1383, 1995.

Chung JA, Cummings JL. Neurobehavioral and neuropsychiatric symptoms in Alzheimer's disease: characteristics and treatment. *Neurologic Clinics,* 18(4):829–846, 2000.

Center for Medicare and Medicaid Services (CMS). *National Health Care Expenditures Projections: 2000–2010. Table 3:* Center for Medicare and Medicaid Services. Available at: http://www.hcfa.gov/stats/NHE-proj/proj2000/proj2000.pdf 2001. Accessed January 7, 2002.

Cochrane AL. *Effectiveness and Efficiency. Random Reflections on Health Services.* London: Nuffield Provincial Hospital Trust (Reprinted in 1989 is association with the BMJ, reprinted in 1999 for Nuffield Trust by the Royal Society of Medicine Press, London).

Cohen D, Cairl R. Mental health care policy in an aging society. In: Levin BL, Petrila J (eds). *Mental Health Services: A Public Perspective.* New York: Oxford University Press, pp. 301–319, 1996.

Colenda CC, Bartels SJ, Gottlieb GL. The North American system of care. In: Copeland J, Abou-Saleh M, Blazer D (eds). *Principles and Practice of Geriatric Psychiatry*, 2nd ed. London: Wiley, pp. 689–696, 2002.

Coyne JC, Brown G, Datto C, et al. The benefits of a broader perspective in case-finding for disease management of depression: early lessons from the PROSPECT Study. *International Journal of Geriatric Psychiatry*, 16(6):570–576, 2001.

Cummings NA. Behavioral health in primary care: dollars and sense. In: Cummings NA, Cummings JL, Johnson JN (eds). *Behavioral Health in Primary Care: A Guide for Clinical Integration.* Madison, WI: Psychosocial Press, pp. 3–21, 1997.

Demmler J. *Utilization of Specialty Mental Health Services by Older Adults: National and State Profiles.* Alexandria, VA: National Technical Assistance Center for State Mental Health Planning, 1998.

Dixon L, Postrado L, Delahanty J, et al. The association of medical comorbidity in schizophrenia with poor physical and mental health. *Journal of Nervous and Mental Disease*, 187(8):496–502, 1999.

Doody RS, Stevens JC, Beck C, et al. Practice parameter: management of dementia (an evidence-based review): report of the Quality Standards Subcommittee of the American Academy of Neurology. *Neurology*, 56(9):1154–1166, 2001.

Druss BG, Bradford WD, Rosenheck RA, et al. Quality of medical care and excess mortality in older patients with mental disorders. *Archives of General Psychiatry*, 58(6):565–572, 2001.

Druss BG, Rohrbaugh RM, Rosenheck RA. Depressive symptoms and health costs in older medical patients. *American Journal of Psychiatry*, 156:477–479, 1999.

Eng C, Pedulla J, Eleazer GP, et al. Program of all-inclusive care for the elderly (PACE): an innovative model of integrated geriatric care and financing. *Journal of the American Geriatrics Society*, 45(2):223–232, 1997.

Feldman PH, Nadash P, Gursen M. Improving communication between researchers and policy makers in long-term care: or, researchers are from Mars; policy makers are from Venus. *The Gerontologist*, 41(3):312–321, 2001.

Florio ER, Jensen JE, Hendryx M, et al. One-year outcomes of older adults referred for aging and mental health services by community gatekeepers. *Journal of Case Management*, 7(2):74–83, 1998.

Frank R, McGuire T, Bae J, et al. Solutions for adverse selection in behavioral health care. *Health Care Financing Review*, 18(3):109–122, 1997.

Frank R, McGuire T, Newhouse J. Risk contracts in managed mental health care. *Health Affairs*, 14(3):50–64, 1995.

Friedland DJ, Go AS, Davoren JB, et al. *Evidence-Based Medicine: A Framework for Clinical Practice.* Stamford, CT: Appleton and Lange, 1998.

Gatz M, Smyer MA. The mental health system and older adults in the 1990s. *American Psychologist*, 47(6):741–751, 1992.

Giron MS, Wang HX, Bernsten C, et al. The appropriateness of drug use in an older nondemented and demented population. *Journal of the American Geriatrics Society*, 49(3):277–283, 2001.

Gold M. Medicare + Choice: an interim report card. *Health Affairs*, 20(4):120–138, 2001.

Goldman W, McCulloch J, Cuffel B, et al. More evidence for the insurability of managed behavioral health care. *Health Affairs*, 18(5):172–181, 1999.

Goldman W, McCulloch J, Sturm R. Costs and use of mental health services before and after managed care. *Health Affairs*, 17(2):40–52, 1998.

Gottlieb GL. Financial issues. In: Sadavoy J, Lazarus LW, Jarvik LF (eds). *Comprehensive Review of Geriatric Psychiatry*, 2nd ed. Washington, DC: American Psychiatric Press, pp. 1065–1089, 1996.

Granholm E, McQuaid JR, McClure FS, et al. A randomized controlled pilot study of cognitive behavioral social skills training for older patients with schizophrenia. *Schizophrenia Research*, 53(1–2):167–169, 2002.

Gray GV, Brody DS, Hart MT. Primary care and the de facto mental health care system: improving care where it counts. *Managed Care Interface*, 13(3):62–65, 2000.

Greenwald J. Mental health parity not as costly as feared. *Business Insurance*, 34(31):16–17, 2000.

Guyatt G, Rennie D. *Users' Guides to the Medical Literature: A Manual for Evidence-Based Clinical Practice / the Evidence-Based Medicine Working Group*. Chicago: AMA Press, 2002.

Health Care Financing Administration. *Medicare 2000: 35 Years of Improving Americans' Health and Security*. Washington, DC: Health Care Financing Administration, Department of Health and Human Services, 2000a.

Health Care Financing Administration. *A Profile of Medicaid: Chartbook 2000*. Washington, DC: Health Care Financing Administration, Department of Health and Human Service, 2000b.

Hennessy KD, Goldman HH. Full parity: steps toward treatment equity for mental and addictive disorders. *Health Affairs*, 20(4):58–68, 2001.

Herbert PB, Young KA. The Americans with Disabilities Act and deinstitutionalization of the chronically mentally ill. *Journal of the American Academy of Psychiatry and the Law*, 27(4):603–613, 1999.

Higgins ES. A review of unrecognized mental illness in primary care. Prevalence, natural history, and efforts to change the course. *Archives of Family Medicine*, 3(10):908–917, 1994.

Holder HD, Blose JO. Changes in health-care costs and utilization associated with mental-health treatment. *Hospital and Community Psychiatry*, 38(10):1070–1075, 1987.

Institute for Health and Aging. *Chronic Care in America: A 21st Century Challenge*. Princeton, NJ: Robert Wood Johnson Foundation, 1996.

Institute of Medicine. *Crossing the Quality Chasm: A New Health System for the 21st Century*. Washington, DC: Institute of Medicine, 2001.

Jeste DV, Alexopoulos GS, Bartels SJ, et al. Consensus statement on the upcoming crisis in geriatric mental health: research agenda for the next 2 decades. *Archives of General Psychiatry*, 56:848–853, 1999.

Jeste DV, Gladsjo JA, Lindamer LA, et al. Medical comorbidity in schizophrenia. *Schizophrenia Bulletin*, 22(3):413–430, 1996.

Jones A. The National Nursing Home Survey: 1999 summary. *Vital and Health Statistics*, 13(152):2002.

Kales HC, Blow FC, Copeland LA, et al. Health care utilization by older patients with co-existing dementia and depression. *American Journal of Psychiatry*, 156(4):550–556, 1999.

Kane RL. Managed care as a vehicle for delivering more effective chronic care for older persons. *Journal of the American Geriatrics Society*, 46(8):1034–1039, 1998.

Kane RL, Kane RA, Finch M, et al. S/HMOs, the second generation: building on the experience of the first social health maintenance organization demonstrations. *Journal of the American Geriatrics Society*, 45(1):101–107, 1997.

Kaplan MS, Adamek ME, Calderon A. Managing depressed and suicidal geriatric patients: differences among primary care physicians. *Gerontologist*, 39(4):417–425, 1999.

Katzelnick DJ, Kobak KA, Greist JH, et al. Effect of primary care treatment of depression on service use by patients with high medical expenditures. *Psychiatric Services*, 48(1): 59–64, 1997.

Kidder SW, Kalachnik JE. Regulation of inappropriate psychopharmacologic medication use in U.S. nursing homes from 1954 to 1997: part II. *Nursing Home Medicine*, 7(2):56–62, 1999.

Koranyi EK. Morbidity and rate of undiagnosed physical illnesses in a psychiatric clinic population. *Archives of General Psychiatry*, 36(4):14–19, 1979.

Lebowitz BD, Pearson JL, Schneider LS, et al. Diagnosis and treatment of depression in late life. Consensus statement update. *Journal of the American Medical Association*, 278(14):1186–1190, 1997.

Lenze EJ, Rogers JC, Martire LM, et al. The association of late-life depression and anxiety with physical disability: a review of the literature and prospectus for future research. *American Journal of Geriatric Psychiatry*, 9(2):113–135, 2001.

Levit K, Smith C, Cowan C, et al. Inflation spurs health spending in 2000. *Health Affairs*, 21(1):172–181, 2002.

Livingston G, Manela M, Katona C. Depression and other psychiatric morbidity in carers of elderly people living at home. *British Medical Journal*, 312:153–156, 1996.

Luber MP, Meyers BS, Williams-Russo PG, et al. Depression and service utilization in elderly primary care patients. *American Journal of Geriatric Psychiatry*, 9(2):169–176, 2001.

Lyness JM, Caine ED, King DA, et al. Psychiatric disorders in older primary care patients. *Journal of General Internal Medicine*, 14(4):249–254, 1999.

Ma CA, McGuire TG. Costs and incentives in a behavioral carve-out. *Health Affairs*, 17(2):53–69, 1998.

Marwick S. Parity for mental health and substance abuse treatment. *Journal of the American Medical Association*, 279(15):1151, 1998.

Mechanic D. Approaches for coordinating primary and specialty care for persons with mental illness. *General Hospital Psychiatry*, 19(6):395–402, 1997.

Miller R, Luft H. Does managed care lead to better or worse quality of care? *Health Affairs*, 16(5):7–25, 1997.

Mollica RL, Riley T, Kane RA, et al. *Managed Care, Medicaid and the Elderly: An Overview of Five State Case Studies*. Portland, ME: University of Minnesota National Long Term Care Resource Center, National Academy for State Health Policy, 1996.

Moore MJ, Zhu CW, Clipp EC. Informal costs of dementia care: estimates from the National Longitudinal Caregiver Study. *Journal of Gerontology: B: Psychological Science and Social Science*, 56(4):S219–S228, 2001.

Mulsant BH, Stergiou A, Keshavan MS, et al. Schizophrenia in late life: elderly patients admitted to an acute care psychiatric hospital. *Schizophrenia Bulletin*, 19:709–721, 1993.

Mumford E, Schlesinger H, Glass G, et al. A new look at evidence about reduced cost of medical utilization following mental health treatment. *American Journal of Psychiatry*, 141(10):1145–1158, 1984.

Narrow WE, Rae DS, Robins LN, et al. Revised prevalence estimates of mental disorders in the United States: using a clinical significance criterion to reconcile 2 survey's estimates. *Archives of General Psychiatry*, 59(2):115–123, 2002.

National Conference of State Legislatures. *State Laws Mandating or Regulating Mental Health Benefits*. Available at http://204.131.235.67/programs/health.mentalben.htm Accessed August 21, 2002, 2002a.

National Conference of State Legislatures: *Pharmaceuticals Accessed*. Available at: http://www.ncsl.org/programs/health/pharm.htm Accessed August 21, 2002, 2002b.

National Council for Community Behavioral Healthcare. *Olmstead: Department of Health and Human Services Urges Implementation of Olmstead*. National Council for Community Behavioral Healthcare. Available at: http://www.nccbh.org/html/policy/archives/olmstead.htm Accessed August 21, 2002

National Council for Community Behavioral Healthcare. *Parity. Mental Health Parity Law Skirted in Private Sector; Policy Report, June 2000.* National Council for Community Behavioral Healthcare. Available at: http://www.nccbh.org/html/policy/archives/parity.htm Accessed August 21, 2002.

National Institute of Mental Health. *Bridging Science and Service.* Rockville, MD: National Institute of Mental Health, 1999.

O'Donnell BF, Drachman DA, Barnes HJ, et al. Incontinence and troublesome behaviors predict institutionalization in dementia. *Journal of Geriatric Psychiatry and Neurology,* 5(1):45–52, 1992.

Office of the Inspector General (OIG). *Mental Health Services in Nursing Facilities* (OIG-02-91-00860). Rockville, MD: OIG, Department of Health and Human Services, 1996.

Office of the Inspector General (OIG). *Medicare Payments for Psychiatric Services in Nursing Homes: A Follow-up* (OIE-02-99-00140). Rockville, MD: OIG, Department of Health and Human Services, 2001a.

Office of the Inspector General (OIG). *Psychotropic Drug Use in Nursing Homes* (OEI-02-00-00490). Rockville, MD: OIG, Department of Health and Human Services, 2001b.

Office of the Inspector General (OIG). *Medicare Part B Payments for Mental Health Services* (OEI-03-99-00130). Rockville, MD: OIG, Department of Health and Human Services, 2001c.

Olfson M, Pincus HA. Outpatient mental health care in nonhospital settings: distribution of patients across provider groups. *American Journal of Psychiatry,* 153(10):1353–1356, 1996.

Oxman TE, Dietrich AJ. The key role of primary care physicians in mental health care for elders. *Generations,* 11:59–65, 2002.

Pacala JT, Boult C, Hepburn KW, et al. Case management of older adults in health maintenance organizations. *Journal of the American Geriatrics Society,* 43:538–542, 1995.

Pacula RL, Sturm R. Mental health parity legislation: much ado about nothing? *Health Services Research,* 35(1):263–275, 2000.

Pratt SI, Bartels SJ, Mueser KT, et al. Psychosocial rehabilitation in older adults with SMI: a review of the research literature and suggestions for development of rehabilitative approaches. Under review.

Reichman WE, Coyne AC, Borson S, et al. Psychiatric consultation in the nursing home. *American Journal of Geriatric Psychiatry,* 6(4):320–327, 1998.

Riley T, Rawlings-Sekunda J, Pernice C. Medicaid managed care and mental health. In: Horvath J, Kaye N (eds). *Medicaid Managed Care: A Guide for States. Challenges and Solutions: Medicaid Managed Care Programs Serving the Elderly and Persons with Disabilities,* 3rd ed., Volume IV, Portland, ME: National Academy for State Health Policy, pp. 79–101, 1997.

Robins LN, Locke BZ, Regier DA. An overview of psychiatric disorders in America. In: Robins LN, Regier DA (eds). *Psychiatric Disorders in America: The Epidemiologic Catchment Area Study.* New York: Free Press, pp. 328–366, 1991.

Sackett DL, Rosenberg WM, Gray JA, et al. Evidence based medicine: what it is and what it isn't. *British Medical Journal,* 312(7023):71–72, 1996.

Schulz R, Beach SR. Caregiving as a risk factor for mortality: the caregiver health effects study. *Journal of the American Medical Association,* 282(23):2215–2219, 1999.

Semke J, Jensen J. High utilization of inpatient psychiatric services by older adults. *Psychiatric Services,* 48(2):172–176, 1997.

Shea DG. Parity and prescriptions: policy developments and their implication for mental health in later life. *Generations,* 26(1):83–89, 2002.

Shea DG, Streit A, Smyer MA. Determinants of the use of specialist mental health services by nursing home residents. *Health Services Research*, 29(2):169–185, 1994.

Simon GE, Ormel J, VonKorff M, et al. Health care costs associated with depressive and anxiety disorders in primary care. *American Journal of Psychiatry*, 152(3):352–357, 1995a.

Simon GE, VonKorff M, Barlow W. Health care costs of primary care patients with recognized depression. *Archives of General Psychiatry*, 52:850–856, 1995b.

Smyer MA, Shea DG, Streit A. The provision and use of mental health services in nursing homes: results from the National Medical Expenditure Survey. *American Journal of Public Health*, 84(2):284–286, 1994.

Snowden M, Roy-Byrne P. Mental illness and nursing home reform: OBRA-87 ten years later. *Psychiatric Services*, 49(2):229–233, 1998.

Strain JJ, Lyons JS, Hammer JS, et al. Cost offset from a psychiatric consultation-liaison intervention with elderly hip fracture patients. *American Journal of Psychiatry*, 148(8):1044–1049, 1991.

Stuart B, Shea D, Briesacher B. Dynamics in drug coverage of Medicare beneficiaries: finders, losers, switchchers. *Health Affairs*, 20(2):86–99, 2001.

Sturm R. How expensive is unlimited mental health care coverage under managed care? *Journal of the American Medical Association*, 278(18):1533–1537, 1997.

Sturm R, Pacula RL. State mental health parity laws: cause or consequence of differences in use. *Health Affairs*, 18(5):182–192, 1999.

Sturm R, Pacula RL. Mental health parity and employer-sponsored health insurance in 1999/2000. *Psychiatric Services*, 51(11):1182–1192, 2000.

Takamura J. Getting ready for the 21st century: the aging of America and the Older Americans Act. *Health and Social Work*, 24(3):232–238, 1999.

Tariot PN, Podgorski CA, Blazin L, et al. Mental disorders in the nursing home: another perspective. *American Journal of Psychiatry*, 150(7):1063–1069, 1993.

The Cochrane Collaboration. *Why the "Cochrane" Collaboration?* [Internet]. Available at: http://www.cochrane.org/cochrane/archieco.htm Accessed August 1, 2002.

Thomas CP, Ritter G, Wallack SS. Growth in prescription drug spending among insured elders. *Health Affairs*, 20(5):265–277, 2001.

Torrey WC, Drake RE, Dixon L, et al. Implementing evidence-based practices for persons with severe mental illnesses. *Psychiatric Services*, 52(1):45–50, 2001.

Unützer J, Katon W, Williams JWJ, et al. Improving primary care for depression in late life: the design of a multicenter randomized trial. *Medical Care*, 39(8):785–799, 2001.

Unützer J, Patrick DL, Simon G, et al. Depressive symptoms and the cost of health services in HMO patients aged 65 years and older. *Journal of the American Medical Association*, 277(20):1618–1623, 1997.

Unützer J, Simon G, Belin TR, et al. Care for depression in HMO patients aged 65 and older. *Journal of the American Geriatrics Society*, 48(8):871–878, 2000.

U.S. Department of Health and Human Services (USDHHS): *Mental Health: A Report of the Surgeon General*. Rockville, MD: USDHHS, Substance Abuse and Mental Health Services Administration, Center for Mental Health Services, National Institutes of Health, National Institute of Mental Health, 1999.

Wells KB, Hays RD, Burnam MA, et al. Detection of depressive disorder for patients receiving prepaid or fee-for-service care: results from the Medical Outcomes Study. *Journal of the American Medical Association*, 262(23):3298–3302, 1989.

Williams L. Long-term care after *Olmstead v. L.C.*: will the potential of the ADA's integration mandate be achieved? *Journal of Contemporary Health Law and Policy*, 17(1):205–239, 2000.

Zylstra R, Steitz J. Knowledge of late life depression and aging among primary care physicians. *Aging and Mental Health*, 4(1):30–35, 2000.

Section D

Substance Abuse

12

Epidemiology of Substance Abuse

JOSEPH GFROERER

Substance abuse, including abuse of alcohol and illicit drugs, has been a public health concern in the United States throughout its history. In the late eighteenth century, Dr. Benjamin Rush, surgeon general of the Continental Army and signer of the Declaration of Independence, promoted the view that long-term drinking was harmful, and he was among the first to state that heavy alcohol use is a health disorder (Jaffe, 1995). Opium use was common among American colonists, including Benjamin Franklin, and the health risks of continual opium use were reported in the American Dispensatory of 1818 (Musto, 1991).

The nature and extent of substance abuse have changed dramatically over the past 200 years in terms of the numbers of persons involved, the types of substances abused, and the nation's perception of and response to the problem. Alcohol use was prevalent among all social and age groups during colonial times and in the early 1800s. Concern over alcohol abuse in the early 1800s led to the passing of prohibition laws in a dozen states before 1850, but these laws were repealed after the Civil War. In the late nineteenth century, antialcohol sentiment again grew, leading eventually to national Prohibition between 1920 and 1933 (Jaffe, 1995). After the repeal of Prohibition, alcohol consumption increased throughout the 1930s and 1940s, leveled off in the 1950s, gradually increased during the 1960s and 1970s, and decreased gradually during the 1980s and 1990s (USDHHS, 1987, 1994). The abuse of opiates and cocaine, drugs that were legal and widely available, was a substantial problem in the late nineteenth century, and cocaine abuse was reported to be the most serious drug problem in the United States in 1910. Parallel to the shifting public attitudes toward alcohol, concern over addiction and misuse led to the Harrison Act of 1914, which restricted the availability of cocaine and opiates and contributed to declines in their use (Musto, 1991). Beginning in the mid-1960s, the use of marijuana rose dramatically among young people and was followed by increased use of opiates (primarily heroin), cocaine, hallucinogens, and other drugs.

Fewer than 5% of Americans had ever used illicit drugs in the early 1960s, but by 2000 nearly 40% had used an illicit drug at some time in their lives and nearly 5 million people were in need of treatment for an illicit drug problem (Epstein, 2002; Miller and Cisin, 1980; SAMHSA, 2001).

This chapter presents the most current information on the epidemiology of substance abuse in the United States. First, it describes methods that have been used to study substance abuse, including a summary of the main data source used in the chapter, the National Household Survey on Drug Abuse. Then a variety of descriptive analyses are presented, showing substance abuse patterns by drug and by sociodemographic and geographic characteristics. Finally, the etiology of substance abuse, health-related problems, recent trends, and implications for behavioral health services are discussed.

Evolution of Substance Abuse Epidemiology

Historically, responses to emerging substance abuse problems have often reflected prevailing public attitudes toward the use of these substances. The response has typically been to enact legal restrictions, such as designating previously legal drugs illegal or increasing the penalties associated with the possession, use, or distribution of specific substances. In addition, the association of alcohol and illicit drug use with criminal behavior has been well documented (Harrison, 1992; Nurco et al., 1991; Room, 1983). Media attention to the drug–crime nexus has also contributed to the widespread public perception that substance abuse is more of a criminal justice issue than a public health issue.

Research on the epidemiology of substance abuse has evolved within this context. Much of the research has focused on particular substances, partly due to changing priorities as different substances of abuse increase and decrease in popularity and public attention, but also because the prevention, treatment, and health concerns vary considerably among different substances and over time (Crider and Rouse, 1988; Kozel and Adams, 1985; Kozel et al., 1985; Miller and Kozel, 1991; Schober and Schade, 1991). Research on alcohol abuse and research on illicit drug abuse have been largely independent, undoubtedly because of the different legal status of the substances and the legislation developed to address them. In part because of the criminal justice aspects of substance abuse, much of the epidemiological research has focused simply on use, rather than on problematic levels of use or criteria for a psychiatric disorder (Dawson et al., 1995; USDHHS, 1994; Weinberg et al., 1998). This is less true for alcohol epidemiological studies, which have focused much more on problematic use, health effects of use, and diagnostic measures (Grant, 1996; Grant et al., 1991) than has illicit drug abuse epidemiological research.

Research has progressed during the past 30 years with the increasing availability of population-based data on substance abuse problems, including diagnostic data collected by survey interviewers. The first national survey on illicit drug use was conducted in 1971 (National Commission on Marihuana and Drug Abuse, 1972). The Epidemiologic Catchment Area Study, conducted in five sites from

1980 to 1984, employed a questionnaire that assessed substance abuse disorders among respondents based on *Diagnostic and Statistical Manual of Mental Disorders* (3rd ed.) (DSM-III) criteria (Eaton et al., 1981). Recent research on both alcohol and illicit drug epidemiology has used nationally representative surveys based on DSM-III-R and DSM-IV to study the epidemiology of dependence and abuse (Anthony and Echeagaray-Wagner, 2000; Anthony et al., 1994; Epstein, 2002; Grant, 1996).

Tools Available for Studying the Epidemiology of Substance Abuse

Researchers have suggested using a variety of data sources to study substance abuse epidemiology (Kozel and Adams, 1986; NIDA, 1998; Russell, 1986; Tomas and Kozel, 1991; WHO, 2000). Administrative data and surveys of facilities have been used extensively. For example, data on substance abusers admitted to treatment programs and emergency departments have been analyzed in epidemiological studies of heroin and methamphetamine users (Greenblatt et al., 1995; Kozel et al., 1985). Reports on drug abuse trends in communities rely heavily on treatment admission and emergency department data (NIDA, 2001). Research has been done based on surveys of hospital inpatients treated for alcohol and illicit drug abuse problems (Caces et al., 1995; Gfroerer et al., 1988) and arrestees (Johnson et al., 1998; Martin et al., 2001). Ethnographic studies have also been useful, particularly in studying hard-core drug addicts (Lambert, 1990). Data on alcohol- and drug-related deaths have also been analyzed (Dawson, 2001; Garfield and Drucker, 2001; Kallan, 1998; Stinson and DeBakey, 1992). These are rich sources of information on specific subpopulations of substance abusers, but they are of limited value in describing the substance-abusing population in the United States.

Large nationally representative general population surveys provide a more complete description of the problem, but they are not an efficient way of sampling the most serious substance abusers because of the low prevalence of this problem in the general population. Substance abusers are also believed to be more difficult to capture in household surveys because many heavy users may not be in a stable living situation; if they are, they may be difficult to find at home. Furthermore, because of the sensitivity of the information collected from respondents for epidemiological study, including much of which involves illegal behaviors, the validity of self-reported data on substance use is often in question. This has led to a large body of methodological research on the reliability and validity of self-reported substance use data that generally supports the use of these data for epidemiological research (Harrison and Hughes, 1997; Midanik, 1988; Rouse et al., 1985; Turner et al., 1992).

Several surveys are available for epidemiological analysis. The largest of these, the National Household Survey on Drug Abuse (NHSDA), is used for the analyses presented in this chapter, primarily because of its broad coverage (ages 12 and older), large sample (70,000 per year), and recency of availability (2000 data). The other major ongoing survey of substance use is the Monitoring the Future Survey, an annual survey of about 50,000 eighth, tenth and twelfth graders (Johnston et al., 2001). Supplemental substance abuse data have been collected periodically in major health surveys such as the National Health Interview Survey (Grant et al., 1991) and the National Health and Nutrition Examination Survey. Two surveys designed to obtain comprehensive data on substance abuse and other mental health disorders are the National Comorbidity Survey (NCS) and the National Longitudinal Alcohol Epidemiology Survey (NLAES). The NCS was conducted during 1990–92 with a sample of 8,038 persons aged 15–54 (Anthony et al., 1994). The NLAES was conducted in 1992 with a sample of 42,862 persons aged 18 and older (Grant, 1996). A second, larger NCS began data collection in 2001 and a survey similar to NLAES, the National Epidemiologic Survey on Alcohol and Related Conditions (NESARC), was conducted in 2001 and 2002. Another widely used survey is the National Alcohol Survey (NAS), which surveys about 5000 adults aged 18 and older about once every 5 years. Finally, the National Longitudinal Study of Adolescent Health (Add Health) is a multiphase study of health-related issues that began with a sample of 90,000 youths in 1994, with follow-up interviews done in 1996 and 2001.

Summary of National Household Survey and Drug Abuse Methodology and Definitions

The NHSDA is the primary source of statistical information on the use of substances by the U.S. population. Conducted by the federal government since 1971, the survey collects data by administering questionnaires to a representative sample of the civilian, noninstitutionalized population of the United States aged 12 or older through face-to-face interviews at their place of residence. The survey is sponsored by the Substance Abuse and Mental Health Services Administration (SAMHSA) (SAMHSA, 2001).

Since 1999, the NHSDA interview has been carried out using computer-assisted interviewing (CAI) methodology. The survey uses a combination of computer-assisted personal interviewing (CAPI) conducted by an interviewer and audio computer-assisted self interviewing (ACASI). Use of ACASI is designed to provide respondents with a private and confidential means of responding to questions and to increase the level of honest reporting of illicit drug use and other sensitive behaviors.

The 2000 NHSDA sample consisted of independent multistage area probability samples for each of the 50 states and the District of Columbia. Samples consisted of about 3600 respondents in each of the 8 largest states and about 900 respondents in each of the remaining 42 states and the District of Columbia. This design allows the production of state-level estimates of substance use and abuse, which SAMHSA accomplishes with the use of small area estimation modeling techniques (SAMHSA, 2000a). The design oversampled youths and young adults, so that each state's sample was approximately equally distributed among three major age groups: 12 to 17 years, 18 to 25 years, and 26 years and older.

Nationally, 169,769 addresses were screened for the 2000 survey, and 71,764 persons were interviewed within the screened addresses. The survey was conducted from January to December 2000. Weighted response rates for household screening and for interviewing were 92.8% and 73.9%, respectively.

The questionnaire includes questions about the initiation, recency, and frequency of use of a variety of substances. In the survey, illicit drug use is defined as use of marijuana or hashish, cocaine, hallucinogens, inhalants, or heroin or the nonmedical use of prescription-type drugs (referred to as *psychotherapeutics*). For each substance (alcohol and each category of illicit drug) used within the past year, respondents are asked additional questions designed to ascertain the occurrence during the past year of symptoms of dependence and abuse of the substance, using DSM-IV criteria as the basis (American Psychiatric Association, 1994). Respondents who report at least three of seven dependence criteria for a substance are classified as dependent. Respondents who are not dependent but report at least one of four abuse criteria are classified as abusing the substance. For convenience, substance use disorders (dependence or abuse) are referred to as SUD in this chapter.

An important limitation of the NHSDA data on SUD is that the determination of SUD for individual respondents does not constitute a clinical diagnosis of the disorder. The limited set of questions included in the survey, coupled with the fact that the survey is administered by professional survey interviewers, not psychiatrists or psychologists, introduces some inaccuracies in the determination of SUD for individual respondents. However, the methodology is useful for epidemiological analysis of aggregate data and has been applied to NHSDA data in a number of studies (Epstein, 2002).

Prevalence by Substance

An estimated 14.5 million Americans aged 12 and older had SUD in 2000 (Table 12.1). This represents 6.5% of the population. Alcohol accounts for most of this estimate, with 12.1 million (5.4% of the population). An estimated 4.3 million persons (1.9%) had illicit drug dependence or abuse, including 1.9 million who had both illicit drug and alcohol dependence or abuse. Marijuana accounted for most illicit drug dependence or abuse, with 2.8 million, while psychotherapeutics (1.1 million), cocaine (0.7 million), hallucinogens (0.4 million), and heroin (0.2 million) were the other drugs primarily mentioned.

There is a great deal of overlap in the populations with dependence or abuse of these different substances. Nearly half (46%) of persons with alcohol dependence or abuse had used an illicit drug in the past year, including 16% with illicit drug dependence or abuse and 30% without illicit drug dependence or abuse. Alcohol dependence or abuse is common among persons with illicit drug dependence or abuse: 45% among those with marijuana dependence or abuse, 67% among those with cocaine dependence or abuse, 45% among those with heroin dependence or abuse, 70% among those with hallucinogen dependence or abuse, and 50% among those with psychotherapeutics dependence or abuse. Multiple drug disorders are also common among illicit drug-dependent or -abusing persons. Among persons with a cocaine use disorder, 32% are dependent on or abusing marijuana. Similarly, 41% of persons with a heroin use disorder, 53% of those with a hallucino-

Table 12.1   Prevalence of Substance Dependance or Abuse for Persons Aged 12 or Older, by Substance: 2000

Substance	Number (in 1000s)	Std. Error	% of Pop.	Std. Error	% of Past-Year Users
Any Substance	14,472	(338)	6.5	(0.15)	10.0
Alcohol	12,110	(307)	5.4	(0.14)	8.8
Any illicit drug	4,308	(168)	1.9	(0.08)	17.6
Marijuana	2,840	(119)	1.3	(0.05)	15.3
Cocaine	748	(85)	0.3	(0.04)	22.5
Heroin	185	(43)	0.1	(0.02)	60.1
Hallucinogens	402	(32)	0.2	(0.01)	11.5
Psychotherapeutics	1,084	(101)	0.5	(0.05)	12.4

Source: SAMHSA, Office of Applied Studies, National Household Survey on Drug Abuse, Rockville, MD, 2000.

gen use disorder, and 25% of those with a psychotherapeutics use disorder are dependent on or abusing marijuana.

In comparing the commonly abused substances, it is interesting to compute rates of dependence or abuse in relation to the prevalence of use (Table 12.1). This suggests the relative *abuse potential* of each substance by showing the percentage of persons who currently use the substance that are dependent or abusing the substance. Among past-year users of alcohol, 8.8% are dependent or abusing. Corresponding rates for illicit drugs were 11.5% for hallucinogens, 12.4% for psychotherapeutics, 15.3% for marijuana, 22.5% for cocaine, and 60.1% for heroin.

Another substance with significant health concerns is tobacco. Although this chapter does not address tobacco use, it is important to note that tobacco use (primarily cigarette use) is highly correlated with alcohol and illicit drug abuse. The rate of current cigarette use is 56.6% among the 14.5 million persons with SUD and 22.7% among persons without SUD.

Prevalence by Sociodemographic Groups and Geographic Location

Tables 12.2 and 12.3 show rates of SUD by various sociodemographic characteristics for the population aged 12 and older. Rates of SUD by marital status, education, and employment are shown in Table 12.4 for persons aged 18 to 49. Table 12.5 shows rates of SUD by state, based on small area estimation methods. These data demonstrate that substance abuse is strongly associated with age, gender, race/ethnicity, family income, education, employment, and marital status. Some geographic differences are seen, but these are less striking than the sociodemographic differences.

Age

The rate of SUD among teenagers increases sharply with age from 2.1% among early teens (aged 12 and 13) to 17.3% among late teens (aged 18 to 20). The rate

Table 12.2   Percentages of Persons Aged 12 or Older Reporting Past-Year Dependence or Abuse for Any Illicit Drug or Alcohol, by Age, Gender, and Race/Ethnicity: 2000

	Type of Dependence or Abuse					
	Illicit Drug		Alcohol		Illicit Drug or Alcohol	
Demographic Characteristic	%	Std. Error	%	Std. Error	%	Std. Error
TOTAL	1.9	(0.08)	5.4	(0.14)	6.5	(0.15)
AGE						
12–13	1.5	(0.17)	1.1	(0.13)	2.1	(0.19)
14–15	4.5	(0.28)	4.8	(0.27)	7.3	(0.34)
16–17	7.4	(0.37)	9.7	(0.40)	13.7	(0.50)
18–20	7.7	(0.35)	13.6	(0.43)	17.3	(0.49)
21–25	3.9	(0.21)	12.2	(0.36)	14.0	(0.39)
26–34	1.9	(0.17)	7.4	(0.32)	8.4	(0.35)
35–49	1.3	(0.17)	5.2	(0.34)	6.0	(0.36)
50 or Older	0.3	(0.11)	2.0	(0.26)	2.2	(0.27)
GENDER						
Male	2.4	(0.11)	7.7	(0.25)	8.9	(0.26)
Female	1.5	(0.11)	3.3	(0.14)	4.2	(0.17)
RACE/ETHNICITY						
Non-Hispanic						
White	1.8	(0.08)	5.5	(0.17)	6.6	(0.18)
Black	2.3	(0.24)	4.7	(0.40)	5.9	(0.43)
American Indian or Alaska Native	4.1	(1.02)	7.9	(1.53)	10.0	(1.76)
Native Hawaiian or other Pacific Islander	1.4	(0.78)	2.8	(0.88)	3.5	(1.11)
Asian	0.7	(0.16)	3.3	(0.70)	3.6	(0.72)
More than one race	5.4	(2.13)	6.4	(1.17)	9.8	(2.29)
Hispanic	2.3	(0.25)	5.9	(0.43)	7.0	(0.46)

Source: SAMHSA, Office of Applied Studies, National Household Survey on Drug Abuse, Rockville, MD, 2000.

among young adults aged 21 to 25 is 14.0%, and the rate declines steadily in older age groups. Only 2.2% of the population aged 50 and older are estimated to have SUD. The pattern across age groups is similar for alcohol and illicit drugs.

Gender

Males aged 12 and older are twice as likely as females aged 12 and older to have SUD (8.9% vs. 4.2%). However, this gender difference is not evident among

Table 12.3   Percentages of Persons Aged 12 or Older Reporting Past-Year
Dependence or Abuse for Any Illicit Drug or Alcohol, by Geographic Characteristics and
Family Income: 2000

	Type of Dependence or Abuse					
	Illicit Drug		Alcohol		Illicit Drug or Alcohol	
Characteristic	%	Std. Error	%	Std. Error	%	Std. Error
TOTAL	1.9	(0.08)	5.4	(0.14)	6.5	(0.15)
REGION						
Northeast	2.2	(0.18)	5.3	(0.30)	6.6	(0.32)
Midwest	1.7	(0.13)	5.3	(0.23)	6.2	(0.27)
South	1.6	(0.09)	5.1	(0.25)	5.9	(0.25)
West	2.6	(0.23)	6.1	(0.32)	7.6	(0.38)
COUNTY TYPE						
Large metro	2.1	(0.13)	5.7	(0.22)	6.9	(0.25)
Small metro	1.8	(0.10)	5.3	(0.22)	6.3	(0.22)
250K—1 mil. pop	1.8	(0.12)	5.3	(0.25)	6.2	(0.26)
<250K pop.	1.8	(0.21)	5.6	(0.43)	6.5	(0.47)
Nonmetro	1.6	(0.12)	5.0	(0.28)	5.9	(0.30)
Urbanized	1.8	(0.17)	5.2	(0.46)	6.2	(0.47)
Less urbanized	1.5	(0.18)	4.8	(0.36)	5.7	(0.39)
Completely rural	1.1	(0.24)	5.5	(1.10)	6.0	(1.12)
FAMILY INCOME						
<$20,000	2.8	(0.25)	6.9	(0.34)	8.3	(0.40)
$20,000–34,999	1.9	(0.16)	6.0	(0.36)	7.2	(0.39)
$35,000–49,999	1.7	(0.16)	5.0	(0.34)	6.0	(0.36)
$50,000–74,999	1.8	(0.20)	5.1	(0.34)	6.0	(0.37)
$75,000+	1.4	(0.15)	4.9	(0.34)	5.7	(0.36)

Source: SAMHSA, Office of Applied Studies, National Household Survey on Drug Abuse, Rockville, MD, 2000.

youths aged 12 to 17. In this age group, 7.9% of boys and 7.4% of girls have SUD.
By ages 18 to 25, a significant gender difference is seen (19.9% for men, 10.9%
for women).

Race/Ethnicity

Rates of SUD for the largest racial ethnic groups do not vary much from the
overall national rate (6.6% for whites, 5.9% for blacks, and 7.0% for Hispanics). However, American Indians and Alaska Natives exhibit a significantly higher
rate of SUD (10.0%) than other groups. Conversely, Pacific Islanders (3.5%)
and Asians (3.6%) exhibit rates lower than those of other groups. These
racial/ethnic patterns are generally consistent across age groups, with a couple
of exceptions. Among youths aged 12 to 17, blacks (5.1%) have a significantly
lower rate of SUD than whites (8.3%) or Hispanics (7.8%). Among young adults
aged 18 to 25, blacks (11.3%) and Hispanics (12.1%) both have lower rates than
whites (17.3%).

Table 12.4   Percentages of Persons Aged 18 to 49 Reporting Past-Year Dependence or Abuse for Any Illicit Drug or Alcohol, by Marital Status, Education, and Employment: 2000

Demographic Characteristic	Type of Dependence or Abuse					
	Illicit Drug		Alcohol		Illicit Drug or Alcohol	
	%	Std. Error	%	Std. Error	%	Std. Error
TOTAL	2.4	(0.11)	7.5	(0.20)	8.8	(0.22)
MARITAL STATUS						
Married	0.9	(0.10)	4.5	(0.26)	5.0	(0.27)
Widowed	2.1	(1.41)	10.6	(3.64)	11.3	(3.60)
Divorced or separated	2.3	(0.39)	8.4	(0.72)	9.9	(0.79)
Never married	5.0	(0.22)	12.2	(0.33)	14.8	(0.36)
EDUCATION						
<High school	4.2	(0.36)	10.3	(0.64)	12.1	(0.66)
High school graduate	2.3	(0.17)	7.5	(0.35)	8.8	(0.38)
Some college	2.4	(0.19)	8.1	(0.38)	9.4	(0.41)
College graduate	1.5	(0.23)	5.4	(0.33)	6.4	(0.39)
EMPLOYMENT						
Full-time	1.9	(0.12)	7.4	(0.25)	8.4	(0.27)
Part-time	3.2	(0.31)	7.8	(0.47)	9.7	(0.53)
Unemployed	8.1	(1.06)	12.3	(1.35)	16.5	(1.51)
Other*	2.8	(0.34)	6.6	(0.48)	8.0	(0.55)

*Retired, disabled, homemaker, student, or "other."
Source: SAMHSA, Office of Applied Studies, National Household Survey on Drug Abuse, Rockville, MD, 2000.

Income

Rates of SUD decrease with increasing levels of family income, ranging from 8.3% for families with annual incomes of less than $20,000 to 5.7% for families with incomes of $75,000 or more. The pattern holds for both alcohol and illicit drugs.

Education

Consistent with the pattern for family income, socioeconomic status as measured by level of education is highly correlated with SUD among persons aged 18 to 49. The highest rate of SUD is found among those with the lowest educational attainment. Among persons aged 18 to 49 with less than a high school education, 12.1% have SUD. Among college graduates the rate is 6.4%. The pattern is similar for alcohol and illicit drugs.

Employment

Among persons aged 18 to 49, the unemployed have significantly higher rates of SUD than employed persons. The rate for the unemployed is 16.5%, while rates are 8.4% for the full-time employed, 9.7% for the part-time employed, and 8.0%

Table 12.5   Percentages Reporting Past-Year Illicit Drug or Alcohol Dependence or Abuse for ages 12 and older, by State: 2000

State	Estimate	Prediction Interval	State	Estimate	Prediction Interval
Alabama	6.33	(5.08–7.77)	Montana	7.61	(6.26–9.15)
Alaska	7.85	(6.35–9.59)	Nebraska	7.51	(6.17–9.04)
Arizona	7.43	(5.94–9.15)	Nevada	6.84	(5.59–8.28)
Arkansas	5.98	(4.85–7.29)	New Hampshire	7.06	(5.79–8.51)
California	7.36	(6.45–8.36)	New Jersey	5.65	(4.44–7.07)
Colorado	7.42	(6.08–8.95)	New Mexico	7.92	(6.45–9.60)
Connecticut	8.01	(6.46–9.78)	New York	6.06	(5.23–6.97)
Delaware	6.89	(5.60–8.38)	North Carolina	5.14	(3.95–6.57)
District of Columbia	7.11	(5.72–8.70)	North Dakota	8.29	(6.85–9.92)
Florida	6.45	(5.54–7.45)	Ohio	5.91	(5.16–6.73)
Georgia	6.19	(4.87–7.74)	Oklahoma	6.21	(4.86–7.80)
Hawaii	6.51	(5.16–8.09)	Oregon	7.07	(5.70–8.64)
Idaho	6.51	(5.38–7.79)	Pennsylvania	6.54	(5.67–7.50)
Illinois	6.80	(5.96–7.72)	Rhode Island	7.36	(5.94–9.01)
Indiana	6.15	(5.06–7.38)	South Carolina	5.55	(4.44–6.83)
Iowa	6.04	(4.98–7.24)	South Dakota	7.79	(6.39–9.38)
Kansas	6.71	(5.33–8.31)	Tennessee	6.14	(4.99–7.47)
Kentucky	6.28	(5.19–7.51)	Texas	6.54	(5.67–7.50)
Louisiana	7.50	(6.09–9.11)	Utah	6.21	(4.92–7.72)
Maine	6.09	(4.98–7.36)	Vermont	7.24	(6.01–8.64)
Maryland	6.48	(5.19–7.98)	Virginia	5.60	(4.46–6.91)
Massachusetts	8.26	(6.62–10.16)	Washington	6.94	(5.45–8.69)
Michigan	6.64	(5.87–7.47)	West Virginia	5.16	(4.23–6.24)
Minnesota	6.37	(5.20–7.70)	Wisconsin	6.89	(5.65–8.31)
Mississippi	6.92	(5.46–8.62)	Wyoming	6.75	(5.53–8.14)
Missouri	6.29	(5.14–7.61)			

Note: Estimates are based on a survey-weighted hierarchical Bayes estimation approach, and the prediction (credible) intervals are generated by Markov chain Monte Carlo techniques.

Source: SAMHSA, Office of Applied Studies, National Household Survey on Drug Abuse, Rockville, MD, 2000.

for others (retired, homemaker, student, or other). However, it is important to recognize that in this age group, 81.4% of persons with SUD are employed. Overall, 9.8 million persons aged 12 and older with SUD are employed.

Marital Status

Rates of SUD vary substantially by marital status among persons aged 18 to 49. The lowest rate is found among married persons (5.0%), and the highest rate is found among those who have never married (14.8%). The rate for widowed persons is 11.3%, and the rate for divorced or separated persons is 9.9%.

County Type

There is little variation in rates of SUD across types of counties categorized by metropolitan and urbanization status. This is particularly true for rates of alcohol dependence or abuse. For illicit drugs, rural areas exhibit a lower rate than metropolitan areas (1.1% in completely rural counties, 2.1% in counties in large metropolitan areas, and 1.8% in counties in small metropolitan areas).

Geographic Region

The western region of the United States exhibits the highest rate of SUD (7.6% of persons aged 12 and older). The lowest rate is in the South (5.9%). Rates are 6.6% in the Northeast and 6.2% in the Midwest.

State

Consistent with the regional estimates, rates of SUD are generally higher in western states and lower in southern states (Table 12.5). However, regional estimates mask some interesting state-level variations. The highest rates of SUD are found in North Dakota, a midwestern state (8.29%), Massachusetts, a northeastern state (8.26%), and Connecticut, a northeastern state (8.01%). The four states with the lowest rates of SUD are all in the South (5.14% in North Carolina, 5.16% in West Virginia, 5.55% in South Carolina, and 5.60% in Virginia). However, the District of Columbia, in the South, has a rate of 7.11%. Utah, a western state, has a rate of only 6.21%.

Characteristics of Persons with Substance Abuse Disorder by Type of Substance

It is important to recognize that the preceding analyses, in which overall rates of substance dependence and abuse for all substances are combined and all illicit drugs are combined, can mask some interesting variations in the characteristics of abusers of some substances. Table 12.6 shows the sociodemographic characteristics of abusers of various substances. Except for abusers of heroin and cocaine, illicit drug abusers tend to be younger than alcohol abusers. Illicit drug abusers are slightly more likely to be female than alcohol abusers. This is particularly evident for non-medical psychotherapeutics abusers, half of whom are female, compared to alcohol abusers, of whom only one-third female. Racial/ethnic, income, and population density differences across substance categories are not statistically significant.

Etiology of Substance Use and Substance Abuse Disorder

Research has shown considerable variation in the pathways leading to alcoholism and drug addiction. Studies have identified a number of factors associated with the transition from nonuse to use as well as from use to problematic use or SUD. While the interactions and relative importance of these factors are not fully understood, research clearly shows that the factors vary by substance and by stage. In other words, the factors influencing whether a person begins to use a substance are not the same as the factors that influence whether a person develops SUD. In

Table 12.6   Percent Distributions of Demographic Characteristics of Persons with Substance Dependence or Abuse, by Type of Substance: 2000

Demographic Characteristic	Type of Dependence or Abuse					
	Alcohol	Marijuana	Cocoaine	Heroin	Hallucinogens	Nonmed. Psychotherapeutic
TOTAL	00.0	100.0	100.0	100.0*	100.0	100.0
AGE						
12–17	9.9	27.6	11.4	7.8*	34.3	22.7
18–25	30.5	41.8	30.2	26.6*	54.6	26.9
26 or older	59.6	30.6	58.4	65.6*	11.1*	50.3
GENDER						
Male	68.0	62.9	55.5	52.4*	64.1	50.5
Female	32.0	37.1	44.5	47.6*	35.9	49.5
RACE/HISPANIC ORIGIN						
White (not Hisp.)	74.7	69.8	62.5	71.6*	81.9	73.6
Black (not Hisp.)	9.8	14.1	18.6	11.9*	4.2	9.8
Hispanic	11.7	11.4	14.3	16.5*	6.4	13.6
FAMILY INCOME						
<$20,000	24.8	29.5	37.6*	49.0*	34.0	28.7
$20,000–34,999	21.8	19.2	20.3	11.3*	15.9	21.0
$35,000–49,999	17.2	16.8	14.4	14.8*	21.0	17.4
$50,000–74,999	17.2	19.2	17.9*	3.8*	13.4	15.5*
$75,000+	19.0	15.2	9.9	21.1*	15.7	17.4
COUNTY TYPE						
Large metro	50.9	54.2	53.7	60.9*	47.4	50.6
Small metro	30.3	29.9	31.3	16.5*	37.1	32.3
Nonmetro	18.8	15.9	15.0	22.6*	15.5	17.1

*Low precision.
Source: SAMHSA, Office of Applied Studies, National Household Survey on Drug Abuse, Rockville, MD, 2000.

a summary of several studies of the etiology of drug abuse, Glantz and Pickens (1992) concluded that peer and social factors appear to be more important in the transition from nonuse to use, but progression to SUD is more closely related to biological and psychological factors. Some factors related to initiation and early use include having friends who use substances, having a favorable attitude toward substance use, poor academic achievement, poor relationships with parents, and having parents who use substances. Factors related to the progression to heavy substance use and SUD include early age at first substance use, family history of substance use problems, antisocial personality, having a mental disorder, and aggressive behavior at a young age (Anthony and Petronis, 1995; Gfroerer and Wu, 2002; Grant and Dawson, 1997; Hawkins et al., 1992; Lane et al., 2001; USDHHS, 2000). Roles and responsibilities also play an important part in the transition from use to either heavier use or reduced use or abstinence. Personal milestones such as starting a career, marriage, and parenthood are associated with reductions in substance use (Bachman et al., 1997). This is one reason that the overall rates of substance use and SUD decline with age beyond age 25.

In addition to personal and family factors, other factors associated with substance use and SUD include contextual factors such as community and school characteristics, and laws and norms regarding substance use. For example, increased taxes on alcohol and a higher drinking age have been associated with lower levels of alcohol use and associated consequences (USDHHS, 2000).

Health Problems Related to Substance Abuse

The use and abuse of substances are associated with a variety of health problems. It has been estimated that there were 120,000 preventable deaths in the United States in 1990 attributed to the use of alcohol and illicit drugs (McGinnis and Foege, 1993). This includes 100,000 attributed to alcohol and 20,000 attributed to illicit drugs. Follow-up studies of SUD populations have estimated significantly higher death rates in a 14-year period than among non-SUD populations (Neumark et al., 2000a, 2000b).

Alcohol

There were an estimated 111,000 alcohol-related deaths in 1996. Liver cirrhosis and motor vehicle accidents were the leading causes (NIAAA, 2002). A recent study found an increased risk of death from external causes (unintentional injuries, suicide, and homicide) among heavy drinkers (Dawson, 2001). Because the liver is the primary site of alcohol metabolism, heavy alcohol use is linked with various liver problems, including cirrhosis, fatty liver, hepatitis, and fibrosis. Effects on the brain include alcoholic dementia and general cognitive impairments. Although some studies have found moderate drinking to decrease the risk of coronary heart disease, heavy drinking is related to hypertension, stroke, weakened heart muscle, and arrhythmias. Some cancers have also been associated with heavy alcohol use (USDHHS, 1994, 2000).

Illicit Drugs

Illicit drug–related deaths are primarily due to overdoses. A complete count of illicit drug overdoses for the United States is not available, but medical examiners in 40 metropolitan areas reported nearly 12,000 drug abuse deaths in 1999, and more than 7000 of these were classified as drug-induced overdoses. Since the mid-1980s, the primary drugs involved in drug-related overdoses have been heroin and cocaine (SAMHSA, 2000b). Needle sharing among injection drug users accounts for 25% of the cases of acquired immune deficiency syndrome, resulting in about 5000 deaths per year from 1997 to 2000 (CDC, 2001).

Some studies have found that long-term marijuana use is associated with cognitive impairment among adults (Solowij et al., 2002). Marijuana smokers may be at risk for many of the same health consequences attributed to cigarette use. The amount of tar inhaled by marijuana smokers and the level of carbon monoxide absorbed are three to five times greater than those of tobacco smokers. Medical complications associated with cocaine use include cardiovascular effects (disturbances in heart rhythm and heart attacks), respiratory effects (chest pain and respiratory failure), neurological effects (strokes, seizure, and headaches), and gastrointestinal complications (abdominal pain and nausea). Regularly snorting cocaine can lead to loss of the sense of smell and nosebleeds. The most serious medical consequences of chronic heroin abuse stem from the injection of the drug, the most common mode of administration among addicts. These include scarred and/or collapsed veins, bacterial infections of the blood vessels and heart valves, abscesses (boils) and other soft-tissue infections, and liver or kidney disease. Additives in street heroin also cause problems such as clogged blood vessels and rheumatological problems. Sharing of injection equipment or fluids can lead to some of the most severe consequences of drug abuse. Drugs most commonly injected include heroin and other opiates, cocaine, and methamphetamine. Associated problems include infections with hepatitis B and C, human immunodeficiency virus, and other bloodborne viruses, which drug abusers can then pass on to their sexual partners and children (NIDA, 2002).

Recent Trends in Use

Trend data on the prevalence of SUD are not available, but trends in substance use may suggest future shifts in SUD rates. Per capita consumption of alcohol decreased steadily from 1981 to 1995 but remained at the same level from 1995 to 1998 (NIAAA, 2002). Estimates of the prevalence of alcohol use also suggest no significant changes in rates of current, binge, or heavy alcohol use from 1994 to 1999 for adults and youth (SAMHSA, 2000a). Rates of illicit drug use are less stable. Overall illicit drug use rates for both youth and adults peaked in 1979 and then declined until 1992. Although rates among adults have not changed much since 1992, the rate among youths more than doubled between 1992 and 1995. The percentage of youths aged 12 to 17 using illicit drugs in the past month was 16% in 1979, 5% in 1992, and 11% in 1995. The rate changed little from 1995 to 2000 (SAMHSA 2000b, 2001).

Implications for Substance Abuse Services

Epidemiological research on the use and abuse of substances provides valuable information that guides the design of prevention and treatment programs. It also allows policy makers to effectively target available resources to populations most in need of services. Although SUD is more prevalent among some U.S. population groups than others, no group is unaffected. It encompasses many specific, differing kinds of problems. Comorbidity with other mental disorders is common. Thus, to address SUD effectively, a variety of approaches must be used that match the range of problems and populations affected.

Planning for future service delivery needs to consider the dynamic nature of illicit drug use and abuse. New drug use behaviors continue to emerge, and trends will undoubtedly shift unexpectedly. One important consideration is the potential increase over the next 20 years in the size of the SUD population as the cohorts with high rates of drug use in the 1970s and early 1990s, including the large baby boom cohort, become older (Gfroerer and Epstein, 1998).

REFERENCES

American Psychiatric Association. *Diagnostic and Statistical Manual of Mental Disorders*, 4th ed. Washington, DC: American Psychiatric Press, 1994.

Anthony JC, Echeagaray-Wagner F. Epidemiologic analysis of alcohol and tobacco use: patterns of co-occurring consumption and dependence in the United States. *Alcohol Research and Health*, 24(4):201–208, 2000.

Anthony JC, Petronis KR. Early onset drug use and risk of later drug problems. *Drug and Alcohol Dependence*, 40:9–15, 1995.

Anthony JC, Warner LA, Kessler RC. Comparative epidemiology of dependence on tobacco, alcohol, controlled substances, and inhalants: basic findings from the National Comorbidity Survey. *Experimental and Clinical Psychopharmacology*, 2(3):244–268, 1994.

Bachman JG, Wadsworth KN, O'Malley PM, et al. *Smoking, Drinking, and Drug Use in Young Adulthood: The Impacts of New Freedoms and New Responsibilities*. Mahwah, NJ: Erlbaum, 1997.

Caces MF, Stinson FS, Dufour MC. Trends in alcohol-related morbidity among short-stay community hospital discharges, United States: 1979–93. *NIAAA Surveillance Report No. 36*. Rockville, MD: National Institute on Alcohol Abuse and Alcoholism, 1995.

Centers for Disease Control and Prevention. HIV and AIDS—United States, 1981–2000. *Morbidity and Mortality Weekly Report*, 50(21):430–434, 2001.

Crider RA, Rouse BA (eds). Epidemiology of inhalant abuse: an update. *NIDA Research Monograph 85*, 1988.

Dawson DA. Alcohol and mortality from external causes. *Journal of Studies on Alcohol*, 62:790–797, 2001.

Dawson DA, Grant BF, Chou SP, et al. Subgroup variation in U.S. drinking patterns: results of the 1992 National Longitudinal Alcohol Epidemiologic Study. *Journal of Substance Abuse*, 7:331–344, 1995.

Eaton W, Regier D, Locke B, et al. The epidemiologic catchment area program of the National Institute of Mental Health. *Public Health Reports*, 96(4):319–325, 1981.

Epstein J. *Substance Dependence, Abuse, and Treatment: Findings from the 2000 National Household Survey on Drug Abuse*, Rockville, MD, Substance Abuse and Mental Health Services Administration, 2002.

Garfield J, Drucker E. Fatal overdose trends in major US cities: 1990–1997. *Addiction Research and Theory* 9(5):425–436, 2001.

Gfroerer JC, Adams EH, Moien M. Drug abuse discharges from non-federal short-stay hospitals. *American Journal of Public Health*, 78(12):1559–1562, 1988.

Gfroerer JC, Epstein JF. Marijuana initiates and their impact on future drug use treatment need. *Drug and Alcohol Dependence*, 54:229–237, 1998.

Gfroerer JC, Wu LT. *Initiation of Marijuana Use: Trends, Patterns, and Implications*. Substance Abuse and Mental Health Services Administration, 2002.

Glantz M, Pickens R (eds). *Vulnerability to Drug Abuse*. Washington, DC: American Psychological Association, 1992.

Grant BF. Prevalence and correlates of drug use and DSM-IV drug dependence in the United States: results of the National Longitudinal Alcohol Epidemiologic Survey. *Journal of Substance Abuse*, 8:195–210, 1996.

Grant BF, Dawson DA. Age at onset of alcohol use and its association with DSM-IV alcohol abuse and dependence: results from the National Longitudinal Alcohol Epidemiologic Survey. *Journal of Substance Abuse*, 9:103–110, 1997.

Grant BF, Harford TC, Chou P, et al. Prevalence of DSM-III-R alcohol abuse and dependence, United States, 1988. *Alcohol Health and Research World* 15(1):91–96, 1991.

Greenblatt JC, Gfroerer JC, Melnick D. Increasing morbidity and mortality associated with abuse of methamphetamine—United States 1991–1994. *Morbidity and Mortality Weekly Report*, 44(47):882–886, 1995.

Harrison L, Hughes A (eds). The validity of self-reported drug use: improving the accuracy of survey estimates. *NIDA Research Monograph* 167, 1997.

Harrison LD. The drug-crime nexus in the USA. *Contemporary Drug Problems*, 19(2):203–246, 1992.

Hawkins JD, Catalano RF, Miller JY. Risk and protective factors for alcohol and other drug problems in adolescence and early adulthood: implications for substance abuse prevention. *Psychological Bulletin*, 112(1):64–105, 1992.

Jaffe JH (ed). *Encyclopedia of Drugs and Alcohol*. Volume 1. New York: Macmillan Library Reference USA, Simon & Schuster Macmillan, 1995.

Johnson BD, Thomas G, Golub AL. Trends in heroin use among Manhattan arrestees from the heroin and crack eras. In: Inciardi J, Harrison L (eds). *Heroin in the Age of Crack Cocaine*. Beverly Hills, CA: Sage, 1998.

Johnston LD, O'Malley PM, Bachman JG. *Monitoring the Future: National Survey Results on Drug Use, 1975–2000. Volume 1, Secondary School Students*. NIH Pub. No. 01-4924. Rockville, MD, National Institute on Drug Abuse, 2001.

Kallan JE. Drug abuse–related mortality in the United States: patterns and correlates. *American Journal of Drug and Alcohol Abuse* 24(1):103–117, 1998.

Kozel NJ, Adams EH (eds). Cocaine use in America: epidemiologic and clinical perspectives. *NIDA Research Monograph* 61, 1985.

Kozel NJ, Adams EH. Epidemiology of drug abuse: an overview. *Science*, 234:970–974, 1986.

Kozel NJ, Crider R, Brodsky MD, et al. *Epidemiology of Heroin: 1964–1984*. Rockville, MD, National Institute on Drug Abuse, Division of Epidemiology and Statistical Analysis, 1985.

Lambert EY (ed). The collection and interpretation of data from hidden populations. *NIDA Research Monograph* 98, 1990.

Lane J, Gerstein D, Huang L, et al. *Risk and Protective Factors for Adolescent Drug Use: Findings from the 1997 National Household Survey on Drug Abuse*. DHHS Pub. No. (SMA) 01-3499. Rockville, MD: Substance Abuse and Mental Health Services Administration, 2001.

Martin SE, Bryant K, Fitzgerald N. Self-reported alcohol use and abuse by arrestees in the 1998 arrestee drug abuse monitoring program. *Alcohol Research and Health*, 25(1):72–79, 2001.

McGinnis MJ, Foege WH. Actual causes of death in the United States. *Journal of the American Medical Association* 270(18):2207–2212, 1993.

Midanik L. Validity of self-reported alcohol use: a literature review and assessment. *British Journal of Addictions* 83(9):1019–1029, 1988.

Miller JD, Cisin IH. *Highlights from the National Survey on Drug Abuse: 1979*. DHHS Pub. No. (ADM) 80-1032, 1980. Rockville, MD: National Institute on Drug Abuse.

Miller MA, Kozel NJ (eds). Methamphetamine abuse: epidemiologic issues and implications. *NIDA Research Monograph* 115, 1991.

Musto DF. Opium, cocaine, and marijuana in American history. *Scientific American*, 265(1):40–47, 1991.

National Commission on Marihuana and Drug Abuse. *Marijuana: A Signal of Misunderstanding*. First Report of the National Commission on Marijuana and Drug Abuse. Washington, DC: March 1972.

National Institute on Alcohol Abuse and Alcoholism. Number of deaths and age-adjusted death rates per 100,000 population for categories of alcohol-related mortality, United States and States, 1979–96. Available at: http://www.niaaa.nih.gov/databases/armort01.htm Accessed March 2002.

National Institute on Drug Abuse. *Assessing Drug Abuse within and Across Communities: Community Epidemiology Surveillance Networks on Drug Abuse*. NIH Pub. No. 98-3614. Rockville, MD, National Institute on Drug Abuse, Division of Epidemiology and Prevention Research, 1998.

National Institute on Drug Abuse. *Epidemiologic Trends in Drug Abuse. Volume 1: Proceedings of the Community Epidemiology Work Group. Highlights and Executive Summary, June 2001*. NIH Pub. No. 01-4916A. Rockville, MD: National Institute on Drug Abuse, Division of Epidemiology, Services and Prevention Research, November 2001.

National Institute on Drug Abuse. NIDA Infofacts: Heroin. Available at: http://www.nida.nih.gov/Infofax/heroin.html Accessed March, 2002.

Neumark YD, Van Etten ML, Anthony JC. Drug dependence and death: survival analysis of the Baltimore ECA sample from 1981 to 1995. *Substance Use and Misuse*, 35(3):313–327, 2000a.

Neumark YD, Van Etten ML, Anthony JC. Alcohol dependence and death: survival analysis of the Baltimore ECA sample from 1981 to 1995. *Substance Use and Misuse*, 35(4): 533–549, 2000b.

Nurco DN, Hanlon TE, Kinlock TW. Recent research on the relationship between illicit drug use and crime. *Behavioral Sciences and the Law*, 9:221–242, 1991.

Room R. Alcohol and crime: Behavioral aspects. In: Kadish SH (ed). *Encyclopedia of Crime and Justice*, Volume 1. New York: Free Press, pp. 35–44, 1983.

Rouse BA, Kozel NJ, Richards G (eds). Self-report methods of estimating drug use: meeting current challenges to validity. *NIDA Research Monograph 57*, 1985.

Russel M. The epidemiology of alcoholism. In: Estes N, Heinemann ME (eds). *Alcoholism: Development, Consequences, and Interventions*, 3rd ed. St, Louis, MO: C.V. Mosby, 1986.

Schober S, Schade C (eds). The epidemiology of cocaine use and abuse. *Research Monograph 110*, 1991.

Solowij N, Stephens RS, Roffman RA, et al. Cognitive functioning of long-term heavy cannabis users seeking treatment. *Journal of American Medical Association* 270(18):2207–2212, 2002.

Stinson FS, DeBakey SF. Alcohol-related mortality in the United States, 1979–1988. *British Journal Addictions* 87(5):777–783, 1992.

Substance Abuse and Mental Health Services Administration. *Summary of Findings from the 1999 National Household Survey on Drug Abuse*. DHHS Pub. No. (SMA) 00-3466. H-12. Rockville, MD: Office of Applied Studies, 2000a.

Substance Abuse and Mental Health Services Administration. *Drug Abuse Warning Network Annual Medical Examiner Data 1999*. DHHS Pub. No. (SMA) 01-3491. D-16. Rockville, MD: Office of Applied Studies. 2000b.

Substance Abuse and Mental Health Services Administration. *Summary of Findings from the 2000 National Household Survey on Drug Abuse*. DHHS Pub. No. (SMA) 01-3549. H-13. Rockville, MD: Office of Applied Studies. 2001.

Tomas JM, Kozel NJ. National substance abuse epidemiology initiatives in the United States: what works for what. *Journal of Addictive Diseases* 11(1):5–21, 1991.

Turner CF, Lessler J, Gfroerer JC. *Survey Measurement of Drug Use: Methodological Studies.* Rockville, MD: National Institute on Drug Abuve, DHHS Pub. No. (ADM) 92-1929. 1992.

U.S. Department of Health and Human Services. *Sixth Special Report to the U.S. Congress on Alcohol and Health.* Rockville, MD: National Institute on Alcohol Abuse and Alcoholism, DHHS Pub. No. (ADM) 87-1519, 1987.

U.S. Department of Health and Human Services. *Eighth Special Report to the U.S. Congress on Alcohol and Health.* Rockville, MD: National Institute on Alcohol Abuse and Alcoholism, NIH Pub. No. 94-3699, 1994.

U.S. Department of Health and Human Services. *Tenth Special Report to the U.S. Congress on Alcohol and Health.* Rockville, MD: National Institute on Alcohol Abuse and Alcoholism, NIH Pub. No. 00-1583, 2000.

Weinberg NZ, Rahdert E, Colliver JD, et al. Adolescent substance abuse: a review of the past 10 years. *Journal of the American Academy of Child and Adolescent Psychiatry*, 37(3): 252–261, 1998.

World Health Organization. *Guide to Drug Abuse Epidemiology.* Geneva, Switzerland: Mental Health and Substance Dependence, Department of Non-communicable Disease and Mental Health Cluster, World Health Organization, 2000.

13

The Treatment System for Alcohol and Drug Dependence

DENNIS McCARTY
ELDON EDMUNDSON

Legacies of discrimination in access to health care, social control systems built on incarceration, reliance on self-help, and an emphasis on experiential training provide the context for contemporary alcohol and drug abuse treatment services. Alcoholics and drug addicts were regularly denied care in hospitals (Plaut, 1967) and confined in drunk tanks and county farms as recently as the 1960s and 1970s (President's Commission on Law Enforcement and Administration of Justice: Task Force on Drunkenness, 1967). Men and women in recovery advocated for changes in state and federal legislation and, through grassroots organization and community development, constructed and delivered services for those dependent on alcohol and drugs. Today the treatment system for alcohol and drug dependence is a hodgepodge of financing sources, a patchwork of small, independent, and specialized addiction treatment services, and a loosely organized workforce that includes many individuals with personal experiences of addiction and recovery. As a result, alcohol and drug abuse treatment services are, to a large degree, an idiosyncratic facet of the health care system in the United States.

This chapter provides an overview of the financing and organization of treatment services for alcohol and drug abuse. Unique attributes of the addiction treatment system become apparent when the patterns of expenditures for treating alcohol and drug problems are reviewed and compared with expenditures for mental health treatments and other health care services. An examination of specialty alcohol and drug treatment programs, a description of patient populations, and a review of the substance abuse treatment workforce provide more background for appreciating the distinctive nature of the services. The chapter concludes with a discussion of how the organization and financing of substance abuse treatment affects the potential for integration of care and adoption of evidence-based practices.

Expenditures on Treatment for Alcohol and Drug Problems

A Center for Substance Abuse Treatment estimate indicates that total spending on treatment for alcohol and drug dependence and abuse was about $11.4 billion in 1997 (Coffey et al., 2001; Mark et al., 2000). Although this is a considerable sum, it represents only 14% of the $82.2 billion spent for behavioral health care (services for the treatment of mental health and substance abuse) and a very small 1% of the nation's $1057 billion in total health care expenditures. Comparisons of the treatment providers and the payment sources for addiction treatments versus mental health and total health care services highlight the unique features of the substance abuse treatment system.

Providers and Services

Figure 13.1 summarizes expenditures for substance abuse treatment and shows comparable patterns for mental health and total health care spending. Spending for alcohol and drug abuse treatment is concentrated in hospital care (40%) and specialty substance abuse treatment centers (33%) (Coffey et al., 2001). The proportion of expenditures for hospital services is greater for substance abuse treatment than for mental health care (30%) and for total health care (35%) (Coffey et al., 2001). Hospital expenditures reflect inpatient services for detoxification and withdrawal management. Lengths of stay are brief (typically 4 days or less), but the cost per day for hospital beds is substantial (e.g., $400 per day or more). Figure 13.1 also illustrates that the specialty substance abuse centers provide a range of residential and outpatient services for alcohol and drug dependence but make no contributions to expenditures for mental health and total health care. Thus, specialty centers reflect the historical development of addiction treatment services and remain comparatively isolated from the larger health care system.

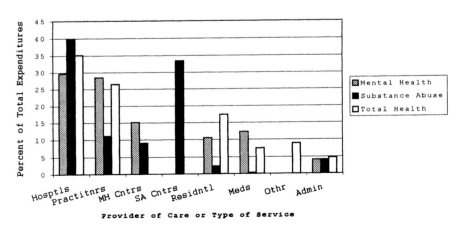

Figure 13.1 Expenditures by provider of care or type of service (percentage of total). (Data from Coffey et al., 2001, pp. 79, 85).

Lack of training and continued stigmatization of people with addictions contribute to the relative absence of physicians, psychologists, and social workers in treatments for alcohol and drug abuse. Physicians and other independent practitioners account for about 11% of expenditures for substance abuse treatment but 28% of mental health and 26% of total health care spending. Multiservice mental health organizations also account for a greater proportion of mental health services (15%) expenditures than for substance abuse treatment (9%). Finally, it is noteworthy that less than 1% of substance abuse treatment expenditures are for prescription drugs (0.3%), while medication accounts for 12.8% of mental health spending and 7.5% of the spending on total health care (Coffey et al., 2001).

Expenditures for alcohol and drug abuse treatment services reflect a reliance on inpatient hospital services, the unique influence of specialty clinics, reluctance among independent practitioners to treat addictions, and a resistance to the use of medications. Thus, the idiosyncratic nature of the substance abuse treatment system begins to emerge. An assessment of payers helps to describe more clearly the current system of care.

Payers

Payment sources for addiction services are summarized in Figure 13.2 (Coffey et al., 2001, p. 82). Private insurance is the largest single category. Alcohol and mental health services, however, receive a lower proportion of private insurance payments (24%) than payments for total health care (33% from private insurance). The disparity reflects historical reluctance among commercial health plans to provide coverage for behavioral health and the persistent lack of parity in the benefits for mental health and substance abuse services.

Most funds spent on services for substance abuse and mental health are from public sources—alcohol and drug treatment (64%) and mental health services

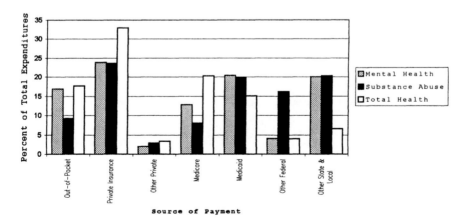

Figure 13.2 Expenditures by source of payment (percentage of total). (Data from Coffey et al., 2001, p. 82).

(57%). Public expenditures also account for a large but smaller portion of the expenditures for total health care (46%) (Coffey et al., 2001). State and local governments contributed more heavily to the financing for mental health and substance abuse treatments (20% of total expenditures) than for total health care (7%). Other federal funds were four times more important to alcohol and drug abuse treatment (16% of expenditures primarily from the federal Substance Abuse Prevention and Treatment Block Grant) than mental health care or total health care (4% of expenditures for each from other federal funds including the Mental Health Block Grant). The Substance Abuse Prevention and Treatment Block Grant has grown over the past 20 years with the expansion of the War on Drugs (U.S. General Accounting Office, 1995, 1996). For federal fiscal year 2000, block grant funding for states and territories was $1.52 billion.

Finally, it is noteworthy that patient out-of-pocket payments are substantially lower for alcohol and drug abuse treatment (9%) than for mental health services (17%) and total health care (18%). This reflects the use of public funds to provide coverage for individuals who would be otherwise uninsured for substance abuse treatment.

The result is a treatment system heavily dependent on public revenues and uniquely dependent on federal block grant funds. Multiple funding streams contribute to fragmentation of service delivery but are also evidence of creative strategies to support substance abuse treatment. The block grant and state revenues flow through state agencies that license and fund services for the treatment of alcohol and drug dependence. States have traditionally funded programs and facilities rather than practitioners. The resulting treatment infrastructure relies on community-based organizations rather than individual practitioners. Data on the treatment programs add detail to the discussion of the addictions treatment system.

Treatment Centers, Workforce, and Patients

Institute of Medicine reviews of alcohol (Institute of Medicine, 1990a) and drug abuse (Institute of Medicine, 1990b) treatment provide excellent overviews of treatment modalities. The substance abuse service system, however, continues to evolve and increasingly reflects a patient population that is dependent on or abusing both alcohol and drugs (McCarty et al., 2000). As a result, most addiction treatment facilities report treating both alcohol and drug dependence. An overview of treatment centers, the workforce, and the patients they serve further illustrates key features of the nation's substance abuse treatment system.

Alcohol and Drug Abuse Treatment Centers

The most comprehensive descriptive data on addiction treatment programs come from a census of known alcohol and drug abuse programs conducted annually by the Substance Abuse and Mental Health Services Administration. The 1997 census (to use data comparable to the expenditure estimates) identified 10,860 facilities (Substance Abuse and Mental Health Services Administration, 1999). Because of changes in census methods and efforts to obtain a more complete universe of centers, the 1999 census reported data on the characteristics of 15,239 programs, but overall trends are similar to those found in the 1997 report (Substance Abuse and Mental Health Services Administration, 2001b).

More than half (54%) of the treatment programs that responded in 1997 identified themselves as providing only services for alcohol and drug abuse (i.e., no medical or mental health services other than addictions treatment (Substance Abuse and Mental Health Services Administration, 1999). These programs are the specialty alcohol and drug abuse treatment settings. In addition, more than one in five programs (21%) were mental health centers and about one in seven (14%) were health care settings. Programs were also located within the criminal justice system (5%) and other service settings (6%) (Substance Abuse and Mental Health Services Administration, 1999).

Most of the substance abuse treatment programs were organized as private nonprofit corporations (60%), but one in four (24%) were private for-profit entities and 17% operated as units of local, state, federal, or tribal government (Substance Abuse and Mental Health Services Administration, 1999). The specialty treatment programs were slightly more likely to be private nonprofit corporations (68%) and less likely to be private for profit (19%).

Facilities that provide alcohol and drug abuse treatments delivered a range of services but focused on assessments for substance abuse (92%) and related counseling services: individual therapy (94%), group therapy (88%), family therapy (73%), and relapse prevention (72%) (Substance Abuse and Mental Health Services Administration, 1999). More than half of the programs also reported providing discharge planning (75%), urine screening for drug use (75%), aftercare counseling (73%), drug and alcohol education (64%), human immunodeficiency virus (HIV) education (58%), self-help groups (56%), health education (53%), and case management (50%). Treatment facilities were less likely to offer medical and support services: medications (40%), parenting skills training 38%), HIV testing (34%), employment counseling (31%), medical care (30%), housing assistance (27%), child care (10%), and family planning (7%). Specialty substance abuse programs were less likely to offer medications (28%) especially compared to mental health organizations (67%) and hospitals (72%) (Substance Abuse and Mental Health Services Administration, 1999, p. 29). Finally, the programs that provide alcohol and drug treatment services tended to have small caseloads. The median daily caseload was 36, and 76% of the facilities served fewer than 100 patients a day (Substance Abuse and Mental Health Services Administration, 1999).

The available information suggests that the programs serving individuals seeking treatment for alcohol and drug dependence are an eclectic group of nonprofit, for-profit, and governmental entities. The largest proportion, however, are the traditional freestanding nonprofit corporations that specialize in treating substance abuse. The programs tend to have small caseloads, and services consist primarily of individual and group therapy, problem assessment, and urine screens for drugs of abuse. For the most part, even though patients have multiple needs, few programs provide ancillary and support services for housing, education, and legal problems. The limited data available on the staff in alcohol and drug abuse programs reinforce impressions about the unique nature of the treatment services.

Workforce

Men and women working in alcohol and drug abuse treatment services reflect a diversity of educational backgrounds and professional training. An analysis of training needs for substance abuse treatment noted 27 professions that were involved directly and indirectly in substance abuse treatment including individuals working in criminal justice, health, mental health, and human services (Lewin-VHI, 1994). The diversity was also observed over time in the 1976 and 1991 censuses of alcohol and drug abuse programs (Brown, 1997). Medical staff—psychiatrists (1%), physicians (1%), and nurses (9%)—represented about 11% of the staff in addiction treatment. Individuals who provide direct care made up the largest portion of the workforce (about 45%)—psychologists (3%), social workers (6%) and counselors (36%). Aides and assistants accounted for 18% of the staff and the remaining 26% had administration and management roles (Brown, 1997).

Because the patients receiving alcohol and drug abuse treatment often have co-occurring problems with criminal justice, employment, mental health, family relationships, housing and other factors that influence functioning, counselors need a wide range of knowledge and skills to address multiple patient needs. Training and sustaining local and national workforces with the capabilities to respond to all of the treatment needs place heavy expectations on education programs to develop counselors with multifaceted skills and to provide continuing education opportunities. Although descriptions of the substance abuse treatment workforce are limited and dated, they are nonetheless informative.

Workforce Characteristics

Analyses of the individuals providing drug and alcohol counseling during the late 1970s and early 1980s suggest that much of the workforce practiced without graduate training; between one in five (Camp and Kurtz, 1982) and one in three counselors (Birch and Davis, 1984) claimed a masters or doctoral degree. Rates of graduate training may have been even lower in programs that were classified as drug treatment (Aiken et al., 1985; LoSciuto et al., 1979). Many of those working without a college degree or a bachelor's degree identified themselves as "in recovery."

A survey of alcohol and drug abuse treatment programs in Massachusetts completed in 1985 found an evolving workforce (Mulligan et al., 1989). Data were obtained from 150 publicly funded alcohol treatment programs, 94 publicly funded drug treatment services, and 18 private chemical dependency treatment centers (86% response rate). When all levels of care were combined, about half of the workforce had graduate degrees, half were women, and half were individuals in recovery. Analyses by level of care, however, found dramatic differences. The most intensive levels of care (detoxification and residential services) were more likely to be staffed with men (50% to 60%), therapists without graduate training (70% to 80%), and individuals in recovery (about 70%). Outpatient services, conversely, were more likely to employ women (about 60%), with masters or doctoral degrees (50% to 80%), and without personal experience with recovery (60% to 90%) (Mulligan et al., 1989).

Subsequent assessments of the workforce in alcohol and drug abuse treatment programs have been limited. Evidence suggests that a shift from inpatient and residential settings to ambulatory services and the growth of managed care has restricted the use of counselors without graduate training and without licenses to practice independently (Steenrod et al., 2001).

Training

Abuse and dependence on alcohol and other drugs affect many facets of functioning, and counselor training and education programs provide basic skills and address interactions among client functioning domains. Colleges and universities shape substance abuse counselor training in a variety of ways—academic certificates as part of academic programs, concentration/emphasis, academic minors and majors, and continuing education. Educational institutions vary in how substance abuse topics are integrated into discipline content areas. Counselor education programs, for example, require specific courses and a majority of content in substance abuse areas (Morgan et al., 1997). Other disciplines (e.g., social work, medicine and psychology) integrate substance abuse topics in general content courses that address specific counseling skills—courses on assessments, ethics, and counseling/therapy skills.

Qualifications, training, and licensure requirements vary among states. Some states require specific degrees before therapists can provide substance abuse counseling. Others require specific coursework and experience but do not require a degree. Entry-level substance abuse treatment professionals can receive course work including field experiences that lead to state certification through formal academic training (at associate, bachelor's, graduate, or certificate levels) and in nonacademic training centers.

Much of the specialized substance abuse training occurs within programs offering associate degrees. The National Association of Alcohol and Drug Abuse Counselors examined programs in 277 colleges and universities; nearly two-thirds (63%) of the substance abuse counseling programs provided associate degrees (www.naadac.org/educate.htm). Similarly, the Northwest Frontier Addiction Technology Transfer Center surveyed 462 treatment programs located in the states of Alaska, Idaho, Washington, and Oregon during 1999; responses were obtained from 197 agencies (43% response rate) (Newby and Gabriel, 2000). Up to three counselors completed the instrument at each agency, and 469 responses were received. Although a low response rate and a relatively uncontrolled method of selecting respondents limit the value of the data, the strong influence of community colleges on development of the substance abuse treatment workforce was apparent. Graduate degrees were common (42%), but nearly one in three (29%) were working without the benefit of a bachelor's degree. More than two of three respondents (69%) reported holding certification in addictions counseling. Nearly half (48%) of those with certifications indicated that the training was provided at a 2-year college.

In short, training for a career in addiction counseling is relatively undeveloped. Practitioners follow many paths toward expertise and experience in counseling men, women, and adolescents with alcohol and drug abuse.

Alcohol- and Drug-Dependent Individuals

The National Household Survey on Drug Abuse (Household Survey) tracks the prevalence and incidence of illicit drug, alcohol, and tobacco use in the United States and can be used to estimate needs for treatment and the demand for treatment services. The 2000 Household Survey reported that 14 million individuals (6.3% of the population 12 years of age and older) used illicit drugs in the 30 days prior to the survey; 104 million (46.6% of the population) drank alcohol in the past month and 12.6 million met criteria for heavy drinking (Substance Abuse and Mental Health Services Administration, 2001a). An estimated 4.3 million individuals (aged 12 and older) were categorized as dependent on or abusing illicit drugs, and another 10.2 million were dependent on or abusing alcohol; the 14.5 million individuals represented about 6.5% of the adult population of the United States (Epstein, 2002).

Most alcohol- and drug-dependent and abusing individuals were not in treatment. About 1 in 6 (17%) of the individuals who needed treatment for problems related to drug use entered care in 2000; similarly, about 1 in 5 (20%) of the individuals with alcohol-related abuse or dependence received treatment (Epstein, 2002). Other estimates suggest that about 44% of the most severely dependent illicit drug users received treatment in the past year (Woodward et al., 1997). The "treatment gap," therefore, exceeds 50% for the individuals with greatest treatment priority and is much higher among alcohol-dependent individuals and individuals with less severe drug problems.

Description of Patients

The annual SAMHSA census of substance abuse treatment facilities includes information about patients. Programs reported 929,086 patients in care on October 1, 1997, and the demographic data outline a patient population of mostly younger white, black, and Hispanic men abusing both alcohol and drugs. (Substance Abuse and Mental Health Services Administration, 1999) About two-thirds of the patients (68%) were men. The proportion of women in drug and alcohol treatment services, however, increased steadily during the 1990s (from 28% in 1990 to 32% in 1997). All races and ethnicities were reported. White (non-Hispanic) patients accounted for 57% of the caseload (a decrease from 62% in 1990), blacks (non-Hispanic) represented 25%, and Hispanics accounted for 14%. Two percent of the patients were American Indians. Young adults (21 to 34 years of age) made up 40% of the patients. Patients less than 21 years of age accounted for 15%, and individuals 45 years of age and older for 16% of the total. Programs reported that 40% of the patients were being treated for both alcohol and drug abuse. Drug abuse only patients accounted for one in three (33%) patients, and alcohol abuse only was reported in about one in four (26%) patients.

Most patients were being treated in outpatient settings (87%), with the remaining patients reported from residential (11%) and hospital inpatient (2%) services. Specialty substance abuse treatment programs were treating about 44% of the patients ($n = 412,577$), and community mental health centers treated 19% ($n = 172,326$). Ten percent of the patients were found in general hospitals. The remaining patients were distributed among solo practitioners (7%), criminal justice programs (6%), psychiatric hospitals (5%), community agencies (3%), community health centers (less than 1%), and multiple or unknown categories (4%). (Substance Abuse and Mental Health Services Administration, 1999).

Implications for Substance Abuse Services

The nation's treatment system for alcohol and drug abuse is relatively isolated from systems of care for health and mental health. There are, consequently, perennial policy issues: (1) a persistent gap in access to care, (2) skepticism about the effectiveness of treatment, (3) limited commercial benefits for alcohol and drug abuse treatment, and (4) poor integration with health care and criminal justice systems. Finally, reliance on a workforce trained in certificate programs may inhibit adoption of emerging behavioral interventions and pharmacotherapies.

Access to Care

The gap between need for care and access to care is a product of patient factors (stigma of addiction and denial about the need for care), financing issues (limited funding and health care coverage for addiction treatments), poor linkages between service systems, and weak screening and referral mechanisms (Substance Abuse and Mental Health Services Administration, 2000). Individuals dependent on alcohol and other drugs frequently may not recognize that they need treatment or may be ambivalent about entering care. One strategy has been to promote outreach and risk reduction. Syringe exchange, for example, promotes the use of sterile equipment for injection drug use and reduces transmission of blood-borne pathogens like HIV and hepatitis C virus. Although controversial, the use of harm reduction interventions seems to be increasing.

Similarly, treatment systems struggle with strategies to engage drug users in care. Motivational interviewing techniques enhance patient motivation and controlled studies consistently find improvements in entry to and retention in care (Miller and Rollnick, 2002; Miller and Wilbourne, 2002; Miller et al., 1994). But facilitation of access and enhanced retention also require improved systems for patient placement (American Society of Addiction Medicine, 1996; Turner et al., 1999), assessment of patients (McLellan et al., 1992), and change in the delivery of services to enhance quality of care (Institute of Medicine, 1997, 1998; McLellan and McKay, 1998; McLellan et al., 1997).

In short, treatment providers and policy makers have much opportunity to improve treatment access and retention through a restructuring of addiction treatment services.

Skepticism About the Value of Treatment

Investigations consistently find that treatment for alcohol and drug dependence is associated with reductions in use and improvements in functioning (Institute of

Medicine, 1990a, 1990b; Simpson, 1997). Comparisons of drug use at intake and 12 months after leaving treatment using data from the Treatment Outcome Prospective Study (TOPS) (intake interviews were completed in 1979 and 1980) and the Drug Abuse Treatment Outcomes Studies (DATOS) (intake interviews conducted in 1991, 1992, and 1993), for example, suggested that about 50% of weekly and daily heroin and cocaine users reported any use at follow-up (Hubbard et al., 2001). The likelihood of use, however, was lower in the (DATOS) cohort (heroin and cocaine = 47% reporting any use) than among patients who partici-pated in the earlier TOPS investigation (heroin = 59%, cocaine = 65%) and sug-gests improvements in the effectiveness of treatment services (Hubbard et al., 2001).

Nonetheless, public and private policy makers continue to question the efficacy of alcohol and drug abuse treatment services. A comparison of treatment outcomes for addiction, asthma, diabetes, and heart disease provides an interesting perspec-tive on efficacy; the analysis found similar rates of treatment compliance (40% to 60%) and readmission to care (about 50%) for each disease (McLellan et al., 2000). The essay suggests that alcohol and drug dependence should be viewed as a chronic illness that requires continued treatment attention and advocates substantive change in the ways care is delivered to provide long-term but low-intensity serv-ices to help patients function and maintain themselves without intensive acute care (McLellan et al., 2000).

Financing and Insurance Parity

Historically, health insurance plans are reluctant to cover treatment for alcohol and drug dependence (Scott et al., 1992). Concern with adverse selection inhibits lib-eral benefits; plans offering better coverage for alcoholism and drug abuse treat-ment services may attract members who need those services and may require ex-pensive services (Frank et al., 1997). To facilitate access to treatment, 41 states mandate coverage for treatment of alcohol and/or drug abuse, but the coverage tends to be limited to $500 of outpatient services (Scott et al., 1992). When avail-able, inpatient benefits are heavily managed, and it may be difficult to fully use the nominal benefit.

The persistent disparity in coverage for alcohol and drug dependence prompted state and federal legislation to require parity—mental health and substance abuse treatment benefits with limits on duration of outpatient and inpatient care similar to the coverage available for most medical services. Current federal legislation, however, excludes treatment for alcohol and drug dependence. Similarly, most states that require parity for mental health treatments do not extend the require-ment to services for substance abuse (Sing et al., 1998). The federal government now requires parity in coverage for services for mental illness, alcohol dependence, and drug dependence in health plans for federal employees. Data are not yet avail-able on the impacts of this requirement for the use of services and adverse selec-tion (for additional discussion of parity, see Chapters 1, 2, 3, and 11 in this volume).

Integration with Health Care

Most individuals with alcohol and drug problems are found in primary care settings rather than specialty clinics and criminal justice systems (Weisner, 2001). Continued reluctance to identify and treat alcohol- and drug-dependent individuals, however, inhibits the integration of substance abuse treatment services with primary care. More integrated services nonetheless continue to promise economic and health care benefits. A recent investigation conducted within a health maintenance organization assigned patients either to a primary care clinician located in the addiction treatment service or to treatment as usual with a primary care clinician not connected with addiction treatment; patients with substance abuse–related medical conditions were more likely to be abstinent 6 months after treatment when primary care was integrated with addiction treatment (69% vs. 55% abstinence) (Weisner et al., 2001). The integrated service was also found to be substantially more cost–effective despite a slightly higher cost (Weisner et al., 2001). Addiction services that are better integrated with primary care thus continue to be an aspiration.

An additional potential benefit from closer integration between substance abuse treatment and primary care is better access to medications. Despite recent advances in the development of pharmacotherapies for alcohol and drug dependence (Garbutt et al., 1999; Institute of Medicine, 1995), adoption of these medications has been slow. Lack of access to primary care clinicians who can write prescriptions inhibits adoption in many freestanding alcohol and drug abuse treatment centers. Policy makers and practitioners will continue to be challenged to find effective strategies for integrating treatment for alcohol and drug problems more effectively with primary care and mental health services.

Coordination with Criminal Justice Systems

Drug users are frequently involved with the criminal justice system, and enforcement and prosecution of drug crimes have burdened courts and corrections departments. Drug courts remove drug offenders from crowded dockets and create a special venue for monitoring offenders and prescribing sanctions designed to promote the use of treatment services and recovery from drug dependence. The authority of the court is used to persuade offenders to choose recovery over continuation of a criminal career. The first drug court began in 1989, and by the end of 2001 the Department of Justice had identified 791 (U.S. General Accounting Office, 2002). Federal funds fueled the tremendous growth of drug courts. Reviews of the management of drug courts, however, continue to find poor data collection and weak evaluation activities (U.S. General Accounting Office, 1997, 2002). As a result, there are little data on the effectiveness of drug courts.

A more recent innovation in linking criminal justice and treatment services is the use of voter referendums to require that drug offenders be offered treatment services rather than incarceration. The initiatives are placed on state ballots, and if voters approve the proposed legislation becomes law—circumventing reluctance in state legislatures to appear weak on crime. In California, the Substance Abuse and Crime Prevention Act of 2000 was passed when 61% of voters supported Proposition 36 in November 2001. The large margin of approval from California voters stimulated similar efforts in other states. The California initiative became effective in July 2001; and data to evaluate its impacts are not yet available.

Evidence-Based Practice

Research is rapidly developing more comprehensive descriptions of the effects of chronic alcohol and drug use on neurobiology and identifying more effective behavioral and pharmacological interventions (Institute of Medicine, 1995, 1996; Leshner, 1999). Program directors and policy makers strive to encourage application of these findings in contemporary treatment services, but community drug and alcohol treatment centers seem to be particularly resistant to the adoption of evidence-based practices (Institute of Medicine, 1998).

Initiatives like the National Institute on Drug Abuse's National Drug Abuse Clinical Trials Network and the Center for Substance Abuse Treatment's Practice Improvement Collaboratives will help research become more relevant to practitioners and encourage practitioners to be more informed about research. The Addiction Technology Transfer Centers will also facilitate identification of practice-relevant research and promote counselor training. Nonetheless, sustained attention is required to support current practitioners and to elevate educational standards for new therapists. The field will continue to be challenged to raise educational expectations and develop a fully professional cadre of practitioners.

Contemporary alcohol and drug abuse treatment services have survived despite limited resources and public ambivalence about the value of addictions treatment. To survive in the next decade, attention will focus on the development of quality improvement strategies to document effectiveness and promote greater accountability. Therapists will enhance their skills, and the field will become more integrated into the health care, mental health, and criminal justice systems. Systematic evolution will promote a continuing role for specialty alcohol and drug abuse treatment programming.

References

Aiken LS, LoSciuto L, Ausetts M. Who is serving drug abuse clients? In: Ashery RS (ed). *Progress in the Development of Cost-Effective Treatment for Drug Abusers.* NIDA Research Monograph 58, DHHS Pub. No. (ADM) 85-1401. Rockville, MD: National Institute on Drug Abuse, 1985.

American Society of Addiction Medicine. *Patient Placement Criteria for the Treatment of Substance Related Disorders: ASAM PPC-2,* 2nd ed., Chevy Chase, MD: American Society of Addiction Medicine, 1996.

Birch and Davis, Inc. *Development of Model Professional Standards for Counselor Credentialing.* Rockville, MD: National Institute on Alcohol Abuse and Alcoholism, 1984.

Brown BS. Staffing patterns and services for the war on drugs. In: Egertson JA, Fox DM, Leshner AI (eds). *Treating Drug Abusers Effectively.* Malden, MA: Blackwell, pp. 99–124, 1997.

Camp JM, Kurtz NR. Redirecting manpower for alcoholism treatment. In: *Prevention, Intervention and Treatment: Concerns and Models.* Alcohol and Health Monograph No. 3, Rockville, MD: National Institute on Alcohol Abuse and Alcoholism, pp. 371–397, 1982.

Coffey RM, Mark T, King E, et al. *National Estimates of Expenditures for Substance Abuse Treatment, 1997.* Rockville, MD: Center for Substance Abuse Treatment, 2001.

Epstein JF. *Substance Dependence, Abuse, and Treatment: Findings from the 2000 National Household Survey on Drug Abuse.* NHSDA Series H-16, DHHS Pub. No. SMA 02-3642. Rockville, MD: Substance Abuse and Mental Health Services Administration, Office of Applied Studies, 2002.

Frank RG, McGuire TG, Bae JP, et al. Solutions for adverse selection in behavioral health care. *Health Care Financing Review,* 18:109–122, 1997.

Garbutt JC, West SL, Carey TS, et al. Pharmacological treatment of alcohol dependence. *Journal of the American Medical Association,* 281:1318–1325, 1999.

Hubbard RL, Flynn PM, Craddock SG, et al. Relapse after drug abuse treatment. In: Tims FM, Leukefeld CG, Platt JJ (eds). *Relapse and Recovery in Addictions.* New Haven, CT: Yale University Press, pp. 109–121, 2001.

Institute of Medicine. *Broadening the Base of Treatment for Alcohol Problems.* Washington, DC: National Academy Press, 1990a.

Institute of Medicine. *Treating Drug Problems.* Washington, DC: National Academy Press, 1990b.

Institute of Medicine. *The Development of Medications for the Treatment of Opiate and Cocaine Addictions: Issues for the Government and Private Sector.* Washington, DC: National Academy Press, 1995.

Institute of Medicine. *Pathways of Addiction: Opportunities in Drug Abuse Research.* Washington, DC: National Academy Press, 1996.

Institute of Medicine. *Dispelling the Myths About Addiction: Strategies to Increase Understanding and Strengthen Research.* Washington, DC: National Academy Press, 1997.

Institute of Medicine. *Bridging the Gap Between Practice and Research: Forging Partnerships with Community-Based Drug and Alcohol Treatment.* Washington, DC: National Academy Press, 1998.

Leshner AI. Science-based views of drug addiction and its treatment. *Journal of the American Medical Association,* 282:1314–1316, 1999.

Lewin-VHI, Inc. *Substance Abuse Training Needs Analysis: Final Report.* Fairfax, VA: Lewin-VHI, Inc., 1994.

LoSciuto LA, Aiken LS, Ausetts MA. Professional and paraprofessional drug abuse counselors: three reports. Rockville, MD: National Institute on Drug Abuse, 1979.

Mark TL, Coffey RM, King E, et al. Spending on mental health and substance abuse treatment, 1987–1997. *Health Affairs,* 19:108–120, 2000.

McCarty D, Caspi Y, Panas L, et al. Detoxification centers: who's in the revolving door? *Journal of Behavioral Health Services and Research,* 27:245–256, 2000.

McLellan AT, Kushner H, Metzger D, et al. The fifth edition of the Addiction Severity Index. *Journal of Substance Abuse Treatment,* 9:199–213, 1992.

McLellan AT, Lewis DC, Obrien CP, et al. Drug dependence a chronic medical illness: implications for treatment, insurance and outcomes evaluation. *Journal of the American Medical Association,* 284:1689–1695, 2000.

McLellan AT, McKay JR. The treatment of addiction: what can research offer practice? In: Lamb S, Greenlick MR, McCarty D (eds). Institute of Medicine, *Bridging the Gap Between Practice and Research: Forging Partnerships with Community-Based Drug and Alcohol Treatment.* Washington, DC: National Academy Press, pp. 147–185, 1998.

McLellan AT, Woody GE, Metzger D, et al. Evaluating the effectiveness of addiction treatments: reasonable expectations, appropriate comparisons. In: Egertson JA, Fox DM, Leshner AI (eds). *Treating Drug Abusers Effectively*. Malden, MA: Blackwell, pp. 7–40, 1997.

Miller WR, Rollnick S. *Motivational Interviewing: Preparing People for Change*, 2nd ed. New York: Guilford Press, 2002.

Miller WR, Wilbourne PL. Mesa Grande: a methodological analysis of clinical trials of treatments for alcohol use disorders. *Addiction*, 97:265–277, 2002.

Miller WR, Zweben A, DiClemente CC, et al. *Motivational Enhancement Therapy Manual: A Clinical Research Guide for Therapists Treating Individuals with Alcohol Abuse and Alcoholism.* Project MATCH Monograph Series, Volume 2. Rockville, MD: National Institute on Alcohol Abuse and Alcoholism, 1994.

Morgan OJ, Tolczko A, Comly E. Graduate training of counselors in the addictions: a study of CACREP-approved programs. *Journal of Addictions and Offender Counseling*, 17:66–76, 1997.

Mulligan DH, McCarty D, Potter D, et al. Counselors in public and private alcoholism and drug abuse treatment programs. *Alcoholism Treatment Quarterly*, 6:75–89, 1989.

Newby M, Gabriel R. *Substance Abuse Treatment Workforce Survey: A Regional Needs Assessment.* Portland, OR: RMC Research Corporation, 2000.

Plaut TFA. *Alcohol Problems: A Report to the Nation by the Cooperative Commission on the Study of Alcoholism*, New York: Oxford University Press, 1967.

President's Commission on Law Enforcement and Administration of Justice. Task Force on Drunkenness: *Task Force Report: Drunkenness.* Washington, DC: U.S. Government Printing Office, 1967.

Scott JE, Greenberg D, Pizarro J. A survey of state insurance mandates covering alcohol and other drug treatment. *Journal of Mental Health Administration*, 19:96–118, 1992.

Simpson DD. Effectiveness of drug-abuse treatment: a review of research from field settings. In: Egertson JA, Fox DM, Leshner AI (eds). *Treating Drug Abusers Effectively*. Malden, MA: Blackwell, pp. 41–73, 1997.

Sing M, Hill S, Smolkin S, et al. *The Costs and Effects of Parity for Mental Health and Substance Abuse Insurance Benefits.* Rockville, MD: Substance Abuse and Mental Health Services Administration, 1998.

Steenrod S, Brisson A, McCarty D, et al. Effects of managed care on programs and practices for the treatment of alcohol and drug dependence. *Recent Developments in Alcoholism: Services Research in the Era of Managed Care*, 15:51–71, 2001.

Substance Abuse and Mental Health Services Administration. *Uniform Facility Data Set (UFDS): 1997—Data on Substance Abuse Treatment Facilities*: Rockville, MD: Substance Abuse and Mental Health Services Administration, Office of Applied Studies, 1999.

Substance Abuse and Mental Health Services Administration. *Changing the Conversation—Improving Substance Abuse Treatment: The National Treatment Plan Initiative.* Rockville, MD: Substance Abuse and Mental Health Services Administration, 2000.

Substance Abuse and Mental Health Services Administration. *Summary of Findings from the 2000 National Household Survey on Drug Abuse.* NHSDA Series H-13, DHHS Pub. No. (SMA) 01-3549. Rockville, MD: Office of Applied Studies, 20011.

Substance Abuse and Mental Health Services Administration. *Uniform Facility Data Set (UFDS): 1999—Data on Substance Abuse Treatment Facilities*: Rockville, MD: Substance Abuse and Mental Health Services Administration, Office of Applied Studies, 2001b.

Turner WM, Turner KH, Reif S, et al. Feasibility of multidimensional substance abuse treatment matching: automating the ASAM Patient Placement Criteria. *Drug and Alcohol Dependence*, 55:35–43, 1999.

U.S. General Accounting Office. *Block Grants: Characteristics, Experience, and Lessons Learned.* Washington, DC: U.S. General Accounting Office, 1995.

U.S. General Accounting Office. *Drug and Alcohol Abuse: Billions Spent Annually for Treatment and Prevention Activities.* Washington, DC: U.S. General Accounting Office, 1996.

U.S. General Accounting Office. *Drug Courts: Overview of Growth, Characteristics, and Results.* Washington, DC: U.S. General Accounting Office, 1997.

U.S. General Accounting Office. *Drug Courts: Better DOJ Data Collection and Evaluation Efforts Needed to Measure Impact of Drug Courts.* Washington, DC: U.S. General Accounting Office, 2002.

Weisner C. The provision of services for alcohol problems: a community perspective for understanding access. *Journal of Behavioral Health Services and Research*, 28:130–142, 2001.

Weisner C, Mertens J, Parthasarathy S, et al. Integrating primary medical care with addiction treatment: a randomized controlled trial. *Journal of the American Medical Association*, 286:1715–1723, 2001.

Woodward A, Epstein J, Gfroerer J, et al. The drug abuse treatment gap: recent estimates. *Health Care Financing Review*, 18:5–17, 1997.

Part III
SPECIAL ISSUES

14

Mental Health Issues in the Criminal Justice System

RANDY BORUM

People with mental health disorders frequently come into contact with the criminal justice system (Borum et al., 1997; Ditton, 1999; Lamb and Weinberger, 1998; Teplin, 1988). In fact, encounters with police (the front line of the criminal justice system) are so common that for people with severe mental illness, they are the norm rather than the exception (Borum, 2000; Clark et al., 1999; Frankle et al., 2001; McFarland et al., 1989). Most of these contacts are precipitated by disruptive behavior or minor infractions that occur because individuals are experiencing psychiatric symptoms or social disruptions related to their disability. They frequently result in arrest, each year causing more than a quarter of a million people with mental illness to be processed through the criminal court system (Ditton, 1999). Many misdemeanants are held in jails; others are charged with more serious offenses and sent to prison. As of 1999, it is conservatively estimated that 123,000 people with severe mental illnesses were lodged in state prisons; at least 14,000 were in federal prison (Beck, 2000); and more than half a million were on probation (Ditton, 1999). Although some people with mental illness do commit offenses for which incarceration is the most appropriate disposition, many are confined as a result of arrests for minor infractions. This outcome is costly and poses a severe challenge to the criminal justice and behavioral health systems.

On the front line, law enforcement officers must spend time processing the arrest and testifying in court. If the subject is arrested and held in jail, the facility must manage more inmates with special mental health needs—a population they already find difficult to serve. Individuals with mental illnesses, while in jail, often become more disconnected from community mental health treatment, may have difficulty getting the proper medication, and may experience a worsening of their symptoms due to lack of treatment and the stress of confinement. When the case is ready for disposition, court systems, including prosecutors, judges, and public defenders, must spend time and resources adjudicating relatively minor offenses. This chapter reviews what is currently known about the prevalence of severe mental illness in U.S. jails and prisons; discusses key legal issues affecting the public care of people with mental health disorders while in correctional confinement; briefly reviews issues related to the availability of mental health services in the criminal justice system; and explains and argues for the use of jail diversion initiatives as a mechanism for primary and secondary prevention of justice system involvement for people with severe mental illnesses.

Prevalence

Police Contacts

People with mental illness frequently report having contact with the police, just as police report having frequent contact with people who have mental illnesses—as many as 7% to 10% of police contacts, according to some estimates (Deane et al., 1998; Janik, 1992).

The rate at which people diagnosed with mental illnesses report being arrested or detained by police is remarkably high. For example, in a study of 360 psychiatric patients seen at an urban outpatient mental health clinical, almost half (48.6%) had a history of arrest. Those patients with a criminal history (average age of 43) had accumulated an average of 6.8 arrests (Frankle et al., 2001). Among 203 people enrolled in a specialized treatment program for dual disorders (mental illness and substance abuse), 83% had contact with the legal system and 44% were arrested at least once over a 3-year follow-up period (Clark et al., 1999).

Some have argued that this inflated rate is confounded with low socioeconomic status because so many people with severe mental disorders live in poverty and high-crime neighborhoods. Interestingly, however, in a survey of members of the Oregon chapter of the National Alliance for the Mentally Ill (a major advocacy organization composed primarily of family members of people with mental illness), more than half reported that their relatives with mental illness had been arrested at least once. The average number of arrests was greater than three (McFarland et al., 1989).

Despite the fact that these arrests are common, the offenses charged typically are minor, including trespassing, disorderly conduct, or other nonserious misdemeanors (Bonovitz and Bonovitz, 1981; Borum et al., 1997; Monahan and Steadman, 1983). This, of course, raises the question of whether people with mental health disorders may be more likely than those without such an illness to be arrested for similar offenses, a process that some have referred to as *criminalization.* The empirical evidence on this point is somewhat mixed.

In a Chicago-based study, trained clinical researchers rode on patrol with police officers and observed over 1000 encounters. In these encounters, police arrested 47% of the subjects with mental illnesses but only 28% of the subjects without mental illness (Teplin, 1984). Teplin interpreted this finding as being consistent with a trend toward criminalization of mental illness. More recently, however, Engel and Silver (2001) examined the question by revisiting data from two large multisite field studies of police behavior and, using multivariate analysis, arrived at a different conclusion. They found that "controlling for a wide range of relevant factors, police are not more likely to arrest mentally disordered suspects" (245). Indeed, one striking finding was that, while suspects with mental illnesses typically were involved in less serious offenses, they were more likely to have a weapon on the scene.

Two clinical factors, however, have been found consistently to increase the risk of arrest—and criminal justice involvement generally—among people with mental health disorders: (1) use or abuse of alcohol and/or other drugs and (2) failure to take their psychiatric medications as prescribed (Borum et al., 1997; Broner et al., 2002; Drake et al., 1993; Lamb and Weinberger, 1998; Munetz et al., 2001; Torrey et al., 1992). Research on individuals who have a severe mental illness shows that those who use alcohol or drugs and do not take their medications are three times more likely to be arrested than others with mental disorder (Borum et al., 1997). Similarly, the reports of family members of people with mental illness suggest that incidents in which people with mental illness are arrested often involve substance abuse and lack of compliance with their prescribed medication (McFarland et al., 1989). Substance abuse and nonadherence with medication regimens also significantly increase the risk of violent behavior (Swartz et al., 1999). Thus, these risk factors clearly mark a subgroup of individuals for whom specialized response and intervention are necessary to reduce recidivism.

Jails and Prisons

The absolute number, rate of admission, and prevalence of people with severe mental illnesses (i.e., schizophrenia, bipolar disorder, and major depression) in U.S. jails and prisons is remarkably high. A review of studies from around the country concluded that 6%–15% of all jail inmates and 10%–15% of all prison inmates have a severe mental illness (Diamond et al., 2001; Lamb and Weinberger, 1998).

Each year, approximately 685,000 people with severe mental illness are admitted to jails in the United States. This means that there are currently more people with severe mental illness in U.S. jails than in state psychiatric hospitals and that they are admitted eight times more often to jails than to hospitals (Torrey et al., 1992).

The rate of mental illness in jail is substantially higher for women than for men (Ditton, 1999; Teplin et al., 1996). Estimates from the U.S. Department of Justice's Bureau of Justice Statistics indicate that approximately 16% of male jail inmates have a mental illness compared to 23% of female inmates (Ditton, 1999). Although some of the early estimates of disorder among incarcerated women came from samples of those referred for evaluation—where rates would obviously be higher (Lamb and Grant, 1983)—subsequent random samples of female inmates show rates of mental disorder that are quite high (Daniel et al., 1988; Teplin et al., 1996; Washington and Diamond, 1985). It should be noted that the estimated prevalence of 6%–15% for mental illness in jail is conservative and accounts for only the three most severe psychiatric diagnoses: schizophrenia, major depression, and bipolar disorder. Perhaps an additional 40% of jail inmates have an anxiety disorder or a less severe mood disorder (Neighbors, 1987), a third of women have post-traumatic stress disorder (Teplin et al., 1996), and as many as a quarter to half or more of male and female jail inmates have an alcohol or drug abuse disorder (Department of Justice, 1984; Guy et al., 1985; Lamb and Grant, 1983; Swank and Winer, 1976; Swartz and Lurigio, 1999; Teplin et al., 1996).

The prevalence at other points in the criminal justice system is equally striking, with nearly 150,000 people with severe mental illnesses located in prisons and another 500,000 under probationary correctional supervision in the community (Ditton, 1999). The gender disparity in estimates of mental illness also persists beyond jails. Estimates of mental illness in state prison inmates were 16% for men and 24% for women. For federal inmates the rates were estimated to be 7% men and 13% for women, and for probationers 15% of men and 22% of women were identified as mentally ill (Ditton, 1999). Moreover, across the genders, three out of four inmates with mental illness had been incarcerated or under criminal justice supervision on at least one prior occasion (Ditton, 1999), suggesting that there is a core subgroup of people with severe mental illness who cycle in and out of the mental health and criminal justice systems—a phenomenon many refer to as the *revolving door.*

Relative to their prevalence in the community, the most severe mental health disorders—particularly bipolar disorder and schizophrenia (and other psychotic disorders)—are substantially overrepresented among people sentenced to state and federal prisons. Indeed, the lifetime prevalence of schizophrenia is often two to three times higher and that of bipolar disorder is three to four times higher than community estimates (Diamond et al., 2001; Lamb and Weinberger, 1998). Moreover, most offenders with one severe primary mental disorder also have at least one other co-occurring (comorbid) psychiatric condition. For example, in a study of nearly 500 Canadian prisoners, more than 90% of those with either major depression or schizophrenia had some co-occurring mental health diagnosis (Cote and Hodgins, 1990). Perhaps not surprisingly, the rate of co-occurring substance abuse among detainees with mental illness is particularly high. Nearly three of out of every four jail inmates with mental illness has a coexisting alcohol or drug abuse problem (Abram and Teplin, 1991), and the proportion is likely as high, or higher, for prison inmates (Cote and Hodgins, 1990; Diamond et al., 2001).

Legal Issues

Many persons with mental illnesses require some degree of medical care to prevent exacerbation or deterioration of their conditions (Cohen, 1998). It is not legally permissible for a correctional facility knowingly to withhold necessary medical care simply because an individual is incarcerated, and thereby has other justifiable restrictions based on his or her rights and liberty (Singer, 1981). Indeed, the U.S. Supreme Court has determined that doing so constitutes "cruel and unusual punishment."

> [D]eliberate indifference to a prisoner's serious medical needs constituted cruel and unusual punishment under the Eighth Amendment and gave rise to a civil rights cause of

action under 42 USCS 1983, regardless of whether the indifference was manifested by prison doctors in their response to the prisoner's needs or by prison guards in intentionally denying or delaying access to medical care or intentionally interfering with treatment once prescribed.

(*Estelle v. Gamble*, 429 U.S. 97, 1976)

Courts have also generally agreed that needs for medical care or treatment arising from mental illnesses are included under this broader rubric of *medical needs*. Indeed, in *Bowring v. Godwin* (551 F.2d 44, 4th Cir. 1977), the Fourth Circuit Court of Appeals stated that they saw "no underlying distinction between the right to medical care for physical ills and its psychological or psychiatric counterpart" (at 226). Subsequently, a number of cases examined the issue of what constitutes adequate or appropriate mental health care in correctional facilities. Perhaps the most specific elucidation and summary of the components were articulated by the court in *Ruiz v. Estelle* (503 F. Supp. 1265,1323, 1980). Drawing on "judicial precedent in previous prison cases, . . . expert testimony in the instant case, and . . . basic principles of minimally adequate care (as applied) to the specific problem of mental health care," the court found six elements necessary to establish "minimally adequate mental health treatment":

• A systematic process for screening and evaluation of inmates for mental illness.
• Availability of treatment that consists of more than segregation and close supervision.
• Participation of a sufficient number of trained mental health professionals.
• Accurate, complete, and confidential records of the mental health treatment process.
• Appropriate supervision and periodic monitoring for prescription and administration of behavior-altering medications.
• A basic program for the identification, treatment, and supervision of inmates with suicidal tendencies.

Mental Health Services

Despite the remarkable prevalence of severe mental illness throughout the criminal justice system and the legal responsibility to provide access to medical care, the system has "traditionally provided little in the way of mental health services" (Roesch et al., 1998). In the mid-1980s, Steadman and colleagues (1989) conducted a survey to assess the nature and scope of mental health services provided in U.S. jails. They found that 70% of jails provided some type of mental health screening. All said they provided access to psychotropic medication when needed, but only 30% provided any psychotherapy or counseling services. Seventy-nine percent of jails had the capacity to use inpatient psychiatric services *outside* the jail, while 21% had the additional ability to provide such services *within* the jail. Smaller jails tended to have fewer mental health services and less access to professional staff than did larger jails. Relatively few facilities provided any coordination with outpatient services for mentally ill inmates after their release.

Approximately a decade later, Steadman and Veysey (1997) conducted a similar survey of over 1000 jails of all sizes nationwide. The results were no more encouraging. While a few more jails (83%) reported having a process for mental health screening, less than a third (27%) provided any counseling/therapy and less than half (42%) provided psychiatric medications. While nearly a quarter still reported having the ability to provide inpatient psychiatric treatment within the jail, only about half (48%) said they had the capacity use to these services outside the jail (Steadman & Veysey, 1997). The use of discharge planning and follow-up case management continued to be very rare in jails of all sizes.

Recent evidence suggests that many people with mental illness may not be receiving adequate mental health treatment or even *any* mental health treatment during incarceration—at least in county detention facilities. Data from the Department of Justice's Survey of Inmates in Local Jails revealed that 34.1% of mentally ill jail inmates receive medication as treatment, and 16.2% of mentally ill inmates receive some type of counseling (Ditton, 1999). Similarly, in a study of incarcerated women in the Chicago area, only 25% of those who were determined to be in need of mental health services ever received any service while in the facility.

Some data suggest, however, that the treatment ratio for those in prisons or on probation may be somewhat better. The 1997 Survey of Inmates in State and Federal Correctional Facilities estimated that 60% of state (60.5%) and federal (59.7%) prison inmates identified as being mentally ill had received some type of mental health service since admission. About half had taken a prescribed medication, and a similar proportion had received counseling or therapy. This ratio for receiving counseling services is nearly three times greater than for inmates in local jails.

For probationers with mental illnesses, the proportion who had received counseling/therapy was similar to that of prison inmates (44%), but the proportion receiving medication (37%) or being admitted overnight to a mental hospital or treatment program (12%) was more similar to that of jail inmates (Ditton, 1999).

Specific Populations

Even among inmates and probationers who receive some type of mental health service, many may not have access to specific services that are appropriate to their status or symptoms (Metzner et al., 1998). Although there are myriad disorders and subgroups that can be identified, two in particular merit consideration: women and persons with co-occurring mental health and substance abuse problems. The prevalence of mental illness is overrepresented in both populations (women and substance abusers) at all points in the criminal justice system. Additionally, a substantial body of research suggests that the treatment needs for these groups may differ from those of other inmates or patients, and that only offering services "as usual" may not be effective (Bartels et al., 1995).

As noted above, the prevalence of mental health disorders among women in the criminal justice system is as great as or greater than it is for men. Moreover, female inmates report very high rates of high-risk health behaviors that are also risk factors for mental health disorders. For example, in one study of women in a county jail, nearly half (43%) reported trading sex for money or drugs, more than half had a history of intravenous drug use, and most had been victims of abuse, either sexually (67%) or physically (79%) (Fickenscher et al., 2001). Nevertheless, some have suggested that women in need of mental health services—more often than not—do not receive them while in jail. In a sample of over 1000 female jail detainees, Teplin and colleagues (1997) found that fewer than one in four (23.5%) of those with an identified need received any services.

The nature, degree, and scope of needed services for female inmates also differ from those of men (Veysey, 1998). Many inmates with mental health disorders require a range of services from multiple systems, especially housing; however, female inmates also report a higher prevalence of health problems requiring care (Lindquist and Lindquist, 1999) and substantial needs for job training, family support, and parenting assistance (Alemagno, 2001).

As noted above, a substantial proportion—probably three out of four—of persons in the criminal justice system with mental health disorders also have co-occurring problems with alcohol or drug use. This is a critical finding for two reasons. First, the co-occurrence of substance use problems dramatically increases the risk of arrest or recidivism (Borum et al., 1997; Broner et al., 2002; Lamb and Weinberger, 1998; Solomon and Draine, 1999; Solomon et al., 1994). Second, a large body of research evidence suggests that people who have both a severe mental illness and a substance use problem need an integrated—rather than an additive or disjunctive—treatment approach to ensure an effective response (Drake et al., 1993, 1998). The nature and intensity of services necessary for adequate treatment are different than those for individuals without co-occurring disorders. Thus, to provide clinically appropriate care and to reduce recidivism, it would be necessary to develop specialized—or at least modified—services for this population.

Essential Ingredients

The three key issues in providing mental health services to offenders in the criminal justice system appear to be (1) screening/identification, (2) tailoring services to needs, and (3) discharge planning with linkage to community services. Appropriate screening is necessary to identify persons in need of services. Once they are identified, the facility or supervising entity is responsible for providing access to necessary medical care. Effective care, however, may require attention to specialized programming. Finally, for those transitioning from a facility or supervised care to the community, it is necessary to plan for discharge and aftercare to ensure continuity of services (Veysey et al., 1997).

Continuity of care and aftercare are critical not only for improving symptoms of psychiatric illness, but also for reducing the risk of recidivism among offenders with mental illnesses (National Commission on Correctional Health Care, 1999; Rice and Harris, 1997; Steadman et al., 1989). In one study, for example, 241 jail inmates who had been diagnosed with a mental disorder were followed for 3 years after their release from the facility. Those who received community-based case management did much better than those who did not. Receiving case management in the community reduced the likelihood of any rearrest and extended community tenure before rearrest (Ventura et al., 1998). Similarly, in a study of jail detainees identified as homeless and having a mental illness, the rate of recidivism was strongly related to how many needed services the individual received. Those receiving fewer services—particularly those pertaining to independent living skills—were at much greater risk of recidivism within 6 months of release (Solomon et al., 1994).

Jail Diversion: Primary and Secondary Prevention

Policy makers have long recognized the need to reduce the prevalence of severe mental illness in the criminal justice system by diverting minor offenders away from incarceration and into mental health treatment (Bengelsdorf et al., 1993). This was a major recommendation of the National Coalition for Jail Reform as early as the 1970s, but its realization did not begin on any scale until the 1990s.

Efforts to redirect offenders with mental illness away from incarceration and into community-based treatment services have been referred to generally as *jail diversion* initiatives. There are two actions that are sometimes confused with jail diversion: (*1*) referral and transfer from the jail to a forensic psychiatric facility for evaluation and (*2*) release of a detainee with mental illness to the community pending trial. Neither of these circumstances is formally considered a jail diversion activity, however, since the defendant remains in the criminal justice system instead of being managed by the community mental health system. There are two major types of jail diversion initiatives: pre-booking (before arrest) and post-booking (after arrest).

Pre-Booking Diversion Strategies

Pre-booking diversion occurs before a subject is arrested or formal charges have been filed. The police officer is the primary decision maker at this point in the process. Because police are often the first line of response for these crisis situations, some have even described their role as that of *gatekeepers* to the mental health system.

In many encounters involving minor offenses committed by people with mental illnesses, law enforcement officers have considerable discretion concerning how the case is to be handled. That is, they may decide whether the subject should be directed into the mental health or the criminal justice system. The American Bar Association's *Criminal Justice Mental Health Standards* posit that "When police custody of a mentally ill or mentally retarded person is based exclusively on either non-criminal behavior or minor criminal behavior, the police should either transport the person to an appropriate facility for evaluation or negotiate a voluntary disposition" (Standard 7-2.5 [a]) (ABA, 1986, p. 40). The success or failure of such a policy, however, depends largely on the degree of cooperation between the law enforcement and mental health systems. The police are unlikely to use a mental health disposition if it is difficult or time-consuming.

In a survey of crisis response services in 69 U.S. communities, law enforcement personnel were found to play a critical role in responding to mental health crises in the community (Stroul, 1993). However, the survey found that although the relationship between the community and the police generally was positive, both entities perceived poor response time to be a significant problem. Officers were frustrated by waiting for crisis staff; likewise, crisis staff felt that they often had to wait excessively for a police response and that mental health calls received lesser priority. In addition, some officers felt lacking in their ability to respond effectively to mental health crises and in their understanding of the intervention process. Many law enforcement agencies have taken active measures to understand and respond to these problems.

A national survey of all major police departments was conducted to determine the nature and type of law enforcement–mental health partnerships that exist for pre-booking diversion. Although 88% provided some training for officers related to mental illness, only 45% of departments reported having some type of specialized response to people with mental illness in crisis. Results suggested that most of these programs conformed generally to one of three models (Deane et al., 1998):

- *Police-based specialized police response*: These models involve sworn officers who have special mental health training, provide the first-line police response to mental health crises in the community, and act as liaisons to the formal mental health system; 3.4% of departments had this type of program.
- *Police-based specialized mental health response*: In this model, mental health professionals (not sworn officers) are employed by the police department to provide on-site and telephone consultations to officers in the field; 11.5% of departments had this type of program.
- *Mental health–based specialized mental health response*: In this more traditional model, partnerships or cooperative agreements are developed between police and mobile mental health crisis teams that exist as part of the local community mental health services system and operate independently of the police department; 30% of departments had this type of program.

A similar survey of law enforcement agencies conducted approximately 5 years later (Hails and Borum, 2003) showed some shifting patterns. In the first survey, slightly less than half (45%) of departments reported having some type of specialized response to people with mental illnesses in crisis, but in the later survey only a third (32%) said they had such a response. The most obvious difference was in the number of agencies using a *mental health–based specialized mental health response* such as the mobile crisis team (MCT) from the local mental health center. This was very common in the earlier survey, with nearly a third of agencies (30%) reporting that they used such teams for calls involving people with mental illnesses. In the later survey, only seven agencies (8%) reported using this form of specialized response.

Mental health MCTs were very popular in the 1960s and 1970s. Geller et al. (1995) surveyed departments of mental health in all 50 states and found that 37 (72.5%) of them had some mobile crisis response capacity. However, in the intervening years, many mental health budgets have been reduced substantially, and there has not been much research to support the effectiveness of MCTs (Fisher et al., 1990). Consequently, they may have been eliminated in some jurisdictions.

Perhaps the most striking finding was that although the proportion of agencies using a *police-based specialized mental health response* model was very similar between the two surveys (12% in 1996 vs. 13% in 1999), the use of a *police-based specialized police response* (such as the crisis intervention team [CIT] model) had increased substantially. At the time of the first survey, only six agencies (3%) had these programs, but—despite a smaller sample—nine agencies (11%) had them in place in 1999. This change is likely due to the increased popularity of the Memphis Police Department's CIT program and its use as a model for police departments nationally (Borum, 2000; Cochran et al., 2000; Dupont and Cochran, 2000). At the time of the first survey, there were only three or four CIT programs in existence. Currently, at least 18 police departments across the United States have adopted—or are implementing—a model of specialized response based on the CIT program (S. Cochran, personal communication, August 22, 2001).

The CIT is a police-based program staffed by police officers with special training in mental health issues. The team operates on a generalist-specialist model, so that CIT officers provide a specialized response to *mental disturbance* crisis calls in addition to their regularly assigned patrol duties. For general patrol, the officers are assigned to a specific area; however, CIT officers have citywide jurisdiction for these specialized calls. The officer may resolve the situation on scene through deescalation, negotiation, and verbal crisis intervention; alternatively, she or he may contact an individual's case manager or treatment provider, provide a referral to treatment services, or transport an individual directly to the psychiatric emergency center for further evaluation (Cochran et al., 2000; DuPont and Cochran, 2000). Results of a preliminary case study on the three models of specialized response suggest that, compared to other programs, the Memphis CIT program has a very low arrest rate for mental disturbance calls, a high rate of use by patrol officers, and a rapid response time and results in frequent referrals to treatment (Steadman et al., 2000).

Post-Booking Diversion Strategies

Post-booking diversion initiatives occur after an arrest has been made and formal charges have been filed; however, the precise point and locus of diversion vary by program. Steadman et al. (1994) have identified three core elements of a formal or informal post-booking diversion program:

1. *Screening* defined groups of detainees for the presence of a mental illness
2. *Evaluation* by qualified mental health professional for those identified in the screening phase
3. *Negotiation* between diversion personnel or the defense attorney and the court or prosecutor to establish a mental health disposition, either in lieu of prosecution or as a condition of reduction in charges or community supervision

Using this working definition, Steadman and colleagues (1994) surveyed 760 U.S. jails, inquiring about the existence of diversion programs. Although 34% of jails reported having some type of jail diversion initiative for inmates with mental illness, only 18% actually had a program that met the basic criteria. Many of those who thought that they had a jail diversion program had no community (non-jail)-based diversion dispositions. That is, some persons were diverted *away* from jail but not *into* alternative services. Based on the result of this survey, the authors estimated that, at that time, only about 50 formal jail-based diversion programs existed in the United States.

In the next phase of their research, Steadman and colleagues (1995) conducted a more detailed inquiry into 21 identified programs that did meet the criteria. All of the 21 identified programs served misdemeanor offenders; however, 15 also served nonviolent felons and 10 even included certain violent felons. The violent felons were more frequently included in programs sponsored by smaller jails. Most of the jail diversion programs were based in mental health centers (75%), although less than half were funded by the state department of mental health. Most programs had at least one assigned staff member, although in a third of the programs they had primarily part-time status. Two-thirds of the program directors rated their programs as moderately effective or very effective.

In examining the factors that distinguished the effective programs, six central features emerged (Steadman et al., 1995):

1. *Integrated services*: Offenders with mental illness typically require services from multiple agencies such as mental health, substance abuse, social service, and housing authorities. When multiple services are coordinated within the auspices of a single entity, this degree of integration meets the offender's needs in a way that is more comprehensive and less redundant. Recent research evidence suggests that integrated mental health–substance abuse treatment is particularly effective in reducing arrests and incarceration for people with co-occurring disorders and in significantly reducing associated costs (Clark, et al., 1999).

2. *Regular meetings of key agency representatives*: The most effective programs were those that involved key stakeholders from multiple agencies early in the planning process and maintained regular contact. Regularly scheduled meetings facilitate the sharing of information and concerns and foster a greater coordination of services.

3. *Boundary spanners*: Another key finding was that program effectiveness was highly reliant on the existence of one or more *boundary spanners*, individuals who serve as a formal link or liaison between the mental health–substance abuse service systems and the criminal justice–judicial systems. These designated individuals must have credibility and competence within both systems to manage critical aspects of ongoing interagency relationships and agreements and to facilitate the resolution of conflicts.

4. *Strong leadership*: The existence of a strong leader for the program was also important. The leader should possess strong communication skills, a working knowledge of local criminal justice and mental health systems, and the ability to identify key players and formal and informal networks in both systems.

5. *Early identification*: The screening phase, to identify detainees with possible mental illness, should occur early in the process of criminal justice contact,

ideally within the first 24–48 hours. This will typically occur in the jail, but it may also be done in the arraignment court.

6. *Distinctive case management services*: The case management effort was identified as one of the most critical elements in creating an effective diversion program. Ideally, the case managers, like the boundary spanners, have an understanding of the mental health and criminal justice systems and an ability
to closely monitor supervisees and maintain regular contact. Steadman and
colleagues (1995) argue that it is helpful if the case management staff is similar to the client population in cultural background and racial composition.
Anecdotal evidence suggests that targeted, intensive case management programs such as Assertive Community Treatment (ACT) may help to reduce
rearrest and reincarceration (Lurigio et al., 2000).

Case Example: Montgomery County Emergency Service

In Montgomery County, Pennsylvania, there is an emergency service that has sponsored a jail-based post-booking diversion program for more than 20 years. In this system, inmates who may have a mental illness are identified either during a weekly
screening conducted by a mental health clinician or during the jail intake process by
correctional officers with special training in the identification of mental health problems. Those individuals identified during the screening are then diverted from jail,
typically through one of three mechanisms, depending on the needs and circumstances in the particular case: (*1*) hospitalization, (*2*) supervised community treatment,
and (*3*) dismissal of charges. If the inmate requires psychiatric hospitalization, he or
she may be transferred to a secure inpatient psychiatric unit operated by the emergency service. If the individual's psychiatric condition is more stable, he or she may
be conditionally released into the community on the condition that he or she will receive mental health treatment. In some cases, the criminal charges may be dropped
altogether to avoid any criminal justice involvement if mental health treatment alone
is determined to have a greater likelihood of success (Solomon and Draine, 1999).

A more recent but fast-growing trend in post-booking diversion is the use of
specialty courts to adjudicate and monitor cases—typically misdemeanors—
involving defendants who may have a serious mental illness (Petrila, 2003; Steadman et al., 2001a; Watson et al., 2001). Although drug courts have existed for
decades, the nation's first mental health court was established in Broward County,
Florida. The Broward County Mental Health Task Force, under the leadership of
Judge Mark Speiser, developed the concept for this court. The court began operation in July 1997, under the supervision of Judge Ginger Lerner-Wren, and only
serves defendants with a mental illness who are charged with nonviolent misdemeanors. The intent of this specialty court is to improve the identification, treatment, and monitoring of individuals with mental illness who enter the criminal
justice system in Broward County. It was believed that by creating a special court
to adjudicate these cases, minor offenders with mental illness would be diverted
quickly from incarceration and that the leverage of ongoing court jurisdiction would
facilitate access and adherence to necessary mental health treatment (Petrila et al.,
2001; Poythress et al., 2002).

Any professional involved in the case can refer a defendant for mental health court jurisdiction. Once referred, a hearing is typically held within 24 hours, at which time the defendant has the opportunity to decline specialty court jurisdiction and return to regular misdemeanor court. The process of hearings is nonadversarial, but the court typically retains jurisdiction and monitors the case through status conferences for up to 1 year. The Department of Mental Health Law and Policy at the Louis de la Parte Florida Mental Health Institute of the University of South Florida is currently conducting a systematic evaluation of the mental health court (Boothroyd et al., 2003; McGaha et al., 2002). Preliminary results suggest that participation in the mental health court, as opposed to a regular misdemeanor court, increases the likelihood that the defendant will make initial contact with treatment services and subsequently receive more of those services (Boothroyd et al., 2003).

Conclusion

People with severe mental health disorders are significantly overrepresented throughout the criminal justice system—from police contact to jails, probation, and prisons. Specifically, the prevalence of severe mental illnesses such as schizophrenia, bipolar disorder, and major depression is three to five times higher than in the community (Diamond et al., 2001; Lamb and Weinberger, 1998; Munetz et al., 2001). Moreover, most persons who have these diagnoses also have serious problems with alcohol and/or illicit drugs. Women in the criminal justice system have at least as many mental health problems as men; however, they also have more health problems and greater needs for supportive services. The number of women in the system is also growing at an alarming rate.

Although correctional facilities are not permitted knowingly to withhold necessary medical care, many inmates who have mental illnesses, especially in jails, do not receive any mental health services and certainly do not receive services appropriate to their specific condition or symptom pattern. The process of managing large numbers of minor offenders with substantial mental health needs in the criminal justice system is costly and burdensome.

Implications for Mental Health Services

As an alternative, many jurisdictions are attempting to reduce recidivism and improve treatment for people with mental illness by diverting those charged with minor crimes away from jail and into the mental health system, where they may receive necessary treatment. Developing an effective system for diverting misdemeanor offenders with mental illness out of jail and into treatment requires a multilayered approach. The foundation of these efforts consists of strong partnerships between the criminal justice and mental health systems and the allocation of mental health resources in a way that views reducing recidivism and criminal justice contact as important treatment-related outcomes (Olivero and Hansen, 1994).

The first element of effective diversion is to develop a strong, comprehensive emergency response. This includes the availability of mental health services during times of crisis, as well as the establishment of a specialized law enforcement response to people with mental illnesses (Steadman et al., 2001b).

The second element, at the post-booking level, is to implement a systematic screening process to identify individuals with a mental illness who are arrested and/or booked into jail. While it may be helpful to have officers make a notation if they book a subject whom they suspect may have a mental illness, it is also necessary to have a more formal screening mechanism to identify those whose symptoms may not be recognized during a field encounter. The local mental health authority can contribute to this effort by developing a case identification system such as the one used in Broward County, Florida, where a representative from the mental health agency obtains the booking roster every morning from the county jail and checks that list against the agency's record of mental health clients. The correctional authority may contribute by conducting a routine screening for mental health problems or taking a treatment history at intake.

The third element is to develop and provide appropriate treatment resources. Successful jail diversion efforts require more than simply diverting an individual with mental illness *away from* jail; he or she must also be directed *into* adequate treatment services. This includes (1) focused, intensive resources for high-risk groups, using program such as ACT, intensive case management, or increased supervision and (2) integrated services for persons with co-occurring mental health and substance use disorders.

Building a strong crisis response capacity, identifying people in need of mental health services, and implementing effective and integrated services are investments in primary and secondary prevention that yield large cost savings in tertiary care (e.g., hospitalization) and incapacitation (e.g., correctional confinement). Moreover, these interventions reduce the likelihood that mental health consumers will become mired in the criminal justice system and substantially increase the likelihood of positive therapeutic outcomes.

REFERENCES

Abram KM, Teplin LA. Co-occurring disorders among mentally ill jail detainees: implications for public policy. *American Psychologist*, 46:1036–1045, 1991.

Alemagno S. Women in jail: is substance abuse treatment enough? *American Journal of Public Health*, 91:798–800, 2001.

American Bar Association. *Criminal Justice Mental Health Standards*. Chicago: American Bar Association, 1986.

Bartels SJ, Drake RE, Wallach MA. Long-term course of substance use disorders among patients with severe mental illness. *Psychiatric Services*, 46(3):248–251, 1995.

Beck A. Prisoners in 1999. *Bureau of Justice Statistics Bulletin*. Washington, DC: U.S. Department of Justice, 2000.

Bengelsdorf H, Church JO, Kaye RA, et al. The cost effectiveness of crisis intervention: admission diversion savings can offset the high cost of service. *Journal of Nervous and Mental Disease*, 181:757–762, 1993.

Bonovitz JC, Bonovitz JS. Diversion of the mentally ill into the criminal justice system: the police intervention perspective. *American Journal of Psychiatry*, 138(7):973–976, 1981.

Boothroyd R, Poythress N, McGaha A, et al. The Broward Mental Health Court: process, outcomes and service utilization. *International Journal of Law and Psychiatry*, 26(1): 55–71, 2003.

Borum R. Improving high risk encounters between people with mental illness and the police. *Journal of the American Academy of Psychiatry and the Law*, 28:332–337, 2000.

Borum R, Swanson J, Swartz M, et al. Substance abuse, violent behavior and police encounters among persons with severe mental disorder. *Journal of Contemporary Criminal Justice*, 13:236–250, 1997.

Broner N, Borum R, Gawley K. Criminal justice diversion of individuals with co-occurring mental illness and substance use disorders: an overview. In: Landsberg G, Rock M, Berg L (eds). *Serving Mentally Ill Offenders: Challenges and Opportunities for Mental Health Professionals*. New York: Springer, 2002.

Clark R, Ricketts S, McHugo G. Legal system involvement and costs for persons in treatment for severe mental illness and substance use disorders. *Psychiatric Services*, 50 (5):641–647, 1999.

Cochran S, Deane M, Borum R. Improving police response to mentally ill people in crisis: crisis intervention teams. *Psychiatric Services*, 51:1315–1316, 2000.

Cohen F. *The Mentally Disordered Inmate and the Law*. Kingston, NJ: Civic Research Institute, 1998.

Cote G, Hodgins S. Co-occurring mental disorder among criminal offenders. *Bulletin of the American Academy of Psychiatry and Law*, 16:333–342, 1990.

Daniel AE, Robins AJ, Reid JC, et al. Lifetime and six-month prevalence of psychiatric disorders among sentenced female offenders. *Bulletin of the American Academy of Psychiatry and Law*, 16:333–342, 1988.

Deane M, Steadman H, Borum R, et al. Police–mental health system interactions: program types and needed research. *Psychiatric Services*, 50:99–101, 1998.

Department of Justice. *1983 Census*. Ottawa: ON: Statistics Canada, 1984.

Diamond P, Wang E, Holzer C, et al. The prevalence of mental illness in prison. *Administration and Policy in Mental Health*, 29:21–40, 2001.

Ditton PM. Mental health and treatment of inmates and probationers. *Bureau of Justice Statistics Special Report*. Washington, DC: U.S. Department of Justice, July 1999.

Draine J, Solomon P. Describing and evaluating jail diversion services for persons with serious mental illness. *Psychiatric Services*, 50:56–61, 1999.

Drake RE, Bartels SJ, Teague GB, et al. Treatment of substance abuse in severely mentally ill patients. *Journal of Nervous and Mental Disease*, 181:606–611, 1993.

Drake RE, Mercer-McFadden C, Mueser K, et al. Review of integrated mental health and substance abuse treatment for patients with dual disorders. *Schizophrenia Bulletin*, 24:589–608, 1998.

Dupont R, Cochran S. Police response to mental health emergencies: barriers to change. *Journal of the American Academy of Psychiatry and the Law*, 28(3):338–344, 2000.

Engel RS, Silver E. Policing mentally disordered suspects: a re-examination of the criminalization hypothesis. *Criminology*, 39(2):225–252, 2001.

Fickenscher A, Lapidus J, Silk-Walker P, et al. Women behind bars: health needs of inmates in a county jail. *Public Health Reports*, 116(3):191–196, 2001.

Fisher WH, Geller JL, Wirth-Cauchon J. Empirically assessing the impact of mobile crisis capacity on state hospital admissions. *Community Mental Health Journal*, 26:245–253, 1990.

Frankle WG, Shera D, Berger-Hershkowitz H, et al. Clozapine-associated reduction in arrest rates of psychotic patients with criminal histories. *American Journal of Psychiatry*, 158:270–274, 2001.

Geller JL, Fisher WH, McDermeit M. A national survey of mobile crisis services and their evaluation. *Psychiatric Services*, 46:893–897, 1995.

Guy E, Platt JJ, Zwerling I, et al. Mental health status of prisoners in an urban jail. *Criminal Justice and Behavior*, 12:29–53, 1985.

Hails J, Borum R. Police training and specialized approaches for responding to people with mental illnesses. *Crime and Delinquency*, 49(1):52–61, 2003.

Janik J. Dealing with mentally ill offenders. *FBI Law Enforcement Bulletin*, 61(7):22–26, 1992.

Lamb HR, Grant RW. Mentally ill women in a county jail. *Archives of General Psychiatry*, 40:363–368, 1983.

Lamb HR, Weinberger LE. Persons with severe mental illness in jails and prisons: a review. *Psychiatric Services*, 49(4):483–492, 1998.

Lindquist CH, Lindquist CA. Health behind bars: utilization and evaluation of medical care among jail inmates. *Journal of Community Health*, 24:285–303, 1999.

Lurigio A, Fallon J, Dincin J. Helping the mentally ill in jails adjust to community life: a description of a post-release ACT program and its clients. *International Journal of Offender Therapy and Comparative Criminology*, 44(5):532–548, 2000.

MaGaha A, Boothroyd RA, Poythress NG, et al. Lessons from the Broward County mental health court evaluation. *Program Planning and Evaluation*, 25:125–135, 2002.

McFarland B, Faulkner L, Bloom J, et al. Chronic mental illness and the criminal justice system. *Hospital and Community Psychiatry*, 40:718–723, 1989.

Metzner J, Cohen F, Grossman L, et al. Treatment in jails and prisons. In: Wettstein R (ed). *Treatment of Offenders with Mental Disorders*. New York: Guilford Press, pp. 211–264, 1998.

Monahan J, Steadman HJ. *Mentally Disordered Offenders: Perspectives from Law and Social Science*. New York: Plenum, 1983.

Munetz M, Grande T, Chambers M. The incarceration of individuals with severe mental disorders. *Community Mental Health Journal*, 37(4):361–372, 2001.

National Commission on Correctional Health Care. *Correctional Mental Health Care: Standards and Guidelines for Delivering Services*. New York: Center on Crime, Communities and Culture of the Open Society Institute, 1999.

Neighbors HW. The prevalence of mental disorder in Michigan prisons. *DIS Newsletter*, 4:8–10, 1987.

Olivero JM, Hansen R. Linkage agreements between mental health and law enforcement agencies: managing suicidal persons. *Administration and Policy in Mental Health*, 24:217–225, 1994.

Petrila J. An introduction to special jurisdiction courts. *International Journal of Law and Psychiatry*, 26(1):3–12, 2003.

Petrila J, Poythress N, McGaha A, et al. Preliminary observations from an evaluation of the Broward County Florida Mental Health Court. *Court Review*, Winter, 14–22, 2001.

Poythress N, Petrila J, McGaha A, et al. Perceived coercion and procedural justice in the Broward Mental Health Court. *International Journal of Law and Psychiatry* 25:517–533, 2002.

Rice ME, Harris GT. The treatment of mentally disordered offenders. *Psychology, Public Policy, and Law*, 3(1):126–183, 1997.

Roesch R, Ogloff JRP, Zapf PA, et al. Jail and prison inmates. In: Bellack AS, Hersen M (eds). *Comprehensive Clinical Psychology: Applications in Diverse Populations* Amsterdam: Elsevier, pp. 85–104, 1998.

Singer R. Providing mental health services for jail inmates: legal perspectives. *Journal of Prison Health*, 1:105–129, 1981.

Solomon P, Draine J. Explaining lifetime criminal arrests among clients of a psychiatric probation and parole service. *Journal of the American Academy of Psychiatry and the Law*, 27(2):239–251, 1999.

Solomon P, Draine J, Meyerson A. Jail recidivism and receipt of community mental health services. *Hospital and Community Psychiatry*, 45:793–797, 1994.

Steadman HJ, Barbera SS, Dennis DL. A national survey of jail diversion programs for mentally ill detainees. *Hospital and Community Psychiatry*, 45:1109–1113, 1994.

Steadman HJ, Davidson S, Brown C. Mental health courts: their promise and unanswered questions. *Psychiatric Services*, 52:457–458, 2001a.

Steadman H, Deane M, Borum R, et al. Comparing outcomes of major models for police responses to mental health emergencies. *Psychiatric Services*, 51:645–649, 2000.

Steadman H, McCarty D, Morrissey J. *The Mentally Ill in Jail: Planning for Essential Services.* New York: Guilford Press, 1989.

Steadman HJ, Morris SM, Dennis DL. The diversion of mentally ill persons from jails to community-based services: a profile of programs. *American Journal of Public Health*, 85(12):1630–1635, 1995.

Steadman H, Stainbrook K, Griffin P, et al. A specialized crisis response site as a core element of police-based diversion programs. *Psychiatric Services*, 52(2):219–222, 2001b.

Steadman H, Veysey B. Providing services for jail inmates with mental disorders. *NIJ Research in Brief.* Washington, DC: U.S. Department of Justice, Office of Justice Programs, April 1997.

Stroul BA. *Psychiatric Crisis Response Systems: A Descriptive Study.* Rockville, MD: National Institute of Mental Health, 1993.

Swank G, Winer D. Occurrence of psychiatric disorders in a county jail population. *American Journal of Psychiatry*, 133:1331–1333, 1976.

Swartz JA, Lurigio AJ. Psychiatric illness and comorbidity among adult male jail detainees in drug treatment. *Psychiatric Services*, 50(12):1628–1630, 1999.

Swartz M, Swanson J, Wagner R, et al. Can involuntary outpatient commitment reduce hospital recidivism? Findings from a randomized controlled trial in severely mentally ill individuals. *American Journal of Psychiatry*, 156(12):1968–1975, 1999.

Teplin LA. Criminalizing mental disorder. *American Psychologist*, 39:794–803, 1984.

Teplin LA, Abram KA, McClelland GM. Prevalence of psychiatric disorders among incarcerated women. *Archives of General Psychiatry*, 53:505–512, 1996.

Teplin LA, Abram KA, McClelland GM. Mentally disordered women in jail: who receives services? *American Journal of Public Health*, 87(4):604–609, 1997.

Torrey EF, Stieber J, Ezekiel J, et al. *Criminalizing the Seriously Mentally Ill: The Abuse of Jails as Mental Hospitals.* Washington, DC: National Alliance for the Mentally Ill and Public Citizen's Health Research Group, 1992.

Ventura LA, Cassel CA, Jacoby JE, et al. Case management and recidivism of mentally ill persons released from jail. *Psychiatric Services*, 49(10):1330–1337, 1998.

Veysey B. Specific needs of women diagnosed with mental illnesses in U.S. jails. In: Levin BL, Blanch AK, Jennings A (eds.) *Women's Mental Health Services: A Public Health Perspective*, Thousand Oaks, CA, Sage, pp. 368–389, 1998.

Veysey B, Steadman H, Morrissey J, et al. In search of the missing linkages: continuity of care in U.S. jails. *Behavioral Sciences and the Law*, 15:383–397, 1997.

Washington P, Diamond RJ. Prevalence of mental illness among women incarcerated in five California county jails. *Research in Community and Mental Health*, 5:33–41, 1985.

Watson A, Luchins D, Hanrahan P. Mental health court: promises and limitations. *Journal of the American Academy of Psychiatry and Law*, 28:476–482, 2001.

15

Racial and Ethnic Minorities

EMILY S. IHARA
DAVID TAKEO TAKEUCHI

The Surgeon General's report, *Mental Health: Culture, Race, and Ethnicity—A Supplement to Mental Health: A Report of the Surgeon General* (2001), finds that racial and ethnic minorities are not only less likely than whites to use services for their mental health problems but are more likely to receive poor quality and inappropriate mental health care (U.S. Department of Health and Human Services [DHHS], 2001). While the findings in the Surgeon General's report are alarming, they are not new. Racial and ethnic disparities in mental health care have been identified and documented for more than 30 years. Although some improvements have been made in the service delivery system, barriers to mental health care persist for racial and ethnic minorities. The report is unique because it is the first time that the high office of the Surgeon General has called attention to mental health issues pertinent to racial and ethnic minorities. This chapter reviews current knowledge about the prevalence of mental disorders, use of services by racial and ethnic minorities, factors explaining the gap between need and care, and the implications for service delivery. A public health model that recognizes the complex interaction of biological, psychological, cultural, economic, and social factors in the environment is particularly useful in our search for a delivery system that promotes mental health and well-being for the entire population.

The Social Context of Minority Mental Health

Race and ethnicity are critical factors in understanding who gets sick, how and where they are treated, and who gets access to quality health care in the United States (Abe-Kim and Takeuchi, 1996; Moscicki et al., 1989; Somervell et al., 1989). These issues are best understood as a reflection of the larger context and structure of our society, specifically how various factors lead to differential outcomes along racial lines. The challenge in understanding the causal pathways and mechanisms by which this occurs is confounded by a lack of clear consensus about definitions, concepts, and measurement of terms such as *race, ethnicity,* and *social class.*

Race and Ethnicity

Despite the use of *race* and *ethnicity* in a wide range of public policy debates, the terms are frequently contested. The popular view of race, also known as *essentialism,* categorizes people into distinct, unambiguous groups based on a set of putative biological traits (e.g., skin color). Essentialism sees racial categories as fixed and constant over time. This view is contrary to current scientific evidence noting limited biological variations across racial groups (Owens and King, 1999). Many social scientists use a more comprehensive definition of race that acknowledges not only the genetic, demographic, and geographical diversity among humans, but also the social and cultural conceptualizations of race and ethnicity (Smelser et al., 2001). The concept of ethnicity is often used interchangeably with race. *Ethnicity* refers to the sense of community or identification with others on the basis of language, nationality, or cultural characteristics (Kaplan et al., 1998). The two concepts, *race* and *ethnicity,* overlap because members of a racial group may share a history and a cultural bond. What separates the two from each other is that race involves distinguishing physical attributes, as seen by group members or others, that make it difficult to change racial identities.

Although race is socially constructed, it does not follow that the concept of race is insignificant. Biological notions of race may not explain much of the variation among groups, but race has both meaning and consequence in a racialized society where race is deeply embedded in the consciousness of individuals, groups, institutions, and policies. Racial categories carry with them implicit and explicit stereotypes about group members, which form the basis for the treatment of individuals within racial groups. Race is particularly meaningful when members of a group are subjected to unequal treatment and access to goods and resources as a result of prejudice and discrimination (Williams, 2000). The concepts of race and ethnicity are used interchangeably throughout this chapter but are meant to capture the historical, political, economic, and social factors that have shaped the minority status of different groups.

Minority Status versus Socioeconomic Position

Considerable debate has taken place over the extent to which disparities in health care use for racial and ethnic minorities can be attributed to minority status or socioeconomic position. The *minority status* argument contends that stratification by race/ethnicity produces inequalities in economic resources, job opportunities, social prestige and influence, and political power. According to this view, racism has been institutionalized by the sanctioning of unequal access to resources and services through policies, priorities, and accepted practices (Sue and Sue, 1999). Institutionalized racism creates obstacles to economic, educational, and occupational parity in American society (Allen and Farley, 1986; Duncan, 1969; Farley, 1984). The discrepancies between minorities and dominant group members create a social environment characterized by alienation, frustration, and powerlessness. Distress, demoralization, and more serious forms of psychopathology are likely to result from this environment (McCarthy and Yancey, 1971; Silberman, 1964). Minority status itself can be considered a stressor, regardless of socioeconomic and demographic predictors of mental health problems (Vega and Rumbaut, 1991).

On the other hand, social class is one of the strongest determinants of variations in health status (Krieger et al., 1997). *Socioeconomic position* refers to interdependent economic relationships based on people's structural location within the economy. A person's social position is represented by the stratified distributions of income, wealth, education, and social status (Krieger et al., 1997). Lower socioeconomic position can lead to higher levels of distress regardless of ethnic minority status (Ilfeld, 1978; Neff, 1985; Roberts and Vernon, 1984; Roberts et al., 1981; Warheit et al., 1975) but, more important, reflects limited access to economic and social resources.

Some researchers argue that minority status and socioeconomic position are not mutually exclusive and that the interaction between the two is especially significant. Neighbors (1990) suggests that, because of their limited access to power and resources, some ethnic minority groups may be more at risk to live in poverty, which in turn increases their chances of developing mental health problems. Socioeconomic position may be part of the causal pathway by which race affects mental health status (Cooper and David, 1986). Socioeconomic differences among the races reflect the impact of economic discrimination by societal structures. The fact that there is considerable error in the measurement of socioeconomic position across racial groups further complicates the issue and points to the need for continued study about how position in social structure may be linked to health status (Krieger et al., 1997).

Demographic Changes

Issues related to race, ethnicity, and socioeconomic position are particularly noteworthy as racial and ethnic minority populations in the United States continue to grow. The total U.S. population in 2000 was 75.1% white, 12.3% African American, 12.5% Hispanic, 3.6% Asian, 0.9% American Indian and Alaska Native, and 0.1% Native Hawaiian and other Pacific Islander[1] (U.S. Bureau of the Census, 2001). Between 1990 and 2000, the white population increased by 5.9% to 211 million people, whereas the growth rates of racial and ethnic minorities were much higher.[2] African Americans have historically been the largest ethnic minority group in the United States. During the 1990s, this population grew by 15.6% to 34.7 million. The Latino/Hispanic population has surpassed African Americans as the largest ethnic minority group; their population has increased rapidly by 57.9% to 35.3 million, due to higher birth and immigration rates. Asian Americans (newly separated from Pacific Islanders in the 2000 Census) grew at the second highest rate of 48.3% to 10.2 million. The American Indian and Alaska Native populations grew by 26.4% to 2.5 million (U.S. Bureau of the Census, 2001). These rapid demographic changes call for continued and improved research of the mental health status of various groups so that our mental health care system can effectively address their needs.

Prevalence of Disorders and Use of Mental Health Services

Much of the research on ethnic minorities and mental health care has focused on the question "Are we providing racial and ethnic minorities with mental health services that are responsive to their needs?" The design and implementation of relevant mental health services requires some estimate of the number of people who are in need of services and how those who receive or seek services differ from those who do not. Ideally, nationally representative studies would yield prevalence rates for each mental disorder within a given minority population for comparison to the U.S. population as a whole. Although such studies are currently in progress, the results are not yet available. However, findings from smaller studies estimate that the overall rate of mental illness for minorities is similar to the overall rate of about 21% across the U.S. population (DHHS, 2001).

Use of mental health services is best predicted by need, but the concept of need can be defined in many ways—for example, as the level of psychological distress, the number of psychiatric symptoms, the psychiatric diagnosis, self-reports of mental health, or limitations in mental health functioning (Greenley and Mechanic, 1976). Need is shaped both by the individual and by his or her social and cultural circumstances. For example, need may indicate the extent to which an individual's psychiatric symptoms disrupt work, school, or other activities on the basis of his or her own conceptions of normal functioning. Need may also reflect the extent to which the external environment (family, community, etc.) cannot tolerate the deviant behavior (Mechanic, 1999).

Although using treatment rates from clinic and hospital records to estimate the prevalence of mental health problems has been a common practice, this method may underestimate actual need because of differences in help-seeking patterns, sources of care, and the tendency by some to present with somatic complaints (Mechanic, 1999). Service use is not an accurate representation of need, particularly for racial and ethnic minorities, many of whom experience barriers to service access and use and may not have contact with conventional treatment facilities. Furthermore, when treatment data are used, factors related to the occurrence of mental disorders are difficult to separate from factors that influence the processes of seeking and receiving mental health care, such as financing options, available transportation, the client's economic status, and the accuracy of the diagnosis (Mechanic, 1999; Williams and Harris-Reid, 1999).

A common method for estimating the prevalence of mental health disorders uses survey research methods to select a sample of residents representative of a total community, regardless of their service use. This method avoids the selection biases associated with treatment studies but presents another challenge of small sample sizes for some minority population groups. Summaries of the use of mental health services and the mental health status for four racial groups will be presented in this section.

African Americans

Findings from treatment studies have shown a consistent pattern of overrepresentation of both inpatient and outpatient mental health care for African Americans (Cheung and Snowden, 1990; Snowden, 1999; Snowden and Cheung, 1990). Although these findings have led to speculation that African Americans have higher rates of mental disorders than whites, community surveys have found both higher and lower rates of mental disorder for African Americans compared to whites (Vega and Rumbaut, 1991). The findings from two of the largest and most comprehensive studies provide evidence that rates of mental illness for African Americans are similar to those of the general population. The Epidemiologic Catchment Area (ECA) Study found that African Americans had rates of major depressive disorder and dysthymia comparable to or lower than those of whites (Robins and Regier, 1991; Somervell et al., 1989). Notable differences in rates for African Americans compared to whites were seen in anxiety disorders, specifically simple phobia, social phobia, and agoraphobia (Brown et al., 1990). However, findings from the National Comorbidity Study (NCS) showed that African Americans living in the community had lower rates of disorder than whites in all of the major classes of disorders, a lower lifetime prevalence of mental illness than whites, and no differences in panic disorder, simple phobia, or agoraphobia (Kessler et al., 1994). Future epidemiological studies may help to resolve these discrepancies.

Asian Americans and Pacific Islanders

Treatment studies have identified a consistent pattern of underuse of inpatient and outpatient mental health care for Asian Americans and Pacific Islanders (Leong, 1986; Matsuoka et al., 1997; Snowden and Cheung, 1990). Accurate prevalence rates of mental disorders have been difficult to estimate for this population due to insufficient sample sizes. Both the ECA and NCS had sample sizes that were too small and not representative of any particular subgroup to make meaningful estimates. However, in several community studies, Chinese, Japanese, Filipino, and Korean Americans in Seattle (Kuo, 1984; Kuo and Tsai, 1986), Korean immigrants in Chicago (Hurh and Kim, 1990), and Chinese Americans in San Francisco (Ying, 1988) had higher scores for depression than whites.

The Chinese American Psychiatric Epidemiological Study (CAPES), conducted in 1993–94, is the largest mental health study to date of any Asian American subgroup. It examined rates of depression among 1747 Chinese Americans in the greater Los Angeles area (Takeuchi et al., 1998). Findings from the CAPES showed lifetime and 12-month rates that were lower than those found in the NCS; however, rates for dysthymia were more similar to estimates from the NCS (Kessler et al., 1994; Takeuchi et al., 1998). Further study of subgroups of Asian American and Pacific Islander populations will provide a better understanding of the role of factors such as generational differences, level of acculturation, and refugee status.

Hispanics/Latinos

Patterns of mental health service use have not been clear for Latinos. Snowden and Cheung (1990) found slight overrepresentation of Latinos compared to whites in state and county mental hospitals but underrepresentation in psychiatric units of general hospitals, Veterans Administration medical centers, and private psychiatric hospitals. Previous studies also show mixed findings. In a review of 17 studies on the use of inpatient care among Mexican Americans, Lopez (1981) found that this group was underrepresented in psychiatric hospitals in 12 studies; the remaining 5 studies showed proportional representation or overrepresentation. Other national studies have shown higher use of inpatient services and lower use of outpatient services for an insured Latino population (Padgett et al., 1994a, 1994b).

Research on the prevalence of mental illness in the Hispanic population does not provide a clear understanding of subgroup differences. In the Hispanic Health and Nutrition Examination Survey (HHANES), which collected data from a large area of the Southwest, some subgroup differences were found. Puerto Ricans in New York City had high rates of depression, and Cubans in Miami had significantly lower rates of depression than other Hispanic groups in the HHANES. These findings must be interpreted with caution because of small sample sizes, high refusal rates, and the lack of comparative data from other U.S. sites (Vega and Rumbaut, 1991).

Although in some studies Mexican Americans had higher rates of depression than whites and African Americans, they had lower rates of depression than other Hispanics in the HHANES (Vega and Rumbaut, 1991). In contrast, the Los Angeles ECA Study, which oversampled Mexican Americans, found that Mexican Americans and whites had similar rates of psychiatric disorder. Important differences were found when the Mexican American group was separated into two subgroups; those born in the United States had higher rates of depression and phobias than those born in Mexico. Vega and colleagues (1998) examined rates of psychiatric disorders of Mexican Americans living in Fresno County, California, and found that approximately 25% of the Mexican immigrants compared to 48% of U.S.-born Mexican Americans had a mental disorder or substance abuse disorder. These findings indicate the importance of further understanding the role of immigration and acculturation, help-seeking behavior, and nativity.

American Indians and Alaska Natives

Similarly, patterns of use for American Indians and Alaska Natives have not been consistent. Data from 1983 (Cheung and Snowden, 1990) showed inpatient and outpatient use for American Indians at rates equal to their proportion in the general population. However, two studies of outpatient use in Seattle found greater than expected use for American Indians and Alaska Natives (O'Sullivan et al., 1989). Almost all the research to date for this population has focused on substance-related disorders; thus conclusions are incomplete without more empirical data about mental health service use (Manson, 2000).

Findings to date on the prevalence of mental disorders have been based on smaller studies of convenience samples or clinic populations. Although limited in their generalizability, these findings suggest that there may be high rates of depression among American Indians; 69% had a definite or probable diagnosis and 32% had moderate or severe psychiatric impairment (Kinzie et al., 1992). Furthermore, there appears to be high comorbidity of alcohol disorders with depression in this population. For example, of those with a history of major depression, 66% also met the criteria for alcohol abuse and dependence (Kinzie et al., 1992).

Recently, the American Indian Services Utilization, Psychiatric Epidemiology, Risk and Protective Factors Project (AI-SUPERPFP) was completed. This large-scale, multistage study of prevalence and use rates of over 3000 individuals in two large American Indian communities will provide substantive knowledge about the need for mental health care among American Indians (DHHS, 2001). Better estimates of prevalence will facilitate the design and implementation of more relevant services for this population.

Future Studies

Several collaborative projects funded by the National Institute of Mental Health (NIMH) are currently underway and will add to our understanding of the prevalence and distribution of mental illness among various minority groups. The National Survey of Health and Stress (NSHS) will interview nearly 20,000 adolescents and adults to estimate the prevalence of mental disorders in the United States. In order to collect data about specific subgroups in the African American, Asian American, and Latino populations, NIMH has also funded two studies—the National Survey of American Lives (NSAL) and the National Latino and Asian American Survey (NLAAS). Substantial portions of the NSHS, NSAL, and NLAAS surveys have been coordinated for the purposes of cross-study comparisons and together will provide one of the most comprehensive sources of symptom patterns, prevalence rates of disorders, access to services, and functioning for different racial and ethnic minority groups and subgroups (DHHS, 2001).

Understanding Differential Use of Mental Health Services

Although use patterns have been used to speculate about the rates of psychopathology among ethnic minority groups, these patterns may more accurately reflect the inappropriateness of existing services, access barriers, fear of institutionalization, limited awareness of or access to existing services, cultural stigma against mental illness, or culture-specific help-seeking behavior (Snowden and Cheung, 1990; Sue and Morishima, 1982; Sussman et al., 1987). Research indicates that there is a gap between need and care for the general population. Over 60% of all individuals with mental health problems never receive professional care, and only about 25% of those who do receive care use specialty mental health services (Kessler et al., 1994). Racial and ethnic minorities are even less likely to use mental health services than whites (Leaf et al., 1985). Use of mental health services is importantly affected by structural factors (e.g., accessibility of the health care system, availability of services, cultural and linguistic appropriateness of services), individual factors (e.g., personal health practices and beliefs, help-seeking behavior, stigma), system factors (e.g., assessment tools, treatment options, alternative treatment systems), and outcomes (e.g., treatment effectiveness, perceived health status). All of these factors influence one another, and race/ethnicity may enter into the process at multiple points. A discussion of all of the factors that influence service use for racial and ethnic minorities is beyond the scope of this chapter. However, essential components, such as accessibility, availability, cultural differences, help-seeking behavior, assessment, and treatment effectiveness will be explored in this section.

Accessibility of Care

Insurance coverage, which is intrinsically tied to socioeconomic position and workforce issues, is one of the most critical components of access to care. Many Americans are unable to afford health insurance or are underinsured, forcing those who do not qualify for low-income health insurance to pay high out-of-pocket costs for care or delay treatment. Racial and ethnic minorities have higher rates of uninsurance than whites (Hargraves, 2000). Nearly 25% of African Americans, 37% of Latinos, 24% of American Indians/Alaska Natives, and 21% of Asian Americans/Pacific Islanders do not have health insurance compared to 14% of whites (Brown et al., 2000). Within subgroup populations, the rate may be even more pronounced. For example, 32% of Korean Americans are uninsured, and 20% of Chinese Americans and Filipino Americans do not have health insurance (Brown et al., 2000).

Income and employment are key factors in access to health insurance because the majority of people get their health insurance through employer-based coverage. Overwhelmingly, those who are uninsured and underinsured are racial and ethnic minorities who are disproportionately represented in marginal and low-wage job sectors. The rate of employer-based coverage is substantially lower for ethnic minorities than for employed whites. Compared with 73% of employed whites, only 53% of African Americans, 43% of Latinos, 64% of Asian Americans and Pacific Islanders, and 51% of American Indians and Alaska Natives have employer-based health insurance (Brown et al., 2000).

An important source of coverage for low-income populations is Medicaid, particularly because Medicaid-funded providers have been more successful in reducing disparities in access to mental health treatment (Snowden and Thomas, 2000). Medicaid covers nearly 21% of African Americans, 18% of Latinos, and 25% of American Indians and Alaska Natives. Attention to mental health coverage in the Medicaid program may help increase access to some low-income racial and ethnic minorities but not to all. Asian Americans and Pacific Islanders have relatively low rates of Medicaid participation compared to whites. This may be explained in part by various barriers to Medicaid enrollment, including the misperception by immigrants that participation in a public program would jeopardize their immigration status (Brown et al., 2000).

Most people who have insurance coverage are enrolled in managed care systems. In 1999, almost 72% of Americans with health insurance were enrolled in managed behavioral health organizations (DHHS, 2001). Managed care has developed in response to the crisis in health care costs and has the potential to improve access, use, and quality of services. However, previously identified barriers to mental health care for racial and ethnic minorities have not necessarily been considered in a systematic manner by managed care models, which may perpetuate the problem or create new barriers to access and treatment (Abe-Kim and Takeuchi, 1996).

Availability of Services

The provider pool may impede ethnic minorities from seeking treatment or remaining in treatment in the conventional mental health system. Minority patients who prefer to see mental health professionals with similar racial and ethnic backgrounds may find it difficult or impossible, because most mental health professionals are white. A 1998 study reports that among clinically trained mental health professionals, only 2% of psychiatrists, 2% of psychologists, and 4% of social workers are African American. There are only 2.0 Hispanic psychiatrists for every 100,000 Hispanics and 1.5 American Indian/Alaska Native psychiatrists for every 100,000 American Indians/Alaska Natives in this country (DHHS, 2001).

Given the verbal nature of mental health services, those with limited English proficiency encounter significant barriers in the mental health system. Insufficient information is available about the language capabilities of mental health providers to have a full understanding of this issue. However, it has been noted that almost one out of every two Asian Americans will have difficulty accessing mental health treatment because they do not speak English or cannot find services that meet their language needs (DHHS, 2001). In 1990, about 40% of Latinos spoke limited English or no English at all. The percentage of Spanish-speaking mental health professionals is not known, but a recent survey found that there were 29 Latino mental health professionals for every 100,000 Latinos in the U.S. population compared to 173 white providers per 100,000 whites (DHHS, 2001). Although continued efforts to increase the pool of minority providers are necessary, the more encompassing concept of *cultural competence* may have better potential to change policies and practices on a systemwide level.

Cultural Factors

Rogler and colleagues (1987) argue that problems attributed to cultural insensitivity are partly due to the incongruence between the characteristics of the mental health system and minority cultures. Specifically, assessment instruments, clinicians, and practices and policies in mental health programs and systems do not adequately address the needs of minority clients. Dropout rates of ethnic minorities are a useful barometer of the responsiveness of mental health services (Neighbors et al., 1992; Sue et al., 1994). For example, African Americans are more likely than whites to terminate treatment prematurely (Sue et al., 1994), indicating that their needs are not being addressed even though they were able to access treatment. In a classic study, Sue and McKinney (1975) found that the dropout rate for ethnic minorities was about 50% compared to 30% of whites. O'Sullivan and colleagues (1989) found that the dropout rate for ethnic minorities had diminished significantly over a 10-year period, during which the mental health system had made significant efforts to hire more ethnic minority service providers and create more ethnic-specific services.

More than 25 years ago, Sue (1977) made a number of recommendations to improve the delivery of mental health services to members of minority groups including (*1*) making changes within existing services, such as hiring more ethnic specialists or training mental health care providers to work with minority groups; (*2*) establishing independent but parallel services specifically devoted to ethnic minorities; and (*3*) creating new and nonparallel services that are culturally relevant. Other researchers have made recommendations based on theory involving cultural match or fit rather than on definitive research findings of treatment outcomes (Sue, 1998).

A combination of such recommendations, greater minority community empowerment through the civil rights movement of the 1960s, and a more widespread acceptance of the inadequacies of the mental health system for ethnic minorities has resulted in some positive changes over recent decades. More ethnic professionals have been hired by community psychiatric clinics in recent years, which in some cases has led to an increase in the use of services among ethnic minorities (DHHS, 2001). This staffing pattern assumes that the presence of more ethnic minority staff will facilitate the use of services by clients with similar backgrounds.

The employment of ethnic minority professionals is related to the more complex issue of cultural similarity. The ability of a therapist (and other staff) to empathize with a consumer plays a critical part in shaping the interaction between the two parties and in defining deviant behavior (Blumer, 1969). When a therapist can take the role of the actor, the interaction is based on a shared understanding (empathy). Empathy is more likely to occur between people or groups of people who are socially or culturally similar (Rosenberg, 1984). Conversely, when a therapist and a consumer are socially or culturally distant, there is less likelihood that the interactions will meet both parties' needs (Scheff, 1984). Matching consumers with therapists on the basis of ethnicity is seen as one method for operationalizing social and cultural similarity.

Although some researchers cite the importance of match, few empirical studies have been conducted and the results of these investigations have been mixed (Jones, 1978; Jones and Matsumoto, 1982; Sue, 1988). Sue and colleagues (1991) conducted one of the first studies of ethnic match and its effect on use and outcome in community mental health clinics. Among Asian Americans and Mexican Americans, ethnic match resulted in reducing premature termination, increasing the length of stay, and, among certain subgroups, improving treatment outcomes. For African Americans, ethnic match resulted primarily in increasing the length of stay. When Asian Americans, particularly those who were unacculturated, saw a therapist who was matched linguistically, ethnically, or both, they generally had better outcomes. Similar effects were found for Mexican Americans, although the results were less dramatic (Sue, 1998). Thus, there is some initial evidence that hiring bilingual and ethnic staff can have important consequences above and beyond improving the representation of ethnic minorities in the community mental health system.

Researchers have also examined the outcomes of ethnic minority clients who used either ethnic-specific services or mainstream services (Takeuchi et al., 1995; Yeh et al., 1994). Ethnic clients who used ethnic-specific services had lower dropout rates and stayed in the programs longer than those who used mainstream services. Cultural match and treatment outcomes are related, but the processes that account for the results are unknown. Sue and his colleagues have continued to study variables at a more micro level by looking at cognitive match. Sue has found that therapist–client matches on goals for treatment and on coping styles were related to better adjustment and more favorable impressions of the sessions (Sue, 1998).

One of the difficulties in studying cultural competence has been the challenge of operationalizing key variables. Efforts have begun on the federal level to operationalize the concept for behavioral health care settings. Various models of cultural competence exist, which compounds the difficulty of measuring cultural competence. One of the most frequently cited models was developed for children and adolescents with serious emotional disturbance (Cross et al., 1989). This model involves five essential elements that contribute to the cultural competence of a system, agency, or professional: valuing diversity, undertaking cultural self-assessment, understanding the dynamics of difference, institutionalization of cultural knowledge, and adaptation to diversity (Isaacs-Shockley et al., 1996). Cultural competence refers to a treatment approach and philosophy that emphasizes the organization and delivery of services that are responsive to the cultural concerns of racial and ethnic minority groups, including their languages, histories, traditions, beliefs, and values. A common theme is that treatment effectiveness for a culturally diverse clientele is the responsibility of the system, not of the people seeking treatment. Achieving cultural competence is a process that occurs over time; simply hiring a minority clinician or providing culturally and linguistically relevant material, while important, does not connote cultural competence. Unfortunately, little empirical data are available that identify the critical components of cultural competence and which factors, if any, actually improve service delivery, use, and clinical outcomes for racial and ethnic minorities (Sue and Sue, 1999; Sue and Zane, 1987). It is hoped that the continued study and refinement of the concept of cultural competence will reveal mechanisms that can assist mental health organizations and providers in their delivery of culturally responsive and competent services.

Help-Seeking Behavior

Once minority consumers navigate access barriers, they seek help at different rates and from different sources. Some minority group members are more likely than whites to delay seeking treatment until symptoms become more severe. For example, Asian Americans who use mental health services have more severe symptoms than whites who use the same services (Bui and Takeuchi, 1992; Durvasula and Sue, 1996). At state and county mental hospitals, Asian Americans have longer inpatient stays than whites (Snowden and Cheung, 1990), perhaps due to the severity of their symptoms. Another indication of treatment delay involves higher use of emergency psychiatric services, or other means of coercive referrals, for African Americans compared to whites (Akutsu et al., 1996; Hu et al., 1991; Rosenfield, 1984; Takeuchi and Cheung, 1998). Furthermore, racial and ethnic minorities are overrepresented in high-need populations—those who are homeless, human immunodeficiency virus (HIV)-positive, incarcerated, or have alcohol or drug problems—and may not receive the mental health care they need in those service delivery systems or may receive inappropriate care.

Although ethnic minorities are less likely than whites to seek help for their mental or emotional problems at all, when they do seek care they appear to turn more often to sources other than mental health providers. For example, Broman (1987) found that although African Americans and whites are equally likely to seek help (e.g., from social services, clergy, or mental health services) for their mental health problems, whites are 1.6 times more likely than African Americans to specifically seek help from mental health resources. Even when controlling for psychiatric symptoms and sociodemographic differences, the percentage of African Americans receiving care from any source was only about half that of whites (Swartz et al., 1998).

The general medical sector is an important pathway to care for mental and emotional problems for the general population (Leaf et al., 1988) and may be even more so for ethnic minorities. In a recent follow-up study at the Baltimore site of the ECA, Cooper-Patrick et al. (1999b) found that the rates of mental health care seeking had increased for all groups. Despite increased use, African Americans continued to be more likely than whites to seek care in the general medical sector for mental health care and less likely to use specialty mental health care. Similarly, Mexican Americans, Asian Americans, and Puerto Ricans are more likely than whites to use the general medical sector for mental health problems and less likely than whites to use mental health specialists (Alegria et al., 1991; Hough et al., 1987; Vega et al., 1998; Zhang et al., 1998). Studies indicate that minorities turn more often to primary care as opposed to specialty care. However, cross-cultural issues may arise in either setting (Cooper-Patrick et al., 1999a), and studies indicate that one-third to one-half of patients with mental disorders go undiagnosed in primary care settings (Williams et al., 1999). Minority patients are at higher risk of missed or incorrect diagnoses of mental disorders in primary care (Borowsky et al., 2000), which can lead to inappropriate or harmful treatments or consequences.

Assessment and Treatment

For minority consumers who do seek care in the specialty mental health sector, issues of differential clinical diagnoses may arise. Clinical diagnoses guide proper treatment, and misdiagnoses may lead to improper care. Misdiagnosis can arise from clinician bias and stereotyping of ethnic and racial minorities. For example, evidence suggests that African Americans are overdiagnosed for schizophrenia and underdiagnosed for affective disorders (Adebimpe, 1981; Neighbors et al., 1989; Snowden and Cheung, 1990). There may be a tendency to label behaviors of some ethnic minority groups *deviant,* even if such behaviors are a normal response to adversity or if culturally normative behavior is wrongly interpreted. Similarly, the needs of some minority groups (e.g., Asian Americans) may go unnoticed if clinicians assume that the population is problem-free. The diagnosis and treatment of mental disorders relies heavily on verbal communication between the patient and clinician about the nature, intensity, and duration of symptoms and the impact on functioning. The potential for miscommunication and misdiagnosis is greater when the clinician and patient come from different cultural backgrounds, even if they speak the same language.

Treatment Effectiveness and Outcomes

A key component of mental health services delivery is the effectiveness of the treatment and whether or not an individual's distress is alleviated. Outcomes and treatment effectiveness may affect an individual's decision to seek treatment or stay in treatment. Controlled clinical trials offer the highest level of scientific rigor for the study of treatment effectiveness, but they have yet to be specified for minority groups. In an analysis of controlled clinical trials used to develop treatment guidelines, the Surgeon General found that very few minorities were included and not a single study that collected data on race and ethnicity analyzed the efficacy of the treatment by ethnicity or race (DHHS, 2001).

Although effective treatments exist for the general population, the influence of social and cultural factors on psychosocial interventions may differentially influence outcomes for ethnic minority groups. Cross-cultural studies have found both similar and different responses to treatment for ethnic minority groups and whites. For example, cognitive-behavioral therapy has been shown to be effective in reducing anxiety for both African American and white children and adults (Friedman et al., 1994; Treadwell et al., 1995). For older Chinese Americans, findings from a pilot study suggest that their response to cognitive-behavioral therapy for depressive symptoms is similar to that of previously studied multiethnic populations (Dai et al., 1999).

Other studies have found different responses to mental health treatment for ethnic minorities. One study of individual outpatient psychotherapy in San Francisco found that Asian Americans had poorer short-term outcomes and were less satisfied with their care than whites (Zane et al., 1994). Another study of interventions for schizophrenia among Latinos found that highly structured family therapy exacerbated symptoms in low-income Spanish-speaking families when compared to less structured case management (Telles et al., 1995).

Definitive conclusions about treatment outcomes and effectiveness for racial and ethnic minorities cannot be made without further research, particularly when considering new approaches or modalities. For example, new innovations in psychopharmacology have produced radical changes in the treatment of mental disorders. An emerging area of research, ethnopsychopharmacology, considers the subtle differences in how medications are metabolized across certain ethnic populations. Lin et al. (1997) found that African Americans and Asian Americans are more likely than whites to metabolize several medications for psychosis and depression at a slower rate. Prescribing the same doses for minority patients that are normally given to whites may lead to more medication side effects and nonadherence to the medication regimen. Within the current environment of managed care and cost containment, research on the most effective treatments for an individual's gender, race, ethnicity, and culture will prove to be beneficial both for the consumer and for the mental health system (for additional discussion on outcomes, see Chapter 9).

Implications for Mental Health Services

Disparities in mental health care and services for racial and ethnic minorities have been well documented, but progress in system reform has been slow. The lack of response to these previously identified problems can be attributed to the inability of researchers and public policy makers to pay systematic attention to the broad issues concerning race. The timing of the Surgeon General's report may reflect the coming of serious responses to problems associated with mental health services delivery in racial and ethnic minority communities.

However, the debate about race and ethnicity has become even more complex in recent years due in part to an increase in the number of people identifying with a multiracial category, recent political efforts to ban the collection of racial and ethnic data, and a widening of inequalities. In such a climate, there may be a tendency to accept uniformly the constraints placed on services that attempt to be *multicultural,* particularly for ethnic minority groups who tend to be politically and often economically disadvantaged. To avoid repeating the past failures of other reforms, the current climate can be viewed as an opportunity to rethink ways to make the mental health system more responsive to ethnic minority concerns.

A public health model provides the most comprehensive framework for mental health services because it addresses discrepancies within the system as well as societal structures and processes that influence the system. Prevention of mental disorders and interventions to promote mental health can be planned for racial and ethnic minorities. Approaches and strategies that increase cultural, linguistic, and geographical access to care need to be combined with efforts to reduce more fundamental financial and structural obstacles to equal access. Within the system, mental health screening tools and greater awareness of mental disorders in primary care settings can help identify racial and ethnic minorities who are unaware of or are reluctant to use specialty mental health services. Furthermore, culturally competent diagnosis, treatment, and delivery of services can affect the perception, the use, and possibly the outcomes of mental health services.

Broader societal factors that are essential to understanding and addressing disparities in the mental health system may bring into question the purpose and scope of ethnic minority mental health services in contemporary society. Chronic social problems such as poverty, racism, and community violence are issues that disproportionately affect racial and ethnic minorities. These factors directly affect access to and use of services but also importantly affect the well-being and mental health of ethnic minority communities. A discussion of ways to improve mental health services is incomplete without a consideration of these factors. Through a constant process of reconceptualization, advocacy, and monitoring, it may be possible to achieve a public health model of mental health services based on a full consideration of how social structure and culture affect mental health (Neighbors et al., 1992; Vega and Murphy, 1990).

Future research challenges include identifying the social structures and processes that help explain why race and ethnicity may be linked to different mental health problems (Vega and Rumbaut, 1991). Understanding the role of the larger social context on mental health status, access to care, service use, and treatment and prevention outcomes requires integrative models that can delineate the interaction of biological, psychological, cultural, economic, and social factors over the life course. Until those factors can be more precisely identified and addressed, we will continue to document racial and ethnic disparities in mental health status and care.

NOTES

1. These percentages are based on those reporting one race (the minimum population) and may underestimate the actual population. The maximum population includes those individuals who identify that race in combination with one or more of the other five races (this does not include the Hispanic population).

2. Individuals could report only one race in 1990 and could report more than one race in 2000. Because of other changes in the questionnaire, the race data for 1990 and 2000 are not directly comparable. The difference in population by race between 1990 and 2000 is due both to these changes and to real changes in the population. These changes do not affect the Hispanic or Latino category.

REFERENCES

Abe-Kim JS, Takeuchi DT. Cultural competence and quality of care: issues for mental health service delivery in managed care. *Clinical Psychology: Science and Practice*, 3:273–295, 1996.

Adebimpe VR. Overview: white norms and psychiatric diagnosis of Black patients. *American Journal of Psychiatry*, 138:279–285, 1981.

Akutsu PD, Snowden LR, Organista KC. Referral patterns in ethnic-specific and mainstream programs for ethnic minorities and whites. *Journal of Counseling Psychology*, 43:56–64, 1996.

Alegria M, Robles R, Freeman DH, et al. Patterns of mental health utilization among island Puerto Rican poor. *American Journal of Public Health*, 81:875–879, 1991.

Allen WR, Farley R. The shifting social and economic tides of Black America, 1950–1980. *Annual Review of Sociology*, 12:277–306, 1986.

Blumer H. *Symbolic Interactionism.* Englewood Cliffs, NJ: Prentice Hall, 1969.

Borowsky SJ, Rubenstein LV, Meredith LS, et al. Who is at risk of nondetection of mental health problems in primary care? *Journal of General Internal Medicine*, 15:381–388, 2000.

Broman CL. Race differences in professional help seeking. *American Journal of Community Psychology*, 15:473–489, 1987.

Brown DR, Eaton WW, Sussman L. Racial differences in prevalence of phobic disorders. *Journal of Nervous and Mental Disease*, 178:434–441, 1990.

Brown ER, Ojeda VD, Wyn R, et al. *Racial and Ethnic Disparities in Access to Health Insurance and Health Care*. Los Angeles: UCLA Center for Health Policy Research and the Henry J. Kaiser Family Foundation, 2000.

Bui KV, Takeuchi DT. Ethnic minority adolescents and the use of community mental health care services. *American Journal of Community Psychology*, 20:403–417, 1992.

Cheung FK, Snowden LR. Community mental health and ethnic minority populations. *Community Mental Health Journal*, 26:277–291, 1990.

Cooper RS, David R. The biological concept of race and its application to public health and epidemiology. *Journal of Health Politics, Policy and Law*, 11:97–116, 1986.

Cooper-Patrick L, Gallo JJ, Gonzales JJ, et al. Race, gender, and partnership in the patient–physician relationship. *Journal of the American Medical Association*, 282:583–589, 1999a.

Cooper-Patrick L, Gallo JJ, Powe NR, et al. Mental health service utilization by African Americans and whites: the Baltimore Epidemiologic Catchment Area follow-up. *Medical Care*, 37:1034–1045, 1999b.

Cross T, Bazron B, Dennis K, et al. *Towards a Culturally Competent System of Care: A Monograph on Effective Services for Minority Children Who Are Severely Emotionally Disturbed*. Washington, DC: Georgetown University Child Development Center, National Technical Assistance Center for Children's Mental Health, 1989.

Dai Y, Zhang S, Yamamoto J, et al. Cognitive behavioral therapy of minor depressive symptoms in elderly Chinese Americans: a pilot study. *Community Mental Health Journal*, 35:537–542, 1999.

Duncan OD. Inheritance of poverty or inheritance of race? In: Moynihan DP (ed): *On Understanding Poverty: Perspectives from the Social Sciences*. New York: Basic Books, pp. 85–110, 1969.

Durvasula RS, Sue S. Severity of disturbance among Asian American outpatients. *Cultural Diversity and Mental Health*, 2:43–52, 1996.

Farley R. *Blacks and Whites: Narrowing the Gap?* Cambridge, MA: Harvard University Press, 1984.

Friedman S, Paradis CM, Hatch M. Characteristics of African-American and white patients with panic disorder and agoraphobia. *Hospital and Community Psychiatry*, 45:798–803, 1994.

Greenley JR, Mechanic D. Social selection in seeking help for psychological problems. *Journal of Health and Social Behavior*, 17:249–262, 1976.

Hargraves MA. Uninsurance and its impact on access on health care: what are the challenges for policy? In: Hogue C, Hargraves MA, Scott-Collins K (eds). *Minority Health in America: Findings and Policy Implications from the Commonwealth Fund Minority Health Survey*. Baltimore: Johns Hopkins University Press, pp. 142–159, 2000.

Hough RL, Landsverk JA, Karno M, et al. Utilization of health and mental health services by Los Angeles Mexican Americans and non-Hispanic whites. *Archives of General Psychiatry*, 44:702–709, 1987.

Hu T-W, Snowden LR, Jerrell JM, et al. Ethnic populations in public mental health: services choice and level of use. *American Journal of Public Health*, 81:1429–1434, 1991.

Hurh WM, Kim KC. Correlates of Korean immigrants' mental health. *Journal of Nervous and Mental Disease*, 178:703–711, 1990.

Ilfield FW. Psychological status of community residents along major demographic dimensions. *Archives of General Psychiatry*, 35:716–724, 1978.

Isaacs-Shockley M, Cross T, Bazron BJ, et al. Framework for a culturally competence system of care. In: Stroul BA (ed). *Children's Mental Health: Creating Systems of Care in a Changing Society*. Baltimore: Paul H. Brookes, pp. 23–29, 1996.

Jones EE. Effects of race on psychotherapy process and outcome: an exploratory investigation. *Psychotherapy: Theory, Research and Practice*, 15:226–236, 1978.

Jones E, Matsumoto D. Psychotherapy with the underserved: recent developments. In: Snowden L (ed). *Reaching the Underserved: Mental Health Needs of Neglected Populations*. Beverly Hills, CA: Sage, pp. 207–228, 1982.

Kaplan JS, Chang D, Abe-Kim J, et al. Ethnicity and mental health. In: Friedman HS (ed). *Encyclopedia of Mental Health, Volume 2*. San Diego, CA: Academic Press, pp. 161–172, 1998.

Kessler RC, McGonagle KA, Zhao S, et al. Lifetime and 12-month prevalence of DSM-III-R psychiatric disorders in the United States: results from the National Comorbidity Survey. *Archives of General Psychiatry*, 51:8–19, 1994.

Kinzie JD, Leung PK, Boehnlein JK, et al. Psychiatric epidemiology of an Indian village: a 19-year replication study. *Journal of Nervous and Mental Disease*, 180:33–39, 1992.

Krieger N, Williams DR, Moss NE. Measuring social class in U.S. public health research: concepts, methodologies, and guidelines. *Annual Review of Public Health*, 18:341–378, 1997.

Kuo W, Tsai Y. Social networking hardiness and immigrants' mental health. *Journal of Health and Social Behavior*, 27:133–149, 1986.

Kuo WH. Prevalence of depression among Asian-Americans. *Journal of Nervous and Mental Disease*, 172:449–457, 1984.

Leaf PJ, Bruce ML, Tischler GL, et al. Factors affecting the utilization of specialty and general medical mental health services. *Medical Care*, 26:9–26, 1988.

Leaf PJ, Livingston MM, Tischler GL, et al. Contact with health professionals for the treatment of psychiatric and emotional problems. *Medical Care*, 23:1322–1337, 1985.

Leong FTL. Counseling and psychotherapy with Asian-Americans: review of the literature. *Journal of Counseling Psychology*, 33:196–206, 1986.

Lin KM, Cheung F, Smith M, et al. The use of psychotropic medications in working with Asian patients. In: Lee E (ed). *Working with Asian Americans: A Guide for Clinicians*. New York: Guilford Press, pp. 388–399, 1997.

Lopez S. Mexican Americans' usage of mental health facilities: underutilization reconsidered. In: Baron A (ed). *Explorations in Chicano Psychology*. New York: Praeger, pp. 139–164, 1981.

Manson S. Mental health services for American Indians and Alaska Natives: need, use, and barriers to effective care. *Canadian Journal of Psychiatry*, 45:617–626, 2000.

Matsuoka JK, Breaux C, Ryujin DH. National utilization of mental health services by Asian Americans/Pacific Islanders. *Journal of Community Psychology*, 25:141–146, 1997.

McCarthy JD, Yancey WL. Uncle Tom and Mr. Charlie: metaphysical pathos in the study of racism and personal disorganization. *American Journal of Sociology*, 76:648–672, 1971.

Mechanic D. *Mental Health and Social Policy: The Emergence of Managed Care*, 4th ed. Boston: Allyn & Bacon, 1999.

Moscicki EK, Locke BZ, Rae DS, et al. Depressive symptoms among Mexican Americans: the Hispanic Health and Nutrition Examination Survey. *American Journal of Epidemiology*, 130:348–360, 1989.

Neff JA. Race and vulnerability to stress: an examination of differential vulnerability. *Journal of Personality and Social Psychology*, 49:481–491, 1985.

Neighbors HW. The prevention of psychopathology in African Americans: an epidemiologic perspective. *Community Mental Health Journal*, 26:167–179, 1990.

Neighbors HW, Bashshur R, Price R, et al. Ethnic minority mental health service delivery: a review of the literature. *Research in Community and Mental Health*, 7:55–71, 1992.

Neighbors HW, Jackson JS, Campbell L, et al. The influence of racial factors on psychiatric diagnosis: a review and suggestions for research. *Community Mental Health Journal*, 25:301–311, 1989.

O'Sullivan MJ, Peterson PD, Cox GB, et al. Ethnic populations: community mental health services ten years later. *American Journal of Community Psychology*, 17:17–30, 1989.

Owens K, King MC. Genomic views of human history. *Science*, 286:451–453, 1999.

Padgett DK, Patrick C, Burns BJ, et al. Ethnic differences in use of inpatient mental health services by blacks, whites, and Hispanics in a national insured population. *Health Services Research*, 29:135–153, 1994a.

Padgett DK, Patrick C, Burns, BJ, et al. Ethnicity and the use of outpatient mental health services in a national insured population. *American Journal of Public Health*, 84:222–226, 1994b.

Roberts RE, Stevenson JM, Breslow L. Symptoms of depression among Blacks and Whites in an urban community. *Journal of Nervous and Mental Disease*, 169:774–779, 1981.

Roberts RE, Vernon SW. Minority status and psychological distress reexamined: the case of Mexican Americans. *Research in Community and Mental Health*, 4:131–163, 1984.

Robins LN, Regier DA. *Psychiatric Disorders in America: The Epidemiological Catchment Area Study*. New York: Free Press, 1991.

Rogler LH, Malgady RG, Costantino G, et al. What do culturally sensitive mental health services mean? The case of Hispanics. *American Psychologist*, 42:565–570, 1987.

Rosenberg M. A symbolic interactionist view of psychosis. *Journal of Health and Social Behavior*, 25:289–302, 1984.

Rosenfield S. Race differences in involuntary hospitalization: psychiatric vs. labeling perspectives. *Journal of Health and Social Behavior*, 25:14–23, 1984.

Scheff T. *Being Mentally Ill: A Sociological Theory*, 2nd ed. Chicago: Aldine, 1984.

Silberman C. *Crisis in Black and White*. New York: Random House, 1964.

Smelser NJ, Wilson WJ, Mitchell F (eds). *America Becoming: Racial Trends and Their Consequences*. Washington, DC: National Academy Press, 2001.

Snowden LR. African American service use for mental health problems. *Journal of Community Psychology*, 27:303–313, 1999.

Snowden LR, Cheung FK. Use of inpatient mental health services by members of ethnic minority groups. *American Psychologist*, 45:347–355, 1990.

Snowden LR, Thomas K. Medicaid and African American outpatient treatment. *Mental Health Services Research*, 2:114–129, 2000.

Somervell PD, Leaf PJ, Weissman MM, et al. The prevalence of major depression in black and white adults in five United States communities. *American Journal of Epidemiology*, 130:725–735, 1989.

Sue DW, Sue D. *Counseling the Culturally Different: Theory and Practice*, 3rd ed. New York: Wiley, 1999.

Sue S. Community mental health services to minority groups. *American Journal of Psychology*, 32:616–624, 1977.

Sue S. Psychotherapeutic services for ethnic minorities: two decades of research findings. *American Psychologist*, 43:301–308, 1988.

Sue S. In search of cultural competence in psychotherapy and counseling. *American Psychologist*, 53:440–448, 1998.

Sue S, Fujino DC, Hu L-T, et al. Community mental health services for ethnic minority groups: a test of the cultural responsiveness hypothesis. *Journal of Consulting and Clinical Psychology*, 59:533–540, 1991.

Sue S, McKinney H. Asian Americans in the community mental health care system. *American Journal of Orthopsychiatry*, 45:111–118, 1975.

Sue S, Morishima J. *The Mental Health of Asian Americans*. San Francisco: Jossey-Bass, 1982.

Sue S, Zane NW. The role of culture and cultural techniques in psychotherapy: a critique and reformulation. *American Psychologist*, 42:37–45, 1987.

Sue S, Zane NW, Young K. Research on psychotherapy on culturally diverse populations. In: Bergin A, Garfield S (eds). *Handbook of Psychotherapy and Behavior Change*, 4th ed. New York: Wiley, pp. 783–817, 1994.

Sussman LK, Robins LN, Earls F. Treatment-seeking for depression by black and white Americans. *Social Science and Medicine*, 24:187–196, 1987.

Swartz MS, Wagner HR, Swanson JW, et al. Comparing use of public and private mental health services: the enduring barriers of race and age. *Community Mental Health Journal*, 34:133–144, 1998.

Takeuchi DT, Cheung M-K. Coercive and voluntary referrals: how ethnic minority adults get into mental health treatment. *Ethnicity and Health*, 3:149–158, 1998.

Takeuchi DT, Chung RC-Y, Lin K-M, et al. Lifetime and twelve-month prevalence rates of major depressive episodes and dysthymia among Chinese Americans in Los Angeles. *American Journal of Psychiatry*, 155:1407–1414, 1998.

Takeuchi DT, Sue S, Yeh M. Return rates and outcomes from ethnicity-specific mental health programs in Los Angeles. *American Journal of Public Health*, 85:638–643, 1995.

Telles C, Karno M, Mintz J, et al. Immigrant families coping with schizophrenia: behavioural family intervention v. case management with a low-income Spanish-speaking population. *British Journal of Psychiatry*, 167:473–479, 1995.

Treadwell KRH, Flannery-Schroeder EC, Kendall PC. Ethnicity and gender in relation to adaptive functioning, diagnostic status, and treatment outcome in children from an anxiety clinic. *Journal of Anxiety Disorders*, 9:373–384, 1995.

U.S. Bureau of the Census. *Census 2000 PHC-T-1: Population by Race and Hispanic or Latino Origin for the United States: 1990 and 2000*. Washington, DC: U.S. Bureau of the Census, 2001. Available at: www.census.gov/population/www/cen2000/phc-t1/ Accessed December 5, 2001.

U.S. Department of Health and Human Services. *Mental Health: Culture, Race, and Ethnicity—A Supplement to Mental Health: A Report of the Surgeon General*. Rockville, MD: U.S. Department of Health and Human Services, Substance Abuse and Mental Health Services Administration, Center for Mental Health Services, 2001.

Vega WA, Kolody B, Aguilar-Gaxiola S, et al. Lifetime prevalence of DSM-III-R psychiatric disorders among urban and rural Mexican Americans in California. *Archives of General Psychiatry*, 55:771–778, 1998.

Vega WA, Murphy JW. *Culture and the Restructuring of Community Mental Health*. Westport, CT: Greenwood, 1990.

Vega WA, Rumbaut R. Ethnic minorities and mental health. *Annual Review of Sociology*, 17:351–383, 1991.

Warheit GJ, Holzer CE III, Arey SA. Race and mental illness: an epidemiological update. *Journal of Health and Social Behavior*, 16:243–256, 1975.

Williams DR. Race, stress and mental health. In: Hogue C, Hargraves M, Scott-Collins K (eds). *Minority Health in America*. Baltimore: Johns Hopkins University Press, pp. 209–243, 2000.

Williams DR, Harris-Reid M. Race and mental health. In: Horwitz AV, Scheid Tl (eds). *A Handbook for the Study of Mental Health: Social Contexts, Theories, and Systems*. Cambridge: Cambridge University Press, pp. 295–314, 1999.

Williams JW, Rost K, Dietrich AJ, et al. Primary care physicians' approach to depressive disorders: effects of physician specialty and practice structure. *Archives of Family Medicine*, 8:58–67, 1999.

Yeh M, Takeuchi DT, Sue S. Asian-American children treated in the mental health system: a comparison of parallel and mainstream outpatient service centers. *Journal of Clinical Child Psychology*, 23:5–12, 1994.

Ying Y. Depressive symptomatology among Chinese-Americans as measured by the CES-D. *Journal of Clinical Psychology*, 44:739–746, 1988.

Zane N, Enomoto K, Chun C-A. Treatment outcomes of Asian- and White-American clients in outpatient therapy. *Journal of Community Psychology*, 22:177–191, 1994.

Zhang AY, Snowden LR, Sue S. Differences between Asian- and White-Americans' help-seeking and utilization patterns in the Los Angeles area. *Journal of Community Psychology*, 26:317–326, 1998.

16

The Public Health Implications of Co-Occurring Addictive and Mental Disorders

FRED C. OSHER

Despite increasing evidence that outcomes for persons with co-occurring addictive and mental disorders improve when care is provided in a comprehensive and integrated fashion (Drake et al., 1998, 2001), access to effective service remains elusive to most individuals with these conditions (U.S. DHHS, 1999). It is estimated that up to 10 million people in the United States meet criteria for co-occurring disorders in any given year (CMHS, 1997). Without adequate treatment, we can predict a continuation of poor adjustment and a suboptimal quality of life in this group (Osher and Kofoed, 1989).

Clinicians, health care administrators, families, and consumers are frustrated because not enough is being done to address the needs of persons with co-occurring disorders. These groups witness the revolving door experience of these individuals as they cycle in and out of costly and inappropriate treatment settings such as emergency rooms and jails and are consistently overrepresented in surveys of homeless populations. This chapter highlights the negative outcomes associated with co-occurring disorders, the need for assessment and the heterogeneity of the population with co-occurring disorders, evidence-based practices and treatment principles associated with positive outcomes, barriers to service delivery, and implications for behavioral health services efforts to address the needs of persons with co-occurring mental and addictive disorders.

Negative Outcomes

Substance abuse among persons with mental illness has been associated with negative outcomes such as increased vulnerability to relapse and rehospitalization (Brady et al., 1990; Carpenter et al., 1985; Caton et al., 1993; Haywood et al., 1995,

Lyons and McGovern, 1989; Negrete et al., 1986; Seibel et al., 1993); more psychotic symptoms (Carey et al., 1991; Drake et al., 1989; Osher et al., 1994); greater depression and suicidality (Bartels et al., 1992); violence (Cuffel et al., 1994; Yesavage and Zarcone, 1983); incarceration (Abram and Teplin, 1991; Bureau of Justice Statistics, 1999); inability to manage finances and daily needs (Drake and Wallach, 1989); housing instability and homelessness (Caton et al., 1994; Drake and Wallach, 1989; Osher et al., 1994); noncompliance with medication regimens and other treatments (Alterman et al., 1982; Drake et al., 1989; Miller and Tanenbaum, 1989; Owen et al., 1996); increased vulnerability to human immunodeficiency virus (HIV) infection (Cournos and McKinnon, 1997; Cournos et al., 1991) and hepatitis (Rosenberg et al., 2001); lower satisfaction with familial relationships (Dixon et al., 1995); increased family burden (Clark, 1994); and higher service use and costs (Bartels et al., 1993, Dickey and Azeni, 1996).

Negative outcomes of substance use disorders among persons with mental illness are not consistent across studies, and establishing causality is complicated by several factors. Comparing persons with severe mental illness who abuse substances with those who do not assumes that the two groups are otherwise equivalent, and clearly they are not. In the first place, the substance-abusing patients are more likely to be young and male (Mueser et al., 1990, 1992). They may also be different from patients who never abused substances prior to the onset of symptoms. For example, between-group differences have been described in the age of onset of the mental disorder (Breakey et al., 1974), in premorbid functioning (Arndt et al., 1992), in premorbid sexual adjustment (Dixon et al., 1991), and in family history of substance use disorders (Noordsy et al., 1994). Finally, medication and treatment noncompliance, homelessness, and other social problems of psychiatric patients who abuse substances may account for their poor adjustment (Drake and Wallach, 1989; Osher et al., 1994). Despite the difficulty in establishing causality, the negative outcomes associated with the presence of co-occurring disorders in traditional treatment settings suggest that nontraditional treatment approaches are required.

The Relationship Between Substance Use and Psychiatric Disorders and the Role of Assessment

It is important to recognize the complex interaction of substance use and psychiatric disorders. Sorting out the interaction is a sophisticated assessment task that may lead to the classification outlined by Lehman et al. (1989), who identified six possible relationships: (*1*) acute and chronic substance abuse may produce psychiatric symptoms; (*2*) substance withdrawal can cause psychiatric symptoms; (*3*) substance use can mask psychiatric symptoms; (*4*) psychiatric disorders can mimic symptoms associated with substance use; (*5*) acute and chronic substance abuse can exacerbate psychiatric disorders; and (*6*) the two types of disorders can exist simultaneously and independently, with a negative synergy. This author suggests modifying the sixth category to read "acute and chronic psychiatric disorders can exacerbate the recovery process from addictive disorders." In this classification scheme, the first two relationships do not qualify as co-occurring disorders but require addiction interventions. The third and fourth relationships are not co-occurring disorders either and require mental health treatment. It is only the last two categories that qualify as co-occurring disorders, and they require integrated treatment strategies.

Determining the nature of the relationship between substance use and abnormalities in mood, thinking, and behavior is a complex yet critical task. It is predicated on the assumption that clinicians in either mental health or addiction services actively search for the relationship. This must become a routine process in any behavioral health treatment setting. Epidemiological data provide compelling reasons for the importance of assessment (see Chapter 8). First, substance use disorders and psychiatric disorders occur at high rates. The Epidemiologic Catchment Area (ECA) study (Regier et al., 1990) assessed psychiatric and substance use disorders in over 20,000 persons living in the community and in various institutional settings and found that persons with a psychiatric disorder, especially those with a severe mental illness, were at increased risk for developing a substance use disorder over their lifetime. For example, persons with schizophrenia were more than four times as likely to have had a substance use disorder during their lifetime as persons in the general population, and those with bipolar disorder were more than five times as likely to have had such a diagnosis. Second, persons with co-occurring disorders frequently seek help. The 1992 National Longitudinal Alcohol Epidemiologic Survey (Grant, 1997) found that dually diagnosed persons were five times more likely to seek services than singly diagnosed respondents, and similar findings in the National Comorbidity Survey (Kessler et. al, 1996) support this bias. Kessler and associates (1996) reported that 19% of alcohol-dependent and 26% of drug-dependent individuals without a co-occurring mental disorder received treatment in a 12-month period, but in the presence of a co-occurring disorder the rates increased to 41% and 63%, respectively. Large numbers of individuals with co-occurring disorders are likely to enter treatment and require accurate assessment.

Heterogeneity of the Population with Co-Occurring Disorders

Treatment planning and policy development require an accurate description of the problem to be addressed. Despite considerable progress in assessment tools and strategies, the identification and characterization of persons with co-occurring disorders remains a difficult task (Lehman, 1996). While the assessment process is complex and can be protracted, the identification of individuals with co-occurring disorders is simply an early step in designing an appropriate response to their needs. It is critical that the *heterogeneity* of the population be acknowledged. Any substance of abuse can be combined with any mental disorder to meet criteria under this umbrella term. These two dimensions can be crossed with any set of demographic variables (age, gender, and/or culture) to create additional subgroups with special needs. If the frequent presence of other medical comorbidities is added, the classification of co-occurring disorders gains additional complexity. These interacting variables underline the adage that "if you've seen one person with co-occurring disorders, you've seen one person with co-occurring disorders."

For clinical and organizational purposes, the separation of persons with co-occurring disorders into subgroups based solely on diagnosis or demographics will not lead to effective matching to treatment. Arguably the most important dimension to consider is the degree of dysfunction the two disorders produce in an individual. One useful model was developed in New York and endorsed by both the National Association of State Mental Health Program Directors and the National Association of State Alcohol and Drug Abuse Directors (NASMHPD and NASADAD, 1999). Rather than focus on diagnoses, the model uses two dimensions—the severity of the mental illness and the severity of the addiction—to define four subgroups of dually diagnosed individuals in a two-by-two matrix. The model then assigns responsibility to (1) primary care providers with consultation from behavioral health specialists (for persons with low severity on each dimension), (2) one of the specialty sector systems (for persons with either severe mental illnesses or severe alcohol or drug abuse) with collaboration from the other specialty sector, or (3) a set of providers providing integrated care to the most disabled consumers. The advantages of this model are that it encompasses the heterogeneity of the dual diagnosis population, it assigns responsibility for providing some degree of care to dually diagnosed individuals to every system, and it is flexible enough to be adapted to most service settings. Significant overlap between systems is inherent in the model, and it corresponds more realistically to the multiple pathways used by dually diagnosed persons to access care.

Evidence Based Treatment

Given the high prevalence rates and the high morbidity and mortality associated with co-occurring disorders, the identification of effective interventions has gained both immediacy and a growing database. For the past 15 years, extensive efforts have been made to develop integrated models of care that bring together mental health and substance abuse treatment. The reported studies have focused primarily on individuals with serious mental illnesses and co-occurring substance use disorders. Recent evidence from more than a dozen studies shows that comprehensive integrated efforts help persons with dual disorders reduce substance use and attain remission (Drake et al., 1998). Integrated approaches are also associated with a reduction in hospital use, psychiatric symptomatology, and other problematic negative outcomes. Comprehensiveness was the critical component in successful interventions. Those programs that simply added a group or short-term treatment intervention to existing programming suffered high dropout rates and had little overall impact on either rates of substance abuse or psychiatric symptomatology. Comprehensive approaches were defined by the inclusion of a staged approach to care, with motivational interventions, assertive outreach, intensive case management, individual counseling, long-term interventions, and family interventions. Positive outcomes included high rates of engaging and retaining patients in care, reduced hospital use, reduced substance use, and increased abstinence. This research base has allowed the development of treatment principles associated with positive outcomes.

Treatment Principles

While historically mental health and substance abuse approaches to care are different, principles of care within the two fields converge on respect for the individual, reaching out to engage those who cannot yet trust, and the importance of community, family, and peers to recovery. The American Association of Community Psychiatrists used the existing evidence base shaped by the experience of developing effective systems of care to develop the following principles (AACP, 2000). These principles serve to bridge the gap between the service orientations and characterize an effective system of care for persons with co–occurring disorders. They can be used for both planning and evaluation purposes.

Acceptance

In a consumer/family-oriented system, for persons with co–occurring disorders the service goal is to ensure that each clinical contact is welcoming, empathic, hopeful, culturally sensitive, and consumer centered. Special efforts should be made to engage persons who may be unwilling to accept or participate in recommended services or who do not fit into the available program models.

Accessibility

In an accessible system for persons with co–occurring disorders, 24-hour crisis services are available to provide competent assessment and intervention for psychiatric and substance symptomatology in any combination. Arbitrary barriers to immediate evaluation (e.g., alcohol levels below legal intoxication limits) are not present.

Integration

There must be an integrated conceptual framework for designing a comprehensive service system for persons with co–occurring disorders. That is, treatment addresses two or more interwoven chronic disorders. This can be achieved by implementing the following procedures: (1) develop a common language for describing the target population; (2) develop a common methodology for describing categories of integrated services in the system based on the severity or disability of the individual; (3) ensure that each disorder receives specific and appropriately intensive primary treatment that takes into account the complications resulting from the co–occurring disorders; (4) identify a primary clinician for each individual who has the responsibility of coordinating ongoing treatment interventions for both disorders. While no specific model should be assumed to be generalizable across systems, the common goal should be to comprehensively address consumers' needs within one setting by one set of providers. Successful integrated efforts will reduce conflicts between providers, eliminate administrative barriers to care, and assist the consumer by providing a consistent message about recovery principles (Minkoff, 1989).

Continuity

Psychiatric and substance use disorders, regardless of severity, tend to be persistent and recurrent. These disorders co-occur with sufficient frequency that a continuous, integrated approach to assessment and treatment is required, regardless of the location of the initial clinical presentation. A goal of the service system is to provide persons with co-occurring disorders early access to continuous, integrated treatment relationships that can be maintained over time through multiple episodes of acute and subacute treatment.

Individualized Treatment

Any psychiatric disorder and any substance use disorder may co-occur in any person, regardless of age, gender, or socioeconomic status. Effective responses must be tailored to the needs of the consumer instead of requiring consumers to fit the specifications of the program. Integrated, continuous treatment relationships should be developed to support the consumer with a balance of appropriate case management and care. The system should be created using existing services and programs as much as possible, with matching of program to individual needs to ensure opportunities for meaningful choice and empowerment at each point during the course of treatment.

Comprehensiveness

Persons with co-occurring disorders have broad primary care and behavioral health treatment, social service, and housing needs. Therefore, the shared mission of the system must be to provide a broad range of necessary services. Some programs within this system will be fully integrated; other programs will be primarily psychiatric, with substance disorder capability or enhancement, or vice versa; and some programs will have minimal behavioral disorder expertise (e.g., housing programs) and require cross-training and collaboration.

Emphasis on Quality

The system of care should be designed in accordance with established national standards for serving persons with co-occurring disorders in public managed care systems (e.g., Center for Mental Health Services Workforce competencies for dual diagnosis treatment in managed care systems: CMHS, 1998). When evidence for the effectiveness of interventions has been established, these best practices should be introduced into the system of care. The development of standardized assessment tools across all clinical settings will enhance quality evaluation efforts. In addition, the identification of objectives or quality monitors (structure, process, and outcome) as markers for successful implementation is a critical step.

Responsible Implementation

There must be an implementation plan that identifies priorities for and barriers to change and recommends strategies to overcome such barriers. The plan should be derived from (1) identification of existing services for persons with co-occurring disorders and specification of the role of those services in the system of care; (2) identification of significant gaps in existing services, which require new services, programs, and/or funding to address those gaps; (3) development of a process to modify policies, procedures, regulations, or laws in order to create flexible funding streams; and (4) creation of an infrastructure empowered to oversee and direct the implementation process.

Optimism and Recovery

A growing evidence base suggests that persons with co-occurring disorders who receive care based on the aforementioned principles have positive outcomes. This is contrary to prevailing attitudes among administrators, providers, families, and consumers. This nihilism serves the systems goals poorly. The problem can be addressed by disseminating available evidence and data. Every person, regardless of the severity and disability associated with his or her co-occurring disorders, is entitled to experience the promise and hope of recovery.

While there is general acceptance of these principles, very few systems are in the process of delivering services consistent with them. Why?

Barriers to Service Delivery

For persons with co-occurring disorders, barriers to accessing comprehensive care embracing the principles outlined above are formidable. This is primarily due to the fragmentation of existing service systems for people with numerous and complex clinical, social, and legal problems. The linkage of mental health and addiction service systems has wavered over time, and despite an understanding of the utility of coordination, these systems are currently predominantly separate. This nonintegration of mental and addictive services exists at both administrative and clinical levels.

Barriers to Administrative Integration: A Federal Case Study

A brief review of the evolution of federal programs for mental health and addiction services can illustrate the development of nonintegrated services and the negative impact on all levels of service delivery. The Mental Health Act of 1946 created the National Institute of Mental Health (NIMH), which assumed responsibility for mental health, alcohol, and drug issues. In the 1960s, in addition to its mental health focus, NIMH actively advocated for more community-based clinics for alcohol treatment. When Congress enacted the Narcotic Addict Rehabilitation Act in 1966, NIMH was authorized to make grants to establish community-based drug treatment programs, and it supported numerous therapeutic communities and methadone maintenance programs. The NIMH findings contributed to a growing awareness of the inadequate capacity for treating the disease of alcoholism and the enormous social costs of the burgeoning drug epidemic in the late 1960s. Passage of decriminalization laws in the late 1960s redirected responsibility for addictions from the criminal justice to the health sector.

In 1970, the Comprehensive Alcoholism Prevention, Treatment and Rehabilitation Act (PL 91-616) was passed by Congress to support increased and improved services for people with alcoholism. The act also created a federal agency, the National Institute on Alcohol Abuse and Alcoholism (NIAAA), to administer, among other programs, a formula grant that allocated money to the states based on population and need. In 1972, the Drug Office and Treatment Act (PL 92-255) authorized the establishment of the National Institute on Drug Abuse (NIDA) and created an analogous formula grant program for this agency to administer. An unintended effect of these positive developments for the alcohol and drug fields was to formalize separation from, and competition with, the mental health establishment (i.e., NIMH). In addition, NIDA and NIAAA joined labor unions and state insurance commissions to promote insurance coverage for the treatment of alcohol and drug dependence. This successful effort, coupled with the new formula grant monies, resulted in a dramatic expansion of both private and public substance abuse employee assistance and chemical dependency programs in the 1970s.

Opening the floodgates to addictive disorder treatment dramatically increased the demand for care. Unfortunately, resources did not increase with this demand. Federal dollars for mental health and substance abuse treatment during the Ford, Carter, and Reagan administrations, adjusted for inflation, did not grow, and state and local governments experienced declining federal support (Baumohl and Jaffe, 1995). In response to widespread resource limitations, a narrowing of target populations and benefit limitations became management strategies of states to achieve cost containment. Considerable effort was placed on defining eligibility for services, the goal being the identification of the *purest* target population, thereby keeping available resources for narrowly defined purposes. In the context of this burgeoning demand for substance abuse and mental health treatment, with diminished resources, the exclusion of individuals with co-occurring disorders became commonplace. Parallel pressure was felt at the service level. Staff time became limited, and individuals with co-occurring disorders were viewed as too labor intensive. It was during the early 1980s that the needs of individuals with co-occurring disorders began appearing in the mental health and addiction literature (Drake et al., 1995; Pepper et al., 1981).

In the most recent of a series of federal agency reorganizations, the Substance Abuse and Mental Health Services Agency (SAMHSA) was created in 1992. It consists of the Center for Substance Abuse Prevention, the Center for Substance

Abuse Treatment (CSAT), and the Center for Mental Health Services (CMHS). The enabling legislation also separated the alcohol and drug portion of the block grant (administered by CSAT) from the mental health portion (administered by CMHS). While SAMHSA was officially authorized to oversee strategies to serve dually diagnosed individuals, to date it has not prioritized this objective and has done little to resolve the categorical nature of the missions of its three centers (Osher and Drake, 1996). Congress has called for a report from SAMHSA (2002), which details the agency's response to the needs of persons with co-occurring disorders.

These separate administrative structures and funding sources serve to reinforce the separation of mental health and addiction systems. Because substance abuse and mental health programs continue to be licensed and monitored under separate authorities, there is virtually no opportunity to comingle funds (Ridgely and Dixon, 1995). Even where it is conceivable to blend monies, conflicting rules and regulations create powerful disincentives not to do so. The prospect of multiple audits from multiple authorities is daunting. This case study illustrates how federal policy has promoted a separation of administrative functions, policies, and practice implemented by either state, local, or private alcohol, drug, or mental health agencies.

Barriers to Clinical Integration: Lack of Cross-Training

With increased national attention on treating addictive disorders in the late 1960s and early 1970s, coupled with the expansion of treatment facilities, the need for human resource development became paramount. Responsibility for addictions services was in flux. Not until new theoretical models posited biological underpinnings to addictions did the traditional health system begrudgingly reconsider its role in providing addiction treatment. Jellinek's seminal work, The *Disease Concept of Alcoholism* (1960), is credited with providing a renewed rationale for medical personnel to treat alcoholism. Short-term inpatient stays with long-term Alcoholics Anonymous/Narcotics Anonymous outpatient fellowship became the modal treatment across the country during the 1960s. Thus, even though addiction treatment returned to medical settings, it remained separate from mental health services. Through grants and contracts, NIAAA and NIDA sponsored *manpower training*, with the goal of producing a large pool of practitioners around the country to positively affect current treatment efforts (Deitch and Carlton, 1992). Training in mental health was not typically a part of these efforts.

Recognizing that large numbers of people with addictive disorders were entering mental health treatment settings, academic psychiatric training centers found themselves under increasing pressure to insert addiction training into the curriculum, and specialty physician organizations such as the American Society of Addiction Medicine were founded. In 1989, the Accreditation Counsel for Graduate Medical Education required all psychiatric residents to receive training in addiction psychiatry. While these developments were welcome, they did not focus on the needs of individuals with co-occurring disorders, and integrated approaches were not emphasized.

While the alcohol and drug field moved to professionalize its human resources, distrust of the *medicalization* of addictions surfaced. To many, the use of mind-altering medications was antithetical to a drug-free lifestyle and was often seen as a misguided shortcut to requisite abstinence. Battle lines were drawn as to whether psychiatric symptoms were simply the result of alcohol and drug abuse or whether this abuse was only a self-medication strategy for the underlying mental disorder. Such conflicts were played out in the treatment planning for dually diagnosed individuals in a way that precluded coordinated approaches. Clinicians with expertise in addictions and consumers recovering from co-occurring disorders, who would improve the quality of care, are routinely excluded from jobs in the mental health system (Drake et al., 2001).

These different treatment philosophies and lack of cross-training result in inaccurate assessments, underrecognition of co-occurring disorders, and failure to implement appropriate interventions. Ongoing stereotyped attitudes derived from a common lack of information and understanding between the fields continue to create barriers to care.

Implications for Mental Health Services

While it is possible to identify principles of care, it is more difficult to determine which practitioners within the existing service systems should be responsible for implementing these principles and engaging the person with co-occurring disorders in treatment. Persons with co-occurring disorders may seek help from mental health, substance abuse, or primary health care providers. The systems that support these providers have historically operated independently of one another, with separate philosophies, administrative oversight, and financial support (Ridgely et al., 1990). Both public and private sector initiatives over the past 20 years have reinforced the separation of these systems (Osher and Drake, 1996) while persons with co-occurring disorders continue to flood clinical settings.

The debate surrounding appropriate models of care and the locus of responsibility for providing care is often acrimonious as administrators and policy makers struggle to stretch scarce resources over the spectrum of care required for effective treatment of singly diagnosed populations. Failure to remove these barriers to care ensures that access to effective, integrated care is unavailable. In order to move the debate forward, there must be a shared language and vision for how to provide care to dually diagnosed individuals. Using the framework outlined in the New York model can serve as the basis for state and local strategies to ensure that the needs of persons with co-occurring disorders are addressed. The appropriate domain for service delivery and the eligibility criteria for various service settings will vary, depending on existing resources and programmatic structure. It is important to develop strategies for persons with co-occurring disorders who have severe mental illnesses different from those for all persons with co-occurring disorders. To date, there has been better research and knowledge generation on care for persons with more severe illnesses.

Various mechanisms can be used to ensure accountability and manage client flow. These include interagency agreements, joint program development, cross-training of providers, and the specific identification of individuals with co-occurring disorders as a priority population within all strategic planning initiatives (Ridgely and Dixon, 1995). At the community and program levels, Minkoff (1997) has outlined a process for implementing integrated services. This starts with the development of an integrated philosophy among all relevant stakeholders—from consumers to administrators. After agreement on an integrated mission and some principles of care, an assessment of current organizational capacity is performed and service gaps are identified. Participants then prioritize modest steps toward creating a continuum of assessment and treatment services using evidence-based practices. Ongoing psychiatric and addiction training is provided to all staff. Minkoff emphasizes the importance of leadership at all levels and the utility of ongoing process and outcome evaluation.

Conclusions

The mental health and addiction fields share a history of stigma and discriminatory financing practices despite having positive outcome data on treatment effectiveness every bit as good as data on somatic health services (NIMH, 1993). In addition, providing services to dually diagnosed individuals with complex biopsychosocial needs is necessarily costly. These costs are present when spending on behavioral health care has declined as a percentage of overall health spending over the past decade (U.S. DHHS, 1999). But the fact that integrated approaches with demonstrated effectiveness for those with co-occurring disorders are not widely available cannot be explained solely on the basis of scarce resources. Not providing high-quality care is ultimately more costly in terms of both dollars and quality of life. The failure to offer more comprehensive care for persons with co-occurring disorders is a failure in clinical and administrative leadership.

Principles of care within mental health and addiction fields converge on respect for the individual, belief in the human capacity to change, and the importance of community, family, and peers to the recovery process. Our consumers do not have the opportunity to separate their addiction from their mental illness. Why should we do so administratively and programmatically?

REFERENCES

Abram KM, Teplin LA. Co-occurring disorders among mentally ill jail detainees. *American Psychologist*, 46:1036–1045, 1991.

Alterman AI, Erdlen DL, LaPorte DJ, et al. Effects of illicit drug use in an inpatient psychiatric population. *Addictive Behaviors*, 7:231–242, 1982.

American Association of Community Psychiatrists. *Position Statement on Co-Occurring Disorders*, 2000. Available at: http://www.comm..psych.pitt.edu Accessed January 15, 2002.

Arndt S, Tyrrell G, Flaum M, et al. Comorbidity of substance abuse and schizophrenia: the role of pre-morbid adjustment. *Psychological Medicine*, 22:379–388, 1992.

Bartels SJ, Drake RE, McHugo GJ. Alcohol abuse, depression, and suicidal behavior in schizophrenia. *American Journal of Psychiatry*, 149:394–395, 1992.

Bartels SJ, Teague GB, Drake RE, et al. Substance abuse in schizophrenia: service utilization and costs. *Journal of Nervous and Mental Disease*, 181:227–232, 1993.

Baumohl J, Jaffe JR. *Encyclopedia of Drug and Alcohol*, New York: Macmillan, 1995.

Brady K, Anton R, Ballenger JC, et al. Cocaine abuse among schizophrenic patients. *American Journal of Psychiatry*, 147:1164–1167, 1990.

Breakey WR, Goodell H, Lorenz PC, et al. Hallucinogenic drugs as precipitants of schizophrenia. *Psychological Medicine*, 4:255–261, 1974.

Bureau of Justice Statistics, U.S. Department of Justice. *Corrections Facts at a Glance*. Revision, 1999. Available at: http://www.ojp.usdoj.gov/bjs/glance/corr2.txt Accessed January 15, 2002.

Carey MP, Carey KB, Meisler AW. Psychiatric symptoms in mentally ill chemical abusers. *Journal of Nervous and Mental Disease*, 179:136–138, 1991.

Carpenter MD, Mulligan JC, Bader IA, et al. Multiple admissions to an urban psychiatric center: a comparative study. *Hospital and Community Psychiatry*, 36:1305–1308, 1985.

Caton CLM, Shrout PE, Eagle PF, et al. Risk factors for homelessness among schizophrenic men: a case-control study. *American Journal of Public Health*, 84:265–270, 1994.

Caton CLM, Wyatt RJ, Felix A, et al. Follow-up of chronically homeless mentally ill men. *American Journal of Psychiatry*, 150:1639–1642, 1993.

Center for Mental Health Services. *Addressing the Needs of Homeless Persons with Co-Occurring Mental Illness and Substance Use Disorders*. Rockville, MD: Substance Abuse and Mental Health Services Administration, U.S. Department of Health and Human Services, 1997.

Center for Mental Health Services. *CMHS Managed Care Initiative: Report of the Panel on Co-occurring Psychiatric and Substance Disorders*. Rockville, MD: Substance Abuse and Mental Health Services Administration, U.S. Department of Health and Human Services, 1998.

Clark RE. Family costs associated with severe mental illness and substance use: a comparison of families with and without dual disorders. *Hospital and Community Psychiatry*, 45:808–813, 1994.

Cournos F, Empfield M, Horwath E, et al. HIV seroprevalence among patients admitted to two psychiatric hospitals. *American Journal of Psychiatry*, 148:1225–1230, 1991.

Cournos F, McKinnon K. HIV Seroprevalence among people with severe mental illness in the United States: a critical review. *Clinical Psychology Review*, 17:259–269, 1997.

Cuffel BJ, Shumway M, Chouljian TL. A longitudinal study of substance use and community violence in schizophrenia. *Journal of Nervous and Mental Disease*, 182:342–348, 1994.

Deitch DA, Carleton SA. Education and training of clinical personnel. In: Lowinson JH, Ruiz P, Millman RB (eds.). *Substance Abuse: A Comprehensive Textbook*. Baltimore: Williams & Wilkins, pp. 970–982, 1992.

Dickey B, Azeni H. Persons with dual diagnosis of substance abuse and major mental illness: their excess costs of psychiatric care. *American Journal of Public Health*, 86:973–977, 1996.

Dixon L, Haas G, Weiden PJ, et al. Drug abuse in schizophrenic patients: clinical correlates and reasons for use. *American Journal of Psychiatry*, 148:224–230, 1991.

Dixon L, McNary S, Lehman A. Substance abuse and family relationships of persons with severe mental illness. *American Journal of Psychiatry*, 152:456–458, 1995.

Drake RE, Essock SM, Shaner A, et al. Implementing dual diagnosis services for clients with severe mental illness. *Psychiatric Services*, 52:469–476, 2001.

Drake RE, Noordsky DL, Ackerson T. Integrating mental health and substance abuse treatments for persons with severe mental disorders. In: Lehman AF, Dixon L (ed.). *Dou-

ble Jeopardy: Chronic Mental Illness and Substance Abuse. New York: Harwood Academic Publishers, pp. 251–264, 1995.

Drake RE, Mercer-McFadden C, Mueser KT. A review of integrated mental health and substance abuse treatment for patients with dual disorders. *Schizophrenia Bulletin,* 24:589–608, 1998.

Drake RE, Osher FC, Wallach MA. Alcohol use and abuse in schizophrenia: a prospective community study. *Journal of Nervous and Mental Disease,* 177:408–414, 1989.

Drake RE, Wallach MA. Substance abuse among the chronic mentally ill. *Hospital and Community Psychiatry,* 40:1041–1046, 1989.

Grant BF. The influence of co-morbid major depression and substance use disorders on alcohol and drug treatment: results from a national survey. In: Onken LS, Blaine JD, Genser S (eds). *Treatment of Drug Dependent Individuals with Co-Morbid Mental Disorders.* Research Monograph 172. Rockville, MD: National Institute on Drug Abuse, pp. 4–15, 1997.

Haywood TW, Kravitz HM, Grossman JL, et al. Predicting the "revolving door" phenomenon among patients with schizophrenic, schizoaffective, and affective disorders. *American Journal of Psychiatry,* 152:856–861, 1995.

Jellinek EM. *The Disease Control of Alcoholism.* New Haven: Hillhouse Press, 1960.

Kessler RC, Nelson CB, McGonagle KA, et al. The epidemiology of co-occurring addictive and mental disorders: implications for prevention and service utilization. *American Journal of Orthopsychiatry,* 66(1):17–31, 1996.

Lehman AF. Heterogeneity of person and place: assessing co-occurring addictive and mental disorders. *American Journal of Orthopsychiatry,* 66(1):32–41, 1996.

Lehman AF, Myers CP, Corty E. Assessment and classification of patients with psychiatric and substance abuse syndromes. *Hospital and Community Psychiatry,* 40:1019–1030, 1989.

Lyons JS, McGovern MP. Use of mental health services by dually diagnosed patients. *Hospital and Community Psychiatry,* 40:1067–1068, 1989.

Miller FT, Tanenbaum JH. Drug abuse in schizophrenia. *Hospital and Community Psychiatry,* 40:847–849, 1989.

Minkoff K. An integrated treatment model for dual diagnosis of psychosis and addiction. *Hospital and Community Psychiatry,* 40:1031–1036, 1989.

Minkoff K. *Integration of Addiction and Psychiatric Services: Managed Mental Health Care in the Public Sector.* Amsterdam: Harwood Academic, 1997.

Mueser KT, Yarnold PR, Bellack AS. Diagnostic and demographic correlates of substance abuse in schizophrenia and major affective disorder. *Acta Psychiatrica Scandinavica,* 85:48–55, 1992.

Mueser KT, Yarnold PR, Levinson DF, et al. Prevalence of substance abuse in schizophrenia: demographic and clinical correlates. *Schizophrenia Bulletin,* 16:31–56, 1990.

National Association of State Mental Health Program Directors and National Association of State Alcohol and Drug Abuse Directors. *National Dialogue on Co-occurring Mental Health and Substance Use Disorders,* Washington, DC: NASMHPD/NASADAD, 1999.

National Institute of Mental Health. *Health Care Reform for Americans with Severe Mental Illnesses: A Report of the National Advisory Council.* Rockville, MD: National Institute of Mental Health, 1993.

Negrete JC, Knapp WP, Douglas DE, et al. Cannabis affects the severity of schizophrenic symptoms: results of a clinical survey. *Psychological Medicine,* 16:515–520, 1986.

Noordsy DL, Drake RE, Biesanz JC, et al. Family history of alcoholism in schizophrenia. *Journal of Nervous and Mental Disease,* 182:651–655, 1994.

Osher FC, Drake RE. Reversing a history of unmet needs: approaches to care for persons with co-occurring addictive and mental disorders. *American Journal of Orthopsychiatry*, 66(1):4–11, 1996.

Osher FC, Drake RE, Noordsy DL, et al. Correlates and outcomes of alcohol use disorder among rural outpatients with schizophrenia. *Journal of Clinical Psychiatry*, 55:109–113, 1994.

Osher FC, Kofoed LL. Treatment of patients with psychiatric and psychoactive substance abuse disorders. *Hospital and Community Psychiatry*, 40:1025–1030, 1989.

Owen RR, Fischer EP, Booth BM. Medication noncompliance and substance abuse among patients with schizophrenia. *Psychiatric Services*, 47:853–858, 1996.

Pepper B, Kirshner MC, Ryglewicz H. The young adult chronic patient: overview of a population. *Hospital and Community Psychiatry*, 32:463–467, 1981.

Regier DA, Farmer ME, Rae DS, et al. Comorbidity of mental disorders with alcohol and other drug abuse. *Journal of the American Medical Association*, 264:2511–2518, 1990.

Ridgely MS, Dixon L. Financing and policy issues in dual diagnosis. In: Lehman A, Dixon L (eds). *Double Trouble: Chronic Mental Illness and Substance Abuse.* New York: Harwood Academic, 1995.

Ridgely M, Goldman H, Willenbring M. Barriers to the care of persons with dual diagnoses—organizational and financing issues. *Schizophrenia Bulletin*, 16(1):123–132, 1990.

Rosenberg SD, Goodman LA, Osher FC, et al. Prevalence of HIV, hepatitis B and hepatitis C in people with severe mental illness. *American Journal of Public Health*, 91(1): 31–37, 2001.

SAMHSA. Report to Congress on the Prevention and Treatment of Co-occurring Substance Abuse Disorders and Mental Disorders. Rockville, MD: Center for Mental Health Services, SAMHSA, 2002 available http://www.samhsa.gov/centers/clearinghouse/clearinghouses.html Accessed July 15, 2003.

Seibel JP, Satel SL, Anthony D, et al. Effects of cocaine on hospital course in schizophrenia. *Journal of Nervous and Mental Disease*, 181:31–37, 1993.

U.S. Department of Health and Human Services. *Mental Health: A Report of the Surgeon General.* Rockville, MD: Substance Abuse and Mental Health Services Administration, Center for Mental Health Services, 1999.

Yesavage JA, Zarcone V. History of drug abuse and dangerous behavior in inpatient schizophrenics. *Journal of Clinical Psychiatry*, 44:259–261, 1983.

17

Advances in Psychopharmacology and Pharmacoeconomics

ALEXANDER L. MILLER
M. LYNN CRISMON
CATHERINE S. HALL
C. BRUCE BAKER

This chapter addresses three aspects of the field of psychopharmacology that, directly or indirectly, have a very large impact on the design and delivery of mental health services to the seriously and persistently mentally ill population. In each area we will highlight the evidence and considerations that should be helpful to policy planners and administrators as they organize systems of care and deal with physicians and consumers.

First is a review of recent advances in medications. The costs of primary drug treatments for schizophrenia, major depressive disorder, bipolar disorder, and dementia have risen dramatically in the past decade. Efforts to ration and limit this growth have, at most, delayed it in some sectors of health care. What are the characteristics of these new medications that have created such huge demand? Why are they better? Why are there so many new antidepressants and antipsychotics, for example? Clearly, the answers to these questions must take into account the enormous marketing clout of the pharmaceutical industry, but it would be a mistake to ignore the pharmacological evidence and clinical trial data that have earned these drugs Food and Drug Administration (FDA) approval and widespread acceptance by clinicians and consumers alike.

Second is a discussion of recent efforts to make drug prescribing more systematic and more uniform through the adoption of medication algorithms and guidelines at the organizational level. The emphasis here will be on identifying the types of guidelines that have been developed, their target populations, and the barriers to their implementation.

Lastly, we will present some of the key issues and major findings in the new and expanding field of pharmacoeconomics. In most health care organizations the pharmacy budget is treated as an independent entity in which the major controllable costs are acquisition of medications and personnel. In reality, there is a growing body of evidence that medication selection and consumer adherence to medication regimens can have a very large impact on use of expensive services, such as hospitalization, and on consumer satisfaction.

New Medications for Major Mental Illnesses

The past two decades have seen the introduction of many new medications for treatment of psychiatric disorders. These new treatments share two characteristics: they have been rapidly and widely accepted for use in the United States and they are significantly more expensive than their predecessors. In this section, the newer medications are compared to older agents used to treat the same condition from a pharmacological perspective. Four classes of medications are discussed: antidepressants, antipsychotics, mood stabilizers, and cognition enhancers. Medications will be compared on dimensions of efficacy, safety and tolerability, and potential to cause drug–drug interactions.

An important initial distinction to make is between the efficacy and effectiveness of a medication. *Efficacy* refers to results of controlled clinical trials, whereas *effectiveness* refers to performance in real-world settings. Effectiveness is affected by a host of factors that have much less impact on efficacy trials (e.g., ease of taking the medication, tolerability of side effects) or that may cause patients to be excluded from clinical trials (e.g., unstable medical illnesses, substance abuse). Efficacy studies may show no differences between treatments, but their effectiveness in general use is quite different because of these factors.

Antidepressants

The advent of fluoxetine (Prozac), the first antidepressant capable of limiting its effects to serotonin, in the late 1980s revolutionized the treatment of depression and introduced a new period of drug development (Judd, 1998). Before fluoxetine, [the first selective serotonin reuptake inhibitor (SSRI)], antidepressants belonged to one of two classes: tricyclic antidepressants (TCAs) and monoamine oxidase inhibitors (MAOIs). The SSRIs that have been FDA approved for the treatment of depression are fluoxetine (Prozac), paroxetine (Paxil), sertraline (Zoloft), and citalopram (Celexa). In addition to the SSRIs, the past decade has witnessed the further development of antidepressants that affect reuptake of other neurotransmitters in addition to serotonin. These are bupropion (Wellbutrin), venlafaxine (Effexor), nefazodone (Serzone), and mirtazapine (Remeron).

There are no differences in overall efficacy among the available antidepressants. Each has a 60%–70% response rate (Horst and Preskorn, 1998). However, any individual patient may preferentially respond to one agent over another. Some data suggest that venlafaxine and the TCAs may be more effective than other antidepressants in patients with severe depression (Clerc et al., 1994; Perry, 1996). There are also reports that mirtazapine is superior in treating severe depression (Hirschfeld, 1999).

The success of the SSRIs and other new antidepressants relates mainly to their safety, tolerability, and ease of dosing. They are much safer in overdose, a major cause of death in persons taking the older antidepressants. Moreover, they have few of the unpleasant side effects of the older drugs—dry mouth, constipation, urinary retention, and dizziness. Thus, physicians feel more comfortable prescribing them and patients feel more comfortable taking them. The impact of these factors (in addition to the destigmatization of depression) is illustrated in a recent study by Olfson and colleagues (2002). In surveys performed in 1987 and 1997, patients treated for depression in 1997 were found to be almost five times more likely to receive an antidepressant medication than those treated in 1987. The authors attributed the increased use of antidepressants to the improved safety and tolerability profile of the newer medications.

Over time, it has become clearer that the newer agents have their own problematic side effects, particularly the reduction of sexual drive and enjoyment. Many of the marketing efforts of manufacturers have been devoted to asserting claimed advantages in this regard, though the evidence has not always been convincing.

A relatively new area of concern in medicine has been drug–drug interactions, in which one drug inhibits or facilitates the metabolism of another. Inhibition can lead to toxicity, while enhanced metabolism can result in low, ineffective levels of drug. Newer antidepressants differ markedly from one another in their inhibitory effects on different components of the liver's drug-metabolizing system. Some of this emphasis is driven largely by marketing considerations, but there are very real issues here and many reports of toxic and fatal drug–drug interactions caused by SSRIs and other newer antidepressants (Richelson, 1998).

A reasonable conclusion from studies of safety, tolerability, efficacy, and drug–drug interactions is that there is no one best antidepressant. In fact, the evidence strongly favors the conclusion that antidepressant treatment must be tailored to the individual and that having multiple medication options available to the clinician is critical to optimizing treatment.

Antipsychotics

In a landmark study published in 1988 (Kane et al., 1988), clozapine (Clozaril) demonstrated efficacy in treatment-resistant schizophrenia and, by doing so, offered hope to millions of patients with schizophrenia whose symptoms had never responded appreciably to older agents, such as chlorpromazine (Thorazine) and haloperidol (Haldol). Unfortunately, clozapine can cause agranulocytosis, a rare but potentially fatal disorder characterized by a severe deficiency of neutrophils (a type of white blood cell). However, the finding that a medication could have better efficacy than existing treatments greatly stimulated drug development efforts in the antipsychotic arena.

Four additional antipsychotics have come to market since the release of clozapine. These second-generation or *atypical* antipsychotics, have become first-line therapy for patients with schizophrenia in the United States. The second-generation antipsychotics include risperidone (Risperdal), olanzapine (Zyprexa), quetiapine (Seroquel), and ziprasidone (Geodon). Of the newer medications, clozapine has demonstrated the greatest efficacy in the treatment-resistant population, but the risk of agranulocytosis precludes its use as first-line therapy.

Historically, the targets of antipsychotic treatment of schizophrenia have been positive symptoms (hallucinations and delusions). It has become clear, however, that impaired functioning in schizophrenia is more closely related to negative symptoms (e.g., lack of motivation, decreased thought production) and to cognitive deficits. There is evidence that the newer antipsychotics can improve negative symptoms and cognitive deficits more than the older antipsychotics. However, these improvements are often modest relative to the degree of impairment and may be related to their causing less typical side effects (see below) rather than remedying the core deficits of the disorder. In comparing older and newer drugs, other than clozapine, there is little evidence for significant differences in efficacy for positive symptoms.

The undisputed advantage of the newer antipsychotics is better tolerability. They are far less likely to produce distressing side effects (muscle spasms, tremors, restlessness) and tardive dyskinesia (a movement disorder often affecting jaw and face muscles associated with long-term antipsychotic treatment). Thus, patients and clinicians usually prefer the newer agents. As a group, however, they are more likely to cause weight gain, adult-onset diabetes, and hyperlipidemias, all of which are associated with higher medical morbidity and mortality. Moreover, concerns have been raised about their potential (mainly ziprasidone) for causing dangerous cardiac arrhythmias in predisposed individuals. Fortunately, the newer antipsychotics differ from one another in their likelihood of producing these and other side effects, so that clinicians can select antipsychotic therapy for an individual patient based on matching patient characteristics with drug profile. Moreover, at this writing, post-marketing surveillance has not found increased reports of sudden death, a marker for fatal arrhythmias, with ziprasidone.

Schizophrenia is a chronic illness requiring treatment of acute exacerbations and maintenance therapy. As noted later in this chapter, several studies have found long-term advantages for clozapine in maintenance of patients with treatment-refractory schizophrenia. One recent study found a newer antipsychotic (risperidone) to be superior to an older one (haloperidol) for relapse prevention (Csernansky et al., 2002). In terms of both quality of life for patients and costs of illness to society, confirmation of this finding with risperidone and with other newer agents will be important.

Most patients with schizophrenia initially respond to their first medication treatment but, over time, many partially or completely lose this response. Studies with the older agents indicate that if one fails, a second is quite unlikely to succeed. A critical question now is whether these poor responders should immediately go on to clozapine or whether they should be tried on one or more of the newer medications. Studies addressing this question are in progress. Current expert opinion and clinical practice patterns in the United States both favor trying at least two atypical antipsychotics before progressing to clozapine for most patients (Miller et al., 2001).

Mood Stabilizers

The recent history of medication treatment for bipolar disorder differs somewhat from that of the other disorders discussed in this chapter in that most of the newer medications have been developed for epilepsy and secondarily applied to the treatment of bipolar disorder. Moreover, since bipolar disorder has two sets of symptom complexes (mania and depression), both of which have a strong likelihood of recurrence, a particularly high premium is placed on prevention of episodes by maintenance treatment. These circumstances have led to common and frequent use of medication combinations, with a shorter-term component targeting the symptoms of the most recent episode and the longer-term component aiming to stabilize mood once the acute episode resolves. In general, available mood stabilizers are more successful in preventing manic than depressive episodes. For some patients, this means that on medication they no longer have periods of enjoyable euphoria, only episodes of dysphoria. Such patients may decide that the benefits of the mood stabilizers are insufficient and opt to discontinue them or to use them only to control the severity of a manic episode.

The first mood stabilizer, lithium, is still a mainstay in the treatment of bipolar disorder. Lithium is found as a naturally occurring salt. Its properties as a mood stabilizer were first noted in Australia in the 1950s and were systematically studied in large clinical trials in Denmark in the 1960s. The newer agents were found serendipitously in the search for treatments for patients who were poorly responsive to lithium. None of them has been found to be superior to lithium for manic episodes. In fact, strong evidence for anti-manic activity exists only for valproic acid (Depakote, Depakene) and carbamazepine (Tegretol, Carbatrol, Epitol) (Post et al., 1996). For none of them is the evidence for protective value against mood disorder recurrences as strong as the evidence for lithium. Nonetheless, the market share of the newer agents continues to increase and new agents continue to be developed. What, then, are the perceived advantages of the newer agents?

First, lithium is quite toxic to the brain and kidney at levels only two to three times the therapeutic range. Toxic levels can be produced by modest overdoses, by interactions with some commonly used medications [e.g., thiazide diuretics, angiotensin converting enzyme (ACE) inhibitors, and nonsteroidal anti-inflammatory drugs (NSAIDS)], and even by low salt diets. Thus, clinicians tend to favor drugs with less acute toxicity and less risk of dangerous drug–drug interactions. Second, initiation and titration of the newer drugs are somewhat easier than with lithium. Again, this is mainly because of concern about inadvertent lithium toxicity. Third, some of the newer agents, are less likely than others to increase liver metabolism of medications, which is a distinct advantage in many circumstances. Finally, lithium has been off patent for a long time, whereas the other widely used mood stabilizers are still on patent. Hence, prescribers are much more likely to hear about the virtues of the latter.

A quite recent development in the treatment of bipolar disorder has been the reemergence of antipsychotics as first-line medications. Clinicians have known for decades that antipsychotics treat manic episodes and can be useful in maintenance treatment. Use of first-generation antipsychotics for these purposes decreased sharply when it became clear that they often cause tardive dyskinesia with prolonged administration. The newer antipsychotics produce much less tardive dyskinesia, however, and are frequently prescribed for bipolar disorder. One newer antipsychotic (olanzapine) has received FDA approval for treatment of manic episodes, and several of the others are undergoing clinical trials to earn the same indication in their labeling.

In summary, with regard to mood stabilizers, there is good evidence that some patients respond better to one than to another. Thus, formularies need to have a variety of mood stabilizers. Moreover, use of combinations is frequent, with some literature support for this practice (Suppes et al., 2002). On the other hand, for many patients, relapses are frequent and improved maintenance treatments are sorely needed.

Cognition Enhancers

Alzheimer's Disease (AD) is a devastating illness that affects cognition, memory, mood, personality, behavior, and physical abilities. On average, an individual with suspected AD will survive 4–8 years after diagnosis. The *clinical milestones* that a patient can expect to experience include (*1*) progression from mild cognitive impairment to dementia, (*2*) loss of the more complex activities of daily living (ADL) such as ability to pay bills or drive a car, (*3*) emergence of neuropsychiatric symptoms, (*4*) nursing home placement, (*5*) loss of self-care ADL, and (*6*) death (Gauthier, 2001).

In contrast to the other disorders discussed in this chapter, there were no effective treatments for the cognitive decline of AD prior to the introduction of the cholinesterase inhibitors (CIs), which raise the level of acetylcholine by inhibiting its breakdown. Tacrine, the first CI, was developed in the early 1980s but is now rarely used because of its potential to cause liver toxicity, severe gastrointestinal upset, and the need for four times daily dosing. Compared to tacrine, the later CIs—donepezil (Aricept), rivastigmine (Exelon), and galantamine (Reminyl)—can be given once or twice a day and have much lower risks of liver toxicity, and serious gastrointestinal side effects. Currently, these are the agents most commonly used in clinical practice.

The main effect of CIs is to slow the rate of cognitive decline in AD. Thus, they work best if prescribed early in the course of illness. Clinicians and caregivers often have difficulty deciding how long these medications should be continued. Generally speaking, patients should remain on a CI while they are stable but once a patient's condition rapidly declines, the drug should be discontinued. However, some patients experience an even more precipitous decline after the medication has been stopped, and experts think that, after the drug is discontinued, patients deteriorate to the point where they would have been if they had never been treated with a CI (Crismon and Eggert, 1999).

There are no studies that clearly address two clinical questions about CIs. First, are there meaningful differences among them that can guide selection for individual patients? Second, if a patient either responds poorly to one CI or loses his or her response, is it worthwhile trying a different one? The answers to these questions will, when available, have important implications for determining how formularies and medication guidelines deal with the CIs.

In conclusion, while the CIs slow the rate of cognitive decline somewhat, they are far from a cure and the clinical course of AD is progressive. Other medications used in AD include antipsychotics and antidepressants for symptoms of depression, psychosis, and agitation.

Guidelines and Algorithms

Practice guidelines have been developed to address the variance that exists in health care with regard to the treatments provided as well as the outcomes achieved (Gilbert et al., 1998; Rush et al., 1998). In principle, the application of treatment guidelines to improve outcomes should decrease the variance in practices both within and among providers and within an individual patient over time.

Numerous methods have been used to develop practice guidelines. The easiest approach is through the use of informal consensus processes (Mellman et al., 2001; Woolf, 1992). This involves a group of clinicians coming together and deciding on the treatment guidelines that are most appropriate; this method is often applied within individual practices, hospitals, or managed care plans (Woolf, 1992). Potential problems with this method include the fact that the resulting guidelines may or may not be based on research evidence, and financial considerations within the health care organization, personal beliefs, or other considerations may be given precedence over health outcomes. Evidence-based processes use rating systems to evaluate the research literature in a given area (e.g., depression, schizophrenia) (Mellman et al., 2001; Woolf, 1992). In general, rules are applied to rank the quality of the research data (e.g., randomized, controlled trials over epidemiological studies or over case series), and this may be done by evaluating individual studies or by using meta-analyses to analyze the overall results from numerous studies with similar designs. One challenge in using evidence-based processes is to decide on the minimum amount of evidence that will result in a guideline recommendation. Requiring high levels of evidence results in guidelines that are highly supported by research; however, these types of guidelines frequently provide clinicians with minimal guidance for the most important decisions that they must make in providing care to patients. This is the case because inadequate randomized, controlled trials are available to address many clinical decisions. Numerous studies are available comparing all marketed antipsychotics with placebo, as this is required by the FDA in the New Drug Application process. Fewer studies are available comparing one drug within a therapeutic category with another (e.g., different antipsychotics), and these are frequently conducted by pharmaceutical companies to establish a marketing advantage compared with competitor agents. Therefore, the study design may enhance the probability of being able to show either efficacy or side effect advantages for the sponsor's drug.

When one looks at sequential treatment decisions, minimal evidence often exists to support guideline recommendations. For example, no evidence exists to support a sequence of choices (i.e., first drug choice, second antipsychotic to use in nonresponders, etc.) for the second-generation antipsychotics (Miller, 1999). The only evidence in this regard is the fact that clozapine appears to have clinical superiority in individuals with treatment-resistant symptoms, and even here the best evidence is in comparison with traditional antipsychotics (Kane, 1988; Miller, 1999, 2001). For antidepressants, we know from naturalistic studies that approximately 50% of patients who do not respond to the first antidepressant will respond to any randomly chosen second agent. It is also known that lithium augmentation will convert minimal responders into responders in about 50% of cases (Crismon et al., 1999; Rush et al., 1998). However, evidence does not suggest whether it is preferable to change antidepressant monotherapies or use lithium augmentation after an initial suboptimal antidepressant response. Beyond this, minimal research evidence exists to guide sequential treatment recommendations for depression.

Given this dilemma, guideline developers have two options. Either they can develop guidelines based only on evidence, as has been the case with the Cochrane Group guidelines (Geddes et al., 2000) and the Patient Outcomes Research Team (PORT) guidelines for schizophrenia (Lehman and Steinwachs, 1998), or they can develop guidelines based on both evidence and expert opinion. The latter has been the case with the guideline development efforts of such groups as the American Psychiatric Association (APA, 2002) and the Texas Medication Algorithm Project (TMAP) (Crismon et al., 1999; Miller, 1999; Suppes et al., 2002). Since evidence often does not exist to answer important clinical questions, guidelines based only on rigorous evidence provide limited guidance for difficult treatment situations (e.g., treatment-resistant patients, patients with a psychiatric disorder and serious comorbid general medical disorders). Thus, expert consensus can be helpful in filling in the gaps where evidence fails to answer important questions. The dilemma in these efforts is to determine to what extent guideline recommendations should be made in the absence of research evidence. This varies from guideline to guideline, but the approach should be discussed and agreed on by the guideline developers before consensus deliberations begin. The approach to decision making should also be clearly outlined in any guideline publications.

Another type of guideline development is the Expert Consensus Methodology (Frances et al., 1996; McEvoy et al., 1999; Sachs et al., 2000). This approach to guideline development is based on a modification of RAND methodology. First, an expert editorial board reviews the available evidence on a particular topic. Based on this evidence, the expert panel designs a list of questions regarding treatment situations that are not addressed adequately by available evidence. The editorial board then identifies a cadre of 50–100 individuals who are considered experts in the given area, to whom the survey questionnaire is sent for completion. Each item in the questionnaire is rated on a scale of 1 to 9. Nine is considered a treatment of choice; 7 and 8 are first-line treatments; 4–6 are second-line treatments that would sometimes be used; 2 and 3 are considered inappropriate; and 1 is extremely inappropriate. The experts' answers are analyzed based on 95% confidence intervals, and thus first-line versus second-line interventions can be determined based upon confidence interval bars that do not overlap.

Algorithms go beyond guidelines and differ in that algorithms provide a framework for clinical decision making (Rush et al., 1999a; Shon et al., 1999). In doing this, algorithms do not dictate clinical decisions, but instead provide a systematic approach to decision making that should yield similar answers when clinicians are faced with similar clinical situations. Algorithms can be divided into strategies and tactics (Rush et al., 1998, 1999). Strategies are the acceptable treatment regimen options that can be implemented in the care of an individual condition. The strategies are divided into treatment stages; for example, one or more medication regimens may be considered first-line interventions (Fig. 17.1). For patients experiencing inadequate symptom improvement or side effect intolerance with the first intervention, a number of options will be made available as stage 2 treatments. These may include alternate stage 1 interventions, and, depending on the available agents and evidence, other medications may be introduced as well. Depending on the disorder, available agents, research evidence, and philosophy of the expert consensus panel, combination treatments will be introduced at some stage in the algorithm. Again, this variable regarding an adequate level of evidence to make a guideline recommendation is a point on which expert consensus conference philosophy is extremely important in algorithm construction. For example, in the TMAP bipolar algorithm (Suppes, 2002), combination mood stabilizers are introduced early in the algorithm stages, even though the evidence for enhanced efficacy is modest. On the other hand, with only slightly lower levels of evidence, the TMAP schizophrenia expert panel introduced combination antipsychotics in the last stage of the algorithm, that is, for the most treatment-resistant individuals (Miller et al., 1999). Thus, in the absence of high levels of research evidence, the expert panels for treatment of these two different mental disorders have different philosophies regarding the approach to treatment.

The algorithm tactics address how to optimally implement a chosen treatment regimen (i.e., a stage) in an individual patient (Fig. 17.2) (Crismon, 1999; Miller et al., 1999; Rush, 1998; Suppes et al., 2002). Tactics address issues such as initial dose, dose titration, how to monitor the treatment response (e.g., symptoms and side effects), and how long to treat with an individual stage in an inadequately responding patient before deciding to move to another stage. Tactics also address the degree of symptom and functional improvement. Traditionally, treatment for the seriously mentally ill has usually been aimed at keeping the patient out of the hospital or minimizing socially unacceptable behaviors. Treatment for any disease state should be aimed at producing remission of the disorder or, if remission is not possible in an individual patient, at producing the maximum possible symptom and functional improvement. Since this may not be the mainstream philosophy in many public mental health settings, interventions to modify the attitudinal expectations of staff working in this environment are encouraged. Quantitative measurement of symptoms or function is one intervention that can be used to enhance clinicians' awareness of residual symptoms. However, rating scales used in clinical research are typically too long and time-consuming to be used in most clinical practice settings. Brief clinical ratings and self-assessments (when appropriate)

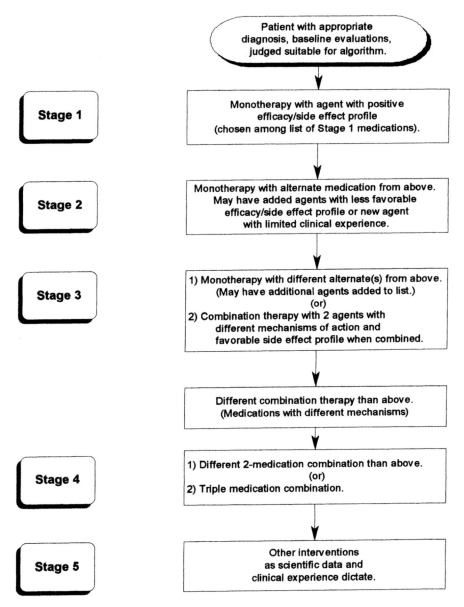

Figure 17.1 Exemplar algorithm showing strategies recommendations.

must be constructed so that quantitative assessment of improvement can occur in clinical care (Crismon, 1999; Miller et al., 1999; Rush, 1988).

The development of a guideline or algorithm is easy compared with actually implementing guidelines within a health care setting. The most common scenario is for guidelines to be developed and disseminated, and then not to be used by health

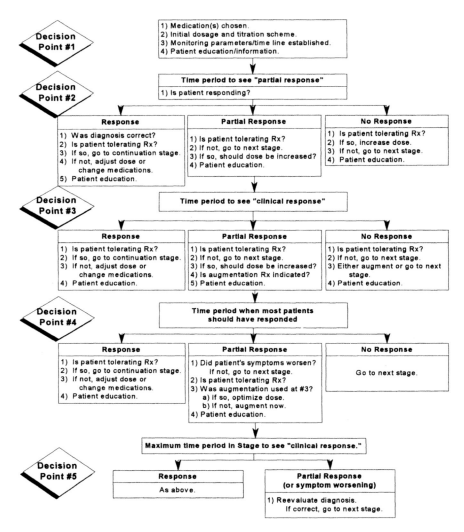

Figure 17.2   Exemplar algorithm showing tactical recommendations.

care providers (Corrigan et al., 2001; Rush, 1999a,b; Torrey, 2001; Trivedi et al., 2000). Ensuring implementation of a treatment guideline within a health care organization is a complex endeavor, and no single intervention will ensure that implementation occurs. Rather, an infrastructure must be put in place to optimize guideline implementation. This implementation infrastructure has been best described as a disease management program (Katon et al., 1995) and consists of four major constructs. First, research evidence (i.e., the guideline) and adequate skills management must be applied to the practice setting. Second, system design issues must be addressed to ensure that work flow processes are appropriate to support implementation; third, patient education programs must be put in place to inform patients and family members about the disease state, available treatment options, and potential outcomes of treatment, and to provide empowerment for the patient and family in receiving care. Lastly, communication systems must be put in place to ensure adequate communication among providers, and between providers and patients/families.

Even within the construct of a disease management program, implementation is not automatic. Clinicians work within health care organizations, and organizations often mold clinician behavior—either intentionally or inadvertently (Adelson et al., 1997; Corrigan et al., 2001; Rosenheck, 2001).

Guideline or algorithm implementation requires a plan for change within an organization. Organizational processes must be designed to achieve a work process that is consistent with implementing the guideline and achieving positive patient outcomes. The first step in this process is to identify individuals within the organization who are willing to become champions for implementation (Rosenheck, 2001). Second, all of the stakeholders who have an interest in the care provided within the organization must be identified. These stakeholders may vary but usually include clinicians, other clinical staff, support staff, administration, patients, family members, advocates, payer groups, and professional organizations (Rush, 1999a,b; Shon et al., 1999).

An implementation team is thus put in place, and planning begins. In doing this, it is important first to identify how the proposed changes are consistent with the goals or ideals of the organization (Rosenheck, 2001). Second, all potential obstacles that may impair implementation must be identified. Once these issues have been addressed, the team develops an implementation plan.

Adequate initial and ongoing training must occur to provide all staff with the necessary knowledge and skills management for implementation. Ongoing technical assistance must be provided to assist staff with implementation. This may consist of in-clinic consultation, call-in technical assistance, focus groups, academic detailing, and data collection and feedback (Trivedi et al., 2000). Computerized feedback systems have been shown to be some of the more effective methods for achieving behavior change. Computerization improves information systems, provides immediate feedback regarding treatment recommendations, and provides the database for quality management activities.

In order to achieve desired levels of implementation, quality management systems must be put in place to drive implementation. These measures are best considered as measures of the alignment of practice behavior with the implemented algorithms; this should be examined at the organizational and provider levels (Adelson et al., 1997; McGrew et al., 1994; Rosenheck, 2001).

Implementation of treatment algorithms is an evolutionary process, and system change does not occur without significant planning or effort. Implementation should be measured in incremental steps so that successes can be realized and plans made for further improvement. Within this context of implementation, evaluation, revision, implementation, and reevaluation, incremental improvements at every step can result in major improvements in the overall quality of care.

Pharmacoeconomics

Pharmacoeconomics can be defined briefly as "the study of economic factors regarding the cost of drug therapy, including their impact on health care systems and society" (Anderson, 2000). The field of pharmacoeconomics has grown tremendously in practical application, number of studies performed, and methodological development in recent years. Pharmacoeconomics is vitally important to policy makers and administrators for at least two reasons. First, it can provide conceptual clarity for decisions about resource allocation. Second, in an increasing number of jurisdictions/contexts, pharmacoeconomic analysis is either required or strongly encouraged by governmental institutions or third-party payers (e.g., Australian Commonwealth Department of Health Housing Community Services, 1995; Finnish Ministry of Social Affairs and Health, 1999; National Institute for Clinical Excellence, 2001; Ontario Ministry of Health, 1994; Portugese Pharmacy and Medicines Institute, 1998; Regence BlueShield, 1997; Ziekenfondraad, 1999).

Pharmacoeconomics covers a wide range of topics and forms of analysis. We limit our discussion to cost–effectiveness analysis of alternative treatments so that the discussion can be more focused and specific.

Despite the promise of cost–effectiveness analysis, several overarching problems/issues are widely recognized. Major issues include incomplete specification of assumptions, value judgments, and methodological choices in the overwhelming majority of studies; multiple disagreements about the underlying methodology; lack of consistency in methodology across studies; controversy about the appropriate role of cost–effectiveness analysis in decision making; and concern that pharmacoeconomic studies present greater than usual opportunities for bias in conducting and reporting research (Gulati and Bitran, 1995; Hillman et al., 1991; Neumann, 1998; Siegel et al., 1996; Udrarhelyi et al., 1992).

These concerns have been strong enough to prompt responses ranging from stricter journal policies for reviewing and accepting pharmacoeconomic studies (Kassirer and Angell, 1994) to multiple large-scale efforts to formulate, disseminate, and sometimes mandate use of guidelines for conducting and/or reporting pharmacoeconomic studies (e.g., Australian Commonwealth Department of Health Housing Community Services, 1995; Belgian Society for Pharmacoepideminology, 1995; Drummond and Jefferson, 1996; Finnish Ministry of Social Affairs and Health, 1999; Government/Pharmaceutical Industry Working Party, 1994; Langley, 1999; Murray et al., 2000; National Institute for Clinical Excellence, 2001; Ontario Ministry of Health, 1994; Pharmaceutical Management Agency Limited, 1999; Pharmaceutical Research and Manufacturers of America 1995; Portugese Pharmacy and Medicines Institute, 1998; Regence BlueShield, 1997; Siegel et al., 1996; Ziekenfondraad, 1999).

To understand both the promise and the issues surrounding cost–effectiveness studies, it is useful to note how such analysis is structured and the controversies arising from the method.

All descriptions of cost–effectiveness analysis do not agree completely (Hjelmgren et al., 2001). The following is one standard description. Cost–effectiveness is represented as a ratio between direct costs (the numerator) and changes in health status (the denominator). Using the example of newer versus older antidepressants, the relative cost–effectiveness would be represented as the incremental or marginal difference in the cost–effectiveness ratios determined for newer versus older antidepressants.

A cost–effectiveness model depends on many parameters, such as the effectiveness of alternative initial treatments, the effectiveness of switching to secondary treatments, the postulated lengths of treatment, and the costs and health effects are included.

The following are the major potential categories of costs and health effects (summarized in Table 17.1). Costs are resources consumed in providing the intervention, in this case treatment of depression, including dealing with side effects and other consequences. Costs are further subdivided into four major categories. The first category encompasses changes in use of health care resources including, for example, medication acquisition cost, physician and other personnel costs, laboratory and other service costs, and appropriately apportioned capital costs such as buildings and equipment. The second category of costs encompasses changes in the use of nonhealth resources including, for example, transportation costs. The final two categories encompass changes in use of informal caregiver time and changes in use of patient time for treatment, respectively.

Health effects are divided into two major categories. The first category, the intrinsic value of changes in health status, refers to the value placed on achieving or avoiding a specific health state. The health state may be characterized using a single domain or multiple domains, for example, including changes in clinical status, functioning, and quality of life. The measurement of outcomes in any one of these domains can range from intermediate outcomes (e.g., changes in depression rating scale scores) to more distal outcomes (e.g., years of life gained). In practice, sometimes when intermediate outcomes are used, the health state and cost–effectiveness ratio is denoted simply in the native units of a single domain (e.g., cost/patient remitted from depression) without assigning value weights. In fuller analyses, the benefits are assigned weights and denominated in more comprehensive generic units that can be compared and combined across domains. The most common generic unit is the quality-adjusted life year (QALY).

Table 17.1 Major Categories of Costs and Health Effects in Cost–Effectiveness Analysis

Category	Examples
COSTS	
Health care resources consumed	Medication acquisition, personnel, capital costs
Non-heath care resources consumed	Transportation
Informal caregiver time	Time diverted to care for patient
Patient time	Time devoted to treatment
HEALTH EFFECTS	
Intrinsic value of changes in health status	Value of achieving/avoiding specific health states
Effects on productivity	Morbidity/mortality effects on work output

The second major category of health effects, productivity effects, refers to resource consumption attributable to changes in productivity caused by changes in morbidity or mortality.

In the most comprehensive cost–effectiveness analysis, these cost and health effects categories would be applied to all sectors of health care even if the specific intervention is in a limited sector (e.g., treatment of depression in the mental health specialty sector). Some analyses are more limited and apply the categories only in the specialty sector.

We should note that *costs* are not the same as *prices*. From an economic perspective, costs refer to the value of the resources consumed in providing/producing a service like treatment of depression, ideally calculated in terms of the consumed resources' next best use, the opportunity cost. The many types of prices that can be assigned to resources, and that are used in most studies, may or may not reflect the economic value of the resources consumed.

The conclusions suggested by any given cost–effectiveness analysis are heavily dependent on each of the factors we have listed: the overall structure of the model, the cost categories and specific cost values used, the health effects categories, the method of measuring health effects, and the weights assigned to outcomes. In addition, the conclusions of the analysis are strongly dependent on the perspective of the analysis (i.e., cost–effective for whom?). The perspective determines which costs, benefits, and outcomes are potentially relevant and what weights are appropriate. Clarity about perspective is critical because, in most contexts, various combinations of cost and benefits are borne by or accrue to different entities. For example, in a highly simplified hypothetical situation, if a health maintenance organization (HMO) pays for prescriptions completely, and if choice of a particular antidepressant results in higher total expenditures for drug purchase but allows patients to be less dependent on family members, the cost is borne by the HMO but the benefit is gained by the patient's family. In this case, the antidepressant might be cost–effective from the perspective of the patient's family, or even from the broader perspective of society, but not from the perspective of the HMO.

Some of the commonly discussed or employed perspectives include a patient or patient/family perspective, an employer or payer perspective, an individual health care institution perspective (e.g., an HMO), a national health care specialty sector perspective (e.g., specialty mental health), a national health care comprehensive system perspective (i.e., including all health care sectors), or a global societal perspective (i.e., including *all* costs and *all* health effects).

There are several controversies surrounding cost–effectiveness studies. Many disputes center on the underlying economic theories. For example, some indirect costs, such as lost productivity, may be based on an economic theory known as *human capital analysis*, which is controversial. Detail on these and other issues can be found in multiple sources (e.g., Drummond et al., 1997; Gold et al., 1996; Luce and Simpson, 1995).

Ironically, given that methodological guidelines were intended to produce consistency across pharmacoeconomic studies, guidelines themselves from different sources are inconsistent on significant issues (Genduso and Kotsanos, 1996; Hjelmgren et al., 2001; Jacobs et al., 1995). For example, some guidelines recognize cost–benefit analysis as an acceptable method (Finnish Ministry of Social Affairs and Health, 1999; Ontario Ministry of Health, 1994; Portugese Pharmacy and Medicines Institute, 1998; Regence BlueShield, 1997), whereas other guidelines do not (Australian Commonwealth Department of Health Housing Community Services, 1995; National Institute for Clinical Excellence, 2001; Ziekenfondraad, 1999).

Even within a given set of guidelines, the clarity and completeness on various issues may be inadequate to yield sufficient direction to improve consistency among studies (e.g., Genduso and Kotsanos, 1996; Hjelmgren et al., 2001; Jacobs et al., 1995). For example, limited or no guidance may be given that would allow consistent assignment of costs or prices (National Center for Pharmacoeconomics in Ireland, 1999).

Individual types of cost–effectiveness study designs carry specific associated limitations (e.g., Drummond et al., 1997; Gold et al., 1996; Hotopf et al., 1996; Woods and Baker, 1997, 2002). For example, retrospective naturalistic studies suffer from the possibility of selection bias due to nonrandom assignment, no direct measurement of clinical outcomes, and a cohort effect, meaning that apparent differences between treatments may be confounded with changing trends in practice over time.

Critiques of cost–effectiveness studies consistently note that their quality is limited. This quality problem is shared by studies published in the academic literature that could use suggested methodology guidelines (e.g., Hotopf et al., 1996; Jones and Cockrum, 2000; Neumann et al., 2000; Woods and Baker, 1997, 2002) and by studies written for governmental agencies that mandate methodology guidelines (e.g., Hill et al., 2000; Rennie and Luft, 2000).

A full description or critique of specific psychopharmacoeconomic studies is beyond the scope of this chapter. Such critiques are available (e.g., Hotopf et al., 1996; Jones and Cockrum, 2000; Neumann et al., 2000; Woods and Baker, 1997, 2002). We present an overview of two case examples to illustrate the principles we have described and to give a sense of how these principles play out differently in different classes of medications. The case examples are for antidepressants and for antipsychotics.

The majority of cost–effectiveness studies with antidepressants have addressed the question of whether SSRIs and other newer antidepressants are more cost–effective than older classes of antidepressants; therefore, our comments focus on these studies.

Any evidence-based general conclusions about whether newer antidepressants are cost–effective must be strongly circumscribed for several reasons. First, there are no published studies on some issues. Second, on issues where there are published studies, there are very few studies based on the strongest research designs (e.g., Hotopf et al., 1996; Woods and Baker, 1997, 2002). Third, even if a given study design is accepted, many of the individual studies have other methodological flaws (e.g., Hotopf et al., 1996; Woods and Baker, 1997, 2002). Fourth, many studies are difficult to evaluate because they do not make their methodology and assumptions fully explicit (e.g., Hotopf et al., 1996; Rennie and Luft, 2000; Woods and Baker, 1997, 2002). Fifth, the studies employ diverse variations on almost all elements of cost–effectiveness analysis, making cross-comparison and aggregate conclusions speculative (e.g., DeVries and Gagnon, 1995; Gold et al., 1996; Hotopf et al., 1996; Rennie and Luft, 2000; Woods and Baker, 1997, 2002).

Only one prospective study has been reported (Simon et al., 1996, 1999). This study was conducted in an HMO in the United States among patients with diagnoses of major depression, minor depression, or dysthymia. Patients were randomly assigned to initial treatment with fluoxetine versus imipramine or desipramine but were allowed to switch treatment subsequently. The 24-month follow-up showed the following: more patients switched from the TCAs to fluoxetine than vice versa, and symptom, functioning, and direct cost outcomes were the same for both groups.

Acknowledging that there is only one prospective study and accepting the caveats previously noted about all of the studies available, one can suggest the following tentative conclusions. From the health care system perspective, first-line use of newer antidepressants in the primary care setting in the United States may be roughly equally effective and cost neutral in terms of direct medical resource costs to the health care system. However, given the many limitations in the quality of the evidence and the specificity of the studies' assumptions, which may not apply to a given health care organization or system, health care organizations or systems would be well advised to carefully check key assumptions, revise studies, or conduct their own studies, depending on the magnitude of the potential consequences flowing from use of the evidence.

Evidence on the psychiatric specialty care sector in the United States and on either primary care or specially care sectors in other countries is too limited to support generalizations. Reviews in other countries have come to the conclusion that TCAs may be more cost–effective in some contexts (e.g., Canadian Coordinating Office for Health Technology Assessment, 1998; Einarson et al., 1995, 1997; Hotopf et al., 1996).

From the global societal perspective, if newer antidepressants in fact are health care resource cost neutral to the health care system, there is a significant chance that these antidepressants are cost–effective to society. However, this conclusion is based more on inference than on available direct evidence. Fewer studies have addressed the societal question. Including the more comprehensive set of variables necessary to address this question is much more difficult, and studies have had limited success in addressing these additional variables (e.g., Hotopf et al., 1996; Woods and Baker, 2002).

Conclusions About Which Model Parameters Are Important

Evidence about which resource inputs and which model parameters generally are important and how they trade off against each other is somewhat more consistent. For example, if one is considering a health care budget rather than a pharmacy budget, in general over shorter time horizons higher acquisition costs of medications may be less important, while over longer time horizons higher acquisition costs may become more important. Cost of treatment failure appears to be a large, often inadequately considered cost that will militate against treatments with high failure rates, whether due to efficacy issues or effectiveness issues such as treatment compliance, even if such treatments have very low medication acquisition costs. These and similar issues have been discussed more fully elsewhere (e.g., Baker and Woods, 2001; Boyer and Feighner, 1993).

Bias

Evidence of sponsorship bias in studies in other areas of medicine (e.g., Gulati and Bitran, 1995; Hillman et al., 1991; Neumann, 1998; Rennie and Flanagin, 1992; Siegel et al., 1996; Udrarhelyi et al., 1992) raises concern over whether this problem also exists with psychopharmacoeconomic studies. We are unaware of any published studies that address this issue. We conducted a quantitative analysis of antidepressant pharmacoeconomic studies (Baker et al., in press). Using contingency table analysis, we investigated several potential associations between industry or nonindustry funding source versus outcomes. We found studies with SSRI manufacture sponsors more likely than those with nonindustry sponsors to report results favoring SSRIs over TCAs. Studies with newer antidepressant sponsors were more likely than studies with nonindustry sponsors to favor the newer antidepressants. Among industry-sponsored studies, those based on simulation models were more likely than those based on administrative databases to report results favoring the sponsors' versus the competitors' drug or drug class. Industry-sponsored studies were more likely than nonindustry-sponsored studies to report outcomes favorable to industry.

With antipsychotics, we focus on studies of clozapine. Clozapine is sufficiently different from other newer antipsychotics, often called *atypical antipsychotics* (e.g., in cost, efficacy, and side effects) that studies of clozapine should be considered separately from studies of other atypical antipsychotics.

The majority of studies have had used a retrospective and/or pre/post *mirror image* design without control groups (reviewed by Zito, 1998). These study designs are subject to numerous limitations. For example, in pre/post designs, patients selected for poor scores in the pre period may appear to improve in the post period simply because they regress to the mean. Some studies have reported results only for clozapine responders (Revicki et al., 1990, 1991). Such study designs markedly underestimate the full cost of treatment to a system.

The best data for specific conclusions come from two prospective studies. The first study was a randomized open label study of treatment-resistant hospitalized patients with schizophrenia in a state mental health system (Essock et al., 1996, 2000). Clozapine-treated patients were compared with patients receiving usual care with conventional antipsychotics. Over the 2-year study period, clozapine patients demonstrated significantly fewer side effects, less disruptive behavior, and a longer time to readmission if discharged. The clozapine patients did not show a greater probability of discharge, lower levels of psychotic symptoms, or less weight gain. Total costs were not significantly different between the two groups. In year 1, the mean cost for the clozapine-treated patients was $1112 greater than that of the conventional group, but in year 2 the mean cost was $7149 less. Cost–effectiveness was calculated for individual outcome measures rather than globally. For those outcome measures on which clozapine was superior to conventional treatment [e.g., extrapyramidal symptom (EPS) free months] it was also more cost–effective, but not for the other outcomes, where clozapine was not superior.

The second study was a randomized, double-blind, multisite study among Veterans Administration (VA), patients stratified for analysis with very high pre-study hospitalization use (mean, 215 days/year) and patients with lower hospitalization use (mean, 58 days/year) (Rosenheck et al., 1997, 1999). Clozapine was compared with haloperidol. Over the 1-year study period, the results were as follows. Among the patients with lower pre-study hospitalization use, the clozapine group versus the haloperidol group showed significantly lower levels of symptoms, no difference in quality of life, lower EPS, and higher QALYs. Among the patients with higher pre-study hospitalization use, the clozapine group versus the haloperidol group showed no difference in symptoms, no difference in quality of life, lower EPS, and higher QALYs. Both high and low pre-study hospitalization use clozapine groups showed absolute savings in total health care costs versus their respective haloperidol groups. The savings for the high hospitalization group were much larger than for the lower hospitalization group ($7134 vs. $759), and neither cost saving was significant due to large variability in costs. Given the higher QALYs and the cost neutrality for both groups, clozapine was considered cost–effective for both groups. However, there are two caveats. First, as the authors noted, these conclusions cannot be generalized across other groups of patients with different hospitalization use histories. The authors estimated that use of clozapine would be cost neutral only for patients incurring $25,000–$60,000/year in inpatient costs. Second, all the cost conclusions are based on the heavily discounted cost of clozapine to the VA, which is markedly lower than the cost to most providers, at least prior to the availability of generic clozapine (Luchins et al., 1998).

The best-designed clozapine studies suggest that clozapine-treated patients may fare better on some clinical outcomes, but the clinical outcomes may vary by patient population. These studies also suggest that clozapine treatment is cost–effective only for populations with high hospitalization rates. Clozapine studies of all designs agree that the biggest contributions to savings come from reduced hospitalization costs. Obviously, this suggests that it will be progressively more difficult to demonstrate cost–effectiveness in populations with lower initial hospitalization use.

Contrasting the cost savings with antidepressant versus clozapine analyses illustrates how seemingly technical issues of cost–effectiveness analysis often implicitly determine much larger issues. First, how a cost–effectiveness analysis weights different inputs (e.g., side effects, reduced symptoms, increased productivity) may favor different medications and different patient populations. With antidepressants, the largest cost savings often come from indirect costs such as increased work productivity. It is unclear whether large increases in work productivity currently can be expected in most antipsychotic-treated populations. With clozapine, the most important cost saving comes from reduced hospital days. Emphasis on work productivity versus hospital costs is likely to favor different populations and different medications.

Second, this difference in sources of savings highlights the way ethical issues are embedded in cost–effectiveness analysis. This case raises one of the underlying ethical controversies in human capital analysis: to what degree should patients' potential and the value of treatment be evaluated in terms of patient work productivity?

Implications for Mental Health Services

The foregoing discussion has important implications for those who pay for medications and regulate their availability in public mental health systems. Each implication will be explicated and discussed below.

First, new medication treatments for serious mental illnesses will continue to be developed in response to a huge demand for improvements in efficacy and tolerability. These new medications will almost certainly be more expensive than the ones they replace. Efforts to control expenses by limiting or impeding access to new medications can delay and slow pharmacy cost increases. This approach, however, risks alienating both consumers and prescribers, who often regard such measures as depriving them of effective treatments and reasonable choices. Moreover, in many instances, it can be shown that there are cost offsets of the more expensive medications, even if the benefits of these offsets are not realized by the organizations that pay for the medications. As a practical matter, it may be advisable for behavioral health care organizations to include front-line clinicians, consumers, and advocates in ongoing problem-solving discussions of resource allocation, including funding for medications.

Second, it seems highly likely that organizations will focus increasingly on maximizing effective long-term use of medications through the adoption of expert guidelines/algorithms and through quality assurance activities that aim to identify and reduce costly and inconsistent practices that lack an evidence base to support them. Essentially, this means taking a disease management approach that attempts to rationally prioritize the sequence of treatments and that promotes prescriber adherence to guidelines on how medications are to be used and how to measure responses to them. Adoption of this approach requires an organizational commitment to creating an infrastructure that will support its implementation. The necessary elements include training of physicians and nonphysicians, monitoring adherence to the guidelines/algorithms, organizing medical records to facilitate adherence, and updating as new knowledge becomes available.

Third, as the science of pharmacoeconomics becomes more exact and more sophisticated, mental health service providers will need to look to its findings to rationally guide changes in their systems of medication management. To do this, they need to understand the strengths and weaknesses of the data and methodologies. Moreover, it seems likely, with the advent of electronic records and internally generated databases, that behavioral health care organizations will be able to begin to track costs and effectiveness within their own systems when new medications or ways of managing medications are introduced.

In sum, medication development, management, and cost–benefit analyses are extremely dynamic areas that have enormous implications for delivery and organization of mental health services. It will be critical for providers of behavioral health services to continually update their practices to incorporate vital new knowledge from these fields. Moreover, a growing body of literature points to the advantages of combined psychopharmacological and psychosocial interventions in a spectrum of psychiatric disorders. To provide these optimal, integrated treatments, many behavioral health care organizations will need to reorganize the ways in which services are delivered, moving away from models based on mental health care professional groups each operating separately in its own domain.

REFERENCES

Adelson R, Vanloy WJ, Hepburn K. Performance change in an organizational setting: a conceptual model. *Journal Continuing Education Health Professions*, 17:69–80, 1997.

American Psychiatric Association. *American Psychiatric Association Practice Guidelines for the Treatment of Psychiatric Disorders*. Washington, DC: American Psychiatric Publishing, 2002.

Anderson DM. Preface. In: Dorland WA (ed.): *Dorland's Illustrated Medical Dictionary*. Philadelphia: WB Saunders, 2000.

Australian Commonwealth Department of Health Housing Community Services. *Guidelines for the Pharmaceutical Industry on Preparation of Submissions to the Pharmaceutical Benefits Advisory Committee*. Canberra, Australia: Commonwealth Department, 1995.

Baker CB, Johnsrud MT, Crismon ML, et al. Quantitative analysis of sponsorship bias in economic studies of antidepressants. *British Journal of Psychiatry*, in press.

Baker CB, Woods SW. Cost of treatment failure for major depression: direct costs of continued treatment. *Administration and Policy in Mental Health*, 28(4):263–277, 2001.

Belgian Society for Pharmacoepideminology. *A Proposal for Methodological Guidelines for Economic Evaluation of Pharmaceuticals*. Brussels: Belgian Society for Pharmacoepideminology, 1995.

Boyer WF, Feighner JP. The financial implications of starting treatment with a selective serotonin reuptake inhibitor or tricyclic antidepressant in drug-naive depressed patients. In: Jonsson B, Rosenbaum J (eds). *Health Economics of Depression*. Chichester, UK: Wiley, pp. 65–70, 1993.

Canadian Coordinating Office for Health Technology Assessment. Selective serotonin uptake inhibitors (SSRIs) for major depression. Part II: the cost effectiveness of SSRIs in treatment of depression. *Evidence-Based Medicine*, 3:87, 1998.

Clerc GE, Ruimy P, Verdeau-Palles J. A double-blind comparison of venlafaxine and fluoxetine in patients hospitalized for major depression and melancholia. The Venlafaxine French Inpatient Study Group. *International Clinical Psychopharmacology*, 9(3):139–143, 1994.

Corrigan PW, Steiner L, McCracken SG, et al. Strategies for disseminating evidence-based practices to staff who treat people with serious mental illness. *Psychiatric Services*, 52:1598–1606, 2001.

Crismon ML, Eggert AE. Alzheimer's disease. In: DiPiro JT, Talbert RL, Yee GC, et al. (eds). *Pharmacotherapy: A Pathophysiologic Approach*. Stamford, CT: Appleton and Lange, pp. 1065–1082, 1999.

Crismon ML, Trivedi M, Pigott TA, et al. The Texas Medication Algorithm Project: report of the Texas Consensus Conference Panel on Medication Treatment of Major Depressive Disorder. *Journal of Clinical Psychiatry*, 60:142–156, 1999.

Csernansky JG, Mahmoud R, Brenner R. A comparison of risperidone and haloperidol for the prevention of relapse in patients with schizophrenia. *New England Journal of Medicine*, 346:16–22, 2002.

DeVries A, Gagnon JP. Cost-effectiveness evaluation in health care: initiative for a standardized methodololgy. *Managed Care Medicine* 2:25–33, 1995.

Drummond MF, Jefferson TO. Guidelines for authors and peer reviewers of economic submissions to the BMJ. *British Medical Journal*, 313:275–283, 1996.

Drummond MF, O'Brien B, Stoddart LG. *Methods for the Economic Evaluation of Health Care Programmes*. Oxford: Oxford University Press, 1997.

Einarson TR, Addis A, Iskedjian M. Pharmacoeconomic analysis of venlafaxine in the treatment of major depressive disorder. *Pharmacoeconomics* 12:286–296, 1997.

Einarson TR, Arikian S, Sweeney S, et al. A model to evaluate the cost-effectiveness of oral therapies in the management of patients with major depressive disorders. *Clinical Therapeutics*, 17(1):136–153, 1995.

Essock SM, Frisman LK, Covell NH, et al. Cost-effectiveness of clozapine compared with conventional antipsychotic medication for patients in state hospitals. *Archives of General Psychiatry*, 57:987–994, 2000.

Essock SM, Hargreaves WA, Covell NH, et al. Clozapine's effectiveness for patients in state hospitals: results from a randomized trial. *Psychopharmacology Bulletin*, 32(4):683–697, 1996.

Finnish Ministry of Social Affairs and Health. *Guidelines for Reparation of an Account of Health Economic Aspects*. Helsinki: Finish Ministry of Social Affairs and Health, 1999.

Frances F, Kahn D, Carpenter D, et al. The Expert Consensus Practice Guideline Project: a new method of establishing best practice. *Journal of Practicing Behavioral Health*, 5:295–306, 1996.

Gauthier S. Alzheimer's disease: current and future therapeutic perspectives. *Progress in Neuro-Psychopharmacology and Biological Psychiatry*, 25:73–89, 2001.

Geddes J, Freemantle N, Harrison P, et al. Atypical antipsychotics in the treatment of schizophrenia: systematic overview and metaregression analysis. *British Medical Journal*, 321:1371–1376, 2000.

Genduso AG, Kotsanos JG. Review of health economic guidelines in the form of regulations, principles, policies and positions. *Drug Information Journal*, 30:1003–1016, 1996.

Gilbert DA, Altshuler KZ, Rago WV, et al. Texas Medication Algorithm Project: definitions, rationale and methods to develop medication algorithms. *Journal of Clinical Psychiatry*, 59:345–551, 1998.

Gold MR, Siegel JE, Russell LB, Weinstein MC (eds). *Cost-Effectiveness in Health and Medicine*. New York,: Oxford University Press, 1996.

Government/Pharmaceutical Industry Working Party. UK guidance on good practice in the conduct of economic evaluations of medicines. *British Journal of Medical Economics*, 7:63–64, 1994.

Gulati SC, Bitran JD. Cost-effectiveness analysis: sleeping with an enemy or a friend? *Journal of Clinical Oncology*, 13(9):2152–2154, 1995.

Hill SR, Mitchell AS, Henry DA. Problems with the interpretation of pharmacoeconomic analyses: a review of submissions to the Australian Pharmaceutical Benefits Scheme. *Journal of the American Medical Association*, 283:2116–2121, 2000.

Hillman AJ, Eisenberg JM, Pauly MV, et al. Avoiding bias in the conduct and reporting of cost-effectiveness research sponsored by pharmaceutical companies. *New England Journal of Medicine*, 324(19):1362–1365, 1991.

Hirschfeld RM. Efficacy of SSRIs and newer antidepressants in severe depression: comparison with TCAs. *Journal of Clinical Psychiatry*, 60(Suppl 14):27–35, 1999.

Hjelmgren J, Berggren F, Andersson F. Health economic guidelines—similarities, differences, and some implications. *Value in Health*, 4(3):225–250, 2001.

Horst WD, Preskorn SH. Mechanisms of action and clinical characteristics of three atypical antidepressants: venlafaxine, nefazodone, bupropion. *Journal of Affective Disorders*, 51:237–254, 1998.

Hotopf MM, Lewis GP, Normand C. Are SSRIs a cost-effective alternative to tricyclics? *British Journal of Psychiatry*, 168(4):404–409, 1996.

Jacobs P, Bachynsky J, Baladi, JF. A comparative review of pharmacoeconomic guidelines. *PharmacoEconomics*, 8:192–199, 1995.

Jones MT, Cockrum PC. A critical review of published economic modelling studies in depression. *Pharmacoeconomics*, 17(6):555–583, 2000.

Judd LL. A decade of antidepressant development: the SSRIs and beyond. *Journal of Affective Disorders*, 51:211–213, 1998.

Kane J, Honigfeld G, Singer J, et al. Clozapine for the treatment-resistant schizophrenic: a double-blind comparison versus chlorpromazine/benztropine. *Archives of General Psychiatry*, 45:789–796, 1988.

Kassirer JP, Angell M. The journal's policy on cost-effectiveness analyses. *New England Journal of Medicine*, 331:669–670, 1994.

Katon W, Von Korf M, Lyn E, et al. Collaborative management to achieve treatment guidelines: impact on depression in primary care. *Journal of the American Medical Association*, 273:1026–1031, 1995.

Langley PC. Formulary guidelines for Blue Cross and Blue Shield of Colorado and Nevada. *PharmacoEconomics*, 16:211–224, 1999.

Lehman AF, Steinwachs DM. Translating research into practice: the Schizophrenia Patient Outcomes Research Team (PORT) treatment recommendations. *Schizophrenia Bulletin*, 24:1–10, 1998.

Luce BR, Simpson K. Methods of cost-effectiveness analysis: areas of consensus and debate. *Clinical Therapeutics*, 17:109–125, 1995.

Luchins DJ, Hanrahan P, Schinderman M, et al. Initating clozapine treatment in the outpatient clinic: service utilization and cost trends. *Psychiatric Services*, 49(8):1034–1038, 1998.

McEvoy JP, Scheifler PI, Frances A. Treatment of schizophrenia. *Journal of Clinical Psychiatry*, 60(suppl 11):4–80, 1999.

McGrew JH, Bond GR, Dietzen, et al. Measuring the fidelity of implementation of a mental health program model. *Journal Consulting Clinical Psychology*, 62:670–678, 1994.

Mellman TA, Miller AL, Weissman E, et al. Evidence based medication treatment for severe mental illness: a focus on guidelines and algorithms. *Psychiatric Services*, 52:619–625, 2001.

Miller AL, Chiles JA, Chiles JK, et al. The TMAP schizophrenia algorithms. *Journal of Clinical Psychiatry*, 60:649–657, 1999.

Miller AL, Dassori A, Ereshefshy L, et al. Recent issues and developments in antipsychotic use. In: Dunner DL, Rosenbaum JF (eds). *Psychiatric Clinics of North America: Annual of Drug Therapy*. Philadelphia: W.B. Saunders, pp. 209–235, 2001.

Murray CJL, Evans DB, Acharya A, et al. Development of WHO guidelines on generalized cost-effectiveness analysis. *Health Economics*, 9:235–251, 2000.

National Center of Pharmacoeconomics in Ireland. *Irish Healthcare Technology Assessment Guidelines (Draft Version 2)*. Dublin: National Center for Pharmacoeconomics in Ireland, 1999.

National Institute for Clinical Excellence. *Revised Guidelines for Manufacturers Sponsors of Technologies Making Submissions to the Institute*. London: National Institute for Clinical Excellence, 2001.

Neumann PJ. Paying the piper for pharmacoeconomic studies. *Medical Decision Making*, 18(Supl 2):S23–S26, 1998.

Neumann PJ, Stone PW, Chapman RH, et al. The quality of reporting in published cost-utility analyses, 1976–1997. *Annals of Internal Medicine*, 132(12):964–972, 2000.

Olfson M, Marcus SC, Druss B, et al. National trends in the outpatient treatment of depression. *Journal of the American Medical Association*, 287:203–209, 2002.

Ontario Ministry of Health. *Ontario Guidelines for Economic Analysis of Pharmaceutical Products*. Toronto: Ontario Ministry of Health, 1994.

Perry PJ. Pharmacotherapy for major depression with melancholic features: relative efficacy of tricyclic versus selective serotonin reuptake inhibitor antidepressants. *Journal of Affective Disorders*, 39:1–6, 1996.

Pharmaceutical Management Agency Limited. *A Prescription for Pharmacoecoomic Analysis (Version1)*. Wellington, New Zealand: Pharmaceutical Management Agency Limited (PHARMAC), 1999.

Pharmaceutical Research and Manufacturers of America. *Methodological and Conduct Principles for Pharmacoeconomic Research*. Washington, DC: Pharmaceutical Research and Manufacturers of America (PhRMA), 1995.

Portugese Pharmacy and Medicines Institute. *Methodological Guidelines for Economic Evaluation Studies on Drugs*. INFARMED: Lisbon, Portugal 1998.

Post RM, Ketter TA, Denicoff K, et al. The place of anticonvulsant therapy in bipolar illness. *Psychopharmacology*, 128:115–129, 1996.

Regence BlueShield. *Guidelines for the Submission of Clinical and Economic Evaluation Data Supporting Formulary Consideration (Version 1.2)*. Seattle: Regence Washington Health, University of Washington, 1997.

Rennie D, Flanagin A. Publication bias: the triumph of hope over experience. *Journal of the American Medical Association*, 267(3):411–412, 1992.

Rennie D, Luft HS. Pharmacoeconomic analyses: making them transparent, making them credible. *Journal of the American Medical Association*, 283(16): 2158–2160, 2000.

Revicki DA, Luce BR, Weschler JM. Cost-effectiveness of clozapine for treatment-resistant schizophrenic patients. *Hospital and Community Psychiatry*, 41:850–854, 1990.

Revicki DA, Luce BR, Weschler JM. Clozapine's cost-benefits: in reply [letter]. *Hospital and Community Psychiatry*, 42:93–94, 1991.

Richelson E. Pharmacokinetic interactions of antidepressants. *Journal of Clinical Psychiatry*, 59 (suppl 10):22–26, 1998.

Rosenheck RA. Organizational process: a missing link between research and practice. *Psychiatric Services*, 52:1607–1612, 2001.

Rosenheck R, Cramer J, Allan E, et al. Cost-effectiveness of clozapine in patients with high and low levels of hospital use. *Archives of General Psychiatry*, 56:565–572, 1999.

Rosenheck R, Cramer J, Xu W, et al. A comparison of clozapine and haloperidol in hospitalized patients with refractory schizophrenia. *New England Journal of Medicine*, 337(12): 809–815, 1997.

Rush AJ, Crismon ML, Toprac M, et al. Consensus guidelines in the treatment of major depressive disorder. *Journal of Clinical Psychiatry*, 59(suppl 20):73–84, 1998.

Rush AJ, Crismon ML, Toprac MG, et al. Implementing guidelines and systems of care: experiences with the Texas Medication Algorithm Project (TMAP*). Journal Practical Psychiatry and Behavioral Health*, 5:75–86, 1999a.

Rush AJ, Rago WV, Crismon ML, et al. Medication treatment for the severely and persistently mentally ill: the Texas Medication Algorithm Project. *Journal of Clinical Psychiatry*, 60:284–291, 1999b.

Sachs GS, Printz DJ, Kahn DA, et al. The Expert Consensus Guideline Series: medication treatment of bipolar disorder. *Postgraduate Medicine* 2000; Apr(spec. no.):1–104.

Siegel JE, Weinstein MC, Russell LB, et al. Recommendations for reporting cost-effectiveness analyses. *Journal of the American Medical Association*, 276(16):1339–1341, 1996.

Shon SP, Crismon ML, Toprac MG, et al. Mental health care from the public perspective: The Texas Medication Algorithm Project. *Journal of Clinical Psychiatry*, 60(Suppl. 3):16–21, 1999.

Simon GE, Heilegenstein JH, Revicki DA, et al. Long-term outcomes of initial antidepressant drug choice in a "real world" randomized trial. *Archives of Family Medicine*, 8:319–325, 1999.

Simon GE, VonKorff M, Heilegenstein JH. Initial antidepressant choice in primary care. Effectiveness and cost of fluoxetine vs. tricyclic antiddepressants. *Journal of the American Medical Association*, 275(24):1897–1902, 1996.

Suppes T, Dennehy EB, Swann AC, et al. Report of the Texas Consensus Conference Panel on Medication Treatment of Bipolar Disorder 2000. *Journal of Clinical Psychiatry*, 63:288–299, 2002.

Torrey WC, Drake RE, Dixon L, et al. Implementing evidence-based practices for persons with severe mental illnesses. *Psychiatric Services*, 52:45–50, 2001.

Trivedi MH, Rush AJ, Crismon ML, et al. Treatment guidelines and algorithms. In: Dunner DL, Rosenbaum JF (eds). *The Psychiatric Clinics of North America Annual Review of Drug Therapy*. Philadelphia: W.B. Saunders, pp. 1–22, 2000.

Udrarhelyi IS, Graham A, Rai A, et al. Cost-effectiveness and cost-benefit analyses in the medical literature: are the methods being used correctly? *Annals of Internal Medicine*, 116:238–244, 1992.

Woods SW, Baker CB. Cost-effectiveness of newer antidepressants. *Current Opinion in Psychiatry*, 10:95–101, 1997.

Woods SW, Baker CB. Cost effectiveness of the newer generation of antidepressants. In: Davis KL, Coyle J, Charney DS, et al. (eds). *Psychopharmacology: The Fifth Generation of Progress*. New York: Raven Press, pp. 1119–1138, 2002.

Woolf SH. Practice guidelines, a new reality in medicine. II. Methods of guideline development. *Archives of Internal Medicine*, 152:946–952, 1992.

Ziekenfondraad. *Dutch Guidelines for Pharmacoeconomic Research*. Amstelveen, Amsterdam: Health Insurance Council (Ziekenfondraad), 1999.

Zito JM. Pharmacoeconomics of the new antipsychotics for the treatment of schizophrenia. *Psychiatric Clinics of North America*, 21(1):181–202, 1998.

Part IV

MANAGING MENTAL HEALTH SYSTEMS

18

Financial Management in Public Mental Health Services: A Strategic and Operational Approach

JAMES E. SORENSEN

Should you read this chapter? It is tempting to skip a chapter on financial management because the topic smacks of dollars and cents and not of more attractive and exciting issues such as clients, services, and treatment outcomes. The temptation may be fatal. *No organization (mental health or otherwise) survives successfully without effective financial management.* Great ideas about mental health must work out financially or they are not likely to work out at all. You do not have to be a financial wizard to understand the basic tools of financial management—tools that ultimately govern your ability to acquire, allocate, and account for resources.

Are you in the target audience? You are the target audience if you *deliver* public mental health services (e.g., mental health program or clinical director), or if you *fund* or *evaluate* public mental health services (e.g., a county mental health administrator or a funding agency at any level of government), or if you want to *learn* about public mental health services.

Why is this chapter relevant to you? Financial constraints and opportunities emerge from (Dixon, 2000; R. Feldman, 2000; S. Feldman, 1992; Kane, 1994; Nauert, 2000; Rosnkjar et al., 2000; Santos, 1997)

- Shifting funding sources (e.g., growth of Medicaid expenditures with cutbacks in federal funds to states and local governments).
- Increasing demands for more organized services (e.g., managed behavioral health care).
- Reorganizing responsibility for the delivery of mental health services (e.g., deinstitutionalization and emergence of community-based programs).

- Developing new service systems (e.g., shift from provider-centered to client-centered services and assertive community treatment).
- Increasing demands for linkages of services with client outcomes and client (family) satisfaction.

Coping with these opportunities and constraints requires a fundamental understanding of the financial management of a public mental health system (Finlay et al., 2000; Frank and McGuire, 1997; Manderscheid and Henderson, 1997; Mazade et al., 1992; McGuire, 1991; Minden and Hassol, 1996; Sorensen, 1989, 1992, 2000a,b; Wagenfeld et al., 1994; *Wall Street Journal*, 1998; Wheeler and Nahra, 2000).

What should you be able to do after reading this chapter? You will be able to assess the strategic management process, comment on the approach to total quality management (Baldrige National Quality Program, 2002; Evans and Lindsay, 2002), and evaluate the relationship of the strategic and operational financial management system to the overall management process. You will be able to review the key performance indicator system and employ the foundations of financial planning and control. You will be able to evaluate costs, budgeting, and cost–outcome and cost–effectiveness. In brief, you will gain a set of fiscal survival skills.

Planning and Performance Information

Management of a public mental health organization requires plans that relate to organizational goals and objectives based on the relative benefits and costs of optional courses of action while maintaining sufficient control to ensure efficiency and effectiveness in pursuing the organization's mission.

Planning information reveals what services the organization will render and to whom and what resources the organization will use to provide these services. Performance information measures how effectively the organization is doing its job and how efficiently the organization is using its resources.

A useful framework for planning and performance emerges from the *Ruiz v. Estelle* (1980) decision identifying six criteria of an adequate mental health system (Diamond et al., 2001, p. 22). While the criteria are focused on health care in correctional settings, the criteria have a striking relevance for all mental health programs:

1. a systematic program for screening and evaluating [clients] to identify those with mental health needs.
2. active treatment and interventions . . .
3. treatment by trained mental health professionals in sufficient numbers to identify and provide individualized treatment to treatable [clients] suffering from serious mental health disorders.
4. accurate, complete, and confidential records of the mental health treatment process
5. appropriate medication practices, and
6. a program for the identification, treatment and supervision of individuals with suicidal tendencies.

Financial Management

Managers of public mental health organizations must acquire and use resources to create effective mental health services at a minimum cost. As part of the general management process, financial management focuses on the analyses, decisions, and actions related to

- acquisition of resources (financing),
- allocation of resources (distribution), and
- accountability for the use of resources (evaluation).

A decision, for example, to develop new programs or service requires financing. The financing decision, in turn, may influence (and may be influenced by) the mix of services and professional staffing. The rate set for services may influence use and third-party payment flows. The amount and kind of service actually received by each client are linked to the financing source and to decisions on which staffs perform what services. The priority established by a state or federal agency for a service may or may not coincide with local priorities, thus slowing or hampering service expansion. Funding sources may require some type of outcome evaluation—what happened to the client? Clarifying the full set of relationships necessary to make optimal decision is difficult.

An Illustration

An illustration may shed light on the complex relationships in financial management.

Financing (or Obtaining the Resources)
To phase up community-based mental health programs and to phase down public psychiatric facilities requires a shift in the funding of public mental systems. To achieve a single stream, funding requires the central funding authority to channel funds to community mental health service. The community services may now have the authority and responsibility for purchasing inpatient services from public psychiatric facilities or from community alternatives.

Distribution (or Allocating the Resources)
New community services may envision home-based crisis stabilization, crisis home care, continuous treatment teams, assertive community treatment (ACT), or intensive case management including varied types of personnel such as a psychiatric nurse practitioner for continuous treatment teams or non–mental health service providers to administer case management services. If a state funding authority places caps on reimbursement (e.g., limits on case management rates), then the amount of service provided may be a function of available funding resources. A state or federal emphasis on crisis response capabilities may be at variance with established local partial hospitalization or day treatment programs.

Evaluation (or Accounting for the Resources)
Public funding sources may require financial reports on how and where the resources were expended. In addition, the agency may require an evaluation of the

customer's satisfaction with the services or some estimate of how well the customer responded to the services (e.g., client level of functioning).

A financial manager may examine some aspect of a decision individually and assume little impact elsewhere. A series of separate decisions may work at cross-purposes and produce bad results. Simple one-by-one financial decisions can wreck effective programs, and financially unsound services and programs providing good client service can scuttle an entire agency. Client service and financial management concerns must merge if public mental health organizations expect to survive in the *long run* (Sorensen, 2000c). A long-run perspective requires strategic financial management to be an integral component of the agency's strategic management.

Financial Management as an Element of Strategic Management: An Overview of Strategic Management

Someone in the financial management of the public mental health sector may wonder about the value of a summary of the strategic management process. Consider, for example, the following questions:

- Is there an appropriate match between financial resources and goals? (This question determines if the organizational resources are being generated and used according to the institution's vision and mission.)
- Do the sources and uses of resources match appropriately? (This question examines how various resources are derived and consumed.)
- Are the financial resources sustainable? (This question probes the stability of revenues, expenses, assets, and liabilities.)

In brief, high-level financial management links to the strategic management process and requires a mutual understanding of both agendas. There is a need "to dance the waltz together."

An integrated model of strategic management involves strategic planning and strategic control. Strategic planning includes formulating and evaluating optional strategies, choosing a strategy, and developing plans for putting it in practice (Dobson and Starkey, 1993; Kaplan and Norton, 1996, 2000). These plans should reflect the values and expectations of the stakeholders, the organization's vision or mission, goals and objectives, external and internal environments of the organization, and major policies (Aaker, 1995; Wheelen and Hunger, 2000). Strategic control means ensuring compliance with the strategic plan (Wheelen and Hunger, 2000).

The vision statement declares key *values or ideals* while the mission statement defines *why* the organization exists and *why* it competes in the public sector. Goals (or the broad directions or results) and objectives (the focus on more specific targets) are *what* the organization wants to accomplish. The formulation of goals and objectives uses an assessment of the organization's environment and resources. Pursuit of organizational goals and objectives leads to the formulation of a strat-

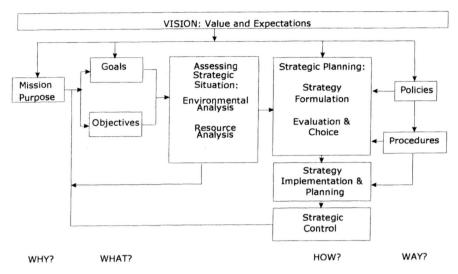

Figure 18.1   Integrated model of strategic management.

egy including a general approach down to specific plans to be implemented. Organizational policies help *to limit choices* among optional strategies, while procedures *guide* the implementation. An illustrative and interactive model appears in Figure 18.1.

The starting point for the formulation of a strategy is the vision statement. As an illustration, West Virginia's vision statement specifies "a community that values and respects people and is responsive to their individual needs, wants and desires for the enrichment of their lives." (West Virginia, 2001, p. 2). Vision statements are general, lofty, and inspiring. The mission statement, on the other hand, focuses more specifically on what the organization tries to do. West Virginia's states, "We ensure that the positive meaningful opportunities are available for persons with mental illness, chemical dependency, developmental disabilities and those at-risk. We provide support for families, providers and communities in assisting persons to achieve their potential and gain greater control over the direction of their future." (West Virginia, 2001, p. 2). West Virginia adds an additional values statement: "We believe in integrity-based leadership that is flexible enough to respond to change that is guided by consumers, employers, and their community" (p. 2). Note that these statements emphasize consumer empowerment, normalization, and client–provider decision making about services to meet consumer needs.

Another example of a vision or mission statement is from the Tennessee PL 99-660 Mental Health Plan (1991) (Yearwood, et al., 1992): The mission statement of the Department of Mental Health and Retardation "is to improve the quality of life for consumers and their families as *they* define quality of life. . . . The Division of Mental Health Services (DMHS) is committed to a mental health delivery system that is centered on the stated needs and preference of primary consumers that is accountable to these individuals and their families, and . . . consumer empowerment through meaningful involvement by consumers in all aspects of planning and providing services. Programs and services supported by the DMHS will assist adults with severe disabling mental illness to control the symptoms of their illness, to develop the skills and acquire the supports and resources they need to succeed where they choose to live, learn, and work. Programs and service supported by the DMHS will assist children and their families in their efforts to remain together and to develop skills and acquire the supports and resources they need to function successfully in the most normalized setting possible. Services will assist adults, children, and their families to maintain responsibility to the greatest extent possible for setting their own goals, directing their own lives, development and acting responsibly as members of the community" (pp. 22, 23).

The foregoing mission statements are about the purpose of the agency. (A mission statement for a health maintenance organization exists in Ludden and Mandell, 1993.) Once the purpose is clear, then the goals (i.e., broad directions and intentions) and objectives (i.e., more specific ends to be met) are next. Illustrative goals for a public mental health agency might be (Yearwood et al., 1992):

1. Design and deliver services guided by the needs and preferences of consumers and family members.
2. Integrate inpatient treatment settings as a flexible backup to comprehensive community support and other mental health services.
3. Allocate most public health financial and human resources to community services focused on persons with serious mental illness.

Objectives are to be written, understandable, challenging, attainable, measurable, and dated (Wheelen and Hunger, 2000). Objectives for the forgoing goals (for several different states) might include the following:

1. For chronically and persistently mentally ill clients, provide an ACT team with in-home stabilization, community-based placements, or brief inpatient treatment and admission to a state institute as a last resort (Santos, 1997).
2. Develop a cost–effective, supported employment program rather than rehabilitative day treatment (Clark et al., 1996, 1998).
3. Develop intensive case management to foster successful community integration using improved housing, improved employment, an increased network of friends, and decreased inpatient admissions treatment (Stroul, 1989).

Generally, goals and objectives provide targets focused on kinds of clients, types and distribution of services, finances, staffing, and growth (or decline).

Assessing the Strategic Situation

Opportunities and threats of the general environment are generally factors over which the organization has little direct control. Generally these include the economy, technology, social factors such as consumer preferences, and political or legal issues. Funding of mental health services in a general national health insurance program, for example, may be beyond the direct influence of most public mental health programs. Another general trend beyond direct control is the shift in the desires of mental health consumers to participate in formulating the type and location of services. Changes and trends in these factors should influence the directions of the strategic plan.

Internal analysis includes the listing of *internal strengths* (e.g., qualified professional staff, good distinctive competence, strong financial position, cost advantages, good image and reputation, demonstrated management, capability for innovation) and *internal weaknesses* (e.g., high cost compared to other providers, weak marketing skills, poor internal information systems, unfocused strategy, lack of shared values).

External opportunities and threats include the listing of *potential opportunities* (e.g., adding new programs, entering new segments or markets, rapid growth in demand, exits of rivals from the market) and *potential threats* (e.g., slower market growth, adverse governmental policies and lower funding, stronger competitive pressures, adverse economic conditions).

Competitive Position Assessment

Assessment should be a careful review of the strengths and advantages and weaknesses and disadvantages to evaluate if the organization's position is improving or slipping and why. Does the organization have a net competitive advantage or disadvantage? How strong is the competitive advantage or how bad is the competitive disadvantage, and how hard will it be to overcome the disadvantage? What are the implications for overall strategy? What are the hurdles the organization will have to overcome in view of the competitive forces, future competitive conditions, and moves of key rivals (University of Denver, 2001)?

Strategy Formulation, Evaluation, and Choice

The organization should define a root strategy, set strategic goals (e.g., five) and key performance objectives (e.g., three to five), and formulate a strategy to achieve the target objectives. The mission statement should indicate what the organization wants to accomplish and the markets it wants to serve.

The overall strategy should indicate the thrust of the business-level strategy (e.g., aggressive grow-and-build, conservative hold-and-maintain, whether major offensive moves should be initiated and if so, what kinds of moves, or whether the emphasis should be on defense and fortification). The business-level strategy should address how to respond to changing mental health industry and competitive conditions, how to compete and how to achieve a stronger position, and the resource allocation priorities within the organization (Sorensen, 1989).

The strategy should develop a competitive approach that will produce a sustainable competitive advantage. Typical options include low-cost service, differentiation of service, or special service niches. The approach pinpoints the competitive advantages the organization should strive for and identifies the acts required to create this advantage. Also included are specific offensive or defensive moves needed as part of the overall competitive approach.

Implementation of the strategic plan comes from the organizational functions of client services, programs, and administration. The analysis of the proposed financial strategy requires a determination of whether all the functional strategies can be funded at reasonable level of costs. Note that the definition of client services, programs, and administration shifts as the organization shifts from a direct public health provider to an administrative unit at a city, county, state, or federal level.

Finally, a review of the strategy should assess if it meets all the industry and organizational strategic issues identified earlier. Recommendations include both short-term and long-term priorities.

Strategic Financial Plans

Most strategic financial plans include a clear statement of the objectives of the entity, along with the costs and financing of the objectives over a specified time period such as 3 years, 5 years, or, in the case of large state agencies, 20 years. The format presented in Figure 18.2 illustrates the basic approach. Specifying objectives, programs, and services requires the *output* of the strategic planning process. Without careful strategic planning, the strategic financial plan cannot take shape.

At this point, reviews and reevaluation of the costs and funding of objectives are possible. If the strategic financial plan is a *rolling* plan (say, a 5-year plan) at the end of each year, the current year is dropped and a new fifth year is added. New information about objectives, programs, and services is added or revised. If, for example, new funding sources appear (or disappear), the information is included in the plan. If the objectives change (e.g., increase, decrease, are eliminated), the appropriate revenue and expense information is included. The power

Variable	T	T+1	T+2	. . .	T+5
Objective/Goal	Expenses				
1. AAA	$ xxx	$ xxx	$ xxx		$ xxx
2. BBB	$ xxx	$ xxx	$ xxx		$ xxx
Total Expenses	$ xxx	$ xxx	$ xxx		$ xxx
Funding	Revenues				
1. YYY	$ xxx	$ xxx	$ xxx		$ xxx
2. ZZZ	$ xxx	$ xxx	$ xxx		$ xxx
Total Revenue	$ xxx	$ xxx	$ xxx		$ xxx
Net Over (Under)					
Recovery (Total Revenue -Total Expense)	$ xxx	$ xxx	$ xxx		$ xxx
Beginning net assets (or fund balance)	+ $ xxx	$ xxx	$ xxx		$ xxx
Ending net assets (or ending fund balance)	= $ xxx	$ xxx	$ xxx		$ xxx

Figure 18.2   Strategic financial plans.

of the strategic financial plan flows from anticipating what is and what might be happening to the organization. If multiple conditions are anticipated, then multiple runs and outputs may be required to provide top managers with an adequate view of the potential future.

Financial Management as an Element of Total Quality Management

Several of the key forces driving total quality management (TQM) (Baldrige National Quality Program, 2002; Evans and Lindsay, 2002; McLaughlin and Kaluzny, 1997; Shuyter and Barnett, 1995) focus on the following:

- Intensifying competition for mental health resources (e.g., pressures to fund other health services or other social services such as education).
- Increasing awareness of the inefficiency in the delivery of mental services (e.g., home-based crisis stabilization is more efficient than inpatient hospitalization).
- The emergence of a new understanding that high quality is possible along with lower costs (e.g., intensive case management can improve the quality of care to a target client group while lowering costs, especially those of inpatient admissions treatment).
- New knowledge about the needs and capabilities of individuals with severe and persistent psychiatric disabilities (e.g., many individuals with severe mental illness and emotional disturbance can maintain jobs, friendships and families).

The *Health Care Criteria for Performance Excellence* (Baldrige National Quality Program, 2002) stimulate an aligned approach to organizational performance management that results in the

- delivery of ever-improving value to patients and other customers and the contribution to improved health care quality;
- improvement of overall organizational effectiveness and capabilities as a health care provider; and
- organizational and personal learning.

The *Health Care Criteria* focus on organizational performance areas including

- patient and other customer-focused results;
- health care results;
- financial and market results;
- staff and work system results;
- organizational effectiveness results, including operational and supplier performance; and
- public responsibility and community health results.

From a practical managerial viewpoint, *quality is ongoing improvement*. The improvement can be incremental (e.g., a modest change) or a breakthrough (e.g., a radical redesign of the delivery of mental health services).

Information Systems and Key Performance Indicators

A significant cornerstone in any approach to financial management is the organizational information system (IS). The information system should produce information that (Chapman, 1976)

- assesses the patterns of service delivery (e.g., who receives how much of what type of services, when, and where?);
- defines how current resources are being acquired and consumed (e.g., what are the major sources of revenue and how are they being spent?);
- provides monitoring aids for various health care providers and managers (e.g., are the admissions appropriate?);
- develops data for multiple reporting requirements (e.g., reporting to funding agencies);
- creates a database for planning (e.g., monitors changing demographics to formulate future program planning); and
- assesses the outcomes of services provided (e.g., level of client functioning, impact of a program on a community).

Significance of Key Performance Indicators in Financial Management

Enhanced financial management results if the outputs of an IS focus on key variables or key performance indicators (KPIs) (also known as *key result areas* or *key success factors*). A similar model is in the Governmental Accounting Standards Board (GASB) *service efforts and accomplishments* reporting or SEA indicators (Bailey, 2002). Identifying KPIs in a public mental health organization requires a thorough understanding of the programmatics and economics of mental health services. Experienced managers are likely to give primary attention to KPIs (Cleverley, 2001). Generally, these indicators are important to the success of the organization, are robust summaries of more complex relationships, are factors requiring managerial action when significant change occurs, and may be sensitive to quick or volatile changes.

One successful approach to multiple multidimensional performance indicators is the Balanced Score Card (BSC) (Kaplan and Norton, 1996, 2000). The BSC assesses KPIs on customers, financial performance, operations, and innovation (or learning). This approach has been successful in the private business sector, and it is now being adapted to health care and education—two of the largest components of our gross domestic product (GDP). Since our focus is strategic financial management, we will narrow our discussion.

One useful approach is to design the KPI around four mixes: revenues, clients, staff, and services (Sorensen et al., 1987). Illustrative ratios include the following:

Revenue Mixes

1. % distribution of revenue by source: $= \dfrac{\text{revenue by source}}{\text{total annual revenue}}$

2. $\dfrac{\text{expense convergence rate by}}{\text{[defined] program element:}} = \dfrac{\text{total standard charges by [defined] program}}{\text{total expenses by [defined] program element}}$

Ratio 1 provides insight into the revenue stream and identifies the sources of revenue of the organization. Ratio 2 examines the convergence of the expenses of a [defined] program element to the value of the services provided. The numerator is the standard charge (or fair market value) of a service multiplied by the number of the services rendered (thus producing the *total standard charges*), while the denominator is the total resource (or expense) consumed by the [defined] program element. Under ideal conditions, the ratio would be 1, thus suggesting that the value of the service (as measured by what is charged for it in the marketplace) is equal to the resources consumed (as measured by its expenses). A quick application of the ratio can find *leaky boats* or program elements that are not carrying their own weight. If program cuts have to be made, the ratio identifies more rational candidates.

Client Mixes

$\dfrac{\text{Client health status by}}{\text{[defined] age group}} = \dfrac{\text{\# of severely mentally ill in [defined] age group}}{\text{totally severely mentally ill}}$

This health status ratio indicates the attention an agency may be directing to varying age groups. For example, are children and geriatric clients present? Are they underrepresented? Does the case finding of geriatric clients deserve more effort? If the denominator comparison was, say, total admissions, a state agency may identify appropriate or inappropriate admission patterns by the service providers it funds.

Staff Mixes

% distribution of clinical staff effort by [defined] program element

$= \dfrac{\text{Total \# of clinical staff hours devoted to [defined] program element}}{\text{Total \# of clinical staff hours devoted to all program elements}}$

This staff ratio reveals the relative distribution of staff effort to [defined] program elements. If the numerator controls for the type of discipline, then the ratio indicates the distribution of disciplines among the program elements.

Service Mixes

1. $\dfrac{\text{Average \# of service units per full-time equivalent (FTE) day by [defined] program element}}{} = \dfrac{\text{Total \# of units of [defined] program element}}{\text{Total FTE days by [defined] program element}}$

$$2. \text{ Cost per unit of service by} \atop \text{[defined] program element} = \frac{\text{Direct + Indirect + Allocated costs of [defined] program element}}{\text{Total units of service of [defined] program element}}$$

Ratio 1 measures the productivity of staff in the varying [defined] program elements. While only measuring how hard the staff is working, it may be useful in comparative assessments to ascertain if the staff is being adequately used. A modification of the ratio is to divide the number of clients attending per day by the number of FTE staff to identify the average attending per day per FTE. In many of the newly emerging programs (e.g., crisis teams), the latter measure is more meaningful.

Ratio 2 is an overall index of resources consumed to production provided for a [defined] program element. Cost per unit can be a useful index of efficiency when compared over time within an agency or when compared to other similar organizations. In some cases, the total cost index may vary between different-sized organizations because of the amount and impact of fixed costs being spread over a smaller or larger number of units of service. Often the cost per unit is the basis for funding negotiations and reimbursement agreements (e.g., Medicaid)

The essence of financial control is the comparison of planned (e.g., budgeted) level of activity with what is actually happening. All the foregoing KPI measures lend themselves to a *budget versus actual* format. For example, if the planned unit cost of service is compared to the actual unit cost of service, the resulting ratio becomes a simplified tool to evaluate the performance of the organization and to detect when appropriate managerial investigations should occur (e.g., the ratio is markedly less or greater than 1, suggestion that the process is out of control).

Management Accounting

Most mental health managers face two difficult questions:

- Are we doing what we should be doing?
- How well are we doing what we do?

Today's complex mental health environment gives neither easy nor clear-cut answers to these questions. The *first* question refers back to our strategic plans and how those translated into a strategic financial plan. Long-term objectives and translation of those objectives into operational financial plans require budgeting tools.

How well the organization is functioning is somewhat easier to assess than whether the objectives are appropriate. Efficiency is the accomplishment of objectives at a minimum cost, while effectiveness measures how well the objectives are achieved. Cost behavior and cost classification, contribution margin analysis, differential analysis, flexible budgeting, and budget variance analysis are the management accounting tools used to address the *second* question.

Cost Behavior

Management accounting examines cost behavior in relation to volume of activity. As volume of activity varies, a cost may increase proportionally to volume (a variable cost), may not change as volume changes (a fixed cost) or may change in stepwise fashion (a step-variable cost) as volume changes. Figure 18.3 portrays these basic cost behaviors including a mixed set of costs. Copying costs, for example, may vary directly with the number of copies produced (e.g., a variable cost), while annual lease payments may remain constant (e.g., a fixed cost), regardless of client volume. The number of administrative assistants may increase as the volume of activity (e.g., number of contracts) changes, and the cost behaves in a stair-step fashion (e.g., step-variable cost) since each assistant can handle a certain number of contracts before another assistant is required.

Revenue Behavior

Management accounting also classifies revenues like costs. Revenues may be variable (e.g., a unit of service provides a specified amount of revenue) or fixed (e.g., categorical funding for a service without regard to volume of service).

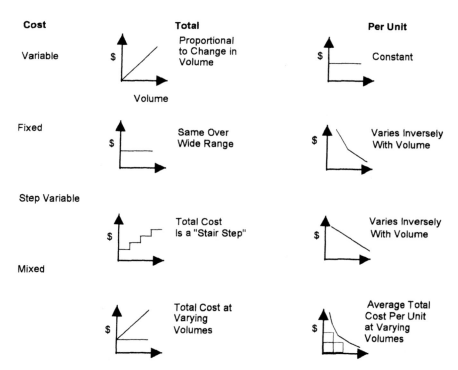

Figure 18.3 Cost behavior.

Breakeven and Beyond

If a manager knows both cost and revenue behavior, she or he can calculate a *breakeven* point where revenues and costs are equal. Basically, revenues are reduced by variable expenses to produce the contribution margin. The contribution margin percentage is the contribution margin divided by the revenue. When the fixed expenses are divided by the contribution margin percentage, the result is the level of revenue required to cover both variable and fixed costs. Assume, for example, that revenues are $1,000,000 and variable costs are $400,000. The contribution margin is $600,000 ($1,000,000 − $400,000 = $600,000) and the contribution margin percentage is 60% ($600,000/$1,000,000). For each dollar of revenue received, 60 cents goes to cover fixed expenses and, after all fixed expenses are recovered, the organization over recovers its costs at 60 cents on the dollar. If the fixed expenses are, say, $600,000, then the required revenue to break even is $1,000,000 ($600,000/.60 = $1,000,000). If the fixed expenses are $660,000, then the organization needs $1,100,000 ($660,000/.60 = $1,100,000). If, on the other hand, the fixed expenses are $540,000, then the required revenue is only $900,000 ($540,000/.60 = $900,000). If the organization receives $1,000,000 with $540,000 of fixed costs, the over recovery is $60,000 ($1,000,000 less variable costs at .40 × $1, 0000,000 equals a contribution margin of $600,000 less fixed costs of $540,000 equals $60,000). A more direct computation is to multiply the revenue *in excess of breakeven revenue by the contribution margin percentage* ($1,000,000 − $900,000 × .6 = $60,000).

The analysis extends to multiple services, programs, and agencies. (See a managerial accounting text for extended applications.)

Cost Distinctions for Planning and Control

Fixed costs are either committed or discretionary. Committed fixed costs may be fundamental (e.g., property taxes, bond interest payments, key personnel) and reflect long-run capacity needs. Typically, these costs are not responsive to short-run variations in activity. Discretionary fixed costs, on the other hand, are periodic costs influenced by top management decisions (e.g., scheduled maintenance, staff training, professional travel) and often bear little relationship to volume of activity. In times of hardship, these costs are subject to reduction, although long-term effects may be negative.

Variable costs are either engineered or discretionary. Engineered costs represent a defined cost to produce a given service or product (e.g., cost of a psychologist to perform testing). Shifts in engineered costs change the resulting service or product (e.g., moving from a Ph.D. to a master's-level psychologist). Discretionary variable costs represent managerial choices that may be altered without producing a fundamental effect on the service or product (e.g., switching from a brand name drug to a generic type).

When management is looking for short-term cost reductions, discretionary variable and discretionary fixed costs become prime targets. Often these costs are subject to reduction without immediate adverse effects, but some, if postponed indefinitely, will produce adverse effects (e.g., training or maintenance).

Differential Costs and Revenues

Often short-term decision making involves asking what the differential effects on costs and revenues are if a program or service is added or dropped. Only the revenues or costs that are expected to change are relevant to the decision. The differential revenues and costs correctly identify the financial effects of a decision. For example, should program B be dropped since it appears to lose $100,000 (all dollar amounts in the analysis below are in thousands)?

	A	B	Totals
+Revenue	$1000	$3000	$4000
−Variable expense	−600	−2000	−2600
=Contribution margin	=400	=1000	=1400
−Fixed expense	−300	−1100	−1400
=New over (under) recovery	=100	=(100)	=0

The differential analysis identifies the differences *without* B as the loss of contribution margin and the continuation of fixed expenses. Dropping program B results in the loss of $1,000,000 of contribution margin and could leave a substantial fixed expense (up to $1,100,000). Instead of breaking even, as shown in the "Totals" column, the agency could face a loss of up to $1,000.000 ($100,000 over recovery from A reduced by the unavoidable fixed expense of B of $1,100,000). In this instance, dropping the service increases the losses of the organization and therefore is *not* the correct decision.

Budgeting

Successful public mental health organizations characterize good operating performance. The cornerstone of success is sound financial planning (Sorensen et al., 1983). The budget process requires planning and encourages better administration. The master budget integrates all the organization's functions into an overall plan and can highlight operating and financial problems early enough for effective remedial action.

Definition

The master budget is a plan of financial operations that provides a basis for the planning, controlling, and evaluation of activities of a public mental health organization. The budget is a quantitative expression of management's plans. The master budget summarizes the objectives of the organization's subunits and quantifies the activities for the next operating cycle (e.g., number of contracts, dollars of funding, levels of client service, number of professional staff, operating expenses)

Human Factors

Top management's view of the budget process influences the attitudes of middle-level managers. If top managers do not give wholehearted support, the budgeting process is not likely to be popular and may be the source of negative attitudes. The budget can help establish goals and objectives in quantitative form, direct behavior, measure results, and identify areas that need management attention. Managers who are expected to use the budget are to be involved in its development. Lukewarm support from the top for a budget process can result in low levels of communication between managers, and with only token participation by line managers the budgeting process fails. Budget failures make the staff wary of efforts to improve managerial effectiveness and efficiency. Budgets can be effective when managers understand and use them, not just execute the mechanics of the process.

Advantages

Skeptics are quick to point out the uncertainties and hard work of budgeting. Ignorance about budgeting may cause negative attitudes; sometime skepticism disguises an unfortunate experience, lack of technical skills, or poor motivation. The benefits of budgeting usually outweigh the costs because budgeting forces managers to think ahead—to anticipate and prepare for changing conditions. Budgets also help managers develop concrete expectations about the future, thus providing standards against which to judge subsequent performance. Budgets help coordinate and communicate plans, and develop congruence between individual and overall organizational goals and objectives.

Budgets measure performance, identify potential problems, and, because they give response, permit corrective actions. Comparisons of actual performance with planned performance give managers attention-directing cues and current readings on performance. These comparisons of actual to planned performance are called *budget variances.*

Types

Budgets focus on time periods or content. Long-range budgets include the acquisition of major new resources such as buildings and equipment and are called *capital budgets.* The master budget covers an organization's financial operation for an operating cycle, usually 1 year, and may be on a yearly basis or continuous. The continuous or rolling budget is updated in monthly or quarterly increments as each month or quarter ends. The rolling budget reflects management's expectations for a year in advance, and the most recent operating experiences can be used to set the budget for the following 12 months. The continuous budget avoids the once-a-year budget preparation scramble and stabilizes planning since new information is added frequently.

Operational Steps

The master budget consists of 10 steps (Sorensen et al., 1983). The manner in which the steps will become operational depends on the type of public mental health organization. The first step, a forecast of activity, is interpreted differently by various public health organizations. For example, a state public mental health agency may be budgeting for state appropriations, while a county mental health agency may be projecting revenues from state or county sources (e.g., taxes) and a county or not-for-profit provider organization may be forecasting levels of service to clients.

Step	Description
1.	*Prepare a yearly forecast of activity by month (or quarter).* Factors influencing the forecast are past levels of activity, growth or decline trends, mandated programs, demographic shifts, seasonal patterns, and changes in public attitudes or awareness.
2.	*Translate the activity forecast into estimates of revenue to be generated.* Distinctions include activities that generate cash immediately and those that result in delayed payments. If services are involved, then prevailing rates (based on experience) should be used unless rates are cost-based, which then requires rates from a cost-finding model discussed later. In several states, providers reimburse on an approved annual budget prorated over the operating cycle. If the prorated amounts are advanced to provide working capital for services, there may be requirements to demonstrate that sufficient services were provided to justify the advance.
3.	*Estimate any other sources of revenue.* Other examples include categorical grants, research grants, and donations; the timing of the revenue uses estimates on monthly (or quarterly) time frame.
4.	*Translate all sources of revenue into estimated cash collections by month (or quarter) by combining steps 2 and 3.* Estimates of cash collections from all sources should link to the planned times of collection. Collections from third-party payers (e.g., Medicaid, insurance) often lag behind the rendering of services. The lags should reflect current collection experiences.
5.	*Estimate the purchases of any services or supplies inventories for each month (quarter).* Purchases are subject to estimation with the following formula: purchases = desired ending inventory + cost of inventory used or sold − beginning inventory. The formula applies to administrative supplies, medications, and so on. The costing of inventory items requires experience and an inflation adjustment factor.
6.	*Estimate the timing and payments for purchases of services and inventories.* If products or services are acquired on account, the bill payment usually lags behind the receipt of the goods or services. Some expenses are a function of activity (e.g., number of grants given, number of clients served), while others are a function of time (e.g., rent, insurance).
7.	*Estimate salary and wage expense disbursements and anticipated increases (or decreases) by month (quarter).*
8.	*Prepare the budgeted statement of operations.* This statement uses the revenue information from steps 2 and 3 along with expenses from steps 5 and 7. If the organization is a nonprofit, additional expenses such as depreciation and uncollectible accounts should be added to complete the list of expenses. In the case of a local or state government, the revenue is recognized on the modified accrual basis, which means cash collections from step 4 (which combines steps 2 and 3) may be sources of the revenue. Expenditures (instead of expenses) are used and should be easily estimated from steps 6 and 7. Usually orders placed, but not received (which may result in encumbrances), are not included as expenditures until the orders are received. The title of the activity summary changes to the Budgeted Statement of Revenues and Expenditures.
9.	*Prepare the budgeted statement of cash receipts and disbursements.* The lag of cash receipts behind activities and cash disbursements for goods and services purchased on account affect expected cash flows and cash balances, especially if a minimum cash balance is desired (or required). Some payments are fixed and will occur at specific intervals (e.g., monthly advances from a state agency, rent expenditure at the beginning of the month, or salary/wage payments every 2 weeks), while others will occur irregularly and in varying amounts (e.g., payments on accounts payable). At this point, financing activities may be considered if there are uneven cash flows resulting in negative cash balances. If the organization or agency can obtain additional funds (e.g., loans or advances), the organization may seek additional funds (e.g., loans or advances) or decide to delay certain payments until cash is available or try to stimulate lagging cash receipts.

Step	Description
10.	*Prepare the budgeted statement of financial position (or balance sheet) and budgeted statement of cash flows (if desired)*. The projected statement of financial position (or balance sheet) draws on the beginning-of-period statement and is adjusted for all the activity described in steps 2 through 9. A sample of the logic to produce specific account balances is described below: • The ending cash position, for example, is the ending balance calculated in step 9. • Receivables start with the beginning balance, are increased by current period additions, and are decreased by current period collections to produce the ending balance. • Inventories commence with the beginning balance, add purchases during the period, and subtract amounts used or sold to produce the ending balance. • Accounts payable starts with the beginning balance, adds current period purchases on account, and subtracts amounts paid on account to create the ending balance. • A similar pattern of computations would produce ending balances for the remaining asset, liability, or equity accounts.

From Sorensen et al. (1983).

Figure 18.4 portrays the budgetary process.

Many times the resources are insufficient to develop and implement the master budget as described above. Another form of budgeting, known as *incremental budgeting* (Herzlinger and Nitterhouse, 1994), appears in public mental health organizations. The analysis starts with existing volumes of activity, revenue, and expenses and then makes *incremental adjustments* for factors such as changes in the volume, efficiency, quality, and prices of good and services. Finally, after all of the foregoing adjustments, the revised totals are multiplied by an inflation percentage

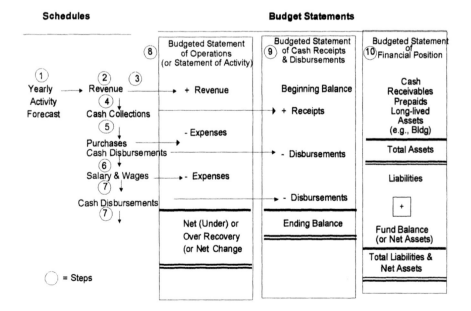

Figure 18.4 Budgetary process flowchart.

expressed as a multiplier (e.g., 5% = 1.05 multiplier) to produce the new budget. An illustrative format follows.

Last Year (*$*)	Volume (*%*)	Efficiency (*$*)	Quality (*$*)	New Prices (*$*)	Revised Totals (*$*)	Inflation (*$*)	New Budget (*%*)
[Volume: xxx					xxx		xxx]
Revenue: $xxx					$xxx		$xxx
Expense: $xxx					$xxx		$xxx
(or expenditure) over (under)							
recovery: $xxx					$xxx		$xxx

[ ] Non-dollar amounts.

Controlling Against the Budget

Budgetary control is a comparison of the planned revenues and expenses (or expenditures in the case of a governmental unit) to the actual revenues and expenses (or expenditures). The difference is a variance. Brackets on a variance usually indicate an unfavorable variance.

If planned revenue is less than expected, it may be as follows:

Budget:	Actual:	Variance:
$50,000,000	$48,000,000	$(2,000,000)

If favorable, then

$50,000,000	$51,000,000	$1,000,000

Expenses (expenditures) may follow the same scheme: An unfavorable variance would appear as follows:

$30,000,000	$31,500,000	$(1,500,000)

If favorable, then

$30,000,000	$28,900,000	$1,100,000

If the variances follow the logic of brackets for unfavorable variances, the variances combine *additively* to identify the *net* effect. In the foregoing example, the two unfavorable variances would combine to a negative impact of ($3,500,000), or if the revenues are favorable ($1,000,000) and the expenses (expenditures) are unfavorable ($1,500,000), the net consequence is an unfavorable ($500,000).

Direct comparison of the original fixed budget and actual results may be misleading if the actual level of activity differs significantly from the planned level of activity. To cope with this issue, a public mental health organization may prepare a *flexible budget*, which changes as activity levels change. A flexible budget, unlike a fixed budget adopted by a governmental unit, is not a form of appropriations, but a plan that can facilitate budgetary control and operational evaluations. A flexible budget allows the organization to prepare several budgets at different levels of activity to identify an acceptable comparative basis of planned activity with actual results.

Cost Accounting (Cost-Finding) and Rate-Setting for Services and/or Programs

Costs are associated with some activity, event, situation, product, or service—in short, with some cost objective. If the cost objective is the unit cost of services (or cost per unit (MacFarland et. al., 1995), competent cost-finding requires 10 procedures (Sorensen, 2000a):

Procedure Number	Description
1.	Identify and document the organizational units and the services (or programs) of each unit of the organization.
2.	Assign the direct salary and wage cost to each organizational unit and to each service (or program).
3.	Determine the cost of fringe benefits (e.g., Social Security, vacation, insurance, education leaves) and assign (estimated) fringe benefits to each organizational unit and to each service (or program).
4.	Assign other direct and traceable expenses to each organizational unit and to each service (or program).
5.	Assign indirect operating expenses by organizational unit and service (or program).
6.	Estimate and assign the value of donated services, supplies, and facilities (e.g., essential volunteers' services or "in kind" expenses) to each organizational unit and to each service (or program).
7.	Assign the costs of administrative and support units to other organizational units and to services (or programs).
8.	Determine the most feasible basis for unitizing the services provided by the organization.
9.	Identify the actual (or estimated, if prospective) annual (or some other period) amount of service for each service (or program).
10.	Compute the unit cost rate for each service (or program) (step 7 divided by step 9).

From Sorensen (2000a).

Figure 18.5 summarizes the 10 cost-finding procedures required to produce unit costs for public mental health services or programs. A federal agency (the Substance Abuse and Mental Health Services Administration or SAMHSA) funded a uniform system of accounting and cost reporting for substance abuse treatment providers (Capital Consulting Corporation, 1993) that embraces the foregoing methodology.

Activity-based costing suggests that costs should be allocated to cost pools and then to specific services. This two-stage allocation procedure can result in improved cost assignments. The costs of the information system (e.g., IS personnel, computer, processing costs) may be collected in a cost pool and then assigned to organizational units based on use (e.g., number of transactions or hours of use). Administrative costs may be collected in a cost pool, for example, and assigned to other organizational units

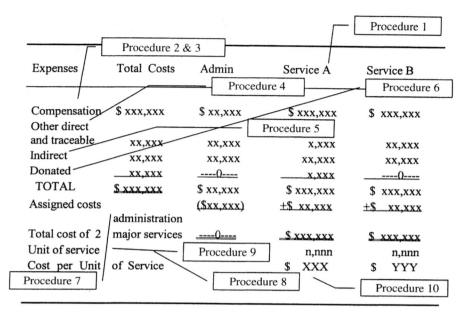

Figure 18.5 Schedule of unit cost procedures.

based on the number of FTE personnel (e.g. two half-time persons equal one FTE) employed in each unit (e.g., if a unit had 100 FTE out of a total of 1000 FTE in the organization, the unit's assignment would be 10 % [100/1000 = .10 or 10%]).

Unit costs are used often for rate-setting, contract negotiation, or highlighting problems in rates or productivity. Comparison of budgeted unit costs to actual unit costs is a KPI cited earlier. Unit costs of comparable organizations can serve as a useful benchmarking process.

Cost–Outcome and Cost–Effectiveness

Cost–outcome assessment is one key to building viable cost–effectiveness analyses to perform program evaluation and to achieve desired accountability (Newman and Sorensen, 1985). Figure 18.6 identifies the major financial, statistical, and evaluation tasks required for cost–outcome and cost–effectiveness analysis.

Starting with total costs of a public mental health organization, costs are refined to the per unit cost of service. Statistical data on professional staff activities are required to assign personnel costs, while information about services (e.g., units of service) is necessary to unitize program and service costs. With unitized costs of service and accumulated services received by specific target groups, total costs for an episode of care may be computed. Evaluation tasks then involve the selection of a target group, pre-intervention assessment, and random assignment of clients to varied treatments or services. After post-intervention measurements, outcomes

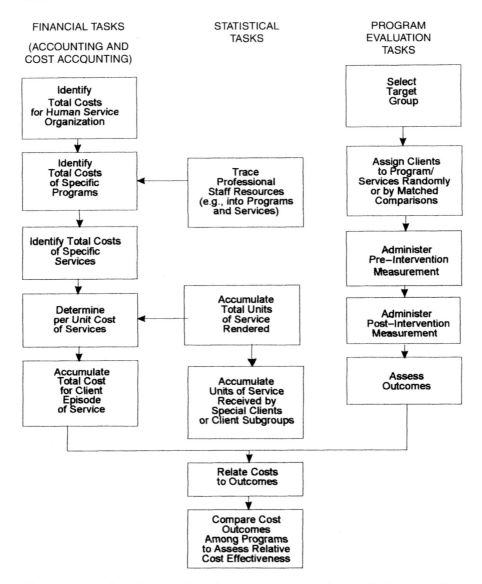

Figure 18.6 Overview of major tasks in cost–outcome and cost–effectiveness studies in a human service organization. (Source: Sorensen et al., 1983)

are assessed. Then costs can be related to outcomes and, if calculated on more than one service, can be comparatively analyzed for assessing the cost–effectiveness of optional approaches for specific target groups (Frishman and Rosenbeck, 1996; Jerrell, 1996; Jerrell et al., 1994, 2000; National Evaluation Data Technical Assistance Center, 1998; Schalock, 2001; Sorensen 2000b; Thornton et al., 1990).

Implications for Mental Health Services

Financial management focuses on the analyses, decisions, and actions related to the acquisition of resources (financing), allocation of resources (distribution), and accountability for the use of resources (evaluation).

Strategic Financial Management

Successful strategic financial management in public mental health is linked critically to the strategic management process. The future of public mental health depends on how effectively the strategic management process of vision, mission, goals, and objectives is understood and applied. Fruitful strategic financial plans depend on assessments of the organization's strategic situation, competitive position, strategy formulation, evaluation, and choice. These long-term plans must have a quality orientation with a focus on ongoing improvement—either incremental or breakthrough improvement. The successful strategic processes focuses on the customer, quality-driven processes, leadership and management, and engagement and commitment of employees.

Operational Financial Management

Operational financial management begins with a focus on KPIs drawn from the IS. The KPI system is a managerial guidance system. Public mental health information systems should be shaped to produce ongoing comparisons between expected and actual KPIs to aid managers in assessing services, how resources are acquired and spent, and program outcomes.

Managers in public mental health organizations should have a basic understanding of cost and revenue behavior, that is, how to assess breakeven operations, cost classification, differential costs, and revenues. The fundamentals of the budgeting process, budget variance analysis, and unit of service costing are needed to assess meaningfully the financial operations of a public mental health organization. Finally, costs and client (program) outcomes should be linked through cost–outcomes and cost–effectiveness analysis to enhance mental health program accountability and effectiveness.

Many public mental health managers emerge from medical, behavioral, and clinical backgrounds, and therefore are not systematically exposed to fundamental strategic and operational financial management skills. It is hoped that this chapter begins to meet this need.

What is the payoff? Managers in public mental organizations with effective strategic and operational financial management can face an uncertain and threating environment with greater confidence and with higher odds of success.

REFERENCES

Aaker D. *Developing Business Strategies.* New York: Wiley, 1995.
Baily L. Service efforts and accomplishments reporting. *HBJ Miller Comprehensive Governmental GAAP Guide.* New York: Harcourt Brace, 2002.

Baldrige National Quality Program. *Health Care Criteria for Performance Excellence.* Gaithersburg, MD: National Institute for Standards and Technology, Technology Administration, Department of Commerce, (http://www.quality.nist.gov), 2002.

Capital Consulting Corporation. *Uniform System of Accounting and Cost Reporting for Substance Abuse Treatment Providers.* SAMHSA contract number 271-91-8327. Fairfax, VA: Capital Consulting Corporation, 1993.

Chapman R. *The Design of Management Information Systems for Mental Health Organizations: A Primer.* DHEW Pub. No. (ADM) 76-333. Washington, DC: U.S. Government Printing Office, 1976.

Clark RE, Bush PW, Becket DR, et al. A cost-effectiveness comparison of supported employment and rehabilitative day treatment. *Administration and Policy in Mental Health,* 24(1):63–78, 1996.

Clark RE, Xie H, Becker DR, et al. Benefits and costs of supported employment from three perspectives. *Journal of Behavioral Health Services and Research,* 25(1):22–34, 1998.

Cleverley WO. Financial dashboard reporting for the hospital industry. *Journal of Health Care Finance,* 27(3):30–40, 2001.

Diamond PM, Wang EW, Holzer CE III, et al. The prevalence of mental illness in prison. *Administration and Policy in Mental Health,* 29(1):21–40, 2001.

Dixon K (ed). Special issue: managed behavioral healthcare. *Administration and Policy in Mental Health,* 28(1):7–59, 2000.

Dobson P, Starkey K. *The Strategic Management Blueprint.* Cambridge, MA: Blackwell Business, 1993.

Evans JR, Lindsay WM. *The Management and Control of Quality, 5th ed.* Cincinnati: South-Western, a division of Thomson Learning, 2002.

Feldman R. The ability of managed care to control health care costs: how much is enough? *Journal of Health Care Finance,* 26(3):8–29, 2000.

Feldman S. Special issue: mental health services in the public sector. *Administration and Policy in Mental Health,* 19(4):209, 1992.

Finlay A, Cosovich C, Gebur S. A national disease registry moves beyond clinical impact, fostering measurable costs savings at the community hospital level. *Journal of Health Care Finance,* 26(3):15–25, 2000.

Frank RG, McGuire TG (eds). Mental health economics (special issue). *Administration and Policy in Mental Health,* 24(4):279–376, 1997.

Frishman L, Rosenheck R. How transfer payments are treated in cost-effectiveness and cost-benefit analyses. *Administration and Policy in Mental Health,* 23(6):533–546, 1996.

Herzlinger R, Nitterhouse D. *Financial Accounting and Managerial Control for Nonprofit Organizations.* Cincinnati: South-Western, 1994.

Jerrell JM. Toward cost-effective care for persons with dual diagnoses. *Journal of Mental Health Administration,* 23(3):329–337, 1996.

Jerrell JM, Hu T, Ridgely MS. Cost-effectiveness of substance disorder interventions for people with severe mental illness. *Journal of Mental Health Administration,* 21(3):283–297, 1994.

Jerrel JM, Wilson JL, Hiller DC. Issues and outcomes in integrated treatment programs for dual disorders. *Journal of Behavioral Health Services and Research,* 27(3):303–313, 2000.

Kane TJ (ed). Community mental health centers. *Administration and Policy in Mental Health,* 21(4):279–352, 1994.

Kaplan RS, Norton DP. *The Balanced Scorecard.* Boston: Harvard Business School Press, 1996.

Kaplan RS, Norton DP. *The Strategy-Focused Organization: How Balanced Scorecard Com-*

panies Thrive in the New Business Environment. Boston: Harvard Business School Press, 2000.

Ludden JM, Mandell LJ. Quality planning for mental health. *Journal of Mental Health Administration,* 20(1):75, 1993.

Manderscheid RW, Henderson MJ. Federal and state legislative and program directions for managed care. In: Mullen EJ, Magnabosco JL (eds). *Outcomes Measurement in the Human Services: Cross-Cutting Issues and Methods.* Washington, DC: NASW Press, pp. 113–123, 1997.

MacFarland BH, Smith JC, Bigelow DA, et al. Unit costs of community mental health services. *Administration and Policy in Mental Health.* 23(1):27–42, 1995.

Mazade N, Wurster C, Lutterman T. Special issue: mental health services in the public sector. *Administration and Policy in Mental Health,* 19(4):211–212, 1992.

McGuire TG. Special issue: the economics of mental health administration. *Administration and Policy in Mental Health.* 18(1):7–8, 1991.

McLaughlin CP, Kaluzny AD. Total quality management issues in managed care. *Journal of Health Care Finance,* 24(1):10–16, 1997.

Minden S, Hassol A. *Final Review of Available Information on Managed Behavioral Health Care.* Rockville, MD: Center for Mental Health Services, 1996.

National Evaluation Data and Technical Assistance Center. *Cost-Benefit of Substance Abuse Treatment: Selected Bibliographies, 1990–1998.* Rockville, MD: Center for Substance Abuse Treatment, Department of Health and Human Services, 1998.

Nauert RC. The new millennium: health care evolution in the 21st century. *Journal of Health Care Finance,* 26(3):1–14, 2000.

Newman F, Sorensen J. *Integrated Clinical and Fiscal Management in Mental Health.* Norwood, NJ: Ablex, 1985.

Rosnkjar S, O'Connell D, Robertson R. Managing care and dollars in the 21st century: recommendations for community mental health systems of care. *Administration and Policy in Mental Health,* 27(4):239–245, 2000.

Ruiz V. Estelle, 503 F. Supp. 1256, 1323 (1980).

Santos AB (ed). Assertive community treatment. *Administration and Policy in Mental Health,* 25(2):101–238, 1997.

Schalock RL. *Outcome-Based Evaluation, 2nd ed.* New York: Kluwer Academic/Plenum, 2001.

Shuyter GV, Barnett JE. Application of total quality management to mental health: a benchmark case study. *Journal of Mental Health Administration,* 22(3):278–285, 1995.

Sorensen JE. Collaboration among state and local mental health organizations: examples of knowledge utilization. *Journal of Mental Health Administration,* 16(1):3–8, 1989.

Sorensen JE. Special issue: financial management in mental health services. *Administration and Policy in Mental Health,* 20(2):71–74, 1992.

Sorensen JE. Cost dynamics of frontier mental health services. *Journal of the Washington Academy of Sciences,* 86(3):143–158, 2000a. Also available at the Frontier Mental Health Resource Center, Western Interstate Conference on Higher Education at www.wiche.edu.

Sorensen JE. Clients' outcomes and costs in frontier mental health organizations. *Journal of the Washington Academy of Sciences,* 86(3):159–177, 2000b. Also available at the Frontier Mental Health Resource Center, Western Interstate Conference on Higher Education at www.wiche.edu.

Sorensen JE. Effective management strategies for frontier mental health organizations. *Journal of the Washington Academy of Sciences,* 86(3):179–187, 2000c. Also available at the Frontier Mental Health Resource Center, Western Interstate Conference on Higher Education at www.wiche.edu.

Sorensen JE, Hanbery G, Kucic A. *Accounting and Budgeting Systems for Mental Health Or-ganizations.* DHHS Pub. No. (ADM) 83-1046. Rockville, MD: National Institute of Mental Health, 1983.

Sorensen JE, Zelman W, Hanbery GW, et al. Managing mental health organizations with 25 key performance indicators. *Evaluation and Program Planning,* 10(3):239–247, 1987.

Stroul BA. Community support systems for persons with long-term mental illness. *Psy-chosocial Rehabilitation Journal,* 12(6):9–26, 1989.

Thornton P, Goldman H, Stegner B, et al. Assessing the costs and outcomes together. *Eval-uation and Program Planning,* 13:231–241, 1990.

University of Denver, College of Business Administration. *Mission and Goals of the College of Business Administration.* Denver: University of Denver, 2001.

Wagenfeld MO, Murray JD, Mohatt DF, et al. *Mental Health and Rural America: 1980–1993, an Overview and Annotated Bibliography.* Rockville: NIH Publ. No. 94-3500, 1994. Office of Rural Health Policy and Office of Rural Mental Health Research.

Wall Street Journal. Study finds mental health spending cut in half over last decade. May 7, 1998, p. B1.

West Virginia Department of Health and Human Resources Behavioral Health Advisory Council. *Strategic Plan 2000 and Beyond.* Charleston, WV, 2001.

Wheelen TL, Hunger JD. *Strategic Management Business Policy,* 7th ed. Princeton, NJ: Prentice Hall, 2000.

Wheeler JRC, Nahra TA. Private and public ownership in outpatient substance abuse treat-ment: do we have a two-tiered system? *Administration and Policy in Mental Health.* 27(4):197–209, 2000.

Yearwood, Johnson, Stanton and Smith, Inc. & Consultants for Community Change, Inc. *p.* Nashville, TN, and South Burlington, VT: Yearwood, Johnson, Stanton and Smith, Inc. and Consultants for Community Change, Inc, 1992.

19

Mental Health Informatics

ARDIS HANSON
BRUCE LUBOTSKY LEVIN

The second half of the twentieth century was marked by striking changes in the way people live, work, and communicate with each other. The twenty-first century brings minimal change to a new era of continuing fiscal constraints and advanced technologies. Although telecommunications has an important and prominent role in society, in knowledge exchange, and in commerce, it is in the field of public health practice that the most remarkable opportunities, as well as challenges, have emerged. The growth of information, the development of communication technology, and the evolving infrastructures to support technology have contributed to dramatic changes in the methods of managing information and its application to improve the quality of health care and health systems performance through new approaches for the delivery of health services.

For example, telecommunication strategies continue to broaden access to health care, health education, and health services delivery for at-risk populations in the United States (Levin and Hanson, 2001). Interest in applying new technologies to public health has increased dramatically, particularly with the expansion of communication satellites, the transition from analog to digital transmission, and the rapid increases in computer hardware and software development. These elements have driven the development of computer-based patient records, personal health information systems, and unified electronic claims systems.

Society has increasingly used the Internet for the transmission of information, education, and clinical care. Technology development has also provided increasing opportunities for health care consumers to access information regarding their care and treatment, allowing consumers to understand and become more knowledgeable about their health status. The application of informatics in mental health services delivery provides similar opportunities to maximize information sharing and to diversify the delivery of mental health services in the United States. For example, these technologies are becoming increasingly available to health providers in the delivery of health services to rural and frontier populations.

This chapter will examine the history of mental health informatics in the United States and the evolution of information systems used in mental health services, as well as selected applications of information and communication technologies to mental health services delivery. In addition, the chapter will present some of the key ethical, confidentiality, and privacy issues involved in the provision of mental health services via these emerging technologies.

Background

Telemedicine

Telemedicine began in the 1960s as physicians who were geographically remote from their patients rendered treatment or provided consultations over the telephone and/or wire services. Although today the principles are largely the same, the technology and milieu of contemporary telemedicine are vastly different. In the age of high-speed data lines, advanced data compression technologies, privatization of defense technologies, and computerization of patient records, clinical outcomes, and physician practices, telemedicine promises to be the next milestone in health care advances.

Telehealth

Telehealth has been described as the use of telecommunications and information technology to provide access to a variety of health activities—assessment, intervention, consultation, education, and information—in a cost–efficient manner when geographic distance separates health care providers and consumers (Angaran, 1999; Nickelson, 1998). Whereas telehealth technologies have included videoconferencing, telephones, computers, the Internet, e-mail, fax, radio, and television, newer technologies are increasingly being introduced and used in health care. More recently, programs are delivering health care using a combination of audio graphic, store-and-forward, and telemetry technologies (the automatic transmission and measurement of data from remote sources by wire, radio, or wireless technologies).

Health Informatics

Health care informatics is the systematic application of information and computer science technology to health care practice, research, and learning (Yasnoff et al., 2000). The term *health informatics* covers a very wide range of applications and research, all dedicated to the improvement of patient care and public health. Health informatics continues to incorporate rapidly changing information environments and to encounter emerging public health issues, some created by the advent of new technological opportunities and others emerging from the application of technology to complex public health problems. For example, applications range from electronic patient records to national health databases in the establishment of clinical guidelines and clinical pathways to care. The key component of informatics is the process of converting data to accessible and usable information that enables improvements in the quality, value, and effectiveness of health services.

Electronic information systems are revolutionizing health care practice, research, and education. Efficient management of information improves patient satisfaction and makes time available for new aspects of practice and for learning. Many health care professionals realize that they need skills in finding and using information and in assessing information systems.

The proliferation of interest in health informatics has centered on the technical and sociological aspects of the medium. It is only recently, however, that legal and regulatory issues have been discussed. In fact, the potential for mass availability of telemedicine and telehealth will likely depend on how the legal and regulatory issues are resolved.

Mental Health Informatics

The rapid development and growth of information and communication technology provides a wealth of opportunities to create new approaches for the delivery of mental health services that can fill the void for current users of the various mental health systems, as well as tap into the mental health market that has not been developed. Mental health informatics is the systematic application of information and computer science and technology to mental health practice and research. Prior to discussing recent technologies used for providing mental health services, we will examine the development of mental health informatics in the United States.

History

Cecil Wittson and staff at the Nebraska Psychiatric Institute first demonstrated the use of technology in mental health care in the United States in the mid-1950s. A small closed-circuit interactive television (IATV) system, originally established for lectures and instructional purposes at the Institute, was expanded as a means of extending mental health services to areas that were remote from psychiatric centers. Therapists led two televised and two nontelevised small groups of patients (Wittson et al., 1961). In 1956, interactive audio links were established to hospitals in Nebraska, Iowa, North Dakota, and South Dakota.

During the 1960s, the use of computers in mental health research was a recurring theme in the literature. Although data analysis was the most popular use of computers, there were emerging discussions on the use of computers in medical diagnosis (Graetz, 1965; Ledley and Lusted, 1960), the use of automated information retrieval for literature reviews (DuBois, 1965; Edmundson and Wyllys, 1961), and the use of systems analysis and research to assist in decision-making systems (Fliege, 1966).

During the 1960s, early mental health information systems were developed at Camarillo State Hospital in California (Graetz et al., 1965) and at the Fort Logan Mental Health Center in Colorado (Truitt and Binner, 1969). In addition, microwave technology was used as a method of consultation between the Dartmouth-

Hitchcock Mental Health Center in New Hampshire and Claremont General Hospital in New Hampshire (Solow, 1971). By 1968, Massachusetts General Hospital was providing emergency mental health consults at the Logan Airport Medical Station using IATV (Dwyer, 1973).

By the 1970s, computer applications had emerged in the field of mental health. First, computers expedited the handling of routine, repetitive tasks. Second, the speed and flexibility of new computer information systems provided timely information on patients, ward rosters, doctor–patient rosters, and drug inventory reports in addition to providing administrative data concerning length of stay and readmission statistics. Third, the transmission of vast amounts of data across geographic distances had improved the clinician's ability to make decisions on patient care.

Also during the 1970s, discussion of the use of computer retrieval services was growing in the professional literature (Markley and Adams, 1973; Peper and Toth, 1971). For example, Chun et al. (1973) reviewed a 20% sample of 15 mental health journals published during 1960–69. They showed approximately 2500 reports of new measures, with 70% of these measures never cited again after publication. A new computerized information retrieval system (National Repository of Social Science Measures) was described as a primary resource in locating the psychological measures. Other literature addressed the use and limitations of online bibliographic resources, as well as the difficulties encountered in staying up-to-date (Beck, 1977; Knapp, 1979; Parr, 1979).

The increased reliance on mental health information databases became critical in the planning, provision, and evaluation of mental health services delivery. By the end of the 1970s, more than three-fourths of all community mental health centers were using some form of computerized management information system (MIS) (Gorodezky and Hedlund, 1982). Although most of these systems offered traditional services (staff activity reporting, patient register, financial and billing systems, and program evaluation) run through a batch process, newer systems included online interactive data entry and retrieval. During this time period, the National Institute of Mental Health (NIMH) was designing a prototype MIS system for community mental health centers (NIMH, 1983; Wurster and Goodman, 1981).

By the 1980s, use of computing in mental health was entering the fourth generation. According to Blum (1983, p. 45), this was "because the Japanese [were] already at work on the fifth generation." Emphasis was placed on the information needs of private practice, current and future trends in microtechnology for clinical applications, organizational issues in implementing computer systems, automated psychological testing, patient assessment and diagnosis, computer-aided education and treatment, accounting systems, and administrative and clinical information management.

The MIS systems were now viewed as an evolving technology for improving emergency mental health services and decision making, for planning alcohol abuse services, for supporting consultation and liaison mental health services, and for behavioral assessment and diagnosis of children with mental disorders. Computer-assisted instruction (CAI) for mental health professionals and mental health consumers was also on the rise. For example, programs were developed to teach clinicians and nurses basic mental health information using short simulated patient interviews, specialized interviewing techniques based on diagnosis or discipline, suicide assessment techniques, or use of antipsychotic medications (Santo and Finkel, 1982; Smith et al., 1980; Van Donegan, 1984; Wolfman, 1980). Continuing professional education was also a growing area (Lynett, 1985), and community mental health public information CAI programs were more prevalent. Abernathy (1979) developed an interactive system that asked for basic individual demographics, gave a short quiz on general mental health knowledge, and gave feedback-correcting misconceptions about mental illness and treatment.

During the 1990s, computing took a quantum leap forward with the development of the World Wide Web (or Web). Computing was no longer limited to local area networks; it now had wide area networks. Although computer-mediated communication, in various forms, was commonly used in disaster management, this decade saw the emergence of wide area computer networks (i.e., the Internet) in disaster management and prevention (Butler and Anderson, 1992). The first directory file structure, Gopher, was ubiquitous and provided easy access to mental health resources set up by professional associations, colleges, and universities. The types of resources found at these sites included links to job listings, electronic journals, and university psychology departments with Internet directories of information. The first Internet-based journal, initially circulated by electronic mail, was *Psycoloquy*, which was also the first electronic journal[1] indexed in PsycINFO.

The Computers in Teaching Initiative Center for Psychology saw the Web as providing support to mental health education by disseminating information, generating and accessing resource materials, and enhancing knowledge exchange (Trapp et al., 1996). The Web also provided a useful forum for dialogue and feedback. For example, Hanover College and the American Psychological Society developed Web-based tutorials in sensation and perception (Krantz, 1995). Welch and Krantz (1996) discussed the development and use of a multimedia primer in auditory perception that included instructional material and acoustical experiments conducted over the Web.

With the advent of graphically based browsers, the use of Internet technology accelerated dramatically. The Internet allows the use of updated full-text resource literature (Buring and Felkey, 2000). The main disadvantage of print resource literature was its lag time; the Internet all but eliminated this disadvantage. Publishers of electronically formatted, fee-based literature, previously available only on CDs or network servers, have been rapidly providing their products in Internet formats, resulting in increased accessibility to updated information from anywhere in the world. Journals, textbooks, medical databases, and media productions, such as video- and audiocasts, are available directly online to researchers, mental health care professionals, and consumers of mental health care services.

The Telecommunications Act of 1996 dramatically altered the communication rates and services potentially available to telehealth and telemental health providers. Approximately $500 million was provided to health care providers, libraries, and schools in rural areas to offset telephone line charges incurred in connecting to the Internet via the Universal Service Fund (CBO, 1998; GAO, 2002). Nevertheless, a continuing issue in the use of telecommunications technology in the health and mental health fields is the ongoing expenditure of time and money for staff training.

Obviously, significant progress has been made over the past half century in the growth of information technology and its applications for health and mental health services delivery. Nevertheless, major issues, including the use of evolving mental health information systems in services delivery models, the ethics of telemental health treatment, and licensing and credentialing, have emerged as important themes in both the academic and popular mental health informatics literature.

Mental Health Information Systems

From Diagnosis to Decision Making

The 1880 U.S. Census captured seven distinct forms of mental illness, making it one of the earliest attempts at federal data collection of mental disorders in the United States. By the turn of the twentieth century, diagnosis was one of the descriptive variables in state mental hospital data, the "Census of Patients in Mental Institutions" (Pollock, 1921). Forty years later, administrators at the Crownsville State Hospital in Maryland were analyzing hospital records of individual first admissions to supply information on specific patients and indicated the existence of trends within one hospital or a group of hospitals (Meyer and Preston, 1948).

In 1949, federal mental health statistical operations were moved to the newly created NIMH. This new institute set up the Model Reporting Area (MRA) Program for Mental Hospital Statistics, a joint endeavor with state mental health agencies, with its focus on state-run facilities. To help create comparable national data collection standards, the NIMH held the first National Conference on Mental Health Statistics in 1951. By 1966, the annual conference was the principal vehicle for consensus building and standards development regarding national mental health data.

However, with the growth of outpatient and community-based mental health services in the late 1950s and early 1960s, the MRA was seriously outmoded. At the 1976 National Conference, NIMH proposed a cooperative mental health statistics program. The Mental Health Statistics Improvement Program (MHSIP) was established, supported within the Division of Biometry and Epidemiology at NIMH. The functions envisioned by MHSIP for federal data focused on planning, evaluation, information production and dissemination, program implementation and management, and policy analysis and development (Patton and Leginksi, 1983). The increased use of human services information systems within the federal government helped support the emphasis on automated information systems. In addition, NIMH began publishing a new series within the Mental Health Service Systems Reports: the FN Series on information systems. Many of the reports on MIS reiterated the need for internal information needs, and external reporting requirements focused on definitions for use within mental health information systems (Baxter, 1980; Carter, 1980; Patton and D'huyvetter, 1980).

In the early 1980s, MHSIP published its first set of data standards based on the mental health organization as the principal reporting unit (Patton and Leginski, 1983), envisioning an orderly flow of information from the local to the state to the national level (Fig. 19.1). There were three minimum data sets: organization data (that included standard organizational data as well as at an area to note linkages among service agencies); patient data (that looked at patient to general population comparisons, patient subgroups, and total patient groups); and personnel data (numbers, disciplines, education, relation to mental health organizations, private practice activities, services, and general demographics). Widely adopted by many states, the MHSIP dataset became a model for the World Health Organization (Manderscheid and Henderson, 1995).

However, by the late 1980s, the changing environment in mental health care required a reconceptulization of why these statistics were collected and how they could be used to improve treatment for mental disorders and increase the quality of life for individuals with mental disorders. During this period, the federal government was distributing block grants for mental health services to states with its new mandate for state mental health planning. As part of this effort, MHSIP developed standards to assess outcome measures (Ciarlo, 1985).

There were also changes in the private sector, as fee-for-service delivery systems were beginning to evolve into managed care delivery systems. In 1989,

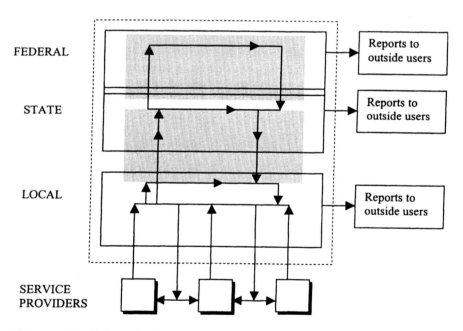

Figure 19.1 Information flow. Upward arrows denote data moving up the statistical reporting chain, and downward arrow denote information coming down the reporting chain. Lateral arrows denote data/information conversion at each level. (Adapted from Patton and Leginski, 1983, p. 29)

MHSIP added two new minimum datasets for financial information and events and updated its original datasets (organizations, human resources, and clients). The clinical event was defined as the basic unit of the system, to which one could link client, provider, and financial information within an organizational framework. A later version of the MHSIP data standards represented a major shift in scope and perspective, and addressed the need for a broadly conceived system of information to support decision making at the service provider level in public and private mental health services systems, including local, state, and federal governments, providers of services, and national organizations (Leginski and Croze, 1989).

During the 1990s, these standards were expanded to include recommended performance measures for programs and new data standards for child mental health programs. Service outcomes also became a priority with the publication of *Caring for People with Severe Mental Disorders: A National Plan of Research to Improve Services* (National Advisory Mental Health Council, 1991). Concurrently, the National Institute on Drug Abuse and the National Institute on Alcohol Abuse and Alcoholism collaborated with states and providers to create a minimum dataset for a client data system for public sector substance abuse treatment programs that was compatible with the MHSIP standard.

Mental health consumers also became more involved in the development of consumer-defined service outcome domains. Working with MHSIP, a consumer workgroup provided input into the National Association of State Mental Health Program Directors State Mental Health Profiling System. The work initiative not only provided a recommended consumer component for the Profiling System, it also pioneered the use of concept mapping in developing consumer measures (Trochim et al., 1993).

By 1995, the shape of health care had changed dramatically. Historically, most state mental health agencies had employed statistical information to plan only for state-operated or -funded programs that did not include nonprofit or private sector mental health organizations or practitioners, primary care organizations or practitioners, social service organizations, or self-help groups. The growth of managed care changed the way states used and shared statistical information. The use of federal waivers to create carve-out programs furthered the transformation of state Medicaid programs into managed care plans operated by private sector management services organizations.

Today's mental health information systems are far more complex than those originally envisioned by NIMH. However, the original intent of an integrated mental health information system still remains the goal. The question then becomes how these new systems, including client information systems (administrative and accounting functions), decision support functions, and outcomes assessments (*report cards* on services, operations, and the quality of mental health care) can best achieve this goal.

Client Information Systems

Mental health and substance abuse organizations have numerous internal and external requests for information. As the scale and complexity of such delivery systems have increased, the use of computer-based information systems has become a necessity. However, the migration from legacy systems to second-generation systems has also become more complicated. Developing second-generation systems to meet current reporting and information needs often reveals the unique data structure and analysis problems of mental health delivery systems. These problems are complicated by regulatory agencies' imposition of external reporting requirements.

Decision Support Functions

Computer-based clinical decision support systems can be broadly or narrowly defined. The broad definition includes any computer system that deals with clinical data or medical knowledge. This definition would include online resources such as databases, journals, textbooks, and clinical reporting systems. A more narrow definition limits the scope of the system to a knowledge-based system that provides patient-specific advice, possibly as simple as a client information system. A knowledge-based system for a clinical decision support system would need to contain medical knowledge to provide clinical consultations; disease profiles; frames with semantic relations to represent clinical findings; production rules with probabilities so that findings are related to diagnoses; a hierarchical classification tree to represent disease categories; heuristic questions to narrow the diagnostic hypotheses; and diagnostic criteria to conclude the clinical investigation (Biczyk do Amaral et al., 1993). With the increased emphasis on evidence-based practice to establish practice guidelines in mental health, decision support tools may help move the focus of treatment models to a disease management model as opposed to a crisis care model.

For example, one California-based provider of mental health services implemented a system that not only documents the progress of treatment for payers, but also helps the organization provide better care by supplying continuous updates on patient status. The system uses two research-based tools that look at critical triggers as well as a patient's overall level of distress (Staff, 2002). Another example is the use of written and computerized decision support aids (DSAs) based on the Agency for Healthcare Research and Quality depression guidelines. Although a written DSA improved diagnostic accuracy, the computerized DSA improved specificity and reduced mental health consultations (Medow et al., 2001).

Buican et al. (1999) stated that clinical decision support systems are the key to optimizing the performance of programs serving the most severely disabled and treatment-resistant patients. Mohan et al. (1998) assessed a personal computer–based decision support system developed for mental health providers in New York State, which enabled administrators to track key indicators of productivity, such as face-to-face time and non-face-to-face time against organizational goals. A key feature of the system was the conversion of raw data into action-oriented information to facilitate problem finding and problem solving.

Outcomes Assessments

White (1998) suggested that there has been an increasing demand for outcomes data from both purchasers of health care and providers. This is especially true within the managed behavioral health care industry. As consumers become more educated about health care and participate more actively in treatment decisions, providers will need to provide report cards so that consumers may assess the quality of medical care and make informed decisions on which treatment provider to use. Therefore, when creating outcomes components in mental health information systems, system designers need to build in patient-reported outcomes data, clinical information, and functional status as components of the system.

With the revolutionary changes in mental health delivery systems, the original intent of the MHSIP data standards continues to influence twenty-first-century standards. From a state perspective, reports will be available that will provide a more complete description of their services. Data will also be available for comparison of programs and services with other states that are similar in size, population, and resources. These standardized datasets will provide a framework for state mental health authorities to work with local agencies to establish data standards within the state. From a federal perspective, state data will meet federal data needs, a major objective of the MHSIP. And from a dual state-federal perspective, data will provide accurate and timely information "snapshots" and trends to inform policy and expenditures for behavioral health delivery systems.

Additional Applications

Services Delivery

Historically, telehealth and telemental health followed the classic medical model of top-down services delivery: from provider to patient. Initially this was accomplished via telecasts, videocasts, the telephone, or other point-to-point or dial-up information exchanges. With the emergence of the Internet, consumers of health and mental health services have increasingly taken advantage of the immediate access to web databases, virtual libraries, conference proceedings, disease-specific sites, and the popular as well as scientific literature in disease prevention, health education, and treatment of somatic and mental disorders. As a result, consumers are increasingly faced with opportunities to make more informed decisions and thus to take more responsibility for their personal health and mental health care (Ferguson, 1998; Spielberg, 1998).

Smith and Allison (1998) reported that between 1993 and 1997, the number of telemedicine programs in the United States grew from 9 to over 100, with most programs providing mental health services. They also highlighted the seven most active telemental health initiatives in America; Oregon's RODEO NET, the University of Kansas Center for Telemedicine and Telehealth, the Menninger Center for Telepsychiatry, Eastern Montana Telemedicine Network, Arizona TeleBehavioral Health Network, VideoLink of St. Peter's (Montana), and the Appal-Link Network of Virginia.

These networks provide a wide range of mental health services, provider education, and administrative functions. For example, RODEO NET, the oldest telemental health program in continuous operation in the United States, is a consortium of nine community mental health programs that serve 13 rural and frontier counties in eastern Oregon. Because of limited telephone transmission technology and access to satellite networks, RODEO NET uses a mixture of telecommunications satellite technology, microwave, video conferencing, frame relay-based data services, and electronic conferencing to provide increased access to mental health services and information for providers, consumers, and their families in rural Oregon.

The University of Kansas Center for Telemedicine and Telehealth, uses communication technology to deliver health and mental health care to medically underserved communities throughout the state of Kansas. This is accomplished by providing wellness and education programs, technical consultation, and research on the effectiveness of health informatics technologies.

The Menninger Center for Telepsychiatry provides specialty consultation services in Kansas and provides distance learning and continuing education to mental health facilities throughout the United States.

The Eastern Montana Telemedicine Network uses two-way interactive video conferencing technology to provide specialty health and mental health services in Montana. The network provides a variety of clinical, educational, administrative, and community development services to the region and throughout the nation.

The Arizona TeleBehavioral Health Network was created by the Northern Arizona Regional Behavioral Health Authority to develop a telemedicine system that would enhance the delivery of behavioral health services throughout the 62,000 square miles of northern Arizona. The Authority contracts with a network of community-based agencies that provide behavioral health services to adults, children, families, and individuals with mental disorders in a rural population of 440,000. The network uses two-way interactive video and audio, tape recordings, and numerous computer applications.

VideoLink of St. Peter's developed an interactive telecommunications system within Montana. It serves a 12-county, 28,509-square-mile area with a population of 190,000. VideoLink uses two-way, interactive compressed video technology within the project's six-site network, including Montana State Hospital and Montana Developmental Center.

Appal-Link Network of Virginia was created to improve access to mental health care in rural and frontier areas of southwest Virginia. It is the first telepsychiatry network in Virginia. The telemental health system uses compressed video and audio transmission over high-speed, enhanced telephone lines.

The above telemental health networks illustrate the vast range of mental health services provided to rural and frontier individuals and communities. These networks also have the capacity to provide education and training for mental health providers and to provide education and coordinate support for consumers and their families.

Education

As telecommunication and information management becomes an integral part of the definition of mental health research and practice, it becomes critical to incorporate an understanding of informatics in all postgraduate mental health training programs. Such a curriculum should include basic tasks of patient care, communication, education, and practice management.

As the structures and knowledge of the mental health service systems change, investment in continued education to update strategic thinking and the analytical competency of mental health professionals is imperative (Clement and Wan, 1997). For example, Lopez and Prosser (1999) recommended changes to graduate education in psychology to aid the preparation of psychologists for dealing with the emergence of organized systems for mental health services.

Academic and continuing professional educational programs must be able to respond to the educational needs of mental health professionals using cutting-edge computer technology for distance learning. Academic courses offered as continuing education classes, online certificate programs, and online degree-granting programs also emphasize these skills. Entwined with these literacy skills are technology skills such as the ability to use e-mail, send and open attachments, and download plug-ins to read, view, or listen to media applications and library skills, such as the ability to formulate a research question, identify the type of literature in which the answer may be found, and effectively negotiate the academic, government, fugitive, or Web-based environments where the information may reside. Varian and Lyman (2000) suggest that information management at the individual, organizational, and societal levels is the next stage of literacy in the information-rich world of the twenty-first century.

For urban mental health professionals, opportunities to gain information and computer literacy skills have been more plentiful. Telecommunications infrastructure development in urban areas has supported multimedia Web-based learning, rapid transmission of text and data, and Internet access via cable. Classes are also available at universities, community colleges, and technical centers, where opportunities have been more common for mental health professionals to interact with colleagues, access libraries online, and create informal support networks.

However, for rural mental health professionals there are numerous problems and obstacles, including the lack of telecommunications infrastructure, professional isolation, and/or lack of peer support from other mental health colleagues (Levin and Hanson, 2001). This isolation also includes lack of access to continuing education, academic and research library resources (online or in situ), as well as the potential to lose specialty skills because of functioning as a health and/or mental health generalist (Levin and Hanson, 2001).

Thus, the use of technology, such as interactive television, audio and audio/video telephone conferencing, fax, and e-mail to teach can create challenging and exciting environments for professionals in the delivery of mental health services.

The increasing computerization of health and mental health care data, combined with the emergence of new telecommunications applications and technologies, creates vast opportunities for the provision of health and mental health care. Some of the ethical, legal, accessibility, and regulatory issues, though, seem to present major challenges for the application of communication and information technology to the delivery of mental health services. The next section is devoted to these ethical and legal issues.

Legal and Ethical Issues

Confidentiality/Access Issues

As medical records move to an electronic format, concerns about patient privacy and data security increase. The behavioral health care industry is moving to electronic patient records, establishing intranets to share information among related health care providers and using the Internet to distribute health information. Therefore, behavioral health care professionals increasingly depend on the availability of computer systems and rely on the accuracy of stored data. As secure, accurate transmission, encryption, and reception of data is paramount, more sophisticated software and hardware solutions are required in the areas of data management, digital imaging, storage and archiving, security, network communications, and infrastructure solutions. Not only patient records require confidentiality and privacy. Personnel files, corporate and human resources records, and research and development formulas are also at risk (Fig. 19.2) (Laske, 1994).

Another key confidentiality concern in the networked environment is the *integrity* of health care information. From a provider perspective, health care data are needed to analyze the outcomes and costs of different treatment plans. From a consumer perspective, health care data are used to generate provider report cards to inform health care users of their health options. The possibility that the user could compromise the integrity of such data, either intentionally, inadvertently, or from sheer negligence, becomes all the more real.

Since current business practices often require the transfer of electronic medical records across state lines, state and federal governments have serious concerns surrounding patient data. The Workgroup on Electronic Data Interchange (WEDI) provides the following example:

> A Florida resident, insured through their employer in Alabama by a carrier in Connecticut, goes to a California clinic for treatment. Prior to treating the patient, the California clinic would electronically request eligibility information through a local Cali-

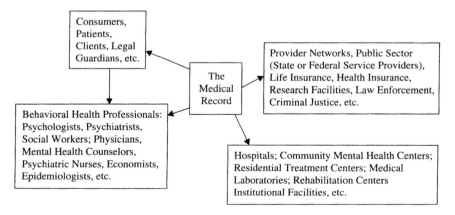

Figure 19.2 Who uses health care information?

fornia clearinghouse, which routes the request to another clearinghouse in New York, who then routes it to yet another clearinghouse in Georgia, who finally routes it to the carrier's eligibility contractor in Tennessee. The eligibility contractor's system then generates a response that reverses the path and is delivered back to the clinic, all within 30 seconds of the California clinic generating the initial request. After treating the patient, the clinic would generate an electronic claim that is transmitted to a clearinghouse in Illinois, that sends it to another clearinghouse in Ohio, that routes it to the insurance carrier in Connecticut. After processing the claim, the insurance carrier could then deliver the EFT [electronic funds transfer] and electronic remittance advice to a clearinghouse in Indiana, that routes it to the clinic's bank in Nebraska who, after balancing with the ERA [electronic record account], deposits the EFT and forwards the ERA on to the clinic for posting.

(WEDI, 1999)

This example is not even a worst-case scenario. Consider that as these transactions pass through 11 states, none of the transacting agencies or organizations knows the route of any of the transactions. To the number of organizations and states involved in this one transaction add the routing of the electronic data through the local telecommunications carrier. Routing these transactions through multiple telecommunications carriers could easily add 10 more states to the transaction path. There is no way for the health care entities to know which state laws are applicable to their transactions.

Finally, because different states have different laws and different levels of protection for this information, it has been difficult to enforce these laws effectively when information was transferred or used out of state (Gobis, 1997). Add to the mix payments from federally funded health and welfare programs, and the number of issues increases exponentially.

In 1996, the Health Insurance Portability and Accountability Act (HIPAA) of 1996 (U.S. Congress, 1996) was passed by Congress to protect individually identifiable health information. As part of the act, the U.S. Department of Health and Human Services recommended that federal law preempt states only when state law would be less protective than the future federal law. The confidentiality protections provided would therefore be cumulative, with federal law providing a minimum level of protection. Although the cost of restructuring the health care industry, as a result of HIPAA, is estimated at more than $43 billion during the next few years, HIPAA should reduce costs for health care organizations by as much as $73 billion each year through electronic dissemination practices and $9 billion annually in administrative overhead (WEDI, 1999). The United States spends approximately 24% of its health care budget for administrative overhead[2] (AMSA, 2003).

At the state level, California's Telemedicine Development Act addresses confidentiality in two ways (California Telemedicine Act, 1996). First, it provides for state law to protect a patient's medical information record transmitted electronically for telemedicine similar to the protection accorded all other medical records. Health and mental health care providers then have certain legal obligations on use, disclosure, confidentiality, retention, maintenance, and access to patient information. Second, the patient must be informed of his or her rights regarding confidential information and the existing legal protections, and verbal and written consent must be obtained from the patient prior to the use of telemedicine.

Liability, Licensing, and Accreditation

As consultations now cross state (and possibly international) borders, states have a direct interest in interstate telehealth licensure. How can regulatory and licensing state agencies protect the health and safety of their citizens? From the agency's perspective, this has been most effectively accomplished by requiring a full license for interstate telemedicine practice. This license holds an out-of-state professional to the same standard of care and legal responsibility in each state in which he or she practices telemedicine. However, for the private practitioner, the cumulative costs of holding licenses in each state would be prohibitive. However, in-state health and mental health professionals could lose a significant patient population if barriers to interstate telemedicine licensure were reduced. Therefore, health and mental health professional associations actively support full licensure requirements for out-of-state health and mental health practitioners.

As shown in the example under "Confidentiality/Access Issues," telecommunication carriers and hardware and software vendors may also need to be licensed, since they too carry confidential health information (Laske, 1997). The Alaska Telehealth Advisory Committee (1999) considered telecommunications providers to be comparable to ambulance services, whose staff must have specific expertise and credentials and whose equipment must comply with specific regulations as well as other elements of service.

There has been a proliferation of state laws and regulations addressing telemedicine licensure for health and mental health professionals. These laws vary widely in their range of options, with nearly 20 states passing laws or regulations stating that the interstate practice of medicine via electronic means (i.e., telemedicine/teleradiology) is illegal unless the distant consultant possesses a license in the patient's state (Sandberg, 1999). According to legal telemedicine precedent, it is the patient's state of residence that matters in issues of licensing, not the state in which the specialist practices and is licensed.

These regulations also affect the use of certain technologies in health care delivery systems, since use of these technologies may not be eligible for reimbursement in evaluation and management (E&M) services (i.e., patient visits and consultations). Many states require that E&M services be in real-time or near real-time (delay counted in seconds or minutes) to qualify as interactive two-way transfer of health data and information between the patient and practitioner. Therefore, many store-and-forward patient visits and consultations are not reimbursable by many federal or state programs. However, in 2000, the Medicare, Medicaid and State Children's Health Insurance Program Benefits Improvement and Protection Act of 2000 (U.S. Congress, 2000) expanded the services Medicare would reimburse for telehealth. The expansion included the following psychiatric services:[3] office and other outpatient consultations; initial inpatient consultations; follow-up inpatient consultations; confirmatory consultations; office and other outpatient services for new and established patients; individual insight-oriented, behavior-modifying, and/or supportive psychotherapy; and pharmacological management. (For more information on implementation, see the Centers for Medicare and Medicaid Services concerning implementation policies for the telehealth provisions in the Benefits and Improvement Protection Act.)

Although most states have dealt with telemedicine licensure through regulations, not legislation, there have been attempts to develop model legislation. The first attempts were made in 1996 by the Association of Telemedicine Service Providers (ATSP) and the Federation of State Boards of Medical Licensure. The ATSP compact focused on reducing the barriers to practicing interstate telemedicine by using a limited license, mutual recognition model, while the Federation model proposed a limited licensing mechanism, permitting telemedical consultations only in remote (i.e., rural or frontier) states. However, the passage of SB600 by Oregon in April 1999, which focused on out-of-state physicians practicing on Oregon patients, is considered a possible model for other licensed professions (Oregon, 1999).

Ethical Issues

Numerous ethical issues were raised in a white paper issued by the Physicians Insurers Association of America (1998). These ethical issues included the use of e-mail to transmit patient data, duty of care and defining the standard of care, accountability if liability arises from a telehealth consultation, jurisdictional differences in liability cases and how they relate to licensure, inclusion of hardware and software vendors and telecommunications carriers in liability cases, and informed consent (if a state deems telehealth consultations experimental in nature).

The eRisk Working Group on Healthcare published their *Guidelines for Online Communications* in November 2002. This group included members from the American Medical Association, other national and regional medical societies, medical malpractice carriers covering more than 70% of insured physicians, and state medical licensing boards. Its guidelines addressed the special concerns and risks of the technology of online communications and considerations for fee-based online consultations. The guidelines include informed consent, highly sensitive subject matter and attendant privacy risks, emergency subject matter, the doctor–patient relationship (liability for only online relationships is a concern), licensing jurisdiction (which may subject the provider to increased risk), and the use or creation of authoritative information. The last guideline advises health care providers that they are responsible for both Web-based and e-mail information that they provide or make available to their patients.

Implications for Mental Health Services

Telecommunication and information technology, including the Internet, holds enormous potential for transforming mental health service delivery systems in the United States. Central to the application of information science and technology to promote mental health and prevent mental disorders in populations is the establishment of an infrastructure to develop comprehensive integrated health surveillance and information systems that bridge programmatic boundaries within communities, provide informatics training for both new and existing health and medical professionals, provide safeguards for the confidentiality and privacy of these information systems, and foster improved exchange of information between health and mental health professionals and their patients (Yasnoff et al., 2000).

Historically, federal and state budgets appropriated funding for health and mental health programs. However difficult it may have been to administer health programs in rural areas prior to online communications networks, provision of services to rural and frontier areas has become more difficult. Criteria for funding have often been based on criteria relevant to urban areas. Allocation of these funds to rural areas may not cover the administrative requirements of the grant.

From an organizational perspective, a continuing issue in the use of telecommunications technology is the ongoing expense of time and money for staff training. This issue has become more complicated with HIPAA regulations for compliance and training of all staff on what their knowledge of HIPAA regulations must be. Training should not be viewed as a one-time expense, as the infrastructure changes over time to keep pace with new regulations and network updates.

Finally, if technology is to become a tool to improve delivery of and access to services for behavioral health, then five issues need to be resolved: reimbursement; licensure; expanded coverage area by Medicare and private health plans; adequate infrastructure in rural and frontier areas; and the costs of technology. *Reimbursement practices* need to be standardized to expedite payment for services and expanded to provide fuller access to essential behavioral health diagnostic, consultative, and clinical services. In addition, federal agencies, such as Medicare, need to move forward to ensure adequate reimbursement for teleconsultations. Although the Centers for Medicare and Medicaid Services issued new rules regarding reimbursement of telehealth services in 2001, many practitioners believe that there is still much more that Medicare could allow, especially in the area of mental health services. *Interstate licensure* is still a contentious issue for states and may require intercession by the federal government, possibly with the creation of a national telemedicine license. However, states and professional boards are reluctant to cede their control over licensure or credentialing to a federal authority. One exception is the National Council of State Boards of Nursing, which has been working with several state boards of nursing and nurse examiners to identify models for regulation of nurses across state lines, with a mutual recognition or reciprocity model.

Although there is federal legislation mandating *Medicare reimbursement* for specific interactive teleconsultations in rural underserved areas, there is no comparable legislation for urban and suburban areas. To include these areas under similar legislation for metropolitan and suburban areas would require congressional action and would only affect federal programs, not private plans. *Adequate infrastructure* in rural and frontier areas is still a significant problem. Although telecommunications networks are ubiquitous in metropolitan and suburban areas, the efforts and cost of "telefying" rural and frontiers areas mirror those of the rural electrification program in the early twentieth century. *Costs of technology* must be added to the infrastructure development costs. For example, teleconferencing units that cost

$300,000 in the early 1990s now cost $10,000. However, for rural and frontier area facilities or single-practitioner settings, this equipment is still not affordable without subsidization from the federal government. Even with subsidies, the costs of maintenance, training, and upgrades still place teletechnologies beyond the reach of many facilities.

There is general agreement in the literature that subsidized transmission costs (Universal Services Fund) should not be depended on for the long term. For planning purposes, telehealth systems must be self-sufficient.

NOTES

1. The article was: Salzinger K. The road from vulnerability to episode: a behavioral analysis. *Psycoloquy* 2(5):NP, 1991.

2. Overhead includes activities such as enrolling beneficiaries in a health plan, paying health insurance premiums, checking eligibility, obtaining authorization for specialist referrals, and filing reimbursement claims. (HCFA Press Office, 1997)

3. Current Procedural Terminology (CPT) codes 99241–99275, 99201–99215, 90804–90809, and 90862.

REFERENCES

Abernathy WB. The microcomputer as a community mental health public information tool. *Community Mental Health Journal* 15(3):192–202, 1979.

Alaska Telehealth Advisory Committee. *Final Report,* 1999. [Electronic resource]. Retrieved February 15, 2002, from http://appliedsci.uaa.alaska.edu/nlm/archive/ATAC%20Final%20Report%206-99.pdf

AMSA. *Frequently Asked Questions Regarding "Single-Payer" Universal Health Care.* [Electronic Resource]. Retrieved March 25, 2003, from http://www.amsa.org/hp/uhcfaqs.cfm

Angaran DM. Tele-medicine and tele-pharmacy: current status and future implications. *American Journal of Health-systems Pharmacy*, 56:1405–1426, 1999.

Baxter JW. *Definitions for Use in Mental Health Information Systems.* Rockville, MD: U.S. Department of Health, Education, and Welfare, Alcohol, Drug Abuse, and Mental Health Administration, National Institute of Mental Health, 1980.

Beck C. Information systems and social sciences. *American Behavioral Scientist*, 20(3):427–448, 1977.

Biczyk do Amaral M, Satomura Y, Honda M, et al. A design for decision-making: construction and connection of knowledge bases for a diagnostic system in medicine. *Medical Informatics (Medicine et Informatique)*, 18(4):307–320, 1993.

Blum BI. Mainframes, minis, and micros: past, present, and future. *Medcomp*, 48:40–48, 1983.

Buican B, Spaulding WD, Gordon B, et al. Clinical decision support systems in state hospitals. *New Directions for Mental Health Services*, 84:99–112, 1999.

Buring SM & Felkey BG. *Internet Research in the New Millennium: A Powerful Tool.* Pharmaco-Informatics Online, http://www.aphanet.org/pInfo/JAPhA_Mar-Apr_2000_Article.htm.

Butler DL, Anderson PS. The use of wide area computer networks in disaster management and the implications for hospital/medical networks. In Parsons DF, Fleischer CM, et al (eds). *Extended Clinical Consulting by Hospital Computer Networks. Annals of the New York Academy of Sciences*, Volume 670. New York: New York Academy of Sciences, pp. 202–210, 1992.

California Telemedicine Act, Cal. S.B. 1665 § 2290.5, 1996.

Carter DE. *A Client-Oriented System of Mental Health Service Delivery and Program Management: A Workbook and Guide.* Rockville, MD: U.S. Department of Health, Education, and Welfare, Alcohol, Drug Abuse, and Mental Health Administration, National Institute of Mental Health, 1980.

Chun K-T, Cobb S, French JR, et al. Storage and retrieval of information on psychological measures. *American Psychologist*, 28(7):592–599, 1973.

Ciarlo, JA. *Assessing Mental Health Treatment Outcome Measurement.* Rockville, MD: U.S. Department of Health and Human Services, Public Health Service, Alcohol, Drug Abuse, and Mental Health Administration, National Institute of Mental Health, Division of Biometry and Epidemiology, 1985.

Clement DG, Wan TT. Mastering health care executive education: creating transformational competence. Journal of Health Administration Education, 15(4):265–274, 1997.

Congressional Budget Office. *Federal Subsidies of Advanced Telecommunications for Schools, Libraries, and Health Care Providers.* Washington, DC: Congressional Budget Office, 1998.

DuBois NS. Documents from two sources are reconciled with a digital computer. *Behavioral Science*, 10:312–319, 1965.

Dwyer TF. Telepsychiatry: psychiatric consultation by interactive television. *American Journal of Psychiatry*, 130(8):865–869, 1973.

Edmundson HP, Wyllys RE. Automatic abstracting and indexing-survey and recommendations. *Commission of the ACM*, 4(5):226–234, 1961.

eRisk (2002). *eRisk Working Group on Healthcare's Guidelines for Online Communications* (November 2002). [Electronic Resource]. Retrieved March 20, 2003 from http://www.medem.com/corporate/corporate_Addendum_A_eRiskGuidelines.cfm#medem_erisk

Ferguson T. Digital doctoring-opportunities and challenges in electronic patient–physician communication. *Journal of the American Medical Association*, 280:1361–1362, 1998.

Fliege S. Digital computers. In Sidowski JB (Ed). *Experimental Methods and Instrumentation in Psychology.* New York: McGraw-Hill, 1966.

General Accounting Office. *Telecommunications: Federal and State Universal Service Programs and Challenges to Funding.* Washington, DC: General Accounting Office, 2002.

Gobis L. An overview of state laws and approaches to minimize licensure barriers. *Telemedicine Today* 5(6):14–15, 18, 1997.

Gorodezky MJ, Hedlund JL. The developing role of computers in community mental health centers: past experience and future trends. *Journal of Operational Psychology*, 13(2): 94–99, 1982.

Graetz RE. Research utilization of patient data files in clinical drug studies. *Behavioral Science*, 10:320–323, 1965.

Graetz RE, Agan ML, Arnsfield PJ, et al. *Psychiatric Data Automation Project: Final Report.* Camarillo, CA: Camarillo State Hospital, 1965.

HCFA Press Office. *Health Insurance Portability and Accountability Act of 1996 Administrative Simplification.* [Electronic Resource]. Retrieved March 19, 2003 from http://www.hhs.gov/news/press/1997pres/970213.html

Knapp SD. Online searching in the behavioral and social sciences. *Behavioral and Social Sciences* Librarian, 1(1):23–36, 1979.

Krantz JH. Linked Gopher and World-Wide Web services for the American Psychological Society and Hanover College Psychology Department. *Behavior Research Methods, Instruments and Computers*, 27(2):193–197, 1995.

Laske C. Legal aspects of digital image management and communication. *Medical Informatics*, 19(2):189–196, 1994.

Laske C. Health care telematics: who is liable? *Computer Methods and Programs in Biomedicine*, 54(1–2):1–6, 1997.

Ledley RS, Lusted JB. Computers in medical data processing. *Operations Research*, 8:299–310, 1960.

Leginski WA, Croze C. *Data Standards for Mental Health Decision Support Systems: A Report of the Task Force to Revise the Data Content and System Guidelines of the Mental Health Statistics Improvement Program*. Rockville, MD: U.S. Department of Health and Human Services, Public Health Service, Alcohol, Drug Abuse, and Mental Health Administration, National Institute of Mental Health, Division of Biometry and Applied Sciences, 1989.

Levin BL, Hanson A. Rural mental health services. In Loue S, Quill BQ (eds). *Handbook of Rural Health*. New York: Plenum, pp. 241–256, 2001.

Lopez SJ, Prosser E. Preparing psychologists: more focus on training psychologists for a future in evolving health-care delivery systems. *Journal of Clinical Psychology in Medical Settings*, 6(3):295–301, 1999.

Lynett PA. The current and potential uses of computer assisted interactive videodisc in the education of social workers. *Computers in Human Services*, 1(4):75–85, 1985.

Manderscheid RW, Henderson MJ. *Speaking with a Common Language: The Past, Present and Future of Data Standards for Managed Behavioral Healthcare*. Rockville, MD: Center for Mental Health Services, Division of State and Community Systems Development, July 1995. Also available online http://www.mentalhealth.org/publications/allpubs/MC95-51/default.asp

Markley RP, Adams RM. The Science Citation Index. *American Psychologist*, 28(6):534, 1973.

Medow MA, Wilt TJ, Dysken S, et al. Effect of written and computerized decision support aids for the U.S. Agency for Health Care Policy and Research depression guidelines on the evaluation of hypothetical clinical scenarios. *Medical Decision Making: An International Journal of the Society for Medical Decision Making*, 21(5):344–356, 2001.

Meyer H, Preston GH. What happens to first admissions to state hospitals. *American Journal of Psychiatry*,104:546–548, 1948.

Mohan L, Muse L, McInerney C. Managing smarter: a decision support system for mental health providers. *Journal of Behavioral Health Services and Research*, 25(4):446–455, 1998.

National Advisory Mental Health Council. *Caring for People with Severe Mental Disorders: A National Plan of Research to Improve Services*. Rockville, MD: U.S. Department of Health and Human Services, Alcohol, Drug Abuse, and Mental Health Administration, National Institute of Mental Health, 1991.

National Institute of Mental Health. *Implementing the NIMH Prototype in a Mental Health Agency*. Rockville, MD: Division of Biometry and Epidemiology, 1983.

Nickelson DW. Telehealth and the evolving health care system: strategic opportunities for professional psychology. *Professional Psychology: Research and Practice*, 29(6):527–535, 1998.

Oregon State Legislature. *Telemedicine Licensure. Senate Bill 600*, 1999.

Parr VH. Online information retrieval and the undergraduate. *Teaching of Psychology*, 6(1):61–62, 1979.

Paton JA, D'huyvetter PK. *Automated Management Information Systems for Mental Health Agencies: A Planning and Acquisition Guide*. Rockville, MD: U.S. Department of Health and Human Services, Alcohol, Drug Abuse, and Mental Health Administration, National Institute of Mental Health, 1980.

Patton RE, Leginski WA. *The Design and Content of a National Mental Health Statistics System*. Rockville, MD: U.S. Department of Health and Human Services, Alcohol, Drug Abuse, and Mental Health Administration, National Institute of Mental Health, 1983.

Peper E, Toth M. How do you get those references for that review paper? *American Psychologist*, 26(8):740, 1971.

Physicians Insurers Association of America. *Telemedicine: A Medical Liability White Paper*. Rockville, MD: Physicians Insurers Association, 1998.

Pollock HM. Patients with mental disease, mental defect, epilepsy, alcoholism and drug addiction in institutions in the United States, January 1, 1920. *Mental Hygiene*, 5:139–169, 1921.

Sandberg LA. Telemedicine continues to wrestle wicked problems: reimbursement, licensure, and bandwidth rules (or is it compliance?). *Health Management Technology*; 20(1):133–134, 1999.

Santo Y, Finkel A. A computer simulation of schizophrenia. In Blum BI (ed). *Proceedings of the Sixth Annual Symposium on Computer Applications in Health Care*. New York: Institute of Electrical Engineers, pp. 737–741, 1982.

Smith HA, Allison RA. *Telemental Health: Delivering Mental Health Care at a Distance*. Rockville, MD: Substance Abuse and Mental Health Services Administration and the Health Resources and Services Administration, 1998.

Smith NJ, Parmar G, Paget N. Computer simulation and social work education: a suitable case. *British Journal of Social Work*, 10(4):491–499, 1980.

Solow C. 24–hour psychiatric consultation via TV. *American Journal of Psychiatry*, 127(12): 1684–1687, 1971.

Spielberg A. Sociohistorical, legal, and ethical implications of e-mail for the patient–physician relationship. *Journal of the American Medical Association*, 280:1353–1359, 1998.

Staff. New tools help behavioral health providers boost quality while documenting value. *Disease Management Advisor*, 8(1):5–8, 2002.

Trapp A, Hammond N, Bray D. Internet and the support of psychology education. *Behavior Research Methods, Instruments and Computers*, 28(2):174–176, 1996.

Trochim W, Dumont J, Campbell J. *A Report for the State Mental Health Agency Profiling System: Mapping Mental Health Outcomes from the Perspective of Consumers/Survivors. Technical Report Series*, Alexandria, VA: National Association of State Mental Health Program Directors Research Institute, 1993.

Truitt EI, Binner PR. The Fort Logan Mental Health Center. In Taube CA (Ed). *Community Mental Health Center Data Systems: A Description of Existing Programs*. Rockville, MD: National Institute of Mental Health, pp. 22–38, 1969.

U.S. Congress. Health Insurance Portability and Accountability Act, PL 104-191, 104th Congress, 1996.

U.S. Congress. *Medicare, Medicaid and SCHIP Benefits Improvement and Protection Act of 2000 (Benefits and Improvement Protection Act)*. PL 106-554, 106th Congress, 2000.

Van Donegan CJ. CAI applications in mental health nursing. *Computers in Psychiatry/Psychology* 6(1):25–26, 1984.

Varian H, Lyman P. *How Much Information?* Available at: http://www.sims.berkeley.edu/how-much-info/index.html 2000. Accessed 3 May 2003.

Welch N, Krantz JH. The World-Wide Web as a medium for psychoacoustical demonstrations and experiments: experience and results. *Behavior Research Methods, Instruments and Computers*, 28(2):192–196, 1996.

White EB. Outcomes: essential information for clinical decision support: an interview with Ellen B. White. Interview by Melinda L. Orlando. *Journal of Health Care Finance*, 24(3):71–81, 1998.

Wittson CL, Affleck DC, Johnson V. Two-way television in group therapy. *Mental Hospitals*, 12(10):22–23, 1961.

Wolfman C. Microcomputer simulated psychiatric interviews used as a teaching aid. *Journal of Psychiatric Education*, 4(3):190–201, 1980.

Workgroup for Electronic Data Interchange. *WEDI Board Submits Preliminary Recommendations on Pending Privacy Regulations,* 1999. [Electronic Resource] Retrieved March 20, 2003 from http://www.wedi.org/public/articles/details%7E25.htm

Wurster CR, Goodman JD. NIMH Prototype management information system for community mental health centers. In O'Neill JT (ed). *Proceedings of the Fourth Annual Symposium on Computer Applications in Medical Care, November 2–5, 1980, Washington, D.C.* New York: Institute for Electrical and Electronic Engineers, pp. 907–912, 1981.

Yasnoff WA, O'Carroll PW, Koo D, et al. Public health informatics: improving and transforming public health in the information age. *Journal of Public Health Management and Practice* 6(6):67–75, 2000.

20

Evaluating Alcohol, Drug Abuse, and Mental Health Services

ROBERT G. ORWIN
HOWARD H. GOLDMAN

While some areas of social programming have undergone relatively little evaluation, this is not true of the delivery of alcohol, drug abuse, and mental health services. From the advent of the community mental health movement through the Robert Wood Johnson and McKinney Act demonstrations of the late 1980s and early 1990s, and most recently the numerous multisite studies sponsored by the Substance Abuse and Mental Health Service Administration (SAMHSA), evaluation has been part of the mental health program development and policy-making process. With increasing competition for shrinking resources and uncertainty over future organization and financing of services, the need for anyone associated with the delivery of services to understand what evaluation can do, how it is done, and how it is used has probably never been greater. This is true whether the individual is a direct service provider, program manager/administrator, policy maker/sponsor, or other stakeholder.

Clearly, there is more to program evaluation than can be covered in this chapter, and our intent in writing it was *not* to train evaluators. The capability to design and conduct a quality evaluation of any complexity requires a high level of technical training and experience. Recognition of this has fostered the development of program evaluation as a profession and the subject of specialization in graduate education curricula. Evaluation professionals with the requisite skills should be consulted before any evaluation is undertaken. This advice applies equally to the planning stages of the evaluation and to the actual assessment of a program's impact.

This chapter will enable the reader to

- understand the various purposes of evaluation;
- understand the social and political context in which evaluation occurs;

- participate in the planning of evaluations;
- request and oversee useful and credible evaluations;
- read, understand, and assess evaluation reports; and
- use evaluation results appropriately.

For readers wishing to learn more about evaluation, the references in this chapter are an excellent place to start. As elsewhere, a well-informed consumer can demand a better product. The more thoroughly program managers, administrators, and policy makers understand the technical, resource, and political issues confronting evaluators, the better equipped they are to ask the right questions and insist on adequate answers.

Basic Concepts and Terms

Program evaluation can be defined as the use of scientific methods to assess the implementation and outcome of programs. This definition is not comprehensive, as it does not encompass every aspect of the enterprise that writers and theorists have associated with the term. However, it does cover the vast majority of the activities that are carried out daily under the name of evaluation. And typically it is what administrators or policy makers mean when they request that a program be evaluated.

A *program* is an intervention or set of activities intended to achieve external *program objectives*—that is, to meet some recognized social need or to solve an identified social problem. For example, a residential treatment program for clients who are homeless and mentally ill with a co-occurring substance abuse problem (i.e., *dual diagnosis*) might be dedicated to reducing alcohol and other drug use, increasing economic and residential stability, improving social functioning, and decreasing costs to the community. It might also have system-oriented objectives, such as better integration of the community network of services.

A program rarely consists of a single activity but more typically comprises a set of *program components*. So the residential program for dually diagnosed clients might include outreach and engagement, transitional housing, a treatment approach, and case management.

Each program component should logically result in a set of *program outputs*, which are the actual services delivered by the program. So the treatment approach mentioned above might include individual and/or group therapy at some level of intensity (e.g., 2 hours/day, 5 days/week) and drug education seminars, plus socialization activities and vocational assistance. Whereas programs and program components are abstractions, their embodiment in program outputs is empirically observable and measurable by the evaluator.

Finally, the effects of the program outputs—whether on people or systems—are the *program outcomes*. Just as the specification of program outputs attempts to turn the abstract notions of programs and program components into a measurable reality, the specification of program outcomes does the same for program objectives. Program objectives are often stated in vague terms, particularly when written into legislation. Clarification and practical definition of objectives—including their mapping into measurable program outcomes—are necessary for both program management and subsequent evaluation. So the above-mentioned objective of decreasing costs to the community might be operationalized as reduced numbers of arrests, psychiatric hospitalizations, and visits to the emergency room.

A *program theory*, sometimes called a *program model*, explains the expected linkages between program components, outputs, and outcomes. Although definitions vary, it is primarily a specification of how the components of the program are supposed to produce or cause their intended effects. Its basis can be medical knowledge, social science theory, services research, or the experience-based consensus of a human service field. A good program theory includes a specification of the mediational mechanisms through which change will occur. Returning to the program for homeless clients with a dual diagnosis, the mediational mechanisms linking outputs to outcomes might include stabilization of psychiatric symptoms and increased personal responsibility.

In the pages that follow, several stages of program evaluation are discussed. *Formative evaluation* provides feedback to program management during the program's early stages on areas of the program needing further development or modification. *Process evaluation* describes the program's implementation and assesses whether the intended services are being delivered to the targeted participants. *Outcome evaluation*, sometimes called *impact evaluation* or *summative evaluation*, determines whether the program achieves its intended objectives.

Purposes of Evaluations

Chelimsky (1978) identified three principal purposes of evaluation: (*1*) more meaningful accountability, (*2*) improved program delivery, and (*3*) addition to the knowledge of the social sciences. In addition, there are what Rutman and Mowbray (1983) call hidden or *covert* purposes for doing evaluation. Each of these is discussed in turn.

Accountability

The demand for accountability has probably been the main impetus behind support for evaluation and the growth of the evaluation field. In this age of taxpayer revolts and record deficits, budgetary restraint has gained the political spotlight as never before. The public and their legislative representatives demand to know if a program "works." If it does, it merits continued or expanded support; if it doesn't, it should be scaled back or even eliminated. Accountability questions include: Has the program been implemented as intended? Is it reaching its target population? Is it achieving its objectives and doing so efficiently? How does it compare in cost and effectiveness to other programs with similar objectives? Are there unintended negative side effects?

At the federal level, the use of evaluation as an accountability tool has frequently been codified into law. For example, the Congressional Budget and Control Act of 1974 authorizes congressional committees to carry out evaluations, contract for them, or require executive branch agencies to perform them. It also requires the General Accounting Office (GAO) to review and evaluate the administration's programs. The GAO itself has seen a tremendous expansion of its mission from simple financial audits to full-blown effectiveness evaluations and policy analyses (Chelimsky, 1992). Another mechanism is the *set-aside*, where funders make the support of programs contingent on periodic evaluation and earmark a certain percentage of program funds for that purpose. In mental health, for example, the 1975 legislation authorizing community mental health centers required centers to set aside 2% of their annual operating expenditures to evaluate the effectiveness of their programs (Rutman and Mowbray, 1983). Still another is *sunset* legislation, where programs are established initially for a specified number of years, after which they must be evaluated and shown to work in order to be reauthorized. It is relatively easy for legislators to insert such mechanisms into statutes. The extent to which they truly instill accountability is a subject of some debate (e.g., there are few instances in which programs have actually been shut down by sunset legislation), but their nominal intent to do so is clear.

Improved Program Delivery

The second purpose—improved program delivery—represents the program manager's perspective. Evaluation provides information for modifying services and their delivery mechanisms in order to increase effectiveness. The customer is typically the program manager, and the sponsorship of the evaluation is internal rather than external. The main rationale for evaluation in this context is that program managers need to know how their programs are being implemented and how that implementation is affecting outcomes. Program delivery questions include: How is the program being implemented? What are the impediments to implementation and how can they be removed? Is the program reaching its target population? Are clients satisfied with the services? Are they staying in the program, and if not, why not? What types of clients appear to benefit most from which services? Should existing services be modified or new services added? Can efficiency be improved?

Clearly, evaluations that are primarily intended to serve program management purposes can also serve accountability purposes, as is evident from the overlap in the questions. But the emphases are different, and more important, the perspectives and intended uses of the results are different. Accountability questions the fundamental value of the program, with the intent of making an informed policy or resource allocation decision about its future. The management perspective is less fundamental; it stipulates the program's value and focuses the evaluation on finding ways to improve it.

Increased Knowledge

The third purpose—producing knowledge for the field—differs from the first two in that the results of the evaluation may not be of immediate actionable use, but may instead lay the foundations for far-reaching program innovations in the longer term. At the far end of this continuum is what Cordray and Lipsey (1986) have called *program research*, whose principal purpose is to develop valid, generalizable knowledge about intervention, the social problems on which intervention is targeted, and the social system within which intervention is implemented. In mental health, Fairweather and his colleagues (1975) spent more than 20 years examining the effectiveness of existing interventions, and developing and testing new ones, for mental patients released from hospitals. Demonstration projects also fall under the knowledge development purpose. For example, the Robert Wood Johnson Foundation's (RWJF) Program on Chronic Mental Illness assessed whether changes in the organization and financing of the system of care, in particular through the creation or strengthening of a local mental health authority, would lead to the development of a comprehensive system of mental health and social welfare services, which in turn would improve the quality of life of persons with severe and persistent mental illness (Goldman et al., 1992). The National Institute on Alcohol Abuse and Alcoholism (NIAAA) McKinney demonstrations assessed the extent to which homeless persons with alcohol and other drug problems could be retained in programs, and the effectiveness of various interventions in reducing alcohol and other drug use, increasing employment and economic security, improving physical and mental health status, and increasing residential stability, as well as collecting lessons learned from the implementation experiences of the projects (NIAAA, 1992). None of these research efforts was intended to lead to a decision about a particular program or policy, either by program managers or by the people to whom they were accountable.

Covert Purposes

Finally, as noted above, there are hidden or covert political purposes for evaluation—to make a program look good, to make it look bad, or to avoid action. They explain in part why program managers are suspicious of and/or nervous about accountability evaluations imposed from outside and why oversight bodies (e.g., the Congress) are skeptical about the objectivity of internal evaluations conducted or sponsored by program managers.

Apart from whether covert purposes are actually operating, the differing perspectives and organizational motives of the insider versus the outsider can influence the scope, design, and execution of the evaluation. Questions that sound identical (e.g., is the program achieving its objectives?) tend to be pursued differently when asked internally versus externally. Miles' law states it best: "Where you stand depends on where you sit" (Miles, 1978). Program managers, and the internal evaluators who report to them, are unlikely to conclude that their program should be terminated. Oversight bodies and their evaluators (e.g., Congress and the GAO) are just as unlikely to conclude that the program is working so well that further oversight is unnecessary. The consumer should recognize that the aspects of the study that one usually reads for—the clarity of the objectives, the rigor of the design, the reliability and validity of the measures, and the statistical appropriateness of the analyses—do not tell the whole story. The institutional affiliation of the evaluator should also be considered.

Planning the Study

After enduring several minutes of verbal pummeling from a congressional committee on the adequacy of weapons testing, a Pentagon official rhetorically asked, "Why is there always enough time to do it over but never enough time to do it right?" The question could as easily be applied to the evaluation of social service programs, except that in evaluation there is rarely the time (or opportunity) to do it over. More often than not, the program will simply surge ahead, limp along, or die an early death without the input to that decision that a high-quality evaluation might have provided. So the evaluator has to get it right the first time. Adequate time for planning at the front end is key to doing that, and should be insisted on by sponsors, managers, and evaluators alike.

In this section, several activities that have proven useful in the planning of evaluations are described: evaluability assessment, logic models, formative studies, and syntheses of prior evaluations. The role and perspectives of competing stakeholders in the planning process is also discussed. We close by describing a recent change in the way SAMHSA funds multisite demonstration programs in an effort to improve evaluation planning and ensure useful results.

Evaluability Assessment

As noted by Weiss (1973), the sins of the program are often visited on the evaluation. When programs are poorly designed, goals are vague, and implementation is poorly managed and disorganized, the evaluation will suffer the consequences. *Evaluability assessment*—a term coined by Joseph Wholey—is a tool to prevent such fiascos from occurring.

Rutman and Mowbray (1983) define evaluability assessment as the front-end analysis that enables managers and evaluators to determine the extent to which the program can appropriately and reasonably be evaluated. Its primary purpose is to ensure that any evaluations conducted will reach their objectives and produce results that are credible and useful. It analyzes the nature of the program, its activities, and its delivery mechanisms, and clarifies its objectives and intended effects in relation to what is being done to achieve them. It also assesses the feasibility of proposed evaluation methodologies. In short, the evaluability assessment establishes the probability of a subsequent evaluation's being successful.

With new programs, evaluability assessment can identify a number of problems. These include poorly defined programs, vague or unrealistic objectives, unintended effects (negative or positive), and the absence of a credible way to approximate what would have happened to the target recipients in the absence of the program. Any of these problems can plague alcohol, drug abuse, and mental health service programs. Vague or nebulous objectives are particularly common (e.g., "improve the quality of life" or "enhance social functioning").

Evaluability assessment is also applied to ongoing programs, to describe how the program is being implemented as a prelude to deciding on how best to evaluate it. Failure to recognize problems of program implementation may result in an evaluation that tests the effectiveness of a program that was never implemented, or at least not implemented to the degree intended. Evaluability assessment can point out some of these problems, leading to a possible decision that the evaluation should focus on understanding the implementation issues rather than on measuring effectiveness. Evaluability assessment of an ongoing program is a close cousin to process evaluation, discussed later.

Techniques have been developed to determine whether a program is evaluable in the senses discussed above (Rutman, 1980; Smith, 1989; Wholey, 1979). In general, they include procedures such as preparing a detailed program description, interviewing program personnel, observing program operations, developing an evaluable program model, determining the key questions and the information needed to answer them, determining the feasibility of evaluation procedures, identifying potential users of the evaluation, and achieving agreement to proceed. A successful evaluability assessment requires the commitment and collaboration of program staff and other stakeholders, in addition to technical expertise and leadership from the evaluator.

Experience has shown that evaluability assessments can increase the probability of achieving useful and credible evaluations. For example, the evaluation of the National Institute of Mental Health (NIMH) Community Support program (Turner and TenHoor, 1978) was initiated with an evaluability assessment (Tessler and Goldman, 1982), and the program director continues to view the evaluability assessment as critical to her understanding of her own program and its evaluation (J. Turner, personal communication, 1993). It can also lead to many incidental benefits to program managers, facilitating improvements in program delivery prior to formal evaluation. Another frequent outcome of evaluability assessment is a decision not to conduct a formal evaluation. There may be too few agreed-upon objectives, no credible design that is administratively feasible, or some other lack of clarity that makes a formal evaluation either impossible or likely to be largely uninformative.

Recognizing this—as well as the reality that programs and evaluations can encounter unanticipated structural problems that time and money cannot solve—SAMHSA recently began funding its multisite demonstrations in two phases (the Homelessness Prevention, Supportive Housing, Women and Violence, and Homeless Families demonstrations are examples of this practice). Phase I is a "getting ready" period (typically 2 years) that includes program development, articulation, and process evaluation at the site level and the collaborative planning of the outcome evaluation at the cross-site level. The latter includes development of the cross-site logic model, instrument protocols, eligibility criteria, and so forth. Phase II is the cross-site outcome evaluation itself (typically 3 years). However, a site's transition to Phase II is not automatic. Rather, Phase I sites have to compete among themselves with a new application, and the application review process is, in large part, an evaluability assessment. Here, sites have to provide evidence that the resources they are requesting will lead to scientifically valid and policy-relevant results. Some of the ways to do this are discussed in subsequent segments of this section.

Stakeholder Perspectives

Evaluation is part of the policy process and therefore part of the political process. As Berk and Rossi (1990) note, the outcome of an evaluation can be expected to attract attention from whoever holds stakes in the outcome. Rossi and Freeman (1993) identify 10 distinct stakeholder groups with an interest in the process and its results:

- Policy makers and decision makers: those responsible for deciding whether a program is to be instituted, continued, discontinued, expanded, or curtailed;
- Program sponsors: organizations that initiate and fund the program to be evaluated;
- Evaluation sponsors: organizations that initiate and fund the evaluation (sometimes identical to program sponsors);
- Target participants: program participants who receive the intervention services being evaluated;
- Program management: persons responsible for overseeing and coordinating the program;
- Program staff: persons responsible for actual delivery of services;
- Evaluators: persons responsible for the design and/or conduct of the evaluation;
- Program competitors: organizations that compete with the program for available resources;
- Contextual stakeholders: local government officials or agencies and political influentials situated in the program's environment;
- Evaluation community: other evaluators who read evaluations and pass judgment on their technical quality.

Three other groups of stakeholders have become increasingly vocal in the community mental health movement. The first are national advocacy groups such as the National Alliance for the Mentally Ill, the National Mental Health Association, and the National Association of Psychiatric Survivors. These groups typically have no direct involvement in the funding or management of programs or their evaluations, but aspire to represent the target recipients who are unable to represent themselves effectively in the political arena (e.g., persons who are homeless and mentally ill). The second are local opposition groups, who simply object to the program's placement in their community (the "not in my back yard" or NIMBY syndrome). They typically protest that it will increase crime, lower their property values, or simply decrease their aesthetic quality of life. These groups have proven quite effective in using both the courts and the media to delay or even prevent the implementation of programs for clients with mental illness and substance abuse problems. The third and newest group, which is actually an outgrowth of the first, is consumers providing direct and continuing input to major evaluation projects. Over the past 5 years, it has become increasingly the norm in multisite demonstrations sponsored by SAMHSA to have consumer representatives at the site and cross-site levels. These individuals advise on all aspects of the studies (research questions, logic models, measures, data interpretation, etc.) and frequently have full voting rights on cross-site steering committee decisions.

The strains that result from conflicting stakeholder interests can be reduced in part by anticipating and planning for them; in part they come with the territory and must be accepted and lived with. A common yet particularly trying conflict occurs when the results of the evaluation do not support the policies of its sponsors or the programs they advocate and the sponsors then turn on the evaluators. The first author bore frequent witness to this phenomenon during his 6-year tenure with the GAO conducting evaluations for the Congress. The sponsoring member or committee chair rarely denounced the report publicly (to do so would confirm the initial bias long suspected by the opposition); more often, the report was quietly buried or subtle pressure was applied to recast the conclusions. The latter can be a particularly wrenching experience for evaluators, particularly if it is their first exposure to the political process.

The evaluation's methodology must be all the more airtight when stakeholder conflicts guarantee that the report will be attacked. Slipshod procedures will surely become apparent to critics, who will be combing the report for evidence of their occurrence. The methodology will be attacked in well-conducted studies too because no study is without methodological flaws. While social scientists can usually distinguish between a serious and a trivial flaw, the public opinion to which a critic is playing may not. Still, it is worthwhile to spend extra resources on a strong, quantitatively based design when attack is imminent. As Chelimsky (1987) observed, it is rarely prudent to enter a burning political debate armed only with a case study.

In planning any evaluation, it is wise to consider the range of stakeholders that are affected by or affect, in one way or another, either the program or the evaluation, or both. Identifying the stakeholders and thinking through a strategy for building consensus and minimizing discord among them is generally a worthwhile investment. Often this requires careful prior negotiations with each group on program objectives, the design of the evaluation, commitment of required resources, and use of the evaluation results. Not surprisingly, the complexity is greater in a multisite project. In this context, Leff and Mulkern (2002) discuss the continual need for cross-site study governance (typically called the *steering committee*) to balance scientific and participatory principles. On the positive side, multisite investigators cite participatory processes as contributing to the values base (Babor et al., 2002) or view the participatory process as creating an *invisible college* (Boruch et al., 1976) in which participants share knowledge and expertise. On the negative side, the participatory process is inefficient and time-consuming (Cook et al., 2002; Rog and Randolph, 2002). In addition, it is seen as sometimes leading to decisions in which the methods chosen to execute the scientific requirements are driven by the capacities of the least capable sites (Rog and Randolph, 2002). Better site selection and study planning can address these issues, if not eliminate them, and the past decade has seen considerable progress on this front.

Logic Models

Logic modeling is a graphic technique for displaying the causal relationships or logical linkages between the context and resources devoted to a programmatic effort, the activities supported by the effort, and the outcomes intended as consequences of these activities. Logic models, which can serve different purposes at different stages, can provide a useful guide to the planning and implementation of evaluations. They can be corrected, modified, and differentiated as the program proceeds through implementation. They can also play a crucial role in planning client-level and system-level outcome analyses. When logic models are periodically updated throughout implementation, they are also a principal product of the evaluation and a practical tool in the generalization of implementation results.

For an evaluation of a multisite program, logic models can be constructed for individual sites' programs or for the program as a whole. Figure 20.1 shows the logic model from a therapeutic community (TC) program for addicted women with children funded under the SAMHSA Homeless Families demonstration program. Consistent with the general TC approach, the main therapist is the community itself; the staff and senior residents serve as role models. In addition, each resident is given work assignments that help maintain the community, and as she progresses in her treatment she is given more responsible jobs. The program does not use a traditional TC confrontation approach to group therapy, but instead uses what the program director terms a "carefrontation" approach, grounded in recent research suggesting that a more caring and supportive group process is more effective with this population. As clients proceed through the program, they develop greater identification with the staff and senior residents, their self-efficacy increases, a positive expectancy develops, and—as illustrated in the model—they become more knowledgeable about the process of addiction and how to avoid relapse. As illustrated, this triggers a positive learning feedback loop that produces the desired treatment outcomes listed in the model.

Figure 20.2 shows the generic cross-site logic model from the same demonstration. This is structured somewhat differently, in that it attempts to capture the

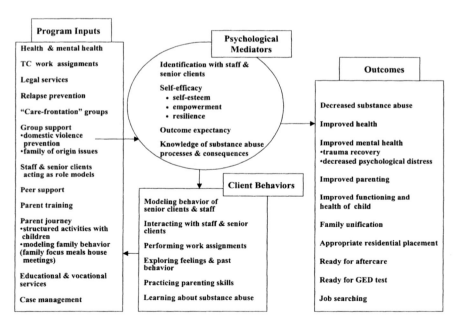

Figure 20.1   Program logic model for the Veritas Young Mothers' Program core treatment phase. GED: general educational development; TC: therapeutic community.

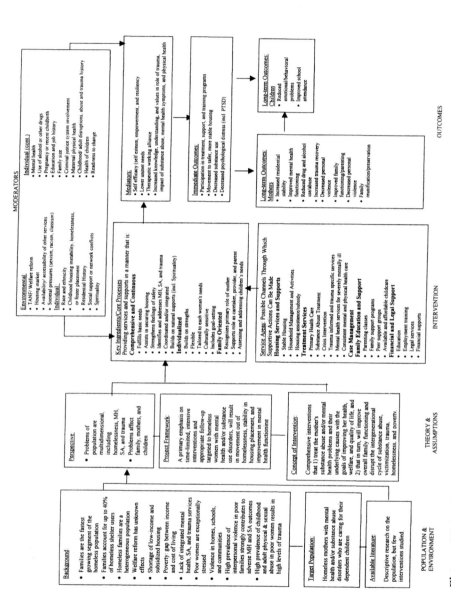

Figure 20.2 Cross-site homeless families program logic model. MH: mental health; PTSD: posttraumatic stress disorder; SA: substance abuse; TANF: Temporary Assistance to Needy Families.

logic of the myriad interventions, settings, and research designs spread over 14 projects nationally. Note the two boxes in the middle: "Key Ingredients/Core Processes and Service Areas: Possible Channels Through Which Supportive Actions Can Be Made." These were continually stressed at grantee meetings to ensure that the essence of the forest was not lost in the complexity of the trees.

Logic models have their limitations. The most important of these is that it is easy for a logic model to oversimplify a program's theory. Evaluators must be careful to capture the nuances and details of program logic through repeated contact and discussion, and not to be satisfied with quick agreement by program developers who may agree just to get on with the real business of program implementation. Reality often is not logical. Change often is not rational. A logic model is just a model—a device to identify the steps and processes of intended change—a benchmark for comparing what was planned with what was accomplished.

Program Templates

Program templates (Scheirer, 1996) are a tool for implementation assessment and formative evaluation and a recent extension of logic models. A program template is a matrix format for specifying the components of an intervention and comparing the elements intended to be implemented at a particular site with those actually implemented. Templates were intended to make it easier for evaluators and program managers to specify *best practice* or other external standards for programs, compare the components of a particular program with these standards, and then summarize what was learned in monitoring about the process and extent of program implementation. Although the method as practiced tends to keep the assessments at the level of qualitative summaries in a table, Lamberti and Katzenmeyer (1996) address ways of transforming qualitative data from templates into quantitative codes to describe multiple programs within a large-scale study. Thus, though templates were originally developed as formative evaluation tools, they are beginning to be used in cross-site comparisons and other comparative analyses.

Formative Studies

It has been repeatedly shown that innovative programs take time to develop and mature (Goldman et al., 1992; Orwin et al., 1994b; 1998; Ridgely and Willenbring, 1992). Successful implementation requires extensive program planning, model development, and start-up time, especially when integrating services provided by diverse agencies with different ideologies, treatment practices, and organizational cultures. As discussed earlier, it may also require protracted negotiations with stakeholders and a full-scale evaluability assessment before the program even opens its doors. Extensive time for planning prior to program startup is invaluable but does not obviate the need for a maturation period after startup to overcome initial barriers and fine-tune the intervention.

Formative studies assess the conduct of programs during these early stages and provide feedback to program management on areas of the program needing further development or modification. Formative studies also provide the opportunity to *pretest* the evaluation procedures and instruments. Many programs fail because insufficient time and resources were invested in formative efforts either in the design phase or during early periods of operation. Attempting to conduct an outcome evaluation on a still-developing program is frustrating for both evaluators and program staff and limits what can be concluded, generalized, and contributed to the field.

Formative studies vary in their rigor and sophistication, but simple studies are frequently sufficient to uncover the problems an intervention will face and identify ways to overcome them. Rossi and Freeman (1993) describe a typical formative study that was conducted on a representative sample of targeted participants for a community mental health program. The intervention design required weekly attendance at meetings; therefore, it was necessary to assess whether participants would comply. Careful records were kept of the various means of recruiting clients, the proportion who attended for the full 8-week program, and those who dropped out. Dropouts were interviewed to determine their reasons for not completing the program and to find ways to improve retention. In the NIAAA Cooperative Agreement Program, a formative pilot study in one of the projects for dually diagnosed clients revealed that while almost all prospective clients agreed to participate in the study, only about half ever showed up (McGlynn et al., 1993). The concern was that not all clients were making an informed, noncoerced decision to participate. In the main study, a 2-week cooling-off period was instituted for prospective clients to consider whether they truly wished to enroll. The no-show rate fell accordingly.

A recommended formative study for any program where the size or participation rate of the target population is at all in doubt is a *pipeline* study. A pipeline study typically focuses on the points of entry of clients into the system and the points at which constriction of flow occur. It often requires interviewing staff at each potential referral site (jails, shelters, etc.). Such a study can answer a number of useful questions, such as what proportion of the qualifying population will actually be identified and selected as eligible and willing to participate, and how and where in the pipeline cases are excluded. A pipeline study is generally necessary to assess whether required sample sizes can realistically be achieved, particularly in substance abuse treatment evaluations (Ashery and McAuliffe, 1992). In conducting one, it is critical to ask specific questions of referral agency staff about any estimated numbers they provide. Considerable leakage can occur between the *estimated* number of *potential* eligibles and the *actual* numbers of *true* eligibles that are successfully contacted, screened, agree to participate, assigned, and show up for the program.

In a multisite program, it is sometime possible to pilot test the program or the evaluation instruments at one or a few sites prior to full implementation at all sites. In the NIAAA Cooperative Agreement Program, for example, the early starter projects provided feedback to the national evaluators on problems with the baseline assessment instrument. Solutions were discussed and agreed upon, and then formally disseminated to the other projects (Cordray et al., 1991).

Syntheses of Prior Evaluations

In the past 10–15 years, the venerable literature review has given ground to newer, more quantitative techniques for systematically synthesizing the literature in a particular content area. Quantitative synthesis is a generic methodological approach to summarizing the collective evidence from multiple primary research studies. Its most distinctive features are (*1*) the statistical transformation of results from each primary study into a common metric, (*2*) the aggregation of the results into summary statistics, and (*3*) systematic examination of the variation across primary studies (e.g., in client characteristics, treatments, and settings) and their relationship to outcomes. The most well-known version of quantitative synthesis is called *meta-analysis,* introduced by Glass (1976).

Syntheses are usually done to answer outcome-related research questions and, as discussed later, are one strategy for conducting an outcome evaluation. They can also be useful for planning purposes, however, because they provide a database analogous to those used for estimating expectancies in actuarial tables (Cordray and Orwin, 1983). The basic notion is to establish a set of statistics that indicate the prevalence of specific evaluation-related events. Just as insurance companies establish rates for premiums based on expected incidences, evaluators can use expectancies derived from previous studies to support resource allocation decisions for the evaluation. Cordray and Sonnefeld (1985) applied this technique to the planning of a multisite evaluation of the effects of early initiation of psychosocial services on hospital length of stay.

A key assumption is that the set of synthesized studies cover the range of research conditions that are likely to be encountered in the new evaluation being planned. As with simulations, this makes it more useful in an area where a good deal of empirically based knowledge is available and correspondingly less useful in an area where little is known.

Evaluation Design

The planning phase should solidify the basic scope and objectives of the evaluation. The evaluation design turns the broad-brush strokes from the planning process into a detailed operational guide for conducting the evaluation. For example, if the agreed-upon program objectives include reduction in psychiatric symptomatology, then the evaluation design should specify the measurement instruments that will reliably and validly determine whether such reductions occurred and by how much. It should also specify how often and at what intervals clients will be assessed and what mechanisms will be put in place to ensure that high rates of follow-up are obtained. Or, if the plans called for establishing a nonequivalent comparison group (i.e., a group selected by means other than random assignment), the design should specify how this group will be selected, how it is likely to differ from the targeted group, and the extent to which these differences can be accommodated in the analyses. These are just a few of the details that an evaluation design should cover. Others will be noted in the sections below. Optimally, the detailed design should be completed and approved before the evaluation begins. In practice, time pressures often preclude this.

Process Evaluation

Program evaluation is typically concerned with the assessment of program impact, but it is also concerned with assessing the implementation processes of the program. In essence, process evaluation attempts to describe how the program is being carried out, including whether it is being carried out as planned. There are numerous reasons why programs for persons with mental illness and/or alcohol and other drug problems are *not* implemented as planned. Typical startup problems include NIMBY issues (described earlier), unanticipated legal difficulties in obtaining or renovating facilities, and recruitment and staffing difficulties.

When projects do finally initiate their service interventions, deviations from original plans are not unusual. In the NIAAA Cooperative Agreement Program, for example, interorganizational dynamics and resource limitations in the external environment resulted in significant changes in the original program design of several projects. One project for dually diagnosed clients originally planned to refer clients in one of its two treatment conditions to other community agencies and self-help groups for alcohol and other drug treatment services. But long waiting lists and eligibility restrictions limited client access to these resources, so the program design was redefined to focus instead on the clients' social support networks. Another project decided to discontinue its plans to develop a new drop-in center after encountering difficulties in subleasing the facility from another community treatment agency. Deviations from the program as planned are not necessarily negative. Where uncontrollable external events intrude on the program (e.g., a major shift in a city's shelter policy), adaptive changes to the original plan are both appropriate and necessary. Even in the absence of such intrusions, post-startup discoveries of a better way to do things are common.

Perspectives on Process Evaluation

As with the purposes of evaluation described earlier, the reasons for and uses of process evaluation depend in part on where you sit. Therefore, process evaluation will be described from three different perspectives: the sponsor's, the manager's, and the evaluator's.

Sponsor Perspective

Program sponsors and some other stakeholders typically take an accountability perspective. Process evaluation serves a program monitoring function. Government sponsors and funding groups, including Congress, operate in a fish bowl. Their actions are visible to the legislative groups that authorize and appropriate programs, government oversight agencies like the Office of Management and Budget (OMB) and GAO, and, of course, the mass media. State governments and large cities have analogous oversight groups. Privately funded programs attract less scrutiny, but executives of private foundations are accountable to their boards of trustees. Finally, the stakeholder groups who support the program will want assurances that the program is being adequately implemented, and stakeholder groups who oppose the program will be equally vigilant for their own purposes.

Consequently, sponsors require evidence that the program they funded was in fact implemented and implemented as intended. Questions include: Are funds being expended properly? Are the appropriate types and quantities of services being delivered? Are they reaching the people they are intended to reach? Sponsors need this information to defend the program from its critics, as well as to support decisions on whether the program should be continued, expanded, or contracted.

Manager Perspective

Managers are less concerned with making decisive judgments about the program and more concerned with improving program operations. In order to administer and manage a social services program efficiently, program managers need regular feedback on who is being served, the services being provided, and their associated costs. For them, process evaluation is a necessary tool for documenting the operational effectiveness of the organization, requesting further support, and defending the organization's performance (Rossi and Freeman, 1993). It is *also* necessary to incorporate corrective measures if needed.

Monitoring from a management perspective is particularly important early in the program. In this sense, the program monitoring function of process evaluation is a continuation of the formative study from the planning phase described earlier. Gross problems—such as the complete inability to retain clients in the program—tend to surface early. Monitoring remains important beyond the development stage, however, although the mix of problems to look for may change. For example, staff burnout and turnover become an issue, and the intensity of service provision may actually *decrease* as the program matures, that is, the initial enthusiasm for a new project may give way to the tendency to standardize and bureaucratize human service programs (Ridgely and Willenbring, 1992). Other problems that may have been present from the beginning may not be statistically *detectable* until later, such as whether the eligibility criteria are succeeding in meeting the coverage goals.

Evaluator Perspective

From the evaluator's perspective, there is little point in assessing the impact of a program if it has not been implemented, and implemented with some resemblance to the original design. If plans exist to estimate the benefits or effectiveness of the program relative to its cost, the evaluator also needs information on resource expenditures. Finally, the status of the evaluation itself must be monitored to track and redress any degradation of the research design in the field (Cordray et al, 1991). Process evaluation can supply information on all of these fronts.

In the absence of program process information, the evaluator is left with the dreaded "black box." If the program shows signs of effectiveness, there is no basis to determine which components were effective, who they were most effective for, in what "dose," or why. Consequently, there is no way to describe the program for others to replicate in the future. This can be particularly problematic in mental health services programs, where the interventions can be vaguely defined to begin with (e.g., case management). If the program shows *no* signs of effectiveness, there is no way to determine whether the negative findings were due to poor implementation of the program, poor implementation of the evaluation (e.g., the comparison group inadvertently received the same services as the target group), or poor program theory. Without these basic distinctions, there is little of use to be concluded from the evaluation. This harsh lesson—learned and relearned at substantial cost—also figured prominently in the previously described decision by SAMHSA to fund multisite demonstration grantees in two phases.

Characterizing the Implementation Process

Most measures of process are straightforward. For example, service use records are frequently employed to track the number of clients served and to quantify level and type of service delivery. Numbers do not tell the whole story, however, in process evaluation as elsewhere. The narrative implementation history of new programs, particularly the barriers to implementation and ways in which program staff overcame them, can be valuable to practitioners in other settings who wish to replicate the program. Without prodding, however, many ingenious solutions never make it into print. In the authors' experience, program staff is far better at *doing* what they do than at articulating it, so the responsibility for documenting it for others falls to the process evaluation. Many practical lessons—such as how to minimize NIMBY problems when setting up organized congregate living facilities for homeless persons in recovery—have been documented and disseminated in this way.

The implementation history can inform the outcome evaluation as well, permitting the evaluator to pry open the black box still further. The evaluator can use this information to construct a key event chronology, that is, events with the potential to affect client outcomes. For example, the addition of a new program component midstream (e.g., aftercare) represents an increase in the "dose" of that treatment, and it is potentially possible to attribute changes in outcomes to the new component. Such analyses can be particularly useful in evaluations that do not have strong comparative designs (discussed below).

Finally, the lessons learned from implementation histories increase understanding of the field. In addition to serving the immediate practical purposes of practitioners, they increase the knowledge base for the future, consistent with the knowledge-building purpose of evaluations described earlier. Among the broad lessons learned from the NIAAA Community Demonstration Program about implementing alcohol, drug, and mental health services for homeless persons with substance abuse problems were (*1*) that shelter, sustenance, and security needs of the clients should be met first and the treatment needs addressed second; (*2*) the need to reconcile structure and flexibility in residential programming; (*3*) the importance of a well-defined organizational structure; (*4*) the need for transportation services to link residences with treatment centers; and (*5*) the need to recognize and overcome weaknesses in the community network of services (NIAAA, 1992). A variety of lessons about implementing case management programs were learned as well.

Assessing Fidelity

Methods for assessing program fidelity have seen exciting progress in recent years. Because developments have proceeded largely independently in mental health and substance abuse, we discuss the two separately.

Mental Health

Considerable efforts have gone into developing quantitative measures of program implementation or service fidelity in mental health, particularly for persons with severe mental illness (SMI). Much of this activity was spurred by a desire to define operationally and measure empirically the critical dimensions of the widely acclaimed assertive community treatment (ACT) model (Teague et al., 1998), initially developed in the 1970s (Stein and Test, 1980). Brekke (1987) used staff time logs incorporating categories of activity that were specifically matched to critical aspects of the intervention. Jerrel and Hargreaves (1991) developed the Community Program Philosophy Scale to measure a wide range of community support programs through staff ratings of a program's values and practices. Specifically related to ACT, McGrew et al. (1994) surveyed experts on the model to identify its critical ingredients. Perhaps the best-developed work in this area is that of Teague and colleagues. Teague et al. (1995) drew from the literature on ACT to identify 13 key dimensions of program implementation in the study of an ACT-like intervention for dually diagnosed individuals. Dimensions reflected features of the general ACT model and a particular model of integrated treatment for the dual disorders. In applying it, they found that differences in program fidelity across experimental and control conditions were most pronounced for the more structurally constrained features, such as, caseload size. Greater model *drift* was observed for more discretionary features, such as overall treatment approach. The Dartmouth ACT Scale (DACTS) extends the original approach, deriving 26 program criteria for fidelity to ACT from multiple sources (Teague et al., 1998). A formal test of construct validity was conducted by using the scale to examine four groups of programs known to have varying degrees of fidelity to the ACT model. The highest-fidelity group registered as such on the scale, as did the lowest (the two middle groups did not differ significantly). The DACTS scale has since been used for training as well as fidelity assessment, including a version modified for use in the ACCESS evaluation (R. Calsyn, personal communication to J. Sonnefeld, August 2000).

For the Community Mental Health Service (CMHS)-sponsored multisite evaluation of supported housing, the evaluators developed a highly innovative way of assessing fidelity, in part because collaborative apparatus represented by the cross-site steering committee was involved at every step (Rog and Randolph, 2002). The major policy is whether a supported housing approach is more effective than other housing approaches in helping persons with SMI achieve residential stability and improve their level of functioning. A specific model of housing was delineated by CMHS in the 1997 Guidance for Applicants (GFA), outlining the features that defined its specific model of supported housing. The Steering Committee developed a fidelity framework that incorporated those elements considered critical to the supported housing model, as well as others useful in describing the comparison models. It defined each of these major components or dimensions of the housing, provided measurement indicators for each dimension, and described the measurement outcomes necessary to have a *fidelity fit* on each dimension. Each indicator was operationalized at a conceptual level using a 5-point scale, with a rating of 5 generally being closest to the ideal model of supported housing and 1 being furthest away. Instruments were developed to collect data from program management, staff and resident perspectives. Site-specific nuances in some of the terms used, such as *case manager* or *housing program staff*, required flexibility in defining what was meant by these terms at the individual sites to ensure uniformity and quality of data collected across the sites.

The fidelity data have strengthened the multisite evaluation in a number of ways. First, they tested the supported housing programs against an ideal, determining the extent of fidelity fit. Second, the assessment of supported housing fidelity revealed that in reality, there was a continuum of supported housing rather than a fit to an ideal model. Finally, the dimensional approach to measuring the housing permits an examination of the role of key housing ingredients in predicting resident outcomes. Knowing what specific features (such as having the right of tenure and having housing choice) relate to outcomes could guide the work of practitioners in refining existing housing programs to maximize their effects.

Substance Abuse

Historically, the specificity of treatment models in substance abuse has lagged behind that in mental health, so it is not surprising that fidelity assessment has lagged as well. This situation is now changing, however. Investigators in NIAAA's Project MATCH, a multisite clinical trial testing the effect of clinician matching of clients to three different treatment models, recognized the need to ensure a faithful rendering of each treatment model if the results were to be interpretable (Carrol, 1997; Carrol et al, 1994; Mattson et al., 1998). Both NIAAA and the National Institute of Drug Abuse (NIDA) have manualized some of the most popular treatment models for alcohol and other drugs, respectively (e.g., cognitive-behavioral, 12-step, and motivational enhancement). All this represents progress to the evaluator, but only so much. Substance abuse treatment is a complicated business. Operationalizing fidelity as exposure, even a quality-assured exposure guided by manualization, training, and monitoring, may work to a degree if the substance abuse treatment protocol is the sum total of the intervention. It is not sufficient, however, for the more comprehensive interventions that research and practice have shown are necessary for special populations, such as homeless alcoholics, clients with a concomitant SMI (dually diagnosed), court-referred clients, or crack-addicted women with children seeking escape from violent relationships (Orwin, 2000). Often, of course, several of these complications may be present in the same client, further complicated by low education, legal problems, poor social functioning, and learning disabilities.

Other fidelity tools have been developed and used by independent investigators for various purposes. In the alcohol field, Kaskutas et al. (1998) developed a Social Model Philosophy Scale (SMPS) to classify the extent to which a given treatment program follows a social model approach to treatment. The final version of the SMPS contains 33 questions for use in residential programs divided into six conceptual domains: physical environment, staff role, authority base, view of substance abuse problems, governance, and community orientation. Overall internal reliability is high (alpha = .92), with subscale alphas ranging between .57 and .79., and test-retest analyses showed that the information obtained from the SMPS is consistent across time, administrators, and respondents. Although not designed to distinguish philosophies other than social model, early results suggest that the SMPS may also be used to classify other program philosophies. One such use was in the

50-site Center for Substance Abuse Treatment (CSAT) evaluation of residential treatment for women with children and post-partum women (Brady et al., 1999).

In the NIAAA Cooperative Agreement Program, implementation scales were developed from provider and self-report data on services (Orwin et al., 1998). The utility of the implementation scales was demonstrated for three purposes: (*1*) comparing interventions across sites—which were stronger, which were most faithful to their program model, and which were relatively free of cross-group contamination, (*2*) comparing groups within sites, thereby assessing whether proposed contrasts were implemented and maintained as intended, and (*3*) comparing groups over time, thereby assessing whether interventions increased in strength and fidelity over time and whether these increases were linkable to program events. The strength and fidelity scales were also used in the cross-site outcome evaluation (Cordray et al., 1995) to help ascertain whether observed outcomes were attributable to the interventions or to one or more methodological artifacts.

Assessing Context

Programs do not function in isolation; rather, they function in the context of a network of services in the broader community. Such contextual factors play a potentially important role, since the effectiveness of an intervention cannot be isolated from the specific environmental context in which it was effective. In the evaluation of alcohol, drug abuse, and mental health services, this has been most evident when programs included case management components, as they commonly do. A key component of case management is to provide the linkage with the environmental context (i.e., the service network). This has led some writers (e.g., Ridgely and Willenbring, 1992) to suggest that the effectiveness of case management may have more to do with the environment than with the functions of the program per se. Yet case management has often been adopted in community contexts where service networks for the target population were entirely lacking (Stein, 1992) or as a substitute for those services (Goldman et al., 1992). Under such circumstances, it is hardly surprising that it appears ineffective.

Clearly, service environments differ across communities. Some are service-rich, others service-poor. And while the existing service network unquestionably influences the effectiveness of any new program added to it, ferreting out the nature of the influence, and even its direction, can be a complex undertaking (Orwin et al., 1994c). The implication for process evaluation is that collecting data on the program itself is not sufficient; data describing the program environment are necessary as well. This is particularly the case for multisite evaluations of nominally similar interventions where cross-site comparisons of outcomes are planned.

Outcome Evaluation

After a program has been fine-tuned, had its operational "kinks" ironed out, and reached an acceptable level of maturity and stability, the question of its effectiveness remains. Unless programs have demonstrable effects, it is hard to defend sustaining or expanding them.

The fundamental challenge of most outcome evaluation is to persuasively demonstrate that observed changes in the target participants are caused by the program and cannot be plausibly accounted for in other ways. Evaluations, which possess this quality, are said to have *internal validity*. So-called threats to internal validity are nuisance factors that lead to alternative explanations for the observed relationship between program and outcome. For example, comprehensive programs for persons in recovery from alcohol and other drug problems frequently include a vocational component. The evaluation of such programs might assess changes in employment status as a way to determine if the vocational component was effective. This assessment is complicated by the fact that other factors might be operating in the community during the evaluation period, which can also affect employment opportunities, such as a plant closing. Unless the evaluation design includes a provision for ruling out the impact of the plant closing (discussed below), the effects of the program and the plant closing are said to be *confounded*, that is, there is no clear way to disentangle them. The particular threat to internal validity in the example is called *history*; a litany of other threats are described in detail elsewhere (e.g., Cook and Campbell, 1979).

Assuming that all plausible threats to internal validity can be ruled out and a causal inference drawn that the program increased employment in the community where it was studied, that still might not be sufficient for a policy maker who needs to know whether funding the program in *other* communities might yield a similar effect. An evaluation is said to possess *external validity* if the causal relationships it demonstrated can be generalized to and across other persons, settings, and times. Returning to the example, assume that the evaluation of the comprehensive program for recovering persons was designed in such a way that the plant closing could not have threatened internal validity (e.g., through random assignment, as described below). Still, the plant closing may have been such an unusual and powerful event that it caused the effects of the program to be atypical—different from the expected effects in other communities or even in the same community had the evaluation been conducted at a different time. Alternatively, the participants could have had more education, or more economic resources to fall back on, than might have been the case in other communities.

Both types of validity are important in principle, and their relative importance in a given evaluation will depend on that evaluation's priorities. Much of the art of designing outcome evaluations lies in establishing acceptable trade-offs between the two.

Strategies for Assessing Outcomes

Space does not permit an adequate exposition of the full range of design strategies for assessing impact. However, numerous works are available that cover the topic in depth (e.g., Cook and Campbell, 1979; Fink, 1993; Mohr, 1992; Rossi and Freeman, 1993). The abbreviated treatment below follows that of Rossi and Freeman (1993), who divided the strategies into two categories: evaluation of *partial coverage* programs—those that are delivered to a sample of the target population—and evaluation of *full coverage* programs—those that are delivered to all, or nearly all, eligible recipients. The utility of this division is twofold: (*1*) it is comprehensive, in that it encompasses virtually any type of program that might be evaluated, at any stage in its life cycle, and (*2*) it drives home the most severe restriction on the choice of evaluation strategy: whether the program is being delivered to all or just a subset of its target population. For programs with total coverage, such as long-standing, ongoing, fully implemented programs (e.g., major federal entitlements), it is usually impossible to identify a sufficient sample of individuals who are *not* receiving the program yet who in essential ways are comparable to those who *are*. In contrast, programs that are just starting, or that are to be tested on a trial basis (e.g., demonstration programs) will *not* ordinarily be delivered to the entire target population. This increases the design options substantially.

Partial Coverage Strategies

Partial coverage strategies include randomized experiments, regression-discontinuity designs, and the use of matched or statistically equated constructed controls.

Randomized Experiments. The basic procedures of a randomized program evaluation mirror those of a laboratory experiment. In the simplest case, target participants are randomly assigned to two groups. One group is designated the control or comparison group and receives no treatment beyond the usual services already available to them. The other group is designated the experimental group and receives the innovative program. Outcomes are then observed in both groups, and differences between them are attributed to the net effect of the innovative program. Multiple experimental groups are also possible, with each receiving a different "dose" or a different mix of program components. The great strength of the design is that, when successfully implemented, it removes the possibility of systematic pretreatment differences across groups. This eliminates the source of most threats to internal validity, thereby permitting observed outcomes to be causally attributed to the program. The randomized experiment is a powerful instrument in the evaluators' toolbox, and there are many successful examples of its use in the evaluation of alcohol, drug abuse, and mental health services (e.g., Dennis, 1990; Test and Burke, 1985).

However, there are some threats to internal validity that experiments do not rule out, particularly if the experiment cannot be successfully maintained (Cook and Campbell, 1979). They are difficult to pull off, and history shows that they can easily fail if not applied judiciously (Orwin et al., 1994c). While a randomized experiment is the optimal strategy for establishing causality, that does not mean that it is always or even usually the best choice. As noted by Rutman and Mowbray (1983), the option should be considered in light of (*1*) the extent to which the information for decision making requires relatively unequivocal findings about cause and effect; (*2*) the funds available (experiments are not cheap); (*3*) the time frame for the evaluation (experiments take time to plan and mount, and are not well suited to *quick turnaround* studies); and (*4*) the applicable constraints—technical, political, legal, ethical, and administrative. There is a large literature on the legal, ethical, and administrative issues in randomized experiments for readers interested in these issues (e.g., Boruch, 1976; Cook and Campbell, 1979; Fetterman, 1982).

Finally, randomized designs can force some loss of generalizability (i.e., external validity). For example, it is sometimes suspected that clients who are willing to participate in a randomized study differ in important ways from the target population at large. Often this proposition can be tested empirically (see, e.g., Collins and Elkin, 1985). Other problems can occur if referral agencies object to random assignment, because they can undermine the flow of clients into the study (Lam et al, 1994).

The rest of the partial coverage design strategies are sometimes called *quasi-experiments* (Cook and Campbell, 1979). They approximate experiments, in that they rely on comparisons between two or more groups to estimate net effects, and attempt to approximate what an experiment does: rule out alternative explanations to the program. The essential difference is that assignment to groups is nonrandom.

Regression-Discontinuity Designs. Where true experiments are not feasible, *cutoff score* or *regression discontinuity* designs (Trochim 1990) can be an attractive alternative. This class of designs employs an assignment process based on clients' need for treatment, as determined by their scores on pretreatment measures. Because the source of the nonequivalence between treatment and comparison groups is known—namely, the cutoff rule used to assign clients to groups—analyses can correctly adjust for the nonequivalences and produce unbiased estimates of the treatment effect, even without random assignment. The especially attractive feature of these designs is that the determination of need for treatment may include clinical ratings by program staff about a prospective client's suitability or need for treatment. Therefore, regression discontinuity designs come closest to randomized experiments in their ability to produce unbiased effect estimates *and* remove a common objection to random assignment in treatment settings.

However, the strategy can be employed only when the assignment rules are precise, fully explicit, and uniformly administered. If, for example, the rule is to assign clients to treatment based on their score on a standard psychiatric rating scale, then other, nonquantifiable factors (e.g., subjective judgment) *cannot* be considered in the decision without undermining the design. This and some thorny analysis issues (Trochim, 1990) have inhibited widespread adoption of the design. Regression discontinuity has seen some use in the evaluation of alcohol, drug abuse, and mental health services, although its use is still relatively rare.

Matched or Statistically Equated "Constructed" Control Groups. Often a subset of the target population is selected to receive the program, usually by the sponsors or through other means outside the control of the evaluator. Alternatively, the subset might consist of participants who volunteer (i.e., self-select) for the program. The advantage of allowing program recipients to select their own mix of program offerings is that the program is not altered for the sake of the evaluation. Service providers like that feature, as do some evaluators, who argue that more intrusive designs create an artificial program environment that threatens external validity (e.g., Conrad and Conrad, 1994). However, the reasons for being involved in some components and not in others are related to preexisting differences between clients. Therefore, the success or failure of a component may be due primarily to the characteristics of the clients who chose (or were referred to) particular services rather than to the component itself. This particular threat to internal validity is called *selection bias* or *self-selection*. It is often countered through the use of a matching strategy or statistical controls.

Under a matching strategy, the evaluator selects an unserved subset of the target population, which resembles the served group as much as possible in relevant ways (e.g., socioeconomic status, diagnosis, treatment history). The subset may be chosen from existing intact institutions (e.g., for a program being delivered in a psychiatric hospital, another psychiatric hospital in an adjacent community). Alternatively, it may be chosen from unserved individuals from the program setting, or from multiple settings who are considered roughly comparable to the program participants.

An alternative to matching is the use of statistical controls to equate program participants and nonparticipants. Outcomes for the two groups are compared, controlling for differences between groups as identified by a designated set of control variables or *predictors*, using one or more multivariate statistical techniques. The intent is to do with statistics what could not be done by design—remove the effect of pretreatment differences between groups.

In order to be interpretable, most nonrandom design strategies such as matching and statistical controls require the reliable measurement of all preexisting differences between participants that might influence their performance on outcome measures. They also require that each of these differences be properly *modeled* in the statistical analysis. The elegance of the randomized experiment is that it requires none of this (although some of it is still recommended for reasons not covered here). Given that random assignment is frequently not appropriate or feasible, however, modeling techniques are becoming increasingly important evaluation tools. Specifically, the adaptation of *propensity scoring* (Rosenbaum and Rubin, 1984) and related *balancing* technologies such as weighted distance matching (Cologne and Shibata, 1995) is a major development in the evolution of quasi-experimental analysis. The logic is as follows: The propensity (i.e., the probability) of each client to be in the treatment group rather than in the comparison group is estimated based on a set of covariates that are thought to be related to group membership. Estimation of propensity scores can be done in multiple ways (e.g., logistic regression, probit models, classification trees). Within the group of individuals who have the same treatment propensity, associations between outcome and treatment are free of confounding. This is as if treatment had been randomly assigned to individuals as in a designed experiment. Propensity scoring frees the regression modeling process—the traditional tool for applying statistical controls and adjustments—from its usual limitation of reliance on a small number of covariates and simplistic functional forms (e.g., linear main effects only). Rather, a complex model with interactions and higher-order terms can be fit at the propensity scoring stage without concern about overfitting (too many predictors), since the goal is simply to obtain the best estimated probability of group assignment from the observed covariates. When subsequently included in the regression model, the propensity score carries all the information from the complex covariate model in a single variable, consuming only one degree of freedom. It also avoids the potentially adverse effects of multicollinearity (highly correlated covariates destabilizing the model) on the stability of the estimates, regardless of the degree of correlation that exists among the covariates. There are additional technical advantages we will not describe here that improve confidence in treatment effect estimates relative to prior methods (Rubin, 1997, is a good introduction for interested readers). Still, propensity scores are no panacea; like traditional methods for removing group nonequivalence, propensity score methods can only adjust for confounding covariates that are observed and measured. This is always a limitation of nonrandomized studies compared with randomized studies, where the randomization tends to balance the distribution of all covariates, observed and unobserved. Tests can be devised to determine the robustness of the conclusions to potential influences of unobserved covariates, which are more applicable in some circumstances than others (Lin et al., 1998).

Full Coverage Strategies

Full coverage strategies include simple before-and-after studies, cross-sectional studies for nonuniform programs, panel studies for nonuniform programs, and interrupted time series analyses.

Simple Before-and-After Studies

The essential feature of the one-group before-and-after approach is the assessment of participants at two points in time, once prior to and once after exposure to the program. The difference between the two measurements, or *change score,* is the program's estimated net effect. Despite simplicity and intuitive appeal, these are among the weakest approaches for evaluating outcomes. Unless there is powerful theory to specify precisely the amount of change that would have occurred in the absence of the program, there is essentially no way to rule out alternative explanations for the observed change. No theory of that quality exists with regard to the effects of alcohol, drug abuse, and mental health services programs.

Complicating things is the fact that people and systems do change on their own. In fact, controlled studies of substance abuse treatment typically show that the usual-services control group also improves from pretest to posttest (e.g., Orwin et al., 1994c). There are a number of reasons why this might happen, but the most obvious one is that clients do not enroll in the study (or get referred) at random points in their lives. Rather, they tend to enroll after "hitting bottom," and by agreeing to participate in the study, they are already showing at least minimal motivation to do something about it. While some may continue to get worse (or even die), it is only natural to expect that most will be doing somewhat better 6–12 months later, regardless of their group assignment.

Cross-Sectional Studies for Nonuniform Programs. While some full-coverage programs deliver a roughly uniform set of components to all participants, there are others in which the component mix varies. State-administered federal programs such as the Mental Health Block Grant are an example. The effects of these variations can potentially be estimated with cross-sectional surveys that measure what was received at different sites (as part of the process evaluation) and then by comparing outcomes across sites. This approach is sometimes described as *capitaliz-*

ing on naturally occurring variation (Light and Smith, 1971). It provides an advantage over the one-group before-and-after design, but the uncontrolled differences across sites still render causal inference difficult.

Panel Studies for Nonuniform Programs (Several Repeated Measures). These improve on the cross-sectional variety, because the repeated measures at additional time points allow the evaluator to specify the process by which a program has impact on its target participants. This is one way in which key events in the program's implementation history (described earlier) can be incorporated into the outcome evaluation. If the shifts in the outcome measures can be tied to "dips and peaks" in the program, then confidence in making causal attributions to the program is increased.

Interrupted Time Series Analyses (Many Repeated Measures). Times series analyses extend the panel repeated measures concept further by having many data points preceding and following the onset of the program. The technical procedures involved in analyzing time series data are complex, but the ideas underlying them are quite simple (see McCleary and Hay, 1980, for a good introduction). The preprogram trend is analyzed in order to project what would have happened in the absence of the program. This *projected* trend is compared with the *actual* postprogram trend to estimate the net program effect.

The interrupted time series strategy does not rule out all threats to internal validity, but it is easily the strongest of the full coverage designs. A major advantage over the previous strategies is that the maturational trend in the data can be assessed prior to program onset. Returning to the point about clients tending to enroll in treatment programs after hitting bottom, the preprogram time series would allow this bias to be directly observed and ruled out if not present.

Most works on time series analysis recommend having at least 50–100 preintervention measurements at equal intervals in order to model preprogram trends stably (Glass et al., 1975; McCleary and Hay, 1980). It is most useful, therefore, for evaluating programs whose outcomes can be assessed with extant social indicators. So, for example, interrupted time series could be used to evaluate the impact of a community drug treatment program on community arrest rates, detoxification program use, or other data that are routinely collected for administrative purposes and therefore available in time series form.

The basic interrupted time series (ITS) model has seen important statistical advances since its introduction in 1975 (Orwin, 1997). These developments, which typically originate in econometrics, are rather technical and their description is beyond the scope of this chapter. However, they are important to evaluators and policy makers because they expand the range of time series to which ITS analysis can be applied. Consequently, they expand its utility and versatility in addressing policy questions as they arise.

Use of Multiple Strategies

In practice, evaluators need not confine themselves to a single design strategy for evaluating outcomes. For example, the coupling of randomized with nonrandomized designs has long been recommended (e.g., Boruch, 1975). Evaluators of alcohol, drug abuse, and mental health services programs can frequently find themselves in situations where random assignment to a no-treatment control group is infeasible but random assignment to different program *components* is acceptable. An experimental comparison of the program components can then be implemented, *nested* within a quasi-experimental test of the full program. In the NIAAA Cooperative Agreement Program, the coupling of randomized with nonrandomized designs was quite common (5 projects out of 14) (Orwin et al., 1994a).

Design elements from partial coverage and total coverage strategies can be coupled as well. An interrupted time series design nested within a quasi-experiment (i.e., time series on two groups, only one of which received the program) is particularly powerful. Coupling the strategies described above with more qualitative methods, such as case studies and ethnographic interviews, can be invaluable for putting "flesh on the statistical bones."

Synthesis Strategies: Combining Results from Multiple Evaluations

Earlier, the use of quantitative synthesis techniques in the planning stages of an outcome evaluation was described. Under certain circumstances, the synthesis can serve as the outcome evaluation itself. Syntheses are particularly useful when, for whatever reason, new data collection is not feasible. Syntheses of mental health interventions have been common for decades, whereas syntheses of alcohol and other drug treatments are more recent (Wilson, 2000). For example, Orwin et al. (2001a) conducted the first meta-analysis of the women's treatment literature, focusing on the effectiveness of women-only programs. Three types of contrasts were found in the literature: (*1*) women-only versus no-treatment controls, (*2*) women-only versus mixed-gender programs, and (*3*) enhanced versus standard women-only programs. Outcomes were positive across all three contrast types and eight measurement domains. The results therefore made a compelling argument for women-only treatment programming. The enhanced versus standard treatment contrasts showed the largest effects of the three contrast types, suggesting that women-focused enhancements to treatment as usual may yield the best return on investment in women-only treatment programming.

Synthesis techniques can be and have been applied to large-scale national programs as well. The GAO's original evaluation synthesis method (U.S. GAO, 1983) is a cluster of techniques through which information from existing studies can address evaluation questions of interest. These methods were expanded later to include prospective evaluations (i.e., evaluating the likely outcomes of proposed programs [U.S. GAO, 1989]) and *cross-design* synthesis—combining of evaluation results from different complementary designs (U.S. GAO, 1992).

The synthesis approach to outcome evaluation has some unique strengths. It can be conducted quickly, and is generally less costly than designing a new evaluation and collecting new data. Moreover, the ability to draw on a large number of studies adds great strength to the knowledge base, particularly when findings are consistent across studies conducted by different analysts using different methods in different settings. No single study, no matter how high in quality, has the same level of credibility and generalizability. The principal limitation of the synthesis approach is its inapplicability to brand new or rapidly changing program areas or to areas where few quality studies have been conducted. In those situations, new data collection is essential.

Synthesis is typically retrospective, culling data from extant work. A prospective variation on synthesis was recently applied to a SAMHSA-sponsored multisite study of homelessness prevention (Banks et al., 2002). This study targeted persons with psychiatric and/or substance use disorders who were formerly homeless or at risk of homelessness and who were engaged with the mental health and/or substance abuse treatment system(s). The prospective component of the analytic strategy borrows heavily from the randomized clinical trial literature, in that decisions on primary outcomes, program-level factors, client-level moderators, and so on are made a priori to keep statistical tests interpretable. No less important, the focus of the analysis on within-site effect sizes preserves site identity while allowing for the testing of multisite hypotheses. This helped secure *buy-off* on the strategy from site-level representatives with concerns about alternative methods (e.g., multilevel modeling) in which data would be pooled across sites. Across all eight sites, the average advantage of the intervention groups over the comparison groups was approximately 12 additional days in stable housing. In addition, the four sites that had a contrast on a *control of housing stock* factor also had a larger mean effect size for days in stable housing than the four sites with no contrast on this factor. As in traditional (retrospective) synthesis, participant-level covariates also were tested as possible moderators, but only gender proved significant, with the effect for control of housing stock being larger for men than for women.

Multilevel Models and Multisite Evaluations

Treatment outcome data from cross-site evaluations are inherently multilevel and hierarchical in that clients are nested within sites. Moreover, the central evaluation questions are rarely limited to the effectiveness of specific programs at specific locations, but rather to a class of programs *like* them to permit generalization. Consequently, cross-site or between-program effects are properly modeled statistically as random rather than fixed. Therefore, a multilevel, random-effects modeling approach is appropriate for analyzing these types of data.

Several different fields have contributed to the development of this approach, from mathematical statistics to demography and epidemiology to survey research, clinical trials, and program evaluation. While the terminology varies according to the field, multilevel models, *hierarchical linear models, random regression models, random coefficient models,* and *mixed model analysis of variance* all refer to the same basic kind of model. They are a class of models designed to account for nested structures in data (e.g. individuals embedded in treatment groups within different settings). In these models, sampling units such as treatment sites are appropriately modeled as random rather than fixed effects, and measurements within these treatment sites may be correlated. Failure to account for this correlation—called the *intraclass correlation* or *design effect*—and the additional variance attributable to random effects can result in underestimated standard errors and spurious statistical significance. Consequently, traditional statistical models that ignore the multilevel structure of the data are likely to produce erroneous results. In addition, multilevel models more adequately address the direct effects of site characteristics on individual behaviors, and interactions between individual and site characteristics, than are typically expressed in the framework of multiple regression and logistic regression. That is, terms can be specified as individual level (level 1), as site level (level 2), or as interactions both within and across levels.

Until a few years ago, a multilevel, random effects analysis required development of special software. Recently, however, programs such as PROC MIXED from SAS, HLM (a stand-alone program), and others have become available that make the use of random effects models more accessible to program evaluators. Moreover, they are flexible enough to accommodate many different statistical assumptions, and provide diagnostic guidance to facilitate choices between model specifications. All of these factors have contributed to their emerging popularity.

Orwin et al. (1999) conducted one of the first multilevel random effects reanalysis of a multisite treatment outcome study in a reanalysis of the National Treatment Improvement Evaluation Study (NTIES). The NTIES was a 5-year longitudinal study of the impact of substance abuse treatment on 5388 clients purposively sampled from CSAT-funded public substance abuse treatment programs. Data were collected from five program modalities: methadone maintenance, nonmethadone outpatient, short-term residential, long-term residential, and correctional. The original analysis had several limitations (see Orwin et al., 1999, for details), each of which could be successfully overcome with the flexibility of multilevel modeling. Results showed a range of significant program-level main effects and interactions between program variables and client-level variables, and also highlighted how these effects and interactions vary across modalities. Though this study was primarily a methods demonstration, it also had substantive implications for policy and practice. In particular, the identification of program characteristics with positive effects and program by client interactions across different modalities and outcomes suggest ways in which the treatment community might refine programs along these dimensions. For example:

- The finding that positive main effects of program characteristics were primarily seen in the nonmethadone outpatient modality suggests that the likelihood of improving client outcomes by manipulating program-level factors (e.g., having a designated case manager and tailoring the program to the population) may be greatest in that modality.
- The finding that frequent, short sessions appeared more beneficial than longer, less frequent sessions in outpatient treatment has implications for structuring outpatient programming.
- The finding that interactions occurred more frequently than main effects suggests that program-level effects are highly contingent on client-level characteristics and modality—confirming that in substance abuse treatment, the question "what works?" is more productively specified as "what works for whom, and in what setting?".

Outcome Measurement

As noted earlier, the specification of program outcomes attempts to turn the abstract notion of program objectives into a measurable reality. The manner in which those outcomes are *measured*, therefore, is a critically important part of any outcome evaluation. A poorly conceptualized measure can completely undermine the value of the evaluation by producing misleading estimates of program effectiveness.

In selecting measures of those outcomes, the evaluator frequently faces many choices, each tempered by practical considerations: cost, access, confidentiality requirements, and the technical issues of reliability and validity. In this section, the concepts of reliability and validity are introduced, and the most common ways of measuring outcomes in evaluations of alcohol, drug abuse, and mental health services are described.

Reliability and Validity

For outcome evaluations to be credible, measures must possess two qualities: reliability and validity. A measure is considered *reliable* if, in a given situation, it produces the same results repeatedly. Reliability is quantified through a reliability coefficient, which ranges from 0 to 1.0. A general rule of thumb is that reliabilities of .80 and above are acceptable for most evaluation purposes (Nunnally, 1978).

Measures of social behavior are typically less reliable than physical measures. For example, a doctor's scale is a more reliable measure of weight than an IQ test is of intelligence. Yet there is considerable variation among social measures as well—IQ tests are more reliable than most diagnostic measures of mental illness or clinical assessments of alcohol and drug use. The effect of unreliability is to weaken and obscure true differences among clients or between different programs. Generally, unreliable measures make programs appear to be less effective than they actually are.

A measure possesses *validity* to the degree that it measures what it purports to measure. To establish validity, the results produced by the measure must be compared with the results of some other clearly defined criterion. To validate a new measure of anxiety, for example, a researcher might begin by asking those scored as anxious if they would rate *themselves* as anxious. Then she might ask other observers who know them well (e.g., clergyman, doctors, schoolteachers). If clients' and observers' ratings were consistent with the new measure's results, the researcher would begin to gain confidence that it was indeed a valid measure.

But some anxious people attempt to conceal their anxiety. They will not rate themselves as anxious and may be adept enough at concealing their inner state that observers fail to perceive it. So the researcher really needs some other, more objective criteria to validate her measure. Anxiety often produces physiological symptoms (heart palpitations, high blood pressure, breathlessness, perspiration) or cognitive disturbances (confusion, memory errors). If the new measure is a valid indicator of anxiety, its results should show a correlation with these standard behavioral indices.

Some mental health measures incorporate explicit recognition of validity concerns. The best known one is the Minnesota Multiphasic Personality Inventory

(Hathaway and McKinley, 1951), which includes four separate validity scales: the question scale, the lie scale, the fake scale, and the correction scale. The question scale reflects the number of items not answered by the respondent and is considered a measure of evasiveness. The lie scale is a measure of credibility in that it detects attempts at faking in the direction of "looking good." The fake scale detects faking in the "looking bad" direction or it can be a sign of respondent confusion. The correction scale measures the defensiveness of the respondent in disclosing information.

As with other aspects of evaluation, the determination of measurement validity has a political dimension, particularly in the absence of a clear validation criterion. Rossi and Freeman (1993) note that the perceived validity of an outcome measure often depends on whether a measure is accepted as valid by the appropriate stakeholders.

Types of Client Outcome Measures

Common ways of assessing client outcomes include self-report measures, service provider observations and ratings, and administrative records. That is, the evaluator can ask the clients, ask others about the clients, or consult other organizational or statistical sources for information about the clients. A final way, mentioned only in passing, is through physiological measures. Alcohol and other drug use can frequently be detected through urine screens, as can noncompliance with a medication protocol among clients who are mentally ill.

Self-Report Measures. Self-report measures are common in evaluations of alcohol, drug abuse, and mental health services, and many have demonstrated high levels of reliability and validity. One of the most widely used interview instruments in substance abuse treatment evaluation is the Addiction Severity Index (ASI), a structured 45-minute clinical research interview designed to assess problem severity in seven areas commonly affected in persons who abuse alcohol and other drugs: medical condition, employment, alcohol use, other drug use, illegal activity, family relations, and psychiatric condition (McLellan et al., 1988). In each of the problem areas, objective questions are asked that measure the number, extent, and duration of problem symptoms in the patient's lifetime and in the past 30 days. The respondent also supplies a subjective rating of the recent severity and importance of each problem area. Other standardized self-report measures are commonly used in mental health evaluation. Some, like the Beck Depression Inventory and the Rosenberg Self-Esteem scale, measure specific symptomatology or personality traits. Others, like the Diagnostic Interview Schedule and the Structured Clinical Interview for the *Diagnostic and Statistical Manual of Mental Disorders* (3rd ed., revised) are more comprehensive diagnostic assessment instruments.

Self-report measures are not without problems and not without their detractors in the field. For example, research has shown that self-reports of drinking and other drug use tend to be biased toward underreporting at pretest, when individuals are still drinking or using other drugs or are in withdrawal (Skinner 1984; Sobell and Sobell 1981). More accurate reports are to be expected later, when clients have been in treatment (Hesselbrock et al., 1983; Polich et al., 1980). Fuller (1988) also pointed out that the increased candor that occurs during treatment cannot be expected to persist at follow-up assessments 6 months or more after discharge if clients have resumed drinking or drug use. With clients who are mentally ill or with chronic late-stage alcoholics, the problems are somewhat different. The distortions are due less to lack of candor than to the cognitive and affective impairments from which these groups often suffer. Many self-report instruments incorporate interviewer ratings of respondent credibility or competence, which mitigate the problems somewhat.

Responses may be further biased by the choice of interviewer. If program staff are used to collect follow-up data, then particularly distressed clients may be more likely to describe especially negative aspects of their lives to a person they believe can help them than to a research assistant who cannot (Aiken and West, 1990). There is also the possibility that program staff, who are not impartial observers, may then inadvertently contribute to the bias in the way they ask the questions and code the responses. Generally, program staff should not be used to conduct the outcome interviews. Rather, this task should go to research assistants under the administrative authority of a research organization.

Service Provider Ratings. Observations and ratings of client status and behavior can also be a useful way to measure outcomes. Raters can be program staff, family members, other clients, or researcher observers. In a treatment program for alcoholics, for example, a principal program objective was the achievement of "stable abstinence" (Dunham and Nisus, 1979), and success or failure in achieving stable abstinence was measured through professional judgments by the treatment staff. The judgments depended in part on length of abstinence and in part on clients' attitudes toward their abstinence, as perceived by the staff.

Unlike self-report measures, observations and ratings are not dependent on candid, competent responses from reluctant or mentally impaired clients. They are vulnerable instead to various forms of rater bias. For example, Modrein et al. (1988) found that clients in an experimental *developmental-acquisition model* of case management showed greater improvement on several dimensions than clients who received usual case management services from a mental health center, including greater improvement in significant others' ratings of *community living skills.* At the same time, ratings of *socialization skills* by case managers showed a striking difference in the opposite direction: experimental group clients were much more likely to be rated as having socialization problems. The apparent explanation was: that the experimental group case managers had much more contact with their clients than the usual care case managers, especially in their community environment. They therefore had more opportunity to observe social behavior and learn of problems in this area. The suggestion that it was the disparities in case managers' knowledge of clients' problems that accounted for the observed differences in the rating scales, rather than actual lower functioning in the experimental group, was supported by differences in the *opposite* direction on ratings on a similar dimension (community living skills) by significant others: when clients' behavior was rated by those who knew them but were not their service providers, the experimental group's ratings showed greater improvement.

Administrative Records. Administrative records can also be useful in evaluating outcomes, particularly when organized into management information systems (MIS). For example, one of the NIAAA Community Demonstration projects obtained relapse information from Department of Public Health MIS data, which contained the history of client treatment in state-supported substance abuse treatment facilities (Argeriou and McCarty, 1991). Unlike the self-report instrument, these data were obtainable on all study clients, including those who were not followed up. Therefore, they were less vulnerable than the self-report data to attrition from measurement, which can distort the results. They also represented an independent, objective source of information on client behavior, free of any self-report or rater biases. These are standard advantages of MIS data, at least for those that are well supported.

However, MIS data also contain potential sources of error and bias. First, there may be matching errors in the identification of project clients in the MIS. Second, and probably more important, state data capture only those relapsing clients who return to publicly funded detoxification centers. Clients who leave the state, become incarcerated, undergo social detoxification, use private treatment facilities, relapse but do not seek treatment, or die are missed. The extent of error and bias in MIS data will vary, so the problems it presents will be greater in some evaluations than in others.

In substance abuse, administrative records are proving particularly useful for *treatment career* research (Hser et al., 1998), which among other things examines the cumulative effects of repeated treatment episodes. Treatment career research explicitly incorporates the contemporary clinical belief that, for many addicted persons, substance abuse is a chronic, relapsing disease, much like diabetes, hypertension, or persistent mental illness (Leshner, 1997). Like other chronic diseases, it is managed by treatment rather than cured. Harm reduction to the addict and society are also part of the equation (e.g., reducing crime). Under this paradigm, relapse is viewed as a normal part of recovery, and treatment recidivism is the rule rather than the exception. In the traditional substance abuse treatment outcome research model, however, participants are baselined, assigned to a treatment or comparison group, and assessed 3–6 months later on outcomes of interest. It has been this way for the past 30 years. With growing recognition of substance abuse as a chronic, relapsing disease, at least for seriously addicted persons, the single-episode, short-term outcome research model is seen as increasingly irrelevant. Though still controversial, the importance of Hser's work and others like it is that it seems to be demonstrating that repeated treatment has cumulative effects, over and above the effects of the individual episodes. If proven, this has enormous implications for how society should view treatment. Consequently, it is critical that substance abuse evaluation be equipped to detect such long-term effects, and administrative data can help. They can provide precise, extensive chronologies on an individual's treatment history, not only in terms of when it occurred but also the length of each episode, the modality or level of care (e.g., short-term residential vs. intensive outpatient), and, in some systems, discharge status (completed, dropped out, incarcerated, etc.). For high treatment users, this level of detail could never be reliably obtained through self-report.

Using a technique called *event history analysis,* Orwin and colleagues are using MIS data from Ohio to empirically classify, predict, and evaluate patterns of multiepisode treatment histories in the Cuyahoga County CSAT Target Cities sample. Transitions between states are the events in the individual's event history, such as, a client stepping down from residential to outpatient treatment. The type of analysis—which could simply not be done without administrative records— makes maximal use of temporal event-based data by incorporating both the timing and sequencing of all state transitions of interest, up to and including (if applicable) death. Preliminary analyses of transitions are quite informative about continuity of care for chronic substance abusers in Cuyahoga County. For example, only 30% of clients who come in for detoxification are successfully placed into treatment. However, almost two-thirds (64%) of clients who enter short-term inpatient treatment are successfully stepped down to a less intensive level of care (Orwin et al., 2001b).

Systems-Level Outcomes

Not all evaluations focus on client-level outcomes. Some focus on changes at the systems level, which may serve as the *agent* of client-level change. The concepts *systems integration* and *systems of care* pervade contemporary thinking about the organization of modern mental health services and their evaluation. Reforming the fragmented delivery system that many attribute to the legacy of deinstitutionalization and the failure of the community mental health centers to treat the chronically or persistently mentally ill has been a major concern of federal policy makers, State mental health directors, clinicians, and prominent advocacy groups for over three decades (Bickman et al., 1999; DHHS, 1992; Frank and Gaynor, 1994; Stroul and Friedman, 1986). With the advent of the block grant and the shift in fiscal control back to the states in the 1980s, systems integration also began to be viewed as a cost-saving device (Morrissey et al., 1994). Some theorists held that it would not only improve services but would also save money by creating a more efficient system that avoided needless duplication and waste (Frank and Gaynor, 1994). To an extent, health care reform and the larger movement toward increased accountability for all public sector expenditures reinforced the view that systems integration was intrinsically cost–effective.

Measures used to assess system-level outcomes in the earlier-described RWJF evaluation included

- *key informant* surveys of agency personnel in community support system agencies about the fiscal, clinical, and administrative aspects of the local mental health programs;
- interorganizational network surveys of the relationships between the organizations in the system, as well as specific attributes of the component organizations including mission, services provided, budget, personnel, and client caseloads;
- site visit reports covering in-person accounts of the more informal aspects of the service system.

A sophisticated set of techniques known as *network analysis* has been developed for the purpose of incorporating these measures into the evaluation of systems-level change (Morrissey, 1992). Network analysis methods provide unique ways to view the different levels of a service system, as well as answer questions about system integration or lack of it (system fragmentation) at the client, program, organization, and systems level. They were successfully employed in the RWJF evaluation (Morrissey et al., 1994) and again in the CMHS-sponsored ACCESS multisite demonstration program for homeless persons who were mentally ill. Results from ACCESS showed that as a group, the sites assigned to receive additional funds for systems integration had greater improvement in the ties between the project agency and others in the local service system, although on average, the systems as a whole did not increase their overall integration (Morrissey et al., 2002). Continuing analyses are examining site-level differences in integration scores and their relationship to other factors on the ground (e.g., amount and type of services received at by clients).

Use of Multiple Measures

Evaluators should use multiple measures in outcome evaluations whenever possible (Cook and Shadish, 1986; Cronbach, 1982). This strategy partially compensates for reliability and validity problems of individual measures and helps balance the influence of biased measures in the overall interpretation. In the multiple measurement of alcohol use, for example, an instrument like the ASI could be employed to measure alcohol use through client self-report, urinalysis screens could measure alcohol use physiologically, and counselors could measure alcohol use by observing clients' behavior. Each of the three measurement modes has contrasting strengths and weaknesses that affect the measurement of alcohol use in a different way.

Evaluations can also measure outcomes at multiple levels. In the evaluation of the RJWF Program on Chronic Mental Illness, for example, the authors examined whether cities could develop mental health authorities and expand the availability of services and housing (system-level outcome), and whether such systems changes would improve the quality of life of individuals with severe mental illnesses (client-level outcome) (Goldman et al., 1990). When the program theory specifies that outcomes at one level mediate outcomes at another, then both must be measured to evaluate the program fully and properly. On this score, lessons and findings from the Program on Chronic Mental Illness figured prominently in the design of the ACCESS multisite evaluation of mental health systems integration for homeless persons with SMI. At the system level, in addition to the interorganizational measures from the network analysis described above, ACCESS staff members conducted annual site visits to compile descriptive and quantitative information about events in the local system and site community that could affect the systems integration process (e.g., agency mergers, state hospital closures, advent of Medicaid managed care). They interviewed ACCESS program staff, state and county officials, and representatives of local service agencies and conducted focus groups with consumer participants in each ACCESS program. The data obtained from these sources helped determine the extent to which each site implemented systems integration activities, as independently rated by each site visit team member, and results showed greater implementation of systems integration strategies by systems integration sites, on average (Morrissey et al., 2002). At the program level, because of concerns raised in the RWJF study and elsewhere about the impact of the lack of effective services on outcomes, an expert in ACT conducted a side study of the extent to which each ACCESS program conformed to the ACT model by using a previously developed multidimensional rating instrument with acceptable psychometric properties (Teague et al., 1998). The study concluded that all sites had fairly high levels of fidelity to the ACT model (R. Calsyn, personal communication to J. Sonnefeld, August 2000) and that ACCESS provided relevant, effective, and conscientiously delivered services. The ACT study in turn was complemented by an independent qualitative assessment of programs in site-level case studies. Finally, extensive data were collected at the client level on problem severity, service receipt, and 3- and 12-month status on psychiatric, residential, substance abuse, and other relevant outcomes. Clients at all sites showed improvement on the standardized outcome measures of psychiatric status, substance abuse, and housing. However, clients at experimental sites showed no greater increase in improvement on measures of mental health or housing outcomes than clients at comparison sites (Rosenheck et al., 2002). This is explained at least partly by the unexpected patterns in systems integration at baseline and the extent to which both experimental and comparison sites implemented the system integration strategies. ACCESS showed, however, that sites that became more integrated had progressively better housing outcomes, regardless of group assignment or implementation strategies.

Assessing Efficiency

In many cases, the knowledge that a program had an effect is insufficient; its results must be judged against its costs. At the federal level, concern over record deficits has focused on budgetary restraint as never before. Recession-diminished revenues, taxpayer revolts, and federal cuts have done much the same at the state level. Consequently, the issue of program costs has become increasingly critical throughout the nation.

Cost questions have figured prominently in the evaluation of alcohol, drug abuse, and mental health services. With deinstitutionalization, for example, the key question for many fiscally strapped policy makers was not whether community mental health programs were *more* effective than hospitalization in caring for the severely and chronically mentally ill, but whether they could provide roughly comparable benefits at lower cost per unit output. The cost of drug treatment, relative to its effectiveness, has also drawn wide attention (e.g., NIDA, 1991).

Evaluations of the relationship of costs to effectiveness are addressing questions of efficiency. There are two related approaches for assessing program efficiency: cost–benefit analysis and cost–effectiveness analysis. Both estimate the monetary value of program delivery, but they differ in their treatment of outcomes. In cost–benefit analysis the outcomes of the program are also converted to monetary terms, while in cost–effectiveness analysis they are not. Both approaches can be problematic because of the numerous assumptions involved, but in general, cost–benefit analysis is more controversial. The requirement to value outcomes in monetary terms is sensible for many technical and industrial projects but not for human service programs. Recent discussions of health care rationing have resurrected the classic cost–benefit question "How can we place a value on human life?", much to the chagrin of policy makers attempting to defend rationing. Of course, defenders of cost–benefit analysis correctly argue that government policies implicitly and inevitably place value on human lives every day (e.g., Thompson, 1980).

Consequently, cost–effectiveness analysis is often seen as a more useful tool than cost–benefit analysis, and its use in the evaluation of alcohol, drug abuse, and mental health services is not uncommon. One possible outcome of cost–effectiveness analysis is that two programs will appear about equally effective but one will be considerably cheaper. For example, Willenbring and Whelan (1991) developed a case management model for chronic public inebriates. The approach was based on the prior finding that traditional approaches to treatment of this target group had little impact on the costly *revolving door* of detoxification, treatment centers, hospitals, and jails. Methods involved changing goals from total rehabilitation within an institution to providing ongoing community support and services coordination for long periods of time. A randomized comparison showed no clear differences in client outcomes on self-report quality-of-life measures (Willenbring and Whelan, 1991). Yet each of the case-managed clients cost an estimated $750 per year less in detoxification costs, $500 per year less in court expenses, and $400 per year less in medical expenses, for a total savings of $1650 per client per year to local government.

Another possible outcome is that two programs will cost about the same, but one will be notably more effective. For example, the Program of Assertive Community Treatment (PACT) was developed in the 1970s to serve deinstitutionalized persons with SMI (Stein and Test, 1980; Weisbrod et al., 1980). The basis of the program, since widely replicated, is assertive outreach and a continuous care team working with both the client and the client's support system. Evaluation of the PACT model has demonstrated patient outcomes that are significantly better than those achieved with traditional care (Olfson, 1990; Stein and Test, 1980), for about the same net cost (Stein, 1987). Consequently, several states began developing mechanisms for reallocating hospital dollars to community care (Stein, 1992).

Cost–benefit analysis of substance abuse treatment has dramatically highlighted the social costs of untreated substance. These include increased emergency room and hospitalization costs and physicians' fees, which in turn increase public expenditures on health care. Alcohol is a contributing factor in many accidents and injuries, leading to further medical costs. It has been estimated that one out of five Medicaid hospital days can be attributable to substance abuse–related morbidity and mortality, a figure representing $8 billion in 1994 (Fox et al., 1995). In addition, alcohol contributes to criminal activity, generating costs associated with victimization, criminal justice administration, and incarceration (Harwood et al., 1988; DHHS, 1993; Koenig et al., 1999). Using national data, the economic cost to society from alcohol abuse and alcoholism was recently estimated at $148 billion (Harwood et al., 1998). Researchers and clinicians continue to debate best practices, which is all well and good, but the evidence that drug treatment decreases social costs and reduces harm to clients and society is not really in dispute.

Some caveats merit mention. First, efficiency assessment is an extension of, rather than an alternative to, impact evaluation. Therefore, unless there are reasonable estimates of the program's net outcomes, neither cost–benefit nor cost–

effectiveness evaluation is possible. Second, it requires technical procedures and a level of methodological sophistication that typically are beyond the resources of many evaluation projects. Third, the requisite cost data are often not fully available or adequate. This can result from measurement problems or confidentiality constraints, as well as conceptual difficulties in defining the universe of relevant costs. Finally, the results can be highly sensitive to the underlying, but often untested, assumptions of the analytic model (Noble, 1977). Despite these caveats, efficiency assessment does provide a rational and potentially reproducible way of estimating program efficiency. At a minimum, it helps to discipline thinking about the inputs, outputs, and outcomes of programs. Used judiciously, it can be a valuable input into the decision-making process of both program sponsors and managers.

What to Expect from an Outcome Evaluation

The sponsor or other consumer of an outcome evaluation has a right to certain expectations on its completion. Specifically, they should expect that

- the study adhered to the plan (any deviations should be documented and justified);
- methodological rigor and quality were maintained (within resource constraints);
- the report is clearly written and extensively documented;
- conclusions and recommendations (if included) are convincingly justified;
- limitations are made explicit.

There are two things they generally should not expect. The first is unequivocal attributions of observed effects to the program. With rare exceptions, only a randomized design can support such claims, and then only if successfully maintained (e.g., no corruption of the randomization, high follow-up rates in all intervention groups). Absent this, any unqualified claims of program effectiveness should be viewed with skepticism.

The second is large program effects. Consumers must recognize that if the magnitude of a social problem is sizable (and mental illness and substance abuse are certainly in this category), then the impact of any intervention designed to affect it—*even an effective one*—is likely to be modest. The Salk vaccine virtually eradicated polio in the United States. No social technology ever has succeeded or will succeed on that scale. The weakness of social interventions is an evaluation fact of life (Lipsey, 1990; Rossi, 1987). Yet much of the political debate over, say, whether the War on Poverty programs were successes or failures has proceeded apace in woeful ignorance of this (or at least cynical disregard). Some see poverty on the street and conclude that poverty programs have failed. In fact, the effectiveness of those programs has been convincingly (albeit quietly) documented (e.g., Schwarz, 1983). It was never realistic to expect them to eliminate poverty, given (*1*) the resources actually allocated, (*2*) the lack of program theory on how to do it, and, most important, (*3*) the weakness of *any* social intervention in the context of all the other social forces shaping the behaviors and fortunes of the targeted participants and the systems that serve them.

A very different story can result when social intervention is sustained and change is tracked over long periods. The extraordinary drop in U.S. adult smoking prevalence over the past three decades was achieved through a 1% to 2% average decline per year (Hornik, 2002). Had the impact of the seminal 1963 Surgeon General's report on smoking and health been evaluated in 1964, however, the conclusion would doubtless have been no detectable effect! Analogously, the full impact of the groundbreaking 1999 Surgeon General's report on mental health (the first in our nation's history) on reducing stigma and removing financial and racial/ethnic barriers to quality treatment may not be known for years or even decades.

The reality that even effective programs produce only modest effects in the short run is one important reason that modern evaluation has grown up around the scientific method. If effects were large, then strong comparative designs to draw causal inferences probably would not be needed, since most threats to internal validity would be overwhelmed by the program effect. Large sample sizes would not be needed either, since their purpose is to provide the statistical power for detecting small effects. Nor would highly reliable measures be needed; the "noise" from unreliable measures—like the threats to internal validity—would be overwhelmed by the program effect. (*Valid* measures would still be needed, however.) Implementation analyses would still be necessary for improving and explaining programs but would be less critical for understanding outcomes. Turgid statistical analyses to model selection bias and otherwise compensate for the inherent limitations of evaluation design and implementation would be largely superfluous.

Implications for Mental Health Services

The implications of evaluation for mental health services delivery are broad. Previous sections described how the activities of program sponsors, managers, researchers, and the entire spectrum of additional stakeholders are influenced by evaluation. This final section focuses more specifically on the *uses* made of evaluations by mental health professionals.

In the end, the worth of any evaluation must be judged by its utility. For this reason, considerable thought and research have been devoted to the use of evaluation results. This section covers the different ways in which evaluations are used in the policy-making process, some factors believed to affect use, and a summary of guidelines for increasing use.

Types of Use

In their review of the literature on use of evaluations, Leviton and Hughes (1981) identified three different ways in which in which evaluations are used. The first is *direct use*, which refers to the documented and specific use of evaluations to support a policy decision. Evaluators typically hope for the world to greet their findings with gratitude and immediately put them to use in this way. Direct use is not the most frequent type, but it does happen. For example, new psychopharmacological agents often are adopted quickly once their efficacy has been demonstrated.

Psychosocial programs, such as PACT, have had a mixed experience with some direct use (as well as misuse; Stein, 1992).

The second type of use, which is also the most common, is *conceptual use*. Conceptual use encompasses the variety of ways in which evaluation has indirect impact. The impact can range from sensitizing persons and groups to current and emerging social problems to influencing future program and policy development. An example from mental health is the widespread discussion and use of the concept of a community support system following the NIMH Community Support Program demonstrations (Tessler and Goldman, 1982).

The third type is called *persuasive use*, which refers to the enlisting of evaluation results to support or refute a political position, whether they are applicable or not. For example, the broad cutting of social programs in the 1980s was frequently defended by the claim that evaluations failed to show clear findings of positive impact. While evaluations do frequently fail to show positive impact, there are numerous reasons for this other than true ineffectiveness (Campbell and Erlebacher, 1970; Lipsey, 1990; Orwin et al., 1994c). Critics of those cuts saw the true motivation for the cuts as ideological and the use of evaluation to support them as somewhat disingenuous. At the GAO, the first author saw numerous distortions of evaluation findings for political purposes, including one incident where a footnote to a report's appendix became a lead bullet in a press release. Persuasive use usually involves interpersonal influence as well, unlike the other two uses.

Factors Affecting Use

Leviton and Hughes (1981) also described five conditions that appeared to consistently affect use:

- Relevance of the evaluation to the needs of potential users;
- Extent of communication between evaluators and users;
- Translation into implications for policy and programs;
- Credibility of evaluation results;
- User commitment or advocacy.

To assess the importance of these conditions and their relative contributions to use, Weiss and Bucuvalas (1980) examined 155 mental health decision makers and their reactions to 50 actual research reports. They concluded that decision makers apply both a *truth test* and a *utility test* to the reports they read. Truth is judged on the basis of research quality and conformity to prior knowledge and expectations. Utility is judged on the basis of feasibility potential and the degree of challenge to current policy. These two dimensions, along with *relevance* (defined as the match between the topic of the evaluation and the decision maker's job responsibilities), constitute the frame of reference within which usefulness is determined.

Increasing Use

From the research on use as well as from real-world experiences of evaluators, a number of guidelines have emerged for increasing use. Solomon and Shortell (1981) have summarized these as follows:

- *Evaluators must understand the cognitive style of decision makers.* A complex piece of analysis will be of no use to a politician who cannot consume such material. Thus, brief reports and oral presentations are often more appropriate than more comprehensive, scholarly expositions.
- *Evaluation results must be timely and available when needed.* Thoroughness and completeness must be balanced against timing and accessibility, despite the risk of criticism from the outside over certain standards of scholarship not being met.
- *Evaluations must respect stakeholders' program commitments.* Commitments made to stakeholders at the planning phase (discussed previously) must be upheld. Otherwise, the stakeholders will likely discount the findings and may actively *discourage* the evaluation's use.
- *Use and dissemination plans should be part of the evaluation design.* Evaluations are most likely to be used if the effort teaches potential users about the strengths and weaknesses of the evaluation, including how the findings can be effectively communicated by decision makers to their constituencies.
- *Evaluations should include an assessment of use.* Evaluators and decision makers should agree not only on the purposes of the study, but also on the criteria by which its successful use may be judged.

Rutman and Mowbray (1983) describe additional steps that program managers must take as evaluation *consumers* if they wish to ensure that any suggestions or recommendations from the evaluation are in fact implemented as prescribed. Specifically, managers should manage the evaluation for *actionable results,* be aware of the practical barriers to change, set priorities for action on the implementation of recommendations, monitor and control progress to ensure that implementation occurs, and feed back the results to sponsors, staff, and interested stakeholders. Each of these actions reflects the managerial view of evaluation as an ongoing, continuing process for seeking improvements in program delivery.

Use in Perspective

When all is said and done, the use of evaluation, even more than its conduct, is an inherently political act. The decision-making process is complex, and the results of an evaluation are only one of the elements contributing to it. Rossi and Freeman (1993) use a courtroom metaphor to describe the evaluator's role. The evaluator is not the judge and jury of a program's worth. Rather, the evaluator is an expert witness testifying to the program's objective effectiveness. The jury of decision makers may give such testimony more weight than uninformed opinion or guesses, but it is they, not the witness, who reach the verdict. The evaluation findings represent one argument in a political system that weighs, assesses, and balances a variety of arguments, juggling the interests of many constituencies before making a decision. To imagine otherwise would be to grant evaluators veto power in the political decision-making process—a wholly unwelcome (indeed, unconstitutional) development, to say the least. Evaluators are best off observing the political action from a distance, "preferably through heavy lenses" (Berk and Rossi, 1990).

REFERENCES

Aiken LS, West SG. Invalidity of true experiments: Self report pretest biases. *Evaluation Review* 14:374–390, 1990.

Argeriou M, McCarty D. *Stabilization Services Project: Final Evaluation Report*. Boston: Submitted to the National Institute on Alcohol Abuse and Alcoholism, 1991.

Ashery RS, McAuliffe WE. Implementation issues and techniques in randomized trials of outpatient psychosocial treatments for drug abusers: recruitment of subjects. *American Journal of Drug and Alcohol Abuse*, 18:305–329, 1992.

Babor TF, Steinberg K, McRee B, et al. Treating marijuana dependence in adults: a multisite, randomized clinical trial. In: Herrell JM, Straw RB (eds). *Conducting Multiple Site Evaluations in Real-World Settings*. New Directions for Program Evaluation, No. 94. San Francisco: Jossey-Bass, pp. 17–30, 2002.

Banks S, McHugo G, Williams W, et al. Use of a prospective meta-analytic approach in a multisite study of homelessness prevention. In: Herrell JM, Straw RB (eds). *Conducting Multiple Site Evaluations in Real-World Settings*. New Directions for Program Evaluation, No. 94. San Francisco: Jossey-Bass, pp. 45–60, 2002.

Berk RA, Rossi PH. *Thinking About Program Evaluation*. Newbury Park CA: Sage, 1990.

Bickman L, Guthrie PR, Foster EM, et al. *Evaluating Managed Mental Health Services: The Fort Bragg Experiment*. New York: Plenum Press, 1995.

Bickman L, Noser K, Summerfet WT. Long term effects of a system of care on children and adolescents. *Journal of Behavioral Health Services & Research*, 26(2):185–202, 1999.

Boruch RF. Coupling randomized experiments and approximations to experiments in social program evaluation. *Sociological Methods and Research*, 4(1):31–53, 1975.

Boruch RF. On common contentions about randomized field experiments. In: Glass GV (ed.). *Evaluation Studies Review Annual* (pp. 158–194). Beverly Hills, CA: Sage Publications, 1976.

Brady TM, Orwin RG, Deang LP, et al. Residential addiction programs for parenting and childbearing women: treatment philosophy and programmatic characteristics. Presented at the annual meeting of the Association for Health Services Research, Chicago, June 27, 1999.

Brekke JS. The model-guided method of monitoring program implementation. *Evaluation Review*, 11:281–300, 1987.

Campbell DT, Erlebacher AE. How regression artifacts in quasi-experimental evaluations can mistakenly make compensatory education look harmful. In: Gage NL (ed). *The Disadvantaged Child*, Volume 3. New York: Brunner/Mazel, pp. 1970.

Carroll KM. *Improving Compliance with Alcoholism Treatment*. Project MATCH Monograph Series Volume 6. Bethesda, MD: National Institute on Alcohol Abuse and Alcoholism, 1997.

Carroll KM, Kadden RM, Donovan DM, et al. Implementing treatment and protecting the validity of the independent variable in treatment matching studies. *Journal of Studies on Alcohol* (Supplement), 12:149–155, 1994.

Chelimsky E. Differing perspectives of evaluation. In: Rentz CC, Rentz RR (eds). *Evaluating Federally Sponsored Programs*. New Directions for Program Evaluation, No. 2, San Francisco: Jossey-Bass, pp. 19–38, 1978.

Chelimsky E. The politics of program evaluation. *Society*, 25(1):24–32, 1987.

Chelimsky E. Expanding evaluation capabilities in the General Accounting Office. In: Rentz CC, Rentz RR (eds). *Evaluation in the Federal Government: Changes, Trends, and Opportunities*. New Directions for Program Evaluation, No. 55. San Francisco: Jossey-Bass, pp. 1992.

Collins JF, Elkin I. Randomization in the NIMH treatment of depression collaborative research program. In: Boruch RF, Wothke W (eds). *Randomization and Field Experimentation.* New Directions for Program Evaluation, No. 28. San Francisco: Jossey-Bass, pp. 27–38, 1985.

Cologne JB, Shibata Y. Optimal case-control matching in practice. 1995 *Epidemiology,* 6(3):271–275, 1995.

Conrad KJ, Conrad KM. Reassessing validity threats in experiments: a focus on construct validity. In: Conrad KJ (ed). *Critically Evaluating the Role of Randomized Experiments in Evaluation.* New Directions for Program Evaluation. San Francisco: Jossey-Bass, pp. 5–26, 1994.

Cook JA, Carey MA, Razzano L, et al. The pioneer: the employment intervention demonstration program. In: Herrell JM, Straw RB (eds). *Conducting Multiple Site Evaluations in Real-World Settings.* New Directions for Program Evaluation, No. 94. San Francisco: Jossey-Bass, pp. 31–44, 2002.

Cook TD, Campbell DT. *Quasi-Experimentation: Design and Analysis Issues for Field Settings.* Chicago: Rand-McNally, 1979.

Cook TD, Shadish WR. Program evaluation: the worldly science. *Annual Review of Psychology,* 37:193–232, 1986.

Cordray DS, Lipsey MW. Program evaluation and program research. In: Cordray DS, Lipsey MW (eds). *Evaluation Studies Review Annual,* Volume 11. Beverly Hills, CA: Sage, pp. 17–44, 1986.

Cordray DS, Orwin RG. Improving the quality of evidence: interconnections among primary evaluations, secondary analysis, and quantitative synthesis. In: Light RJ (ed). *Evaluation Studies Review Annual,* Volume 8. Beverly Hills, CA: Sage, pp. 91–120, 1983.

Cordray DS, Orwin R, Pion G, et al. *Final National Evaluation Plan.* Prepared by R.O.W. Sciences, Inc. and Vanderbilt Institute for Public Policy Studies for the National Institute on Alcohol Abuse and Alcoholism, Rockville, MD, 1991.

Cordray DS, Pion G, Orwin R. Preliminary outcomes from the NIAAA Cooperative Agreement Program for Homeless Persons with Alcohol and Other Drug Problems. Presented at the Annual Convention of the American Psychological Association, New York, August 11–15, 1995, and the joint American Evaluation Association/Canadian Evaluation Society meeting, November 2–5, 1995.

Cordray DS, Sonnefeld LJ. Quantitative synthesis: an actuarial base for planning impact evaluations. In: Cordray DS (ed). *Utilizing Prior Research in Evaluation Planning.* New Directions for Program Evaluation, No. 27. San Francisco: Jossey-Bass, pp. 29–48, 1985.

Cronbach LJ. *Designing Evaluations of Educational and Social Programs.* San Francisco: Jossey-Bass, 1982.

Dennis ML. Assessing the validity of randomized field experiments: an example from drug abuse treatment research. *Evaluation Review,* 14(4):347–373, 1990.

Department of Health and Human Services. *Efforts to Promote Community-Based Service Integration.* Washington, DC: Department of Health and Human Services, 1992.

Department of Health and Human Services. *Alcohol and Health: 8th Special Report to the U.S. Congress on Alcohol and Health.* Rockville, MD: National Institute on Alcohol Abuse and Alcoholism, 1993.

Dunham RG, Nisus AL. Evaluation of treatment programs. *Evaluation Quarterly,* 3:415, 1979.

Fairweather GW, Sanders DH, Tornatzky LG. *Creating Change in Mental Health Organizations.* Elmsford: UK, Pergamon Press, 1975.

Fetterman DM. Ibsen's baths: reactivity and insensitivity. *Educational Evaluation and Policy Analysis,* 4(3):261–279, 1982.

Fink A. *Evaluation Fundamentals: Guiding Health Programs, Research, and Policy*. Newbury Park, CA: Sage, 1993.

Fox K, Merrill JC, Chang HH, et al. Estimating the cost of substance abuse to the Medicaid Hospital Care Program. *American Journal of Public Health*, 85(1):48–54, 1995.

Frank RG, Gaynor M. Fiscal decentralization of public mental health care and the Robert Wood Johnson Foundation Program on Chronic Mental Illness. *The Milbank Quarterly* 72 (1):81–104, 1994.

Fuller RK. Can treatment outcome research rely on alcoholics' self-report? *Alcohol Health and Research World* 12:180–187, 1988.

Glass GV. Primary, secondary, and meta-analysis of research. *Educational Researcher*, 5:3–8, 1976.

Glass GV, Wilson VL, Gottman JM. *Design and Analysis of Time Series Experiments*. Boulder, CO: Associated Universities Press, 1975.

Goldman HH, Morrissey JP, Ridgely MS, et al. Lessons from the program on chronic mental illness. *Health Affairs,* 11(3):51–68, 1992.

Goldman HH, Lehman A, Morrissey J, et al. Design for the evaluation of the Robert Wood Johnson Foundation Program on Chronic Mental Illness. *Hospital and Community Psychiatry* 41(11):1217–1221, 1990.

Harwood H, Fountain D, Livermore G. *The Economic Costs of Alcohol and Drug Abuse in the United States*. Report prepared for the National Institute on Drug Abuse and the National Institute on Alcohol Abuse and Alcoholism, Department of Health and Human Services, NIH Pub. No. 98-4327. Rockville, MD: National Institutes of Health, 1998.

Harwood HJ, Hubbard RL, Collins JJ, et al. The costs of crime and the benefits of drug abuse treatment: a cost-benefit analysis using TOPS data. In: Leukefeld DG, Tims FM (eds). *Compulsory Treatment of Drug Abuse: Research and Clinical Practice*. NIDA Research Monograph 86, Rockville, MD: National Institute of Drug Abuse, pp. 209–235, 1988.

Hathaway SR, McKinley JC. *The Minnesota Multiphasic Personality Inventory*, revised. New York: The Psychological Corporation, 1951.

Hesselbrock M, Babor TF, Hesselbrock V, et al. "Never believe an alcoholic"?: On the validity of self-report measures of alcohol dependence and related constructs. *International Journal of the Addictions* 18:593–609, 1983.

Hornik RC. Evaluation design for public health communications programs. In: Hornik RC (ed). *Public Health Communication: Evidence for Behavior Change*. London: Erlbaum, 2002.

Hser YI, Grella C, Chou CP. Relationships between drug treatment careers and outcomes: findings from the national drug abuse treatment outcome study. *Evaluation Review*, 22:496–519, 1998.

Jerrel J, Hargreaves W. *The Operating Philosophy of Community Programs*. Working Paper No. 18. San Francisco: UCSF Institute for Mental Health Services, 1991.

Kaskutas LA, Greenfield TK, Borkman TJ, et al. Measuring treatment philosophy: a scale for substance abuse recovery programs. *Journal of Substance Abuse Treatment*, 15(1):27–36, 1998.

Koenig L, Denmead G, Nguyen R, et al. The costs and benefits of substance abuse treatment: findings from the National Treatment Improvement Study. Paper presented at the National Evaluation Data Services annual meeting, Rockville, MD, April 1999.

Lam JA, Hartwell S, Jekel J. "I prayed real hard, so I know I'll get in": living with randomization in social research. In: Conrad KJ (ed) *Critically Evaluating the Role of Randomized Experiments in Evaluation*. New Directions for Program Evaluation. San Francisco: Jossey-Bass, pp. 55–66, 1994.

Lamberti MJ, Katzenmeyer C. Transforming qualitative data from templates into quantitative assessment of multisite programs. In: Scheirer MA (ed). A *User's Guide to Program Templates: A New Tool for Evaluating Program Content.* New Directions for Program Evaluation, No. 72. San Francisco: Jossey-Bass, pp. 81–88, 1996.

Leff HS, Mulkern V. Lessons learned about science and participation from multisite evaluations. In: Herrell JM, Straw RB (eds). *Conducting Multiple Site Evaluations in Real-World Settings.* New Directions for Program Evaluation, No. 94. San Francisco: Jossey-Bass, pp. 89–100, 2002.

Leshner AI. Addiction is a brain disease, and it matters. *Science,* 278(5335):45–47, 1997.

Leviton LC, Hughes EFX. Research on the utilization of evaluations: a review and synthesis. *Evaluation Review,* 5(4):525–548, 1981.

Light RJ, Smith PV. Accumulating evidence: procedures for resolving contradictions among different studies. *Harvard Educational Review,* 41:429–471, 1971.

Lin DY, Psaty BM, Kronmal RA. Assessing the sensitivity of regression results to unmeasured confounders in observational studies. *Biometrics,* 54(3):948–963, 1998.

Lipsey M. *Design Sensitivity: Statistical Power for Experimental Research.* Newbury Park CA: Sage, 1990.

Mattson ME, Del Boca FK, Carroll KM, et al. Compliance with treatment and follow-up protocols in project MATCH: predictors and relationship to outcome. *Alcohol Clinical Experimental Research,* 22(6):1328–1339, 1998.

McGlynn EA, Boynton J, Morton SC, et al. Treatment for the dually diagnosed homeless: program models and implementation experience. In: Conrad KJ (ed). *Treatment of the Chemically Dependent Homeless: Theory and Implementation in Fourteen American Projects.* Alcoholism Treatment Quarterly Special Issue, 1993.

McGrew JH, Bond GR, Dietzen LL. Measuring the fidelity of implementation of a mental health program model. *Journal of Consulting and Clinical Psychology,* 62:670–678, 1994.

McLeary R, Hay R Jr. *Applied Time Series Analysis for the Social Sciences.* Beverly Hills, CA: Sage, 1980.

McLellan AT, Luborsky L, Cacciola J, et al. *Guide to the Addiction Severity Index: Background, Administration, and Field Testing Results.* Philadelphia: Veterans Administration Medical Center, 1988.

Miles RE Jr. The origin and meaning of Miles' Law. *Public Administration Review,* 38:399–403, 1978.

Modrcin M, Rapp CR, Poertner J. The evaluation of case management services with the chronically mentally ill. *Evaluation and Program Planning,* 11:307–314, 1988.

Mohr LB. *Impact Analysis for Program Evaluation.* Newbury Park, CA: Sage, 1992.

Morrissey J. *Network Approaches to Mental Health Service System Assessment.* Washington, DC: American Public Health Association, 1992.

Morrissey JP, Calloway M, Bartko WT, et al. Local mental health authorities and service system change: evidence from the Robert Wood Johnson Foundation Program on Chronic Mental Illness. *The Milbank Quarterly* 72(1):48–80, 1994.

Morrissey J, Calloway M, Thakur N, et al. Integration of service systems for homeless persons with serious mental illness through the ACCESS program. *Psychiatric Services,* 53(8):949–957, 2002.

National Institute on Alcohol Abuse and Alcoholism. *Community Demonstration Projects for Alcohol and Drug Abuse Treatment of Homeless Individuals: Final Evaluation Report.* Contract No. ADM 281-88-0003. Rockville, MD: National Institute on Alcohol Abuse and Alcoholism, 1992.

National Institute on Drug Abuse. *Economic Costs, Cost-Effectiveness, Financing, and Com-*

munity Based Drug Treatment. Research Monograph 113. Rockville, MD: U.S. Department of Health and Human Services, 1991.

Noble JH Jr. The limits of cost-benefit analysis as a guide to priority setting in rehabilitation. *Evaluation Quarterly*, 1(3):347–380, 1977.

Nunnally JC. *Psychometric Theory*, 2nd ed. New York: McGraw-Hill, 1978.

Olfson M. Assertive community treatment: an evaluation of the experimental evidence. *Hospital and Community Psychiatry*, 41:634–641, 1990.

Orwin RG. 21 years old and counting: interrupted time series comes of age. In: Chelimsky E, Shadish WR (eds). *Evaluation for the 21st Century: A Resource Book*. Beverly Hills, CA: Sage, pp. 443–466, 1997.

Orwin RG. Assessing program fidelity in substance abuse health services research. *Addiction*, 95(suppl 3):S309–S327, 2000.

Orwin RG, Cordray DS, Huebner RB. Judicious application of randomized designs. In: Conrad KJ (ed). *Critically Evaluating the Role of Randomized Experiments in Evaluation*. New Directions for Program Evaluation, San Francisco: Jossey-Bass, pp. 73–86, 1994a.

Orwin RG, Francisco L, Bernichon T. *Effectiveness of Women's Substance Abuse Treatment Programs: A Meta Analysis*. Prepared under contract by the Battelle Centers for Public Health Research and Evaluation (CPHRE) for the Center for Substance Abuse Treatment, Department of Health and Human Services, Rockville, MD, 2001a.

Orwin RG, Goldman HH, Sonnefeld LJ, et al. Alcohol and drug abuse treatment of homeless individuals: results from the NIAAA Community Demonstration Program. *Journal of Health Care for the Poor and Underserved*, 5(4):326–352, 1994b.

Orwin RG, Iachan R, Ellis B, et al. The National Treatment Improvement Evaluation Study: multilevel reanalysis of treatment outcomes. *Proceedings of the Survey Research Methods Section of the American Statistical Association*, pp. 221–226, 1999.

Orwin RG, McKay JR, Ginexi E, et al. Use of event history analysis to classify, predict, and evaluate patterns of multiple treatment admissions: preliminary findings. Presented at the American Evaluation Association meeting, St. Louis, November 10, 2001b.

Orwin RG, Sonnefeld LJ, Cordray DS, et al. Constructing quantitative implementation scales from categorical services data: examples from a multisite evaluation. *Evaluation Review*, 22(2):245–288, 1998.

Orwin RG, Sonnefeld LJ, Garrison-Mogren R, et al. Pitfalls in evaluating the effectiveness of case management programs for homeless persons: lessons from the NIAAA Community Demonstration Program. *Evaluation Review*, 18(2):153–207, 1994c.

Polich JM, Armor DJ, Braiker HB. *The Course of Alcoholism: Four Years After Treatment*. Santa Monica, CA: RAND Corporation, 1980.

Ridgely MS, Willenbring ML. Application of case management to drug abuse treatment: overview of models and research issues. In: Ashery RS (ed). *Progress and Issues in Case Management*. NIDA Research Monograph No. 127. Rockville, MD: U.S. Department of Health and Human Services, pp. 12–33, 1992.

Rog DJ, Randolph FL. A multisite evaluation of supported housing: lessons learned from cross-site collaboration. In: Herrell JM, Straw RB (eds). *Conducting Multiple Site Evaluations in Real-World Settings*. New Directions for Program Evaluation, No. 94. San Francisco: pp. 61–72, Jossey-Bass, 2002.

Rosenbaum PR, Rubin DB. Reducing bias in observational studies using subclassification on the propensity score. *Journal of the American Statistical Association*, 79:516–524, 1984.

Rosenheck RA, Lam J, Morrissey JP, Calloway MO, et al. Service systems integration and outcomes for mentally ill homeless persons in the ACCESS program. *Psychiatric Services*, 53:958–966, 2002.

Rossi PH. The iron law of evaluation and other metallic rules. In: Miller J, Lewis M (eds).

Research in Social Problems and Public Policy, Volume 4. Grenwich, CT: JAI Press, pp. 3–20, 1987.

Rossi PH, Freeman HE. *Evaluation: A Systematic Approach,* 5th ed. Newbury Park, CA: Sage, 1993.

Rubin DB. Estimating causal effects from large data sets using propensity scores. *Annals of Internal Medicine,* 127(8 pt 2):757–763, 1997.

Rutman L. *Planning Useful Evaluations: Evaluability Assessment.* Beverly Hills, CA: Sage, 1980.

Rutman L, Mowbray G. *Understanding Program Evaluation.* Sage Human Services Guide, Volume 31. Newbury Park, CA: Sage, 1983.

Scheirer MA (ed). *A User's Guide to Program Templates: A New Tool for Evaluating Program Content.* New Directions for Program Evaluation, No. 72, San Francisco: Jossey-Bass, 1996.

Schwarz JE. *America's Hidden Success: A Reassessment of Twenty Years of Public Policy.* New York: W.W. Norton, 1983.

Skinner HA. Assessing alcohol use by patients in treatment. In: Smart RG, Cappell HD, Glaser FB, et al. (eds). *Research Advances in Alcohol and Drug Problems,* Volume 8. New York: Plenum Press, pp. 183–207, 1984.

Smith MF. *Evaluability Assessment: A Practical Approach.* Norwell, MA: Kluwer Academic, 1989.

Sobell LC, Sobell MB. Effects of three interview factors on the validity of alcohol abusers' self-reports. *American Journal of Drug and Alcohol Abuse,* 8:225–237, 1981.

Solomon MA, Shortell SM. Designing healthy policy research for utilization. *Health Policy Quarterly,* 1:261–273, 1981.

Stein LI. Funding a system of care for schizophrenia. *Psychiatric Annals,* 17:592–598, 1987.

Stein LI. On the abolishment of the case manager. *Health Affairs* 11(3):172–177, 1992.

Stein LI, Test MA. Alternatives to mental hospital treatment I: conceptual model, treatment program, and clinical evaluation. *Archives of General Psychiatry* 37:392–397, 1980.

Stroul BA, Freidman RM. *A System of Care for Severely Emotionally Disturbed Youth.* Washington, DC: CASSP Technical Assistance Center, 1986.

Teague GB, Bond GR, Drake RE. Program fidelity in assertive community treatment: development and use of a measure. *American Journal of Orthopsychiatry,* 68(2):216–232, 1998.

Teague GB, Drake RE, Ackerman T. Evaluating use of continuous treatment teams for persons with mental illness and substance abuse. *Psychiatric Services,* 46:689–695, 1995.

Tessler RC, Goldman HH. *The Chronically Mentally Ill: Assessing Community Support Programs.* Cambridge, MA: Ballinger, 1982.

Test MA, Burke SS. Random assignment of chronically mentally ill persons to hospital or community treatment. In: Boruch RF, Wothke W (eds). *Randomization and Field Experimentation.* New Directions for Program Evaluation, No. 28, San Francisco: Jossey-Bass, pp. 81–94, 1985.

Thompson M. *Benefit-Cost Analysis for Program Evaluation.* Beverly Hills, CA: Sage, 1980.

Trochim WM. The regression-discontinuity design. In: Sechrest L, Perrin E, Bunker J (eds). *Research Methodology: Strengthening Causal Interpretations of Nonexperimental Data.* Washington, DC: U.S. Department of Health and Human Services, pp. 119–140, 1990.

Turner J, TenHoor W. The NIMH Community Support program: pilot approach to a needed social reform. *Schizophrenia Bulletin,* 4:319–348, 1978.

U.S. General Accounting Office. *The Evaluation Synthesis.* Institute for Program Evaluation, Methods Paper 1. Washington, DC: U.S. General Accounting Office, 1983.

U.S. General Accounting Office. *Prospective Evaluation Methods: The Prospective Evaluation Synthesis.* GAO/PEMD-Transfer Paper 10.1.10. Washington, DC: U.S. General Accounting Office, 1989.

U.S. General Accounting Office. *Cross Design Synthesis: A New Strategy for Medical Effectiveness Research.* GAO/PEMD-92-18. Washington, DC: U.S. General Accounting Office, 1992.

Weisbrod B, Test M, Stein LJ. Alternative to mental hospital treatment: II. Economic benefit-cost analysis. *Archives of General Psychiatry*, 37:400–405, 1980.

Weiss CH. Between the cup and the lip. *Evaluation*, 1(2):54, 1973.

Weiss CH, Bucuvalas MJ. Truth tests and utility tests: Decision-makers' frames of reference for social science research. *American Sociological Review*, 45:302–313, 1980.

Wholey JS. *Evaluation: Promise and Performance.* Washington, DC: Urban Institute, 1979.

Willenbring ML, Whelan JA. *Community Treatment of the Chronic Public Inebriate: Final Evaluation Report.* Minneapolis: Hennepin County Community Services Department, 1991.

Wilson DB. Meta-analysis in alcohol and other drug abuse treatment. *Addiction*, 95(suppl 3):S419–S438, 2000.

Index